Handbook of
Psychopharmacology

Volume 12

Drugs of Abuse

Handbook of
Psychopharmacology

SECTION I: BASIC NEUROPHARMACOLOGY

Volume 1 Biochemical Principles and Techniques in Neuropharmacology
Volume 2 Principles of Receptor Research
Volume 3 Biochemistry of Biogenic Amines
Volume 4 Amino Acid Neurotransmitters
Volume 5 Synaptic Modulators
Volume 6 Biogenic Amine Receptors

SECTION II: BEHAVIORAL PHARMACOLOGY IN ANIMALS

Volume 7 Principles of Behavioral Pharmacology
Volume 8 Drugs, Neurotransmitters, and Behavior
Volume 9 Chemical Pathways in the Brain

SECTION III: HUMAN PSYCHOPHARMACOLOGY

Volume 10 Neuroleptics and Schizophrenia
Volume 11 Stimulants
Volume 12 Drugs of Abuse
Volume 13 Biology of Mood and Antianxiety Drugs
Volume 14 Affective Disorders: Drug Actions in Animals and Man

Volume 12

Drugs of Abuse

Edited by

Leslie L. Iversen

Department of Pharmacology
University of Cambridge

Susan D. Iversen

Department of Psychology
University of Cambridge

and

Solomon H. Snyder

Departments of Pharmacology and Psychiatry
The Johns Hopkins University
School of Medicine

SPRINGER SCIENCE+BUSINESS MEDIA, LLC

Library of Congress Cataloging in Publication Data

Main entry under title:

Handbook of psychopharmacology.

Includes bibliographies and indexes.
CONTENTS: v. 1. Biochemical principles and techniques in neuropharmacology. —v. 2. Principles of receptor research. — v. 3. Biochemistry of biogenic amines. — v. 4. Amino acid neurotransmitters. — v. 5. Synaptic modulators. — v. 6. Biogenic amine receptors. — v. 7. Principles of behavioral pharmacology. — v. 8. Drugs, Neurotransmitters, and Behavior. — v. 10. Neuroleptics and Schizophrenia. — v. 11. Stimulants. — v. 12. Drugs of Abuse. 1. Psychopharmacology. I. Iversen, Leslie Lars. II. Iversen, Susan D., 1940- III. Snyder, Solomon H., 1938-
[DNLM: 1. Psychopharmacology. QV77 H236]
RC483.H36 615'.78 75-6851

ISBN 978-1-4684-3188-9 ISBN 978-1-4684-3186-5 (eBook)
DOI 10.1007/978-1-4684-3186-5

Originally published by Plenum Press, New York in 1978
Softcover reprint of the hardcover 1st edition 1978

CONTRIBUTORS

ARTHUR E. JACOBSON, *Medicinal Chemistry Section, Laboratory of Chemistry, National Institute of Arthritis, Metabolism, and Digestive Diseases, National Institutes of Health, Bethesda, Maryland*

REESE T. JONES, *Langley Porter Neuropsychiatric Institute, University of California, San Francisco, California*

PETER A. MANSKY, *Department of Psychiatry, Albert B. Chandler Medical Center, University of Kentucky, Lexington, Kentucky*

RICHARD A. MEISCH, *University of Minnesota, Minneapolis, Minnesota*

NANCY K. MELLO, *Alcohol and Drug Abuse Research Center, Harvard Medical School—McLean Hospital, Belmont, Massachusetts*

JACK H. MENDELSON, *Alcohol and Drug Abuse Research Center, Harvard Medical School—McLean Hospital, Belmont, Massachusetts*

ROGER A. NICOLL, *Department of Pharmacology and Physiology, University of California, San Francisco, California*

ROY PICKENS, *University of Minnesota, Minneapolis, Minnesota*

R. DUANE SOFIA, *Biological Research, Wallace Laboratories, Cranbury, New Jersey*

TRAVIS THOMPSON, *University of Minnesota, Minneapolis, Minnesota*

PREFACE

Underlying the design of the *Handbook of Psychopharmacology* is a prejudice that the study of drug influences on the mind has advanced to a stage where basic research and clinical application truly mesh. These later volumes of the *Handbook* are structured according to this conception. In certain volumes, groups of drugs are treated as classes with chapters ranging from basic chemistry to clinical application. Other volumes are assembled around topic areas such as anxiety or affective disorders. Thus, besides chapters on individual drug classes, we have included essays addressing broad areas such as "The Limbic–Hypothalamic–Pituitary–Adrenal System and Human Behavior" and "Peptides and the Central Nervous System."

Surveying these diverse contributions, one comes away with a sentiment that, far from being an "applied" science borrowing from fundamental brain chemistry and physiology, psychopharmacology has instead provided basic researchers with the tools and conceptual approaches which now are advancing neurobiology to a central role in modern biology. Especially gratifying is the sense that, while contributing to an understanding of how the brain functions, psychopharmacology is a discipline whose fruits offer genuine help to the mentally ill with promises of escalating benefits in the future.

L.L.I.
S.D.I.
S.H.S.

CONTENTS

CHAPTER 5

Alcohol and Human Behavior

NANCY K. MELLO and JACK H. MENDELSON

CHAPTER 6

Cannabis: Structure–Activity Relationships

R. DUANE SOFIA

CHAPTER 7

Marihuana: Human Effects

REESE T. JONES

1

DRUG SELF-ADMINISTRATION: AN ANALYSIS OF THE REINFORCING EFFECTS OF DRUGS

Roy Pickens, Richard A. Meisch, and Travis Thompson

1. INTRODUCTION

The behavioral effects of drugs were once viewed as being limited to the changes in responding that occurred directly following drug administration. Drug effects were believed to be relatively stereotyped and to consist of little more than temporary alterations of the biological mechanisms controlling ongoing responding. However, recent research has forced an expansion of this view. At present, behavioral drug actions can be viewed as existing on a continuum. On one extreme are effects that are relatively independent of environmental influences or the temporal relation between drug administration and responding (e.g., effects of *d*-amphetamine on locomotor activity). On the other end of the continuum are drug actions that are intimately dependent on their functional relation to environmental events and/or their temporal relation to responding (e.g., effects of *d*-amphetamine on high-rate versus low-rate schedule-controlled responding).

For heuristic purposes it is useful to distinguish the former classes of drug effects from the latter. Thus, drugs are considered to have *direct* effects on behavior if their action is relatively independent of environmental influences and is limited in time to the drug's active metabolic life. However, drugs may also have *functional* effects on behavior if their action depends

Roy Pickens, Richard A. Meisch, and *Travis Thompson* • University of Minnesota, Minneapolis, Minnesota.

upon the relation of drug administration to responding and/or is inextricably intertwined with other environmental variables regulating behavior. For the purpose of the present paper, we will focus upon those functional actions of drugs that depend upon the temporal relation between drug administration and responding. In such cases, it will be shown that drugs have effects that establish, maintain, and control a wide variety of behaviors and extend well beyond the drug's active metabolic life.

The concept of functional properties of drugs originated in psychology from the experimental analysis of behavior (Thompson and Schuster, 1968). Early in this study, environmental events were recognized as having multiple effects on behavior. While certain stimuli reflexively elicit fixed responses, the same stimulus given in a different relation to behavior may produce different results. For example, aperiodically placing food directly into a hungry animal's mouth causes an increase in salivation but has few other behavioral effects. However, the same food presented immediately following a motor response produces not only salivation (direct effect) but also an increase in probability of recurrence of the motor response (functional effect, due to the relation of food presentation to responding). Thus, while food elicits salivation in both situations, its presentation contingent on a motor response produces an additional behavioral effect, an increase in response probability that persists well after food presentation is discontinued.

As with other stimulus events, drugs can have both direct and functional effects on behavior. Administration of amphetamine without regard to ongoing responding will cause an increase in locomotor activity, but little change in rate of any specific aspect of behavior. However, if the same dose of amphetamine is administered contingent on lever pressing, both locomotion and lever pressing will increase, with lever pressing persisting well after amphetamine presentation is discontinued. Thus, drugs can engender direct changes in behavior following their administration, and also functional changes in behavior depending on the relation of their administration to responding.

These examples, however, illustrate only one of several functional effects of stimuli in the control of behavior. Functional relations are typically involved in establishing new behavior. In respondent conditioning, for example, a neutral stimulus is paired repeatedly with a stimulus eliciting a reflexive response. As a result of the pairing, the neutral stimulus may come to elicit essentially the same behavioral change as produced originally by the eliciting stimulus. In this manner, a number of elicited behaviors can be made conditional on the occurrence of a wide variety of environmental stimuli. By pairing their administration with presentation of a neutral stimulus, drugs have been shown to function effectively as eliciting stimuli with their behavioral effects being conditioned to previously neutral environmental events. For example, when illumination of a stimulus light was paired with intravenous injection of methamphetamine in rats, only methamphetamine initially elicited an increase in motor activity. However, after several light–drug pairings, the light was also shown to produce similar effects (Pickens and Dougherty, 1971). A drug effect was thus being elicited by a previously neutral stimulus, because of the functional relation of that stimulus in the past with drug administration.

In operant conditioning, emitted behavior is controlled by the relation of its occurrence to consequence events. Certain consequences (reinforcers) increase the probability of recurrence of behavior they follow, either by stimulus presentation (positive reinforcement) or stimulus termination (negative reinforcement). Other consequences (punishers) reduce the future probability of the behavior they follow. In addition, because of its functional relation to responding, such behavior comes under the discriminative control of the surrounding stimulus state.

Depending on their relation to responding, drugs have been shown to function both as consequence events and discriminative stimuli in establishing and controlling operant behavior. In discriminative control, behavior learned under a drug state frequently fails to occur when the drug state is removed, and vice versa (Heistad, 1958). Animals have been shown to learn to turn left or right in a T-maze depending on whether drug or saline was administered prior to testing (Overton, 1971). Operant responding can be brought under stimulus control of intravenously administered drugs (Cook *et al.,* 1960; Schuster and Brady, 1964), with such effects resulting from the functional relation of stimulus presentation to drug administration.

As consequence events, drugs have been found to function as positive reinforcers, negative reinforcers, and punishers in the control of operant behavior. Within this area, the preponderance of studies have been on drugs as reinforcers, perhaps because of the more obvious implications of this research for the problems of human drug dependence. In the discussion that follows, the reinforcing effects of drugs will be reviewed, particularly with regard to characteristics and factors that influence such drug–behavior interactions.

2. METHODS OF SELF-ADMINISTRATION

The procedures characteristically employed to study the reinforcing effects of drugs are the self-administration techniques. A variety of such techniques have been developed for oral, intravenous, intraperitoneal, intragastric, inhalation, and intraventricular routes of drug administration. In each case, a specific response (e.g., drinking response, lever press) is followed by drug presentation.

With oral self-administration of drugs, animals receive drugs by drinking from drug solutions. Since many drug solutions appear to have aversive taste, animals typically must initially be induced by environmental contingencies to drink them, either by fluid deprivation, requiring drinking to avoid electric shock or to obtain food, or by using schedule-inducing procedures (Woods and Winger, 1971).

In intravenous studies, animals are equipped with chronic venous catheters that connect via protective tubing and swivel joints to remote infusion pumps. Operation of the pump is controlled by a response by the subject. Responding is programmed to activate the pump and deliver a fixed amount of drug solution through the catheter directly into the animal's bloodstream (Weeks, 1962; Thompson and Schuster, 1964; Deneau *et al.*, 1969). Changes in behavior that occur as a result of the response–drug contingency are used to determine the reinforcing effects of drugs. Similar procedures are employed in intraperitoneal, intragastric, and intraventricular drug self-administration.

More specific descriptions of the apparatus and procedure for studying drug self-administration in animals are given elsewhere, for oral (reviewed by Woods and Winger, 1971; Meisch, 1977), intravenous (reviewed by Pickens and Thompson, 1975), intragastric (Amit and Stern, 1969; Götestam, 1973; Smith *et al.*, 1975; Yanagita and Takahashi, 1973), inhalation (Jarvik, 1967; Pickens *et al.*, 1973; Yanagita *et al.*, 1970), intraperitoneal (Headlee *et al.*, 1955; Davis and Nichols, 1963), and intraventricular (Gustafson, 1974) routes of administration.

3. ESTABLISHING DRUGS AS REINFORCERS

To demonstrate drug-reinforcement effects, it is necessary to show that behavior is being selectively maintained by the contingency between drug administration and responding, and not because of the drug's direct behavioral effects. Drug self-administration by an animal does not necessarily indicate the drug is functioning as a reinforcer. If a drug increases motor activity or exploratory behavior, continued drug self-administration may be a function of these direct effects rather than of drug-reinforcement effects.

This is a particular problem in studies of stimulant drug self-administration. For example, during one such study, lever pressing by rats was established and maintained when each response was followed by a 0.5 mg/kg intravenous injection of cocaine and concurrent illumination of a stimulus light (Pickens and Thompson, 1968). To determine if responding was being maintained by the drug-behavior contingency, a number of experimental manipulations were performed. During one session (Fig. 1A), drug administration was initially made available contingent on lever pressing, then it was presented noncontingent on behavior. The injection pump was disconnected from the response lever and programmed to deliver the same mean number of drug injections as occurred during the preceding self-administration period. Under such conditions, lever pressing was no longer maintained, indicating that drug-induced increases in activity or other direct behavioral

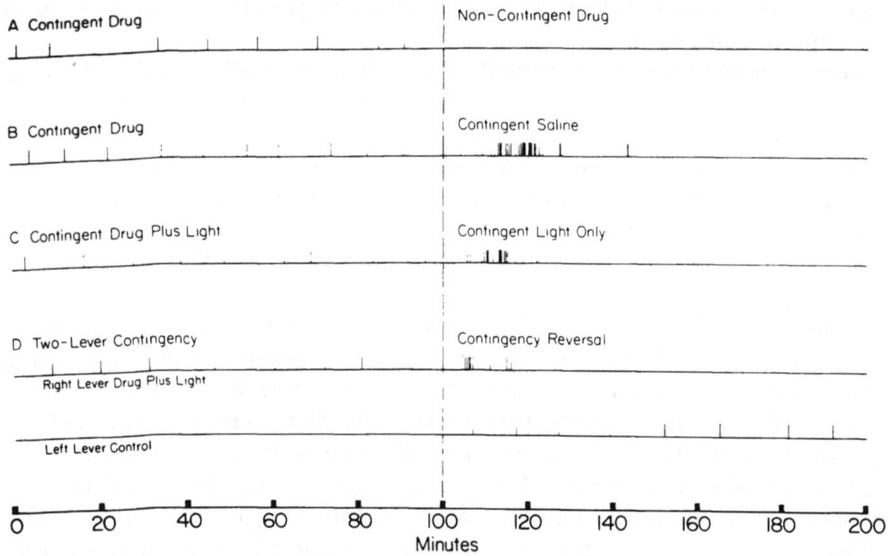

FIG. 1. Effects of drug contingency on responding during intravenous cocaine self-administration in the rat. Each response (vertical line on event record) produced 0.5 mg/kg drug injection and illumination of small stimulus light. Contingency changes were made at dashed vertical line 100 min into each session. See text for details. (From Pickens and Thompson, 1968.)

effects were not engendering responding. Similarly, switching from response-contingent drug injections to response-contingent saline injections (Fig. 1B), or to response-contingent stimulus light illumination alone (Fig. 1C), failed to maintain responding. Finally, when two response levers were added to the test chamber, with one lever delivering response-contingent drug injections and the other having no behavioral consequence, responding occurred only on the drug-contingent lever. However, when these lever contingencies were reversed, lever preference was also reversed (Fig. 1D).

While typically employed to show reinforcing effects of other substances (e.g., food, water) in relatively simple situations (one response/reinforcer presentation), increases in response rate cannot be used to show the reinforcing effects of drugs in such situations, as response rate is also controlled by drug-injection dose. Instead, more complex schedules of drug presentation are employed, with the drug shown to exert schedule control or be selected over vehicle for self-administration. A single cocaine injection after a daily test session has been demonstrated to exert second-order schedule control over lever pressing in monkeys, where every 10th response produced a red light for 2 sec and the first 10-response component completed after 1 hr produced an intramuscular cocaine injection, which occurred with the red light remaining on (Goldberg, 1973*a*). In such procedures, direct drug effects cannot influence responding, since they occur outside the test situation.

With option procedures, animals are at first generally restricted to one and then another solution for self-administration. Later, both solutions are made available and the animal can select between the two. Under such conditions, monkeys have been found to select cocaine or methylphenidate over saline for self-administration (Johanson and Schuster, 1975). Option procedures allow drug-reinforcement effects to be demonstrated independently of response rate, which may be altered or controlled primarily by direct drug effects.

With oral techniques of drug self-administration, responding is influenced by taste as well. Most drug solutions have apparent bitter tastes and animals must be induced to drink them. To determine if the resulting behavior is due to the inducing procedure or to drug-reinforcement effects, responding maintained by presentation of drug solution is typically compared to that of vehicle control. For example, a drug may be drunk because it is placed in a saccharin solution, whose reinforcing efficacy has already been established. After drug experience has been acquired, if more solution is consumed with drug present than without, it is likely the drug *per se* is maintaining responding.

However, the results are more definitive when the inducing conditions are discontinued and the resulting drug intake is compared with baseline or vehicle control. For example, when food-deprived animals are intermittently given small quantities of food on certain schedules, large volumes of water are adjunctively consumed (Falk, 1961). This phenomenon, termed "schedule-induced polydipsia," has been used to induce drinking of large volumes of ethanol and other drug solutions by animals. While drug intake under such conditions is almost always less than water intake (Lester, 1961; Meisch, 1969), when the inducing conditions are discontinued the consumption of drug solutions has been shown to exceed that of water (Freed *et al.,* 1970; Meisch and Thompson, 1971). Figure 2 shows the effects of substituting water for etonitazene as the drinking solution, after etonitazene drinking had first been established using the schedule-inducing procedure. When water replaced etonitazene, responding substantially decreased, and when etonitazene was again replaced, responding returned to its previous level. Thus, in such cases, drinking must be attributed to the reinforcing effects of the drug. In a related procedure, when presses on one lever produced a dipper cup containing water and presses on a second lever produced an ethanol solution, animals responded for ethanol over water, even when the position of the drug and water was alternated between sessions (Meisch and Beardsley, 1975).

Along with helping to overcome the initial aversive properties of drugs, inducing procedures have been employed to establish the self-administration of drugs with relatively weak reinforcing effects. Reinforcing properties of cannabis have been established by allowing monkeys to respond either by

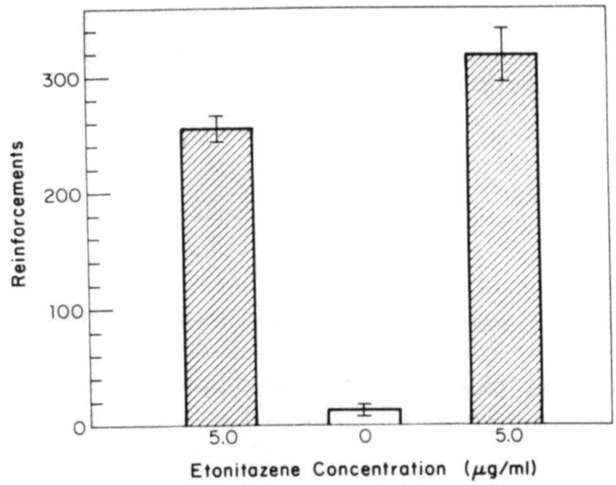

FIG. 2. Etonitazene drinking maintained after schedule-induced polydipsia experience in the rat. Graph shows number of reinforcements obtained as a function of etonitazene (5 μg/ml) or vehicle (water) availability. Each bar is the mean of 25 observations (5 rats × 5 observations). Brackets indicate the average (mean) standard error of the mean for five rats. (Meisch and Stark, unpublished data.)

lever pulling or sucking on a tube containing hashish smoke for food reinforcement. Initially, response requirements were adjusted until about equal amounts of food were obtained by either method. Over time, a preference developed for tube sucking, which was reversed when hashish was removed from the burning chamber and sucking produced heated air only (Pickens *et al.*, 1973).

4. CHARACTERISTICS OF SELF-ADMINISTRATION

As reinforcers, drugs possess characteristics similar to those of other reinforcers, by functioning to strengthen and maintain the behavior leading to their presentation (i.e., self-administration). As with other reinforcers, drugs also differ among themselves in certain unique characteristics related to their direct effects on behavior. Previous reviews have provided a conceptual framework for analyzing the reinforcing and other effects of self-administered drugs (Schuster and Thompson, 1969; Schuster and Johanson, 1974*a*; Thompson and Pickens, 1969, 1975). In the present section, characteristics of performance maintained by the major classes of drugs that function as reinforcers are updated and reviewed. For each drug class, self-administration characteristics are described for the various routes of administration studied. The response patterns generated by conditions of unlimited (24 hr/day) and limited (<24 hr/day) drug access are also included, along with the effects of unit dose of drug on self-administration. Unless otherwise stated, the procedures employed continuous (one response/reinforcement) schedules of drug self-administration.

4.1. Ethanol

4.1.1. Oral

The characteristics of ethanol-maintained responding have been studied in animals previously induced to drink ethanol solutions using the schedule-induced polydipsia procedure. After establishing drinking, food presentation was discontinued and responding delivered dippers of ethanol solution. For both rats and monkeys, ethanol drinking did not occur at a steady rate over limited daily test sessions. In one study with rats, 0.25-ml dippers of 8% (w/v) ethanol were available for drinking over 6-hr experimental sessions. About 40–60% of all drug reinforcements were obtained during the first hour of each session. Thereafter, short bursts of responses alternated with irregular-length periods of no responding (Meisch and Thompson, 1971). A similar temporal distribution of responding was subsequently observed in rats over a wide range (2–32%, w/v) of drinking concentrations, as shown in Fig. 3 (Meisch and Thompson, 1974*a,b*). An initial burst of responding leading to ethanol presentation, followed by shorter bursts during the remainder of the test session, has also been reported with rhesus monkeys previously induced to drink using the polydipsia procedure (Meisch *et al.*, 1975).

With such preparations, ethanol-reinforced responses and ethanol in-

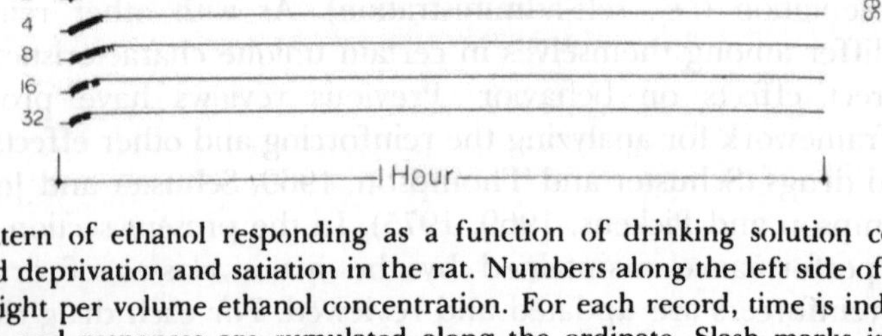

FIG. 3. Pattern of ethanol responding as a function of drinking solution concentration during food deprivation and satiation in the rat. Numbers along the left side of each record indicate weight per volume ethanol concentration. For each record, time is indicated along the abscissa and responses are cumulated along the ordinate. Slash marks indicate 4-sec dipper presentations of 0.25 ml of ethanol solution. Cumulative records presented were selected as being most representative of mean performance over the last five sessions at each concentration. (From Meisch and Thompson, 1974*b*.)

take (mg/kg/body weight) varied separately as a function of reinforcer magnitude. With increases in liquid concentration, responding maintained by ethanol reinforcement initially increased and then decreased, producing an inverted U-shaped concentration–response curve. Peak responding occurred at 4–8% (w/v) concentrations, although responding maintained by 32% (w/v) concentrations significantly exceeded that for water control. Ethanol intake, on the other hand, showed a linear increase with increases in drinking concentration, with intake for 32% (w/v) concentrations being about 10–12 times that for 2% (w/v) concentrations (Meisch and Thompson, 1974*a*, *b*). At an 8% (w/v) concentration, when the dipper volume was increased from 0.17 to 0.274 ml, a linear decrease in response rate along with a linear increase in ethanol intake was obtained. Responding occurred in bursts across the range of volumes. However, as the dipper volume was decreased, responding became more evenly distributed over the session (Henningfield and Meisch, 1975).

4.1.2. Intravenous

Rhesus monkeys initiated intravenous self-administration of ethanol at doses of 200 mg/kg (Deneau *et al.*, 1969). With ethanol available on an unlimited basis (24 hr/day) responding appeared to be confined primarily to the daylight hours. Resumption of drug self-administration in the morning was characterized by an initial marked increase in drug intake. In spite of occurrence of severe withdrawal symptoms, animals periodically abstained from drug self-administrations for 2–4-day periods during chronic drug exposure. Termination of ethanol-reinforced responding by subjects was not observed, however, when drug availability was limited to 3-hr access conditions (Winger and Woods, 1973).

Under limited-access conditions, the temporal distribution of responding during intravenous ethanol self-administration was similar to that during oral self-administration. At 0.2 g/kg/injection, monkeys showed an initial burst of ethanol-reinforced responses, followed later by shorter bursts separated by periods of no responding. With decreases in injection dose, however, responding was distributed more evenly across the 3-hr test session. Whereas drug intake increased when injection dose was increased from 0.05 to 0.075 g/kg, further increases in injection dose up to 0.2 g/kg show no additional increase in drug intake. Between 0.05 and 0.2 g/kg/injection, ethanol intake remained relatively constant (Woods *et al.*, 1971).

4.1.3. Intragastric

With intragastric ethanol self-administration by rats, the effects of infusion dose were similar to those with intravenous injection, with increases in infusion dose resulting in decreases in drug intake (Smith *et al.*, 1976*a*).

4.2. Sedatives

4.2.1. Intravenous

With unlimited drug access, previously drug-naive rhesus monkeys initiated and maintained intravenous self-administration of pentobarbital (3.0–5.0 mg/kg). Drug intake increased gradually over several weeks of testing. Abstinence periods initiated by the subjects were never observed. Self-administration was maintained during the night at approximately one-half of the daytime intake level. Occasionally, self-anesthetization occurred (Deneau *et al.,* 1969; Yanagita and Takahashi, 1973). Intravenous self-administration of diazepam and chlordiazepoxide by previously drug-naive rhesus monkeys has also been reported. With diazepam (0.4 mg/kg), daily drug intake remained relatively constant over 20 weeks of testing. No such abstinence periods or self-anesthetization was observed. With chlordiazepoxide (1 mg/kg), immobility and ataxia were less than with diazepam, and daily drug intake decreased from 10–20 mg/kg to 2–4 mg/kg after 4 weeks of testing (Yanagita and Takahashi, 1973).

In rats previously made tolerant to and physiologically dependent on pentobarbital (150–370 mg/kg/day), responding was initiated by intravenous pentobarbital (3.2 mg/kg/injection). Uniform daily drug-intake rates were observed, with no evidence of periods of abstinence. The lowest injection rate was in the afternoon between noon and 6 :00 p.m., and the highest rate occurred 12 hr later, between midnight and 6 :00 a.m. When the injection dose of pentobarbital was increased, responding decreased but not sufficiently to maintain the same level of drug intake. For example, when injection dose was increased threefold, injection rate was halved, and when injection dose was decreased by one-third, injection rate doubled. Thus, more total drug was taken at the higher than at the lower injection doses (Weeks and Collins, unpublished manuscript).

Methohexital (0.75 to 1.5 mg/kg) was intravenously self-administered by nondependent rats under unlimited-access conditions. When drug access was limited to 6 hr/day, methohexital intake increased with increases in injection dose (1.0–4.0 mg/kg) (Pickens and Muchow, unpublished manuscript).

With drug access limited to daily 3-hr test sessions, intravenous pentobarbital self-administration (0.25 mg/kg) was studied in rhesus monkeys that were not physiologically dependent. There was an initial burst of drug-producing responses during the first 30 min of the test sessions, followed by irregularly spaced responding for the remainder of the session. After a group of injections, animals often showed ataxic movements and appeared to sleep before the lever, but could be easily aroused. Total drug intake increased with increases in injection dose. Pentobarbital intake showed less than a twofold increase across an eightfold change in injection dose (0.25–2.0 mg/kg) (Goldberg *et al.,* 1971*a*).

Also with 3-hr drug access, lever pressing of nondependent monkeys was maintained by intravenous injection of barbital (0.625–10.0 mg/kg), pentobarbital (0.25–4.0 mg/kg), amobarbital (0.25–4.0 mg/kg), thiopental (0.50–4.0 mg/kg), and methohexital (0.125–2.0 mg/kg). For each of the barbiturates, responding at the low and intermediate injection doses occurred in bursts separated by pauses. As the dose increased, the size of the bursts decreased. The initial burst at the beginning of each session was larger than bursts during the middle or latter portions of the sessions. At the higher doses, the response bursts were smaller, with only single or double injections taken. Response rate varied inversely with injection dose, with more total drug being taken at the higher than at the lower injection doses (Winger *et al.*, 1975).

4.2.2. *Intragastric*

Nondependent monkeys intragastrically self-administered pentobarbital (10–40 mg/kg), chlordiazepoxide (10 mg/kg), and oxazolam (10 mg/kg). With pentobarbital, motor impairment and sedation were observed, but self-anesthetization was rare. While intragastric self-administration of chlordiazepoxide and oxazolam was obtained, no marked depressant effects were observed in the animals tested (Yanagita and Takahashi, 1973).

4.3. Opiates

4.3.1. *Oral*

When given a choice between drinking tap water and 0.1% morphine solution under unlimited-access conditions, rhesus monkeys that were not physiologically dependent drank more morphine solution than water (Claghorn *et al.*, 1965). Drug intake increased in roughly stepwise increments over 3–4 months. Each step consisted of approximate 30-day intervals of relatively constant intake separating approximate 1-week intervals of increasing drug intake. More total drug was taken and the animals showed a greater preference for drug over water during the day than at night.

4.3.2. *Intravenous*

Under conditions of unlimited drug access, rhesus monkeys increased their daily intake of morphine (0.5–2.5 mg/kg/injection) steadily for 6–7 weeks and then maintained a fairly stable daily dosage between 50 and 100 mg/kg. Self-administration was limited almost entirely to the daylight period.

Some animals slept from midnight to 8 :00 a.m. while laboratory lights were extinguished. No abstinence periods initiated by the subjects were observed. Reduced food intake and weight loss occurred only during the initial period of increasing drug intake. Intravenous codeine self-administration (0.5–2.5 mg/kg/injection) was also initiated by drug-naive monkeys. The response pattern was similar to that for morphine except no significant decrease in drug intake occurred during the nighttime (Deneau *et al.*, 1969).

With physiologically dependent rats intravenously self-administering morphine (3.2 mg/kg) under unlimited-access conditions, responding occurred on an irregular basis and diurnal variation was evident (Weeks, 1962). When 10 mg/kg morphine was made available on an FR 10 (fixed-ratio) schedule (10 responses/reinforcement), responses were spaced about 2 hr apart. Seldom was more than one injection taken at a time. When the injection dose was decreased to 3.2 mg/kg, however, double and triple injections occurred together (Weeks and Collins, 1968). Under such conditions, sleep, paradoxical sleep, and awake states were monitored by continuous recordings of electroencephalographic and electromyographic activity. With injections occurring about every 2–3 hr, sleep predominated during the 30-min period preceding each injection and wakefulness afterward. The total amount of sleep and paradoxical sleep was within normal limits (Khazan *et al.*, 1967).

In physiologically dependent rats, reducing injection dose by about one-third each morning (from 10.0 mg/kg to 3.2, 1.0, etc.) resulted in respective doubling of the number of injections taken. Thus, a threefold decrease in drug dose produced only a twofold increase in drug intake. More total drug was taken at the higher than at the lower injection doses (Weeks and Collins, 1964).

With morphine available on a limited daily basis, both nonphysiologically dependent rats and monkeys emitted lever-pressing responses maintained by intravenous drug injection. With rats, drug intake was linearly related to injection dose. Over a 10-fold increase in injection dose, drug intake increased by about 3-fold. Methadone intake similarly increased about 8-fold over a 30-fold increase in injection dose (Werner *et al.*, 1976). When morphine was available to monkeys during a 1-hr period every 6th hour of the day, responding produced intravenous drug injection on a VI 2.5-min schedule (where responses are reinforced after varying intervals of time averaging 2.5 min). A curvilinear dose–response function was obtained, with highest response rates occurring at 100 μg/kg/injection and lowest rates occurring at 10 and 1000 μg/kg/injection (Woods and Schuster, 1968).

With codeine available under limited-access conditions on an FR 30 reinforcement schedule, a curvilinear relationship between injection dose and drug intake was found. Maximum intake occurred at 0.03 mg/kg/injection and minimum intakes occurred at 0.001 and 1.0 mg/kg/injection (Downs and Woods, 1974).

Dextropropoxyphene was intravenously self-administered by drug-naive rhesus monkeys when drug availability was limited to 1-hr sessions occurring four times a day. With over a fourfold increase in injection dose (0.5–2.0 mg/kg), drug intake increased about threefold. No periods of abstinence initiated by subjects were seen (Talley and Rosenblum, 1972).

4.4. Stimulants

4.4.1. Intravenous

With drugs available on an unlimited basis, rhesus monkeys initiated intravenous self-administration of cocaine (0.25 and 1.0 mg/kg), *d*-amphetamine (0.1 mg/kg), and caffeine (2.5 and 5.0 mg/kg). With onset of self-administration, cocaine intake increased rapidly but erratically, culminating in convulsions and death within 30 days. When intake was restricted to one dose per hour, responding occurred around the clock usually for 2–5 days, followed by abstinence periods ranging from 0.5 to 5 days. During self-administration periods, the animals showed almost constant choreiform movements, stereotypy, dysmetria, tremors, mydriasis, piloerection, and gross ataxia. Scratching and biting of the skin to the point of digit amputation were also observed. Toxicity increased with increases in daily drug intake. During abstinence periods, the animals slept fitfully and ate frequently. With amphetamine self-administration, behavioral and physiological effects similar to those of cocaine were seen. Self-administration was characterized by irregularity of drug intake and periods of drug responding that continued day and night, interrupted by self-imposed abstinence lasting 1 day to 2 weeks. Toxic effects with amphetamine were less than with cocaine. Intravenous caffeine self-administration produced irregular periods of drug-maintained responding alternating with abstinence. No evidence of toxicity was seen (Deneau *et al.*, 1969).

With rats, onset of intravenous methamphetamine self-administration (0.062–0.5 mg/kg) was characterized by an initial suppression of food and water intake (to 9.8 and 65% of baseline levels, respectively) and a marked increase in motor activity (Fig. 4). Stereotyped head movements and body chewing were observed. After about 5 days, eating and drinking increased and activity decreased. Most animals died within 2 weeks from the start of self-administration, however, with weight losses of 28–42%. Toxicity was greater with the higher injection doses (Pickens *et al.*, 1972). Similar effects have been reported with *d*- and *l*-amphetamine and *l*-methylamphetamine (Yokel and Pickens, 1973*a*; Pickens and Harris, 1968; Pickens *et al.*, 1967).

With unlimited access to amphetamines, periods of uniformly spaced drug responses alternated with periods of drug abstinence (Fig. 5). The amount of time that was spent in drug-intake periods remained relatively constant over the entire period of drug access. Of 12 animals tested, all except one showed drug-intake periods occurring for 63.9 to 80.4% of the

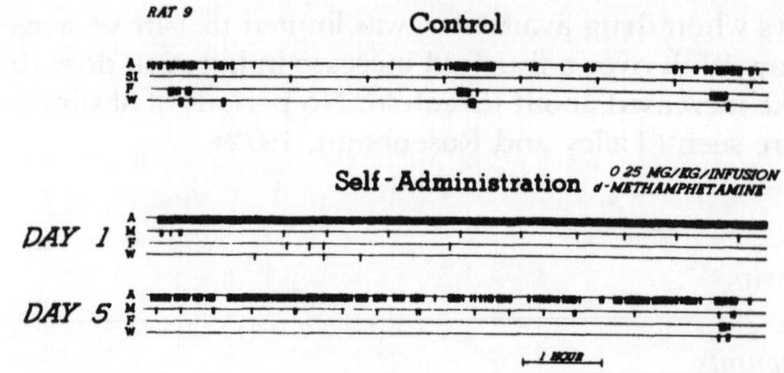

FIG. 4. Motor activity, eating, and drinking in the rat prior to (control), upon initiation of and after 5 days of intravenous methamphetamine self-administration. A, activity, as measured by an ultrasonic activity recorder located within the cage; SI, automatic hourly intravenous saline injection during control procedure (necessary to keep the catheter system patent); F, responses for 45-mg food pellets; W, lick for water; M, lever presses for intravenous 0.25 mg/kg methamphetamine injection. Events records are shown. Each record segment is 8 hr long. (From Yokel and Pickens, 1973*b*.)

total self-administration time. The frequency of alternating between drug-intake and abstinence periods increased, and the lengths of such periods decreased, between the first and second halves of the entire self-administration period (Yokel and Pickens, 1973*b*).

With unlimited access to cocaine, rats also showed alternating periods of drug intake and abstinence, with uniformly spaced lever pressing (Fig. 6) and increased stereotypic activity during drug-intake periods. However, the intake–abstinence cycles were shorter than with the amphetamines, and little evidence of weight loss, overdosage, or toxicity was seen. Rats typically continued to self-administer cocaine without untoward effects until the injection system failed (Pickens and Thompson, 1971).

When cocaine access was limited to daily 6-hr self-administration, rats no longer showed abstinence periods. Drug responding continued throughout the duration of each experimental session. During the first 5 min of each session, response rate was typically higher than during the remainder of the session. In general, the pattern of self-administration was characterized by uniform interresponse times, as was seen during unlimited access to intravenous cocaine (Pickens and Thompson, 1968, 1971; Thompson and Pickens, 1970). Similar effects were also seen in rats with the amphetamines (Yokel and Pickens, 1973*a*) and in monkeys with cocaine, phenmetrazine, pipradrol, and methylphenidate (Wilson *et al.*, 1971). The uniformly spaced responding to intravenous stimulant injection developed within 1–2 days of onset of self-administration and showed little subsequent variability with time (Dougherty and Pickens, 1973*a*).

Under limited-access conditions, increases in stimulant injection dose produced corresponding increases in interval separating drug injections, and decreases in injection dose produced decreases in interinjection interval.

However, total drug intake increased with increases in injection dose. With monkeys, 48-fold increases in injection dose of cocaine (0.025–1.2 mg/kg) produced about 4-fold increases in drug intake; 16-fold increases in injection dose of pipradrol (0.025–0.4 mg/kg) and methylphenidate (0.025–0.4 mg/kg) produced about 4- and 2-fold increases in drug intake, respectively; and 32-fold increases in injection dose of phenmetrazine (0.025–0.8 mg/kg) produced about 6-fold increases in drug intake (Wilson *et al.,* 1971). With rats, 10-fold increases in injection dose of *d*- and *l*-amphetamine (0.25–2.5 mg/kg) produced 3- and 2-fold increases in drug intake, respectively (Fig. 7) (Yokel and Pickens, 1973*a*).

This dose–response relationship may be misleading, however, due to

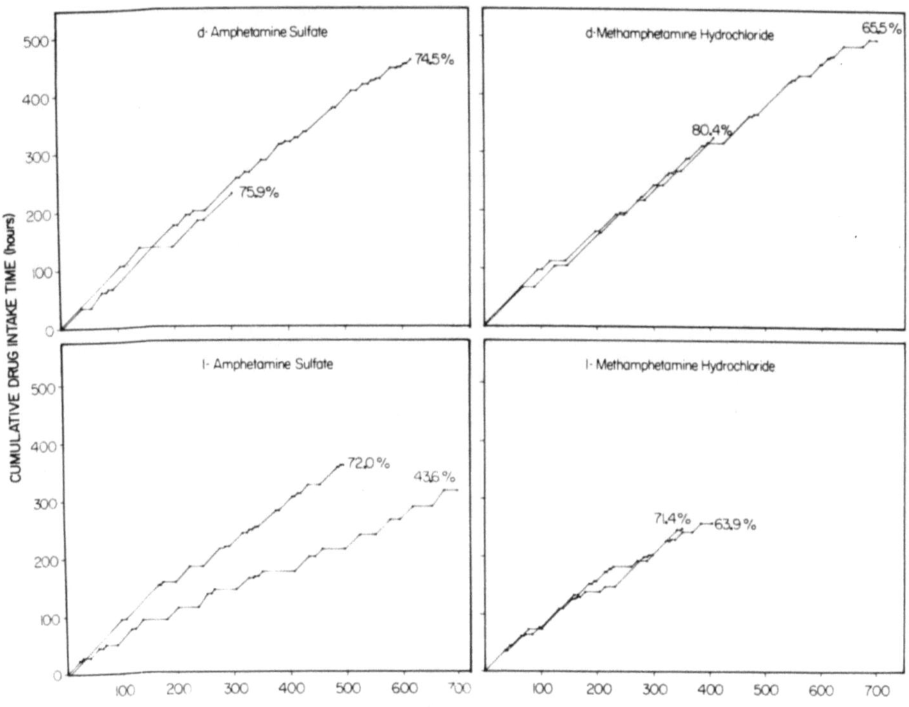

FIG. 5. Alternating periods of drug intake and abstinence in intravenous *d*-methylamphetamine (0.25 mg/kg), *l*-methylamphetamine (2.0 mg/kg), *d*-amphetamine (0.5 mg/kg), and *l*-amphetamine (1.0 mg/kg) self-administration in the rat. Injection doses were selected to produce about equal lever-pressing rates (interinjection intervals) and uniform daily injection volumes. Drug-intake periods are shown as diagonal movement and abstinence periods as horizontal movement of the recording pen. Abstinence periods were defined as periods of at least 2-hr duration without responding. The graphs show the amount of time spent in drug-intake periods (ordinate) during the total time of drug access (abscissa). Data from two animals are presented under each test condition, with data from other subjects falling intermediate to that shown. Figures at the right of each curve represent the percentage of total time spent in drug-intake periods. (From Yokel and Pickens, 1973*b*.)

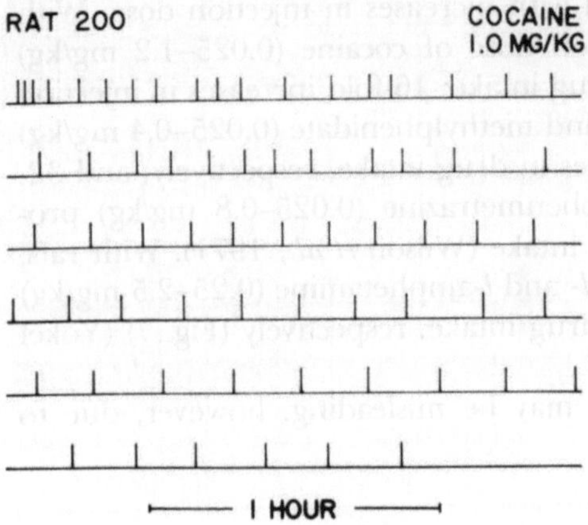

Fig. 6. Temporal distribution of responses during intravenous cocaine self-administration in the rat. With drug available 24 hr/day, event record shows responding during a single drug-intake period lasting 11.3 hr. Each short vertical line indicates drug injection. Note initial clustering of responses and abrupt termination of responding at end of intake period. (From Pickens and Thompson, 1971.)

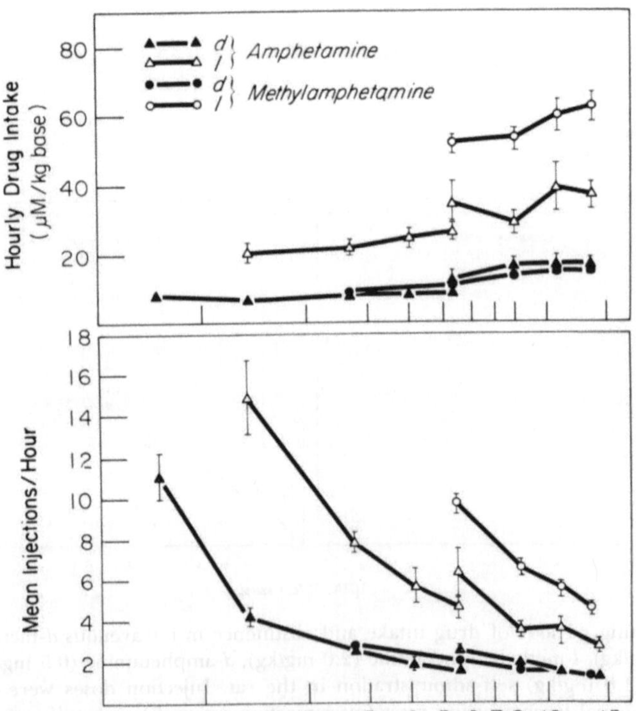

Fig. 7. Mean injection per hour and drug intake per hour as a function of injection dose (one response/injection) during intravenous self-administration of *d*- and *l*-isomers of amphetamine and methylamphetamine in the rat. All values are means ± SE (vertical lines) in micromoles per kilogram of base. SE in some cases is less than point height. (Adapted from Yokel and Pickens, 1973*a*.)

differences in the amount of drug metabolized at the various injection doses. In first-order kinetics, a constant percentage of drug is metabolized per unit time. Thus, while approximately four times more drug would be present in an animal after a 1.0 mg/kg than a 0.25 mg/kg injection, the duration of effect with the 1.0 mg/kg dose will be slightly less than four times as long as with the 0.25 mg/kg dose. While drug intake increases with increases in injection dose, the drug level in the body at the time of responding may, in fact, be constant across all injection doses. Rats were allowed to self-administer ^{14}C-labeled *d*- or *l*-amphetamine in injection doses of 0.25–1.0 mg/kg, and blood samples were obtained from a carotid catheter and analyzed for drug content at the time of responding for an omitted drug injection. No difference in blood level of [^{14}C]amphetamine was found across a range of injection doses (Fig. 8). A similar finding was obtained based on theoretical calculations of whole body levels of amphetamine at the time of responding for successive drug injections (Yokel and Pickens, 1974). These findings suggest that lever pressing maintained by intravenous stimulant injections (i.e., amphetamines and cocaine) is controlled in part by body level of drug. Regardless of injection dose, responding occurs when drug in the body reaches a certain minimum level, which takes longer for the higher than the lower injection doses.

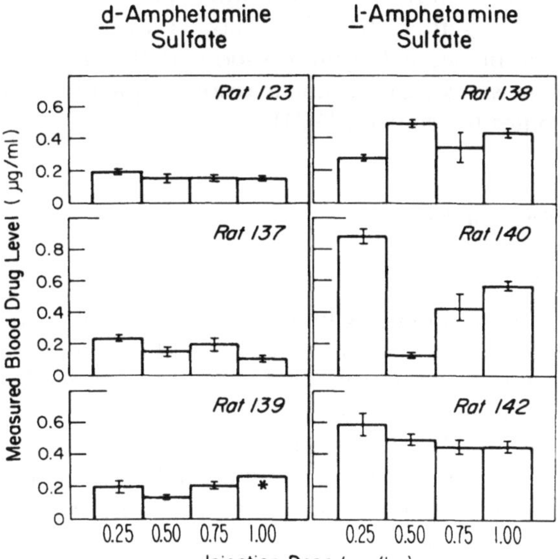

FIG. 8. Mean ± SE of measured blood level (μg/ml) of *d*- and *l*-[^{14}C]amphetamine during intravenous self-administration in the rat. At various times during a 6-hr self-administration, blood samples were obtained when animal responded for omitted drug injection and analyzed for drug content. Across all injection doses, mean blood level for *d*-amphetamine animals was 0.18 μg/ml, while that for *l*-amphetamine animals was 0.48 μg/ml. * = no replication. (From Yokel and Pickens, 1974.)

Another factor that may be related to the highly uniform intervals that separate drug-producing responses in intravenous stimulant self-administration is the direct response-disrupting effects of the drugs. The interinjection interval in cocaine self-administration can be expanded by pretreatment with SKF-525A, an inhibitor of drug biotransformation, and decreased by a series of pretreatments with phenobarbital, which accelerates cocaine metabolism (Dougherty and Pickens, 1974). When rats were trained to lever press on FR 10 schedules of food reinforcement and then given intravenous injections of various doses of cocaine, pauses in responding occurred that were dose related and similar to those obtained during cocaine self-administration (Pickens and Thompson, 1968).

4.4.2. *Intraventricular*

With unlimited drug access, rats with cannulae in left or right cerebral ventricles were found to self-administer *d*-amphetamine intraventricularly (0.1–0.4 mg/kg/injection). All animals showed initial weight loss and stereotypic activity. When drug access was limited to daily 6-hr test sessions, increases in injection dose (0.1–0.8 mg/kg) produced increases in total drug intake. Across an eightfold range of injection doses, a twofold increase in drug intake was obtained. Self-administration was characterized by single responses separated by uniformly spaced intervals. At times, however, several injections occurred together. In rats equipped with both intravenous and intraventricular cannulae, self-administration of 0.5 mg/kg *d*-amphetamine during 12-hr test sessions yielded similar response patterns and rates of drug intake by both routes (Gustafson, 1974).

4.5. Other Drug Classes

4.5.1. *Intravenous*

Drug-naive rhesus monkeys initiated and maintained intravenous self-administration of the dissociative anesthetics phencyclidine and ketamine. With unlimited drug access (50 μg/kg/injection) to phencyclidine, periods of almost complete self-anesthetization were followed by periods in which the animals were only mildly uncoordinated. At night, periods of drug abstinence lasting 3–8 hr almost always occurred. When drug access was limited to 4-hr daily sessions, a higher hourly rate of responding for 50 μg/kg/ injections was found (Balster *et al.*, 1973). With ketamine self-administration in monkeys, response rate was an inverted U-shaped function of injection dose (0.0008 to 1.6 mg/kg). Highest response rate was at 0.0125 mg/kg/ injection. Total drug intake decreased linearly with increases in injection dose. Behavioral effects ranged from light sedation at lower injection doses to heavy sedation and light anesthesia at higher injection doses (Moreton *et al.*, 1975).

4.5.2. Inhalation

Monkeys were found to self-administer chloroform, ether, and lacquer thinner when lever pressing delivered a fixed volume of drug vapor to the animals via a nasal catheter. Daily intake of all compounds was erratic, with periods of drug intake and abstinence during the day. Monkeys typically abstained from midnight to 8:00 a.m. During drug-intake periods, light anesthesia was reached with chloroform but not with ether or lacquer thinner. Ataxia, salivation, and mydriasis were observed with all drugs (Yanagita *et al.*, 1970).

With monkeys trained to smoke hashish by sucking on a tube connected to a burning chamber, drug intake remained relatively constant over 6–8 weeks of testing. Following a period of smoking, the animals appeared relatively inactive and docile. Over the testing period, one animal showed a 38% reduction in food intake, while the second animal's food intake increased by 26%. One animal smoked mostly at night, whereas the other smoked mostly during the middle of the day (Pickens *et al.*, 1973).

5. DRUGS NOT SELF-ADMINISTERED

Not all compounds within the above classes of self-administered drugs maintain responding. Other classes show no evidence of reinforcing effects.

Nalorphine (2.5 mg/kg/injection) was not intravenously self-administered, even after monkeys were given automatic programmed injections every 4 hr for 1 month. Also, under similar conditions, chlorpromazine (0.1 or 0.5 mg/kg/injection) was not self-administered (Deneau *et al.*, 1969). Furthermore, when self-administration was initially established with cocaine, substitution of chlorpromazine (0.05–0.5 mg/kg/injection) suppressed responding below saline-control values (Hoffmeister and Goldberg, 1973).

Fenfluramine, an amphetamine congener with anorexic effects, failed to maintain intravenous self-administration when substituted either for amphetamine in rats (Götestam and Anderson, 1975) or cocaine or methohexital in monkeys (Woods and Tessel, 1974). Tricyclic antidepressants (imipramine, imipramine-*N*-oxide, protriptyline, maprotiline, and iprindole) also failed to maintain self-administration when substituted for 1-1,2-diphenyl-1-dimethylaminoethane-HCl (SPA) in monkeys. Drug-naive animals failed to initiate self-administration with these compounds, although some animals having previous experience in self-administering reinforcing drugs did so, but only at a low level (Yanagita *et al.*, 1972).

Drug-naive monkeys did not initiate intravenous self-administration of acetylsalicylic acid (0.4–5.0 mg/kg/injection) or maintain self-administration when acetylsalicylic acid and other antipyretic analgesics (aminophenazone, phenylbutazone) were substituted for codeine. Mixing such drugs with codeine reduced codeine intake (Hoffmeister and Wuttke, 1973*a*, 1975).

Monkeys failed to initiate intravenous self-administration of mescaline, either before or after 1 month of automatic programmed injection of 1, 5, or 10 mg/kg every 2 hr (Deneau *et al.*, 1969). Monkeys also failed to intravenously self-administer Δ^9-*trans*-tetrahydrocannabinol (0.025–0.3 mg/kg/injection) under similar conditions or following substitution for cocaine during maintained self-administration (Harris *et al.*, 1974), but did so after substitution for phencyclidine in maintained self-administration (Pickens *et al.*, 1973).

Of the drugs not self-administered by animals, a number have been found to function effectively as aversive stimuli, with responding being maintained by the escape or avoidance of drug injection. Drugs that maintained escape–avoidance responding in nonphysiologically dependent monkeys include chlorpromazine, nalorphine, cyclazocine, STP [1-(2,5-dimethoxy-4-methylphenyl)2-propylamine-hydrochloride] and LSD (Hoffmeister, 1975; Hoffmeister and Wuttke, 1973*b*, 1974, 1975). In addition, naloxone maintained escape–avoidance responding in morphine-dependent monkeys (Goldberg *et al.*, 1971*b*; Downs and Woods, 1975). When responding was maintained by intravenous codeine injection, adding naloxone to the codeine solution suppressed responding, indicating a punishment effect (Woods *et al.*, 1975).

6. FACTORS INFLUENCING SELF-ADMINISTRATION

Several other recent reviews have dealt with a broad range of factors influencing drug intake (cf. Wallgren and Barry, 1970). However, for present purposes we will focus on studies specifically dealing with clear-cut demonstration of reinforcing effects of drugs. The influences of drug class, access conditions, unit dose, and route of administration on drug-reinforced behavior have been described above.

6.1. Organismic

Strain differences in ethanol drinking by rats and mice have been well documented (Eriksson, 1968; McClearn, 1968, 1973; Rodgers, 1966, 1967). Sex differences in ethanol drinking by animals have also been observed (Eriksson, 1969). In no case, however, did the high-intake strain drink sufficient ethanol to show behavioral effects or develop physiological dependence (Meisch, 1977).

The tendency for animals to drink drug solutions can be enhanced or impaired by selective breeding. With rats, when high-drinkers were bred with high-drinkers and low-drinkers bred with low-drinkers, offsprings from the two groups differed significantly in morphine intake, and the difference became greater over successively bred generations. Further, the two strains did not differ significantly in quinine intake, suggesting changes in taste sensitivity in general may not be responsible for the results obtained (Nichols and Hsiao, 1967).

6.2. Past History

Past drug experience and behavioral history can influence subsequent self-administration of drugs. For 3 days prior to the start of self-administration, rats were given intravenous injections of either saline or 50, 100, or 300 mg/kg morphine divided into three equal daily doses. When responding produced 1.0 mg/kg intravenous morphine injections, the amount of drug self-administered during the initial acquisition session was directly proportional to the dosage used to induce tolerance (Smith *et al.*, 1976*b*). Initial establishment of physiological dependence also influences later drug self-administration. Rats pretreated with morphine to establish physiological dependence subsequently orally self-administered more morphine solution than animals without the prior drug experience (Cappell and LeBlanc, 1971).

Animals having previous experience with drug self-administration reacquire the behavior more rapidly than animals without such experience (Weeks and Collins, 1968). Furthermore, self-administration of one drug influences subsequent self-administration of other compounds. Following a history of intravenous cocaine, codeine, or pentobarbital self-administration, substitution of *d*-amphetamine produced drug intakes that were dependent on the previous drug experience. At 0.005 mg/kg/injection *d*-amphetamine responding was about five times that of saline control for previous cocaine animals, about the same as saline control for previous codeine animals, and about two times saline control for previous pentobarbital animals (Schlichting *et al.*, 1970). In monkeys having experience with intravenous cocaine or codeine self-administration, substitution of morphine, codeine, pentazocine, propirafumarate, and dextropropoxyphene maintained responding. However, animals with a cocaine history self-administered these compounds less than animals with a codeine history (Hoffmeister and Schlichting, 1972).

6.3. Motivational

Conditions of the organism at the time of testing can influence drug self-administration. Such conditions can be induced by environmental events or current drug state of the organism.

6.3.1. Aversive Stimuli

Aversive stimulation may increase intake of ethanol and sedative drugs by animals. When placed on a shock-avoidance schedule, monkeys increased their ethanol consumption (Clark and Polish, 1960; Mello and Mendelson, 1964). In nonphysiologically dependent rats, amobarbital was intravenously self-administered for several days by animals receiving brief unavoidable electric shocks, but not by animals receiving no shocks (Davis and Miller, 1963; Davis *et al.*, 1968).

6.3.2. Satiation

Self-administration of certain drugs is influenced by the body level of the self-administered drug or similar compound prior to testing. Rats intravenously self-administering methamphetamine were given intraperitoneal injections of saline or various doses of methamphetamine. While saline had no effect, intraperitoneal methamphetamine produced dose-related delays in responding for the next intravenous drug injection, presumably indicating a drug-satiation effect (Pickens *et al.*, 1968).

In physiologically dependent animals, injection of morphine before drinking trials reduced the amount of morphine solution consumed by rats (Stolerman and Kumar, 1970), and the introduction of the synthetic opioid etonitazene into the drinking water of rats reduced the rate of intravenous morphine self-administration (Weeks and Collins, 1964). Monkeys pretreated with morphine or methadone showed decreases in intravenous morphine self-administration that were dose dependent (Thompson and Schuster, 1964; Thompson and Pickens, 1969).

6.3.3. Deprivation

In rats made physiologically dependent on opiates by daily morphine injections, withholding injections for varying intervals produced orderly increases in intake of etonitazene solution over tap water (Wikler *et al.*, 1963). Physiologically dependent monkeys, however, did not show systematic increases in intravenous morphine self-administration with increases in drug deprivation beyond 24 hr (Woods *et al.*, 1973). Responding maintained by intravenous morphine administration in the presence of stimuli originally associated with morphine increased during drug-deprivation periods (Thompson and Schuster, 1964; Woods and Schuster, 1968; Thompson *et al.*, 1971).

Morphine antagonists can also be administered to physiologically dependent animals to produce a drug-deprivation state. Nalorphine administration caused rate of responding maintained by intravenous morphine self-administration by rats to increase (Weeks, 1962). Nalorphine also produced marked increases in responding during the FI component of an FI–FR chain schedule of intravenous morphine self-administration by monkeys (Thompson and Schuster, 1964). Small doses of both nalorphine and naloxone increased intravenous morphine self-administration in monkeys, whereas larger doses decreased self-administration (Goldberg *et al.*, 1971*c*).

6.4. Stimulus Control

6.4.1. Discriminative Stimuli

Environmental stimuli associated with drug self-administration acquire discriminative control over responding, such that their presence or absence in part controls the probability of drug-taking behavior. In experienced animals, the odor of ethanol (Meisch and Thompson, 1973) or the effects of noncontingent drug injection (Stretch *et al.*, 1971; Pickens and Thompson, 1971) precipitated drug self-administration. Such factors were apparently also involved in relapse to drug use following a period of forced drug abstinence (Jones and Prada, 1973). After oral morphine self-administration had been established in one environment, rats were withdrawn and later allowed to reacquire self-administration in either that same environment or a different environment. Reacquisition of oral morphine self-administration occurred more rapidly in the original than in the new environment (Thompson and Ostlund, 1965).

6.4.2. Conditioned Aversive Stimuli

Previously neutral stimuli paired with aversive stimuli acquire conditioned aversive properties. Wikler (1961) has suggested that relapse to opiate use in humans may be related to drug-abstinence symptoms being conditioned to environment events. Presentation of these conditioned stimuli to postaddicts elicits conditioned abstinence symptoms that increase the probability of return to drug use. Conditioned withdrawal has been demonstrated by placing rats in an environment previously associated with drug withdrawal (Wikler, 1965). In physiologically dependent monkeys, a stimulus was paired repeatedly with nalorphine injections that precipitated withdrawal symptoms. Later, presentation of the stimulus alone produced conditioned withdrawal, disruption of food-reinforced responding (Goldberg and Schuster, 1967), and increased intravenous morphine self-administration (Goldberg *et al.*, 1969).

6.4.3. Conditioned Reinforcers

Stimuli paired with administration of reinforcing drugs become conditioned reinforcers, capable of maintaining behavior in their own right. With monkeys, a red stimulus light was paired with drug injection during intravenous morphine self-administration. During extinction morphine was withheld and response rate was found to be higher on days when responding produced red light presentation than when responding had no programmed consequence (Schuster and Woods, 1968). The conditioned-reinforcing effects of stimuli paired with opiate administration have also been demonstrated with rats, involving both oral (Wikler *et al.*, 1971; Stolerman and

Kumar, 1972) and intravenous (Smith and Davis, 1973) drug injection. Conditioned reinforcers to stimuli paired with intravenous amphetamine self-administration have been established (Davis and Smith, 1974*a*). After rats had been given noncontingent pairings of a buzzer with intravenous injection of morphine in doses of 0.0032, 0.032, or 0.3 mg/kg, responding then produced buzzer plus saline injection. The results showed conditioned reinforcing effects to the buzzer–saline presentation, the magnitude of which was directly related to the morphine dose used in the initial pairing (Crowder *et al.*, 1972). Second-order schedule control over responding by a stimulus paired with cocaine injection has also been reported (Goldberg, 1973*b*).

6.5. Reinforcement Schedules

One of the primary determinants of the rate, pattern, and persistence of responding in drug self-administration is the schedule of drug presentation. In general, behavior maintained by drug reinforcers is similar to that maintained by other reinforcers (Thompson and Pickens, 1972; Pickens and Thompson, 1972). However, differences between drug and other reinforcers cannot be accounted for solely in terms of direct drug effects on behavior. For example, the effect of cocaine on behavior maintained by food reinforcement does not resemble that of responding being maintained by cocaine injection, although the same drug dose and reinforcement schedule are employed (Pickens and Thompson, 1968). The schedule effects of drugs as reinforcers reflect both functional as well as direct drug effects on behavior.

In the following sections the definitions of reinforcement schedules are based on those described by Ferster and Skinner (1957) and Thompson and Grabowski (1972).

6.5.1. *Fixed Ratio*

The fixed-ratio schedule has been the most frequently used intermittent schedule in drug self-administration studies, requiring a fixed number of responses for each drug presentation. Responding is typically characterized by break-and-run patterns, with an initial pause after reinforcement followed by high response rate terminating in the next reinforcement.

After rats were induced to drink ethanol using the polydipsia procedure, food reinforcement was discontinued and responding was maintained on geometrically increasing fixed-ratio (FR) schedules of 8% (w/v) ethanol reinforcement. Responding was maintained up to FR 256 (256 responses/reinforcement). The number of responses increased up to intermediate FR values, and decreased thereafter. Most drug-maintained responding occurred at the beginning of each session, followed by a pause and intermittent bursts of responses (Meisch and Thompson, 1973). Similar results have also been obtained with rhesus monkeys (Fig. 9).

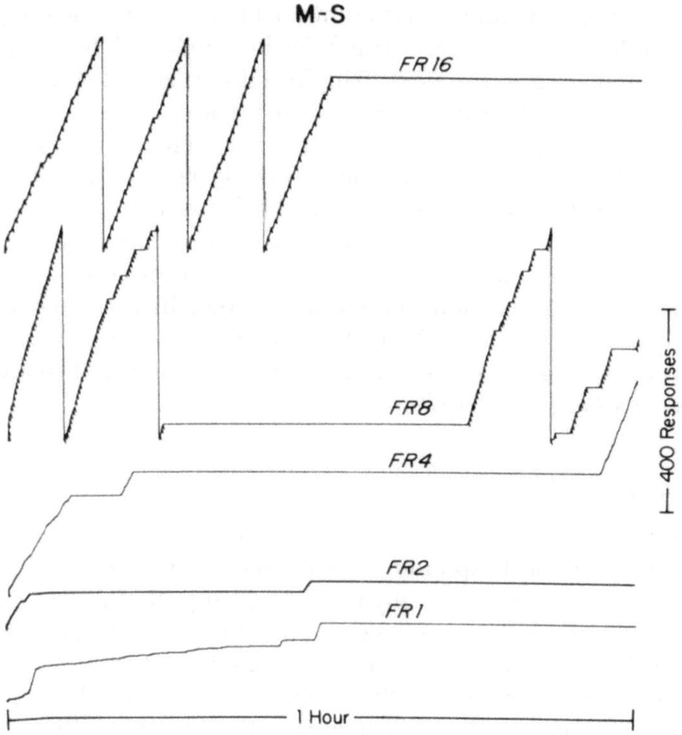

FIG. 9. Fixed-ratio (FR) schedules of ethanol drinking in the monkey where responding was maintained by 8% (w/v) ethanol solution. Responses are recorded cumulatively by upward movement of the recording pen; at FR 8 and FR 16 slash marks indicate ethanol presentation. Note initial burst of responses at all FR values. (Henningfield and Meisch, unpublished data.)

With intravenous pentobarbital self-administration by physiologically dependent rats, increasing the response/reinforcement schedule from FR 1 to FR 5 increased response rate only about twofold and decreased drug intake to less than half the amount of FR 1. Increasing from FR 5 to FR 10 resulted in no change in response rate and a halving of drug intake (Weeks and Collins, unpublished manuscript). In monkeys, while characteristic FR response patterns were seen, increasing response requirement for intravenous pentobarbital (0.25 mg/kg) injections from FR 1 to FR 10 markedly decreased daily drug intake, from about 27 to about 8 mg/kg/session, respectively (Goldberg *et al.*, 1971*a*).

With opiates, increasing response requirement from FR 10 to FR 270 decreased intravenous morphine intake by physiologically dependent rats. At 10 mg/kg/injection mean drug intake at FR 10 was 155 mg/kg/day, and at FR 270 mean drug intake was 40 mg/kg/day, calculated from data provided (Weeks and Collins, 1964).

With stimulants, fixed-ratio schedules of intravenous *d*-amphetamine, methamphetamine, and cocaine self-administration by rats was characterized by dose-dependent pauses after drug injection, followed by high rates of responding terminating in the next drug injection (Fig. 10). Increases in FR value produced corresponding increases in response rate, with the drug intake/hour remaining relatively constant across FR values (Pickens and Harris, 1968; Pickens and Thompson, 1968; Pickens *et al.*, 1967). With cocaine, increasing FR value from FR 5 to FR 20 resulted in a drug-intake decrease from 7.2 to 6.4 mg/kg/hr, respectively, in two animals tested. Higher ratios could be maintained by intermediate and high injection doses than by low injection doses (Pickens and Thompson, 1968). In monkeys, increasing response requirement from FR 1 to FR 10 for intravenous cocaine also had little influence on drug intake, with about the same amount of drug taken at both values (Goldberg *et al.*, 1976).

6.5.2. *Fixed Interval*

On such schedules, the first response after a fixed period of time produces reinforcement. Responding is typically characterized by a scalloped pattern, with response rate gradually increasing up to the time of scheduled reinforcement. Since reinforcer intake is limited to a major extent by fixed-interval (FI) value, response rate is the main datum of study.

Rats orally self-administered ethanol on fixed-interval schedules (0–240 sec). Response rate increased with increases in FI value up to FI 120 sec and decreased thereafter (Fig. 11). When drug sessions were begun with an initial FI 32-min schedule, followed by drug availability on a continuous reinforcement (one response/reinforcement) schedule, responding during the initial FI component produced a scalloped pattern (Meisch and Thompson, 1974*c*).

Fixed-interval schedules of intravenous cocaine self-administration were studied as a function of injection dose and interval duration in rats. Responding was characterized by a scalloped pattern. After drug injection, the pause before initiation of responding was directly related to injection dose and was unaffected by the interval contingency. Overall response rate was inversely related to injection dose, primarily because of dose effects on postreinforcement pause duration (Dougherty and Pickens, 1973*b*). In monkeys, however, response rate for cocaine increased directly with injection dose of 0 to 0.8 mg/kg on an FI 9-min schedule with a limited-hold contingency (Balster and Schuster, 1973). With higher FI values (30 and 60 min) and injection doses (0.5–1.5 mg/kg), response rate decreased with increases in injection dose (Pickens and Thompson, 1972).

6.5.3. *Other Schedules*

Variable-interval and variable-ratio schedules of intravenous cocaine self-administration and chain FI–FR schedules of intravenous morphine self-administration have been described with monkeys (Pickens and Thompson,

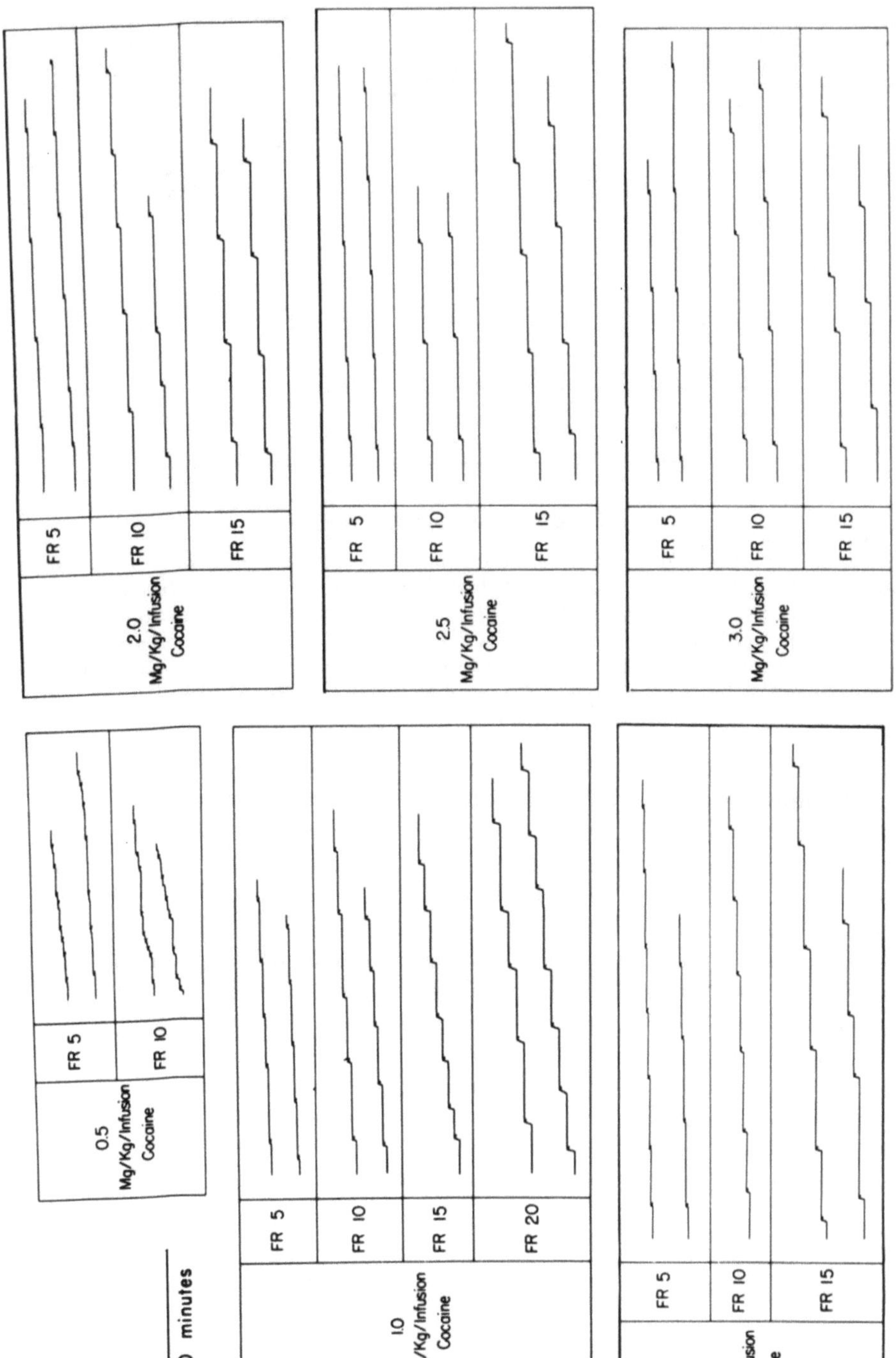

FIG. 10. Fixed-ratio (FR) schedules of intravenous cocaine self-administration in the rat. Responses are recorded cumulatively by upward movement of the recording pen, and slash marks indicate drug injection.

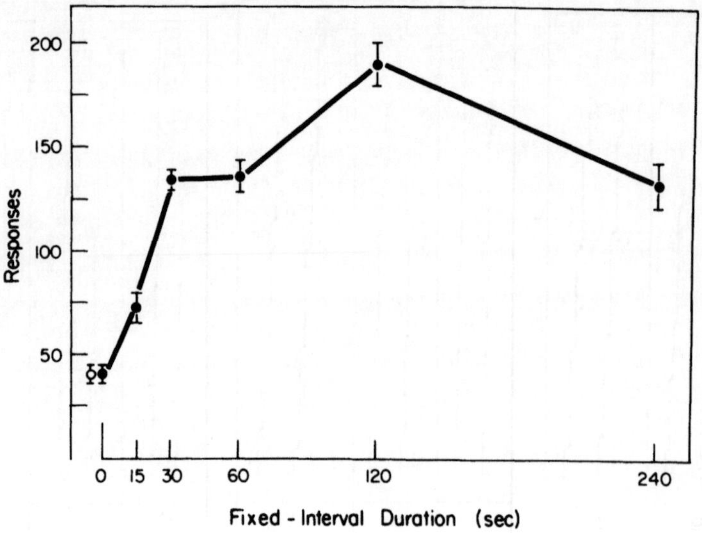

FIG. 11. Response rate in fixed-interval (FI) schedules of oral ethanol self-administration in the rat. Ordinate: responses per 1-hr session; abscissa: FI value in seconds. Each point is the mean for the last five sessions at a particular FI value. Brackets indicate the standard error of the mean. The unfilled circle at FI 0 seconds indicates the number of responses obtained when the rat was returned to FR 1 after completing the test series. The rat weighed 392 g, which was 70% of its free-feeding weight. (From Meisch and Thompson, 1974c.)

1972; Thompson and Schuster, 1964). Responding has also been maintained on second-order schedules of drug presentation in monkeys, in which every tenth response produced a red light for 2 sec and the first such unit completed after 1 hr produced an intramuscular cocaine injection (Goldberg, 1973*a*).

A number of other schedules have been employed to compare the reinforcing efficacy of various self-administered drugs, including progressive-ratio schedules (Griffiths *et al.*, 1975), choice procedures (Findley *et al.*, 1972; Johanson and Schuster, 1975), and concurrent schedules (Iglauer and Woods, 1974; Llewellyn *et al.*, 1976). In general, such studies have shown preferences by animals for certain drugs and injection doses over others, suggesting these techniques may be employed to predict the abuse liability of drugs for humans (Schuster and Johanson, 1974*b*).

7. ELIMINATION OF SELF-ADMINISTRATION

Procedures for eliminating drug-reinforced behavior include satiation, punishment of drug responding, altering stimulus control over responding, reinforcing alternative behavior, and extinction by withholding drug reinforcement or altering the organism biochemically to make drugs less reinforcing (Thompson *et al.*, 1973). Of these, satiation has been discussed previously, while reinforcement of alternative behavior has not been studied in drug self-administration. Stimulus control would involve altering discriminative stimuli, conditioned aversive stimuli, and conditioned reinforcers that control drug-taking behavior (Smith and Davis, 1974*a*; Davis and Smith, 1974*b*).

7.1. Punishment

Rats were trained to intravenously self-administer morphine or *d*-amphetamine on a continuous reinforcement schedule. After responding had been established, each response produced drug injection plus brief electric shock. Within three sessions, responding was suppressed below operant level for both morphine and amphetamine subjects. Removing the shock contingency and giving the subjects 15 "priming" injections failed to reestablish the self-administration over a 3-day test period (Smith and Davis, 1974*b*). In monkeys, responding maintained by intravenous cocaine was made available under two different stimulus conditions on a continuous reinforcement schedule. In one stimulus condition, drug responses were also punished by electric shock. Shocked responses decreased as shock intensity increased. The longer the delay between drug-maintained responding and shock presentation, the less effective was shock in suppressing responding (Grove and Schuster, 1974).

7.2. Extinction

In a procedure similar to that described above, intravenous cocaine self-administration was maintained in monkeys under two stimulus conditions. When drug injection was discontinued in one condition, responding in that condition declined to near-zero levels (Grove and Schuster, 1974). When saline was substituted for drug during self-administration, responding was not maintained (Pickens and Thompson, 1968). However, drug-reinforced responding decreased less rapidly when saline was substituted for drug than when responding had no consequence (Winger *et al.*, 1975). In rats extinguished repeatedly following intravenous *d*- and *l*-amphetamine and *d*- and *l*-methylamphetamine self-administration, the number of responses to extinction did not differ significantly between drugs and doses used, but extinction time was longer for the larger doses and *d*-isomers (Yokel and Pickens, 1976).

A second approach to extinguishing drug-reinforced behavior involves altering the biochemical substrates mediating drug-reinforcement effects. Research in this area has profound significance both for understanding reinforcement processes in general as well as for potential treatment of drug abuse. While cholinergic influences on drug self-administration have been studied (Wilson and Schuster, 1973; Davis and Smith, 1975*a*), most attention has been directed toward dopaminergic and noradrenergic systems of the brain. Compounds that lower brain levels of dopamine and norepinephrine (e.g., α-methyl-*p*-tyrosine) produced changes in intravenous amphetamine self-administration that resembled effects obtained by lowering the self-administration injection dose (Pickens *et al.,* 1968; Wilson and Schuster, 1974), or eliminated self-administration altogether (Davis and Smith, 1972). Similar effects have also been observed on intravenous morphine self-administration (Davis and Smith, 1973). Inhibitors of catecholamine synthesis that selectively deplete norepinephrine but not dopamine (e.g., diethyldithiocarbamate) prevented reacquisition of intravenous morphine and amphetamine self-administration by rats (Davis *et al.,* 1975). However, other investigators have found dopamine-blocking agents, but not norepinephrine-blocking agents, to produce effects that resembled reinforcer reduction or termination in intravenous amphetamine self-administration (Yokel and Wise, 1975). This view is further strengthened by the finding of intravenous self-administration of the dopamine receptor stimulant apomorphine and its disruption by the dopamine receptor blocker pimozide (Baxter *et al.,* 1974). Haloperidol, a dopaminergic blocking agent, decreased morphine self-administration and inhibited amphetamine self-administration, while apomorphine increased responding for morphine self-administration in rats (Glick and Cox, 1975; Davis and Smith, 1975*b*). These findings strongly suggest the involvement of dopaminergic mechanisms in the control of drug-reinforced behavior.

8. CONCLUSIONS

In drug self-administration, behavior is established and maintained by the functional (reinforcing) effects of drugs. However, the response patterns associated with self-administration of different drug classes are modified both by direct drug effects and the influences of environmental variables governing behavior. Such effects interact to determine the general characteristics of drug-taking behavior.

Acknowledgments

The authors thank R. A. Yokel for allowing us to reproduce portions of his research data. Richard A. Meisch is the recipient of a Research Scientist Development Award (No. DA 00007) from NIDA.

9. REFERENCES

AMIT, Z., and STERN, M. H., 1969, Alcohol ingestion without oropharyngeal sensations, *Psychon. Sci.* **15:**162–163.

BALSTER, R. L., and SCHUSTER, C. R., 1973, Fixed-interval schedule of cocaine reinforcement: Effect of dose and infusion duration, *J. Exp. Anal. Behav.* **20:**119–129.

BALSTER, R. L., JOHANSON, C. E., HARRIS, R. T., and SCHUSTER, C. R., 1973, Phencyclidine self-administration in the rhesus monkey, *Pharmacol. Biochem. Behav.* **1:**167–172.

BAXTER, B. L., GLUCKMAN, M. I., STEIN, L., and SCERNI, R. A., 1974, Self-injection of apomorphine in the rat: Positive reinforcement by a dopamine receptor stimulant, *Pharmacol. Biochem. Behav.* **2:**387–391.

CAPPELL, H., and LEBLANC, A. E., 1971, Some factors controlling oral morphine intake in rats, *Psychopharmacologia* **21:**192–201.

CLAGHORN, J. L., ORDY, J. M., and NAGY, A., 1965, Spontaneous opiate addiction in rhesus monkeys, *Science* **149:**440–441.

CLARK, R., and POLISH, E., 1960, Avoidance conditioning and alcohol consumption on rhesus monkeys, *Science* **132:**223.

COOK, L., DAVIDSON, A., DAVIS, D. J., and KELLEHER, R. T., 1960, Epinephrine, norepinephrine, and acetylcholine as conditioned stimuli for avoidance behavior, *Science* **131:**990–991.

CROWDER, W. F., SMITH, S. G., DAVIS, W. M., NOEL, J. T., and COUSSENS, W. R., 1972, Effect of morphine dose size on the conditioned reinforcing potency of stimuli paired with morphine, *Psychol. Rec.* **22:**441–448.

DAVIS, J. D., and MILLER, N. E., 1963, Fear and pain: Their effect on self-injection of amobarbital sodium by rats, *Science* **141:**1286–1287.

DAVIS, J. D., LULENSKI, G. C., and MILLER, N. E., 1968, Comparative studies of barbiturate self-administration, *Int. J. Addict* **3:**207–214.

DAVIS, W. M., and NICHOLS, J. R., 1963, A technique for self-injection of drugs in the study of reinforcement, *J. Exp. Anal. Behav.* **6:**233–235.

DAVIS, W. M., and SMITH, S. G., 1972, Alpha-methyltyrosine to prevent self-administration of morphine and amphetamine, *Curr. Ther. Res.* **14:**814–819.

DAVIS, W. M., and SMITH, S. G., 1973, Blocking of morphine based reinforcement by alphamethyltyrosine, *Life Sci.* **12:**185–191.

DAVIS, W. M., and SMITH, S. G., 1974*a*, Behavioral control exerted by an amphetamine based conditioned reinforcer, in: *Drug Addiction*, Vol. 3, *Neurobiology and Influences on Behavior* (J. M. Singh and H. Lal, eds.), Symposia Specialists, Miami.

DAVIS, W. M., and SMITH, S. G., 1974*b*, Naloxone use to eliminate opiate-seeking behavior: Need for extinction of conditioned reinforcement, *Biol. Psychiat.* **9:**181–189.

DAVIS, W. M., and SMITH, S. G., 1975*a*, Central cholinergic influence on self-administration of morphine and amphetamine, *Life Sci.* **16:**237–246.

DAVIS, W. M., and SMITH, S. G., 1975*b*, Effect of haloperidol on (+) amphetamine self-administration, *J. Pharm. Pharmacol.* **27:**540–541.

DAVIS, W. M., SMITH, S. G., and KHALSA, J. H., 1975, Noradrenergic role in the self-administration of morphine or amphetamine. *Pharmacol. Biochem. Behav.* **3:**477–484.

DENEAU, G. A., YANAGITA, T., and SEEVERS, M. H., 1969, Self-administration of psychoactive substances by the monkey, *Psychopharmacologia* **16:**30–48.

DOUGHERTY, J. A., and PICKENS, R., 1973*a*, Development of temporal patterns of cocaine self-administration, *Proceedings, 81st Annual Meeting of the American Psychological Association*, Montreal, pp. 1003–1004.

DOUGHERTY, J., and PICKENS, R., 1973*b*, Fixed-interval schedules of intravenous cocaine presentation in rats, *J. Exp. Anal. Behav.* **20:**111–118.

DOUGHERTY, J. A., and PICKENS, R., 1974, Effects of phenobarbital and SKF 525A on cocaine self-administration in rats, in: *Drug Addiction*, Vol. 3, *Neurobiology and Influences on Behavior* (J. M. Singh and H. Lal, eds.), Intercontinental Med. Book, New York.

Downs, D. A., and Woods, J. H., 1974, Codeine- and cocaine-reinforced responding in rhesus monkeys: Effects of dose on response rates under a fixed-ratio schedule, *J. Pharmacol. Exp. Ther.* **191**:179–188.

Downs, D. A., and Woods, J. H., 1975, Fixed-ratio escape and avoidance-escape from naloxone in morphine-dependent monkeys: Effects of naloxone dose and morphine pretreatment, *J. Exp. Anal. Behav.* **23**:415–427.

Eriksson, K., 1968, Genetic selection for voluntary alcohol consumption in the albino rat, *Science* **159**:739–741.

Eriksson, K., 1969, Factors affecting voluntary alcohol consumption in the albino rat, *An. Zoo. Fennici* **6**:227–265.

Falk, J. L., 1961, Production of polydipsia in normal rats by an intermittent food schedule, *Science* **133**:195–196.

Ferster, C. B., and Skinner, B. F., 1957, *Schedules of Reinforcement*, Appleton-Century-Crofts, New York.

Findley, J. D., Robinson, W. W., and Peregrino, L., 1972, Addiction to secobarbital and chlordiazepoxide in the rhesus monkey by means of a self-infusion preference procedure. *Psychopharmacologia (Berl.)* **26**:93–114.

Freed, E. X., Carpenter, J. A., and Hymowitz, N., 1970, Acquisition and extinction of schedule-induced polydipsia consumption of alcohol and water, *Psychol. Rep.* **26**:915–922.

Glick, S. D., and Cox, R. D., 1975, Dopaminergic and cholinergic influences on morphine self-administration in rats, *Res. Comm. Clin. Pathol. Pharmacol.* **12**:17–24.

Goldberg, S. R., 1973*a*, Control of behavior by stimuli associated with drug injections, in: *Psychic Dependence* (L. Goldberg and F. Hoffmeister, eds.), Springer-Verlag, Berlin.

Goldberg, S. R., 1973*b*, Comparable behavior maintained under fixed-ratio and second-order schedules of food presentation, cocaine injection or *d*-amphetamine injection in the squirrel monkey, *J. Pharmacol. Exp. Ther.* **186**:18–30.

Goldberg, S. R., and Schuster, C. R., 1967, Conditioned suppression by a stimulus associated with nalorphine in morphine-dependent monkeys, *J. Exp. Anal. Behav.* **10**:235–242.

Goldberg, S. R., Woods, J. H., and Schuster, C. R., 1969, Morphine: Conditioned increases in self-administration in rhesus monkeys, *Science* **166**:1306–1307.

Goldberg, S. R., Hoffmeister, F., Schlichting, V., and Wuttke, W., 1971*a*, A comparison of pentobarbital and cocaine self-administration in rhesus monkeys: Effects of dose and fixed ratio parameters, *J. Pharmacol. Exp. Ther.* **179**:277–283.

Goldberg, S. R., Hoffmeister, F., Schlichting, V., and Wuttke, W., 1971*b*, Aversive properties of nalorphine and naloxone in morphine-dependent rhesus monkeys, *J. Pharmacol. Exp. Ther.* **179**:268–276.

Goldberg, S. R., Woods, J. H., and Schuster, C. R., 1971*c*, Nalorphine-induced changes in morphine self-administration in rhesus monkeys, *J. Pharmacol. Exp. Ther.* **176**:464–471.

Götestam, K. G., 1973, Intragastric self-administration of meduzepam in rats, *Psychopharmacologia* **28**:87–94.

Götestam, K. G., and Anderson, B. E., 1975, Self-administration of amphetamine analogues in rats, *Pharmacol. Biochem. Behav.* **3**:229–233.

Griffiths, R. R., Findley, J. D., Brady, J. V., Dolan-Gutcher, K., and Robinson, W. W., 1975, Comparison of progressive-ratio performance maintained by cocaine, methylphenidate and secobarbital, *Psychopharmacologia* **43**:81–83.

Grove, R. N., and Schuster, C. R., 1974, Suppression of cocaine self-administration by extinction and punishment, *Pharmacol. Biochem. Behav.* **2**:199–208.

Gustafson, L. K., 1974, Intraventricular amphetamine self-administration in the albino rat, unpublished doctoral thesis, University of Minnesota.

HARRIS, R. T., WATERS, W., and MCLENDON, D., 1974, Evaluation of reinforcing capability of delta-9-tetra-hydrocannabinol in rhesus monkeys, *Psychopharmacologia* **37:**23–29.

HEADLEE, C. P., COPPOCK, H. W., and NICHOLS, J. R., 1955, Apparatus and technique involved in a laboratory method of detecting the addictiveness of drugs, *J. Amer. Pharmacol. Assoc.* **44:**229–231.

HEISTAD, G. T., 1958, Effects of chlorpromazine and electroconvulsive shock on a conditioned emotional response, *J. Comp. Physiol. Psychol.* **51:**209–212.

HENNINGFIELD, J. E., and MEISCH, R. A., 1975, Ethanol-reinforced responding and intake as a function of volume per reinforcement, *Pharmacol. Biochem. Behav.* **3:**437–441.

HOFFMEISTER, F., 1975, Negative reinforcing properties of some psychotropic drugs in drug-naive rhesus monkeys, *J. Pharmacol. Exp. Ther.* **192:**468–477.

HOFFMEISTER, F., and GOLDBERG, S. R., 1973, A comparison of chlorpromazine, imipramine, morphine, and *d*-amphetamine self-administration in cocaine-dependent rhesus monkeys, *J. Pharmacol. Exp. Ther.* **187:**8–14.

HOFFMEISTER, F., and SCHLICHTING, U. U., 1972, Reinforcing properties of some opiates and opioids in rhesus monkeys with histories of cocaine and codeine self-administration, *Psychopharmacologia* **23:**55–74.

HOFFMEISTER, F., and WUTTKE, W., 1973*a*, Self-administration of acetylsalicylic acid and combinations with codeine and caffeine in rhesus monkeys, *J. Pharmacol. Exp. Ther.* **186:**266–275.

HOFFMEISTER, F., and WUTTKE, W., 1973*b*, Negative reinforcing properties of morphine antagonists in naive rhesus monkeys, *Psychopharmacologia* **33:**247–258.

HOFFMEISTER, F., and WUTTKE, W., 1974, Self-administration: Positive and negative reinforcing properties of morphine antagonists in rhesus monkeys, in: *Narcotic Antagonists*, Vol. 8 (M. C. Braude, L. S. Harris, E. L. May, J. P. Smith, and J. E. Villarreal, eds.), *Advances in Biochemical Psychopharmacology*, Raven Press, New York.

HOFFMEISTER, F., and WUTTKE, W., 1975, Further studies on self-administration of antipyretic analgesics and combinations of antipyretic analgesics with codeine in rhesus monkeys, *J. Pharmacol. Exp. Ther.* **193:**870–875.

HOFFMEISTER, F., and WUTTKE, W., 1975, Psychotropic drugs as negative reinforcers, *Pharmacol. Rev.* **27:**419–428.

IGLAUER, C., and WOODS, J. H., 1974, Concurrent performances: Reinforcement by different doses of intravenous cocaine in rhesus monkeys, *J. Exp. Anal. Behav.* **22:**179–196.

JARVIK, M. E., 1967, Tobacco smoking in monkeys, *Ann. N.Y. Acad. Sci.* **142:**280–294.

JOHANSON, C. E., and SCHUSTER, C. R., 1975, A choice procedure for drug reinforcers: Cocaine and methylphenidate in the rhesus monkey, *J. Pharmacol. Exp. Ther.* **193:**676–688.

JONES, B. E., and PRADA, J. A., 1973, Relapse to morphine use in dogs, *Psychopharmacologia* **30:**1–12.

KHAZAN, N., WEEKS, J. R., and SCHROEDER, L. A., 1967, Electroencephalographic, electromyographic, and behavioral correlates during a cycle of self-maintained morphine addiction in the rat, *J. Pharmacol. Exp. Ther.* **155:**521–531.

LESTER, D., 1961, Self-maintenance of intoxication in the rat, *Q. J. Stud. Alcohol* **22:**223–231.

LLEWELLYN, M. E., IGLAUER, C., and WOODS, J. H., 1976, Relative reinforcer magnitude under a non-independent concurrent schedule of cocaine reinforcement in rhesus monkeys, *J. Exp. Anal. Behav.* **25:**81–91.

MCCLEARN, G. E., 1968, Genetics and motivation of the mouse, in: *Nebraska Symposium on Motivation* (W. J. Arnold, ed.), Univ. of Nebraska Press, Lincoln.

MCCLEARN, G. E., 1973, The genetic aspect of alcoholism, in: *Alcoholism: Progress in Research and Treatment*, Academic Press, New York.

MEISCH, R. A., 1969, Self-administration of pentobarbital by means of schedule-induced polydipsia, *Psychon. Sci.* **16:**16–17.

MEISCH, R. A., 1977, Ethanol self-administration: Infrahuman studies, in: *Advances in Behavioral Pharmacology* (T. Thompson and P. B. Dews, eds.), Academic Press, New York.

MEISCH, R. A., and BEARDSLEY, P., 1975, Ethanol as a reinforcer for rats: Effects of concurrent access to water and alternate positions of water and ethanol, *Psychopharmacologia* **43:**19–23.

MEISCH, R. A., and THOMPSON, T., 1971, Ethanol intake in the absence of concurrent food reinforcement, *Psychopharmacologia* **22:**72–79.

MEISCH, R. A., and THOMPSON, T., 1973, Ethanol as a reinforcer: Effects of fixed-ratio size and food deprivation, *Psychopharmacologia* **28:**171–183.

MEISCH, R. A., and THOMPSON, T., 1974*a*, Rapid establishment of ethanol as a reinforcer for rats, *Psychopharmacologia* **37:**311–321.

MEISCH, R. A., and THOMPSON, T., 1974*b*, Ethanol intake as a function of concentration during food deprivation and satiation, *Pharmacol. Biochem. Behav.* **2:**589–596.

MEISCH, R. A., and THOMPSON, T., 1974*c*, Ethanol as a reinforcer: An operant analysis of ethanol dependence, in: *Drug Addiction*, Vol. 3, *Neurobiology and Influences on Behavior* (J. M. Singh and H. Lal, eds.), Symposia Specialists, Miami.

MEISCH, R. A., HENNINGFIELD, J. E., and THOMPSON, T., 1975, Establishment of ethanol as a reinforcer for rhesus monkeys via the oral route: Initial results, in: *Experimental Studies of Alcohol Intoxication and Withdrawal*, Vol. 59, *Advances in Experimental Medicine and Biology* (M. M. Gross, ed.), Plenum, New York.

MELLO, N. K., and MENDELSON, J., 1964, Operant performance by rats for alcohol reinforcement, *Q. J. Stud. Alcohol* **25:**226.

MORETON, J. E., MEISCH, R. A., STARK, L., and THOMPSON, T., 1975, Ketamine self-administration in the rhesus monkey, *Neurosci. Abst.* **1:**278.

NICHOLS, J. R., and HSIAO, S., 1967, Addiction liability of albino rats: Breeding for quantitative differences in morphine drinking, *Science* **157:**561–563.

OVERTON, D. A., 1971, Discriminative control of behavior by drug states, in: *Stimulus Properties of Drugs* (T. Thompson and R. Pickens, eds.), Plenum, New York.

PICKENS, R., and DOUGHERTY, J. A., 1971, Conditioning of the activity effects of drugs, in: *Stimulus Properties of Drugs* (T. Thompson and R. Pickens, eds.), Plenum, New York.

PICKENS, R., and HARRIS, W. C., 1968, Self-administration of *d*-amphetamine by rats, *Psychopharmacologia* **12:**158–163.

PICKENS, R., and THOMPSON, T., 1968, Cocaine-reinforced behavior in rats: Effects of reinforcement magnitude and fixed-ratio size, *J. Pharmacol. Exp. Ther.* **161:**122–129.

PICKENS, R., and THOMPSON, T., 1971, Characteristics of stimulant drug reinforcement, in: *Stimulus Properties of Drugs* (T. Thompson and R. Pickens, eds.), Plenum, New York.

PICKENS, R., and THOMPSON, T., 1972, Simple schedules of drug self-administration, in: *Drug Addiction*, Vol. 1, *Experimental Pharmacology* (J. M. Singh, L. Miller, and H. Lal, eds.), Futura, New York.

PICKENS, R., MEISCH, R. A., and DOUGHERTY, JR., J. A., 1968, Chemical interactions in methamphetamine reinforcement, *Psychol. Rep.* **23:**1267–1270.

PICKENS, R., MEISCH, R., and MCGUIRE, L. E., 1967, Methamphetamine reinforcement in rats, *Psychon. Sci.* **8:**371–372.

PICKENS, R., MEISCH, R. A., and DOUGHERTY, JR., J. A., 1968, Chemical interactions in methamphetamine reinforcement, *Psychol. Rep.* **23:**1267–1270.

PICKENS, R., THOMPSON, T., and YOKEL, R. A., 1972, Characteristics of amphetamine self-administration by rats, in: *Current Concepts on Amphetamine Abuse* (E. H. Ellinwood and S. Cohen eds.), U.S. Government Printing Office, Washington, D.C.

PICKENS, R., THOMPSON, T., and MUCHOW, D. C., 1973, Cannabis and phencyclidine self-administration by animals, in: *Psychic Dependence* (L. Goldberg and F. Hoffmeister, eds.), Springer-Verlag, Berlin.

RODGERS, D. A., 1966, Factors underlying differences in alcohol preference among inbred strains of mice, *Psychol. Med.* **28:**498–513.

RODGERS, D. A., 1967, Alcohol preference in mice, in: *Comparative Psychopathology* (J. Zubin and H. Hunt, eds.), Grune and Stratton, New York.

SCHLICHTING, U. U., GOLDBERG, S. R., WUTTKE, W., and HOFFMEISTER, F., 1970, *Proceedings of the Twelfth Meeting of the European Society for the Study of Drug Toxicity* **12:**60–67.

SCHUSTER, C. R., and BRADY, J. V., 1964, The discriminative control of a food-reinforced operant by interoceptive stimulation, *Pavlov J. High. Nerv. Act.* **14:**448–458.

SCHUSTER, C. R., and JOHANSON, C. E., 1974*a*, Behavioral analysis of opiate dependence, in: *Opiate Addiction: Origins and Treatment* (S. Fisher and A. M. Freedman, eds.), V. H. Winston, Washington, D.C.

SCHUSTER, C. R., and JOHANSON, C. E., 1974*b*, The use of animal models for the study of drug abuse, in: *Research Advances in Alcohol and Drug Problems,* Vol. 1 (R. J. Gibbins, Y. Isreal, H. Kalant, R. E. Popham, W. Schmidt, and R. G. Smart, eds.), Wiley, New York.

SCHUSTER, C. R., and THOMPSON, T., 1969, Self-administration of and behavioral dependence on drugs, *Ann. Rev. Pharmacol.* **9:**483–502.

SCHUSTER, C. R., and WOODS, J. A., 1968, The conditioned reinforcing effects of stimuli associated with morphine reinforcement, *Int. J. Addict.* **3:**223–230.

SMITH, S. G., and DAVIS, W. M., 1973, Behavioral control by stimuli associated with acquisition of morphine self-administration, *Behav. Biol.* **9:**777–780.

SMITH, S. G., and DAVIS, W. M., 1974*a*, Interrelationship of exteroceptive and interoceptive stimuli associated with morphine self-administration: Significance to elimination of drug-seeking behavior, in: *Drug Addiction,* Vol. 3, *Neurobiology and Influences on Behavior* (J. M. Singh and H. Lal, eds.), Intercontinental Med. Book, New York.

SMITH, S. G., and DAVIS, W. M., 1974*b*, Punishment of amphetamine and morphine self-administration behavior, *Psychol. Rec.* **24:**432–435.

SMITH, S. G., WERNER, T. E., and DAVIS, W. M., 1975, Technique for intragastric delivery of solutions: Application for self-administration of morphine and alcohol by rats, *Physiol. Psychol.* **3:**220–224.

SMITH, S. G., WERNER, T. E., and DAVIS, W. M., 1976*a*, Comparison between intravenous and intragastric alcohol self-administration, *Physiol. Psychol.* **4:**91–93.

SMITH, S. G., WERNER, T. E., and DAVIS, W. M., 1976*b*, Effects of tolerance on intravenous morphine self-administration behavior, *Physiol. Psychol.* **4:**97–98.

STOLERMAN, I. P., and KUMAR, R., 1970, Preferences for morphine in rats: Validation of an experimental model of dependence, *Psychopharmacologia* **17:**137–150.

STOLERMAN, I. P., and KUMAR, R., 1972, Secondary reinforcement in opioid dependence, in: *Drug Addiction,* Vol. 1, *Experimental Pharmacology* (J. M. Singh, L. Miller, and H. Lal, eds.), pp. 49–59, Futura, Mount Kisco, New York.

STRETCH, R., GERBER, G. J., and WOOD, S. M., 1971, Factors affecting behavior maintained by response-contingent intravenous infusions of amphetamine in squirrel monkeys, *Canad. J. Physiol. Pharmacol.* **49:**581–589.

TALLEY, W. H., and ROSENBLUM, I., 1972, Self-administration of dextropropoxyphene by rhesus monkeys to the point of toxicity, *Psychopharmacologia* **27:**179–182.

THOMPSON, T., and GRABOWSKI, J., 1972, *Reinforcement Schedules and Multioperant Analysis,* Appleton-Century-Crofts, New York.

THOMPSON, T., and OSTLUND, W., JR., 1965, Susceptibility to readdiction as a function of the addiction and withdrawal environments, *J. Comp. Physiol. Psychol.* **60:**388–392.

THOMPSON, T., and PICKENS, R., 1969, Drug self-administration and conditioning, in: *Scientific Basis of Drug Dependence* (H. Steinberg, ed.), J. A. Churchill, London.

THOMPSON, T., and PICKENS, R., 1970, Stimulant self-administration by animals: Some comparisons with opiate self-administration, *Fed. Proc.* **29:**6–11.

THOMPSON, T., and PICKENS, R., 1972, Drugs as reinforcers: Schedule considerations, in: *Schedule Effects: Drugs, Drinking and Aggression* (R. Gilbert and J. D. Keehn, eds.), Univ. of Toronto Press, Toronto.

THOMPSON, T., and PICKENS, R., 1975, An experimental analysis of behavioral factors in drug dependence, *Fed. Proc.* **34:**1759–1770.

Thompson, T., and Schuster, C. R., 1964, Morphine self-administration, food-reinforced, and avoidance behaviors in rhesus monkeys, *Psychopharmacologia* **5**:87–94.

Thompson, T., and Schuster, C. R., 1968, *Behavioral Pharmacology*, Prentice-Hall, Englewood Cliffs, N. J.

Thompson, T., Bigelow, G., and Pickens, R., 1971, Environmental variables influencing drug self-administration, in: *Stimulus Properties of Drugs* (T. Thompson and R. Pickens, eds.), pp. 193–207, Plenum, New York.

Thompson, T., Griffith, R., and Pickens, R., 1973, Drug self-administration by animals: Some implications for human drug dependence, in: *Psychic Dependence* (L. Goldberg and F. Hoffmeister, eds.), Springer-Verlag, Berlin.

Wallgren, H., and Barry, H., 1970, *Actions of Alcohol*, Elsevier, New York.

Weeks, J. R., 1962, Experimental morphine addiction: Method for automatic intravenous injection in unrestrained rats, *Science* **138**:143–144.

Weeks, J. R., and Collins, R. J., 1964, Factors affecting voluntary morphine intake in self-maintained addicted rats, *Psychopharmacologia* **6**:267–279.

Weeks, J. R., and Collins, R. J., 1968, Patterns of intravenous self-injection by morphine-addicted rats, in: *The Addictive States* (A. Wikler, ed.), Williams & Wilkins, Baltimore.

Werner, T. E., Smith, S. G., and Davis, W. M., 1976, A dose-response comparison between methadone and morphine self-administration, *Psychopharmacologia* **47**:209–211.

Wikler, A., 1961, On the nature of addiction and habituation, *Brit. J. Addict.* **57**:73–79.

Wikler, A., 1965, Conditioning factors in opiate addiction and relapse, in *Narcotics* (D. M. Wilner and G. G. Kassebaum, eds.), McGraw-Hill, New York.

Wikler, A., Martin, W. R., Pescor, F. T., and Eades, C. G., 1963, Factors regulating oral consumption of an opioid (etonitazene) by morphine-addicted rats, *Psychopharmacologia* **5**:55–78.

Wikler, A., Pescor, F. T., Miller, D., and Norrell, H., 1971, Persistent potency of a secondary (conditioned) reinforcer following withdrawal of morphine from physically dependent rats, *Psychopharmacologia (Berl.)* **20**:103–117.

Wilson, M. C., and Schuster, C. R., 1973, Cholinergic influence on intravenous cocaine self-administration by rhesus monkeys, *Pharmacol. Biochem. Behav.* **1**:643–649.

Wilson, M. C., and Schuster, C. R., 1974, Aminergic influences on intravenous cocaine self-administration by rhesus monkeys, *Pharmacol. Biochem. Behav.* **2**:563–571.

Wilson, M. C., Hitomi, M., and Schuster, C. R., 1971, Psychomotor stimulant self-administration as a function of dosage per injection in the rhesus monkey, *Psychopharmacologia* **22**:271–281.

Winger, G. D., and Woods, J. H., 1973, The reinforcing property of ethanol in the rhesus monkey: I. Initiation, maintenance and termination of intravenous ethanol-reinforced responding, *Ann. N.Y. Acad. Sci.* **215**:162–175.

Winger, G., Stitzer, M. L., and Woods, J. H., 1975, Barbiturate-reinforced responding in rhesus monkeys: Comparisons of drugs with different durations of action. *J. Pharmacol. Exp. Ther.* **195**:505–514.

Woods, J. H., and Schuster, C. R., 1968, Reinforcement properties of morphine, cocaine, and SPA as a function of unit dose, *Int. J. Addict.* **3**:231–237.

Woods, J. H., and Tessel, R. E., 1974, Fenfluramine: Amphetamine congener that fails to maintain drug-taking behavior in the rhesus monkey, *Science (Washington)* **185**:1067–1069.

Woods, J. H., and Winger, G. D., 1971, A critique of methods for inducing ethanol self-inntoxication in animals, in: *Recent Advances in Studies of Alcoholism* (N. K. Mello and J. H. Mendelson, eds.), United States Government Printing Office, Washington, D. C.

Woods, J. H., Ikomi, F., and Winger, G., 1971, The reinforcing property of ethanol, in: *Biological Aspects of Alcohol* (M. K. Roach, W. M. McIsaac, and P. J. Creaven, eds.), pp. 371–388, Univ. of Texas Press, Austin.

Woods, J. H., Downs, D. A., and Villarreal, J. E., 1973, Changes in operant behavior during deprivation and antagonist-induced withdrawal states, in: *Psychic Dependence* (L. Goldberg and F. Hoffmeister, eds.), Springer-Verlag, Berlin.

WOODS, J. H., DOWNS, D. A., and CARNEY, J., 1975, Behavioral functions of narcotic antagonists: Response–drug contingencies, *Fed. Proc.* **34:**1777–1784.

YANAGITA, T., and TAKAHASHI, S., 1973, Dependence liability of several sedative-hypnotic agents evaluated in monkeys, *J. Pharmacol. Exp. Ther.* **185:**307–316.

YANAGITA, T., TAKAHASHI, S., ISHIDA, K., and FUNAMOTO, H., 1970, Voluntary inhalation of volatile anesthetics and organic solvents by monkeys, *Jap. J. Clin. Pharmacol.* **1:**13–16.

YANAGITA, T., TAKAHASHI, S., and OINUMA, N., 1972, Drug dependence liability of tricyclic antidepressants evaluated in monkeys *Jap. J. Clin. Pharmacol.* **3:**289–294.

YOKEL, R. A., and PICKENS, R., 1973*a*, Self-administration of optical isomers of amphetamine and methylamphetamine by rats, *J. Pharmacol. Exp. Ther.* **187:**27–33.

YOKEL, R. A., and PICKENS, R., 1973*b*, Changes in activity and drug, food, and water intake in 24 hr/day *d*- and *l*-amphetamine and methylamphetamine self-administration by rats, Reports from the Research Laboratories of the Department of Psychiatry, University of Minnesota, Report No. PR-73-1 (March).

YOKEL, R. A., and PICKENS, R., 1974, Drug level of *d*- and *l*-amphetamine during intravenous self-administration, *Psychopharmacologia* **34:**255–264.

YOKEL, R. A., and PICKENS, R., 1976, Extinction responding following amphetamine self-administration: Determination of reinforcement magnitude, *Physiol. Psychol.* **4:**39–42.

YOKEL, R. A., and WISE, R. A., 1975, Increased lever pressing for amphetamine after pimozide in rats: Implications for a dopamine theory of reward, *Science* **187:**547–549.

2

ANALGESICS AND THEIR ANTAGONISTS: STRUCTURE–ACTIVITY RELATIONSHIPS

Arthur E. Jacobson

1. INTRODUCTION

Qualitative theories that attempt to relate molecular structure to analgesic or narcotic antagonist activity have given the contemporary medicinal chemist only slight ability to predict, *a priori*, the analgesic potencies of compounds. The discovery of new types of analgesics by the medicinal chemist has often been serendipitous (Eddy and May, 1973). Other new analgesics were designed through clever rationalizations based on natural products or previously synthesized similar drugs.

Structure–activity relationships among the opiates and other narcotics have generally been limited to compilations of, and comparisons between, the various types of analgesics. These include the opiates and their Diels-Adler products (morphine, etorphine, etc.), morphinans, and 6,7-benzomorphans, among the structurally rigid classes of analgesic; the pethidines, methadones, thiambutenes, benzazocines, and a number of miscellaneous types of compounds (etonitazene, etc.) among the structurally less rigid or acyclic analgesics (Jacobson, 1972; Casy, 1970, 1971; Lewis *et al.*, 1971; Jacobson, *et al.*, 1970; Villarreal, 1970; Thullier *et al.*, 1970; May and Sargent, 1965; Hardy and Howell, 1965; Foldes, 1964; May, 1960; Eddy 1939, 1959; Eddy *et al.*, 1956; Braenden *et al.*, 1955).

Arthur E. Jacobson • Medicinal Chemistry Section, Laboratory of Chemistry, National Institute of Arthritis, Metabolism, and Digestive Diseases, National Institutes of Health, Bethesda, Maryland 20014.

Extensive compilations of the thousands of derivatives of each of the various classes or types of known analgesics have been made several times in the past. This review will include only those compounds that have been used to relate chemical structure and biological activity. The biological activities that we will be concerned with will be, mostly, analgesia mediated by the central nervous system (CNS), the side effects of narcotic analgesics (tolerance, physical dependence, etc.), and the effects of narcotic antagonists.

2. ALKALOIDS DERIVED FROM OPIUM AND THEIR DERIVATIVES

The use of various plants for the relief of pain has been noted among the oldest medical writings. Pain has accompanied man throughout his history, whether or not he has attempted to flee from it, or even to seek it.

It can be argued that pain has served a useful function in survival, through evolutionary mechanisms; animals, in fleeing from painful stimuli, survived and maintained themselves as a species. Indeed, all of the vertebrates that have been examined have been found to have receptors in their brain that can stereospecifically (if not fortuitously) bind analgesics and their antagonists (Terenius, 1973; Pert and Snyder, 1973; Simon *et al.*, 1973). It is difficult for man to be objective about his pain. No doubt, some pain relief can be obtained through psychological mechanisms, as well as through drugs, acupuncture and related techniques, and hypnotism. These effects may be mediated by endogenous opiate-like substances.

Although the witch doctor or a drug placebo can, under certain circumstances, serve to induce analgesia, the isolation of morphine (Fig. 1: 1) from opium, obtained from *Papaver somniferum,* was a major step forward in medicinal chemistry. Morphine was isolated early in the 19th century; its chemical structure was not established until 1925 (Gulland and Robinson). The stereochemistry (Stork and Clarke, 1956; Bentley and Cardwell, 1955; Rapoport and Lavigne, 1953) and absolute configuration (Kalvoda *et al.*, 1955) of the molecule were determined only about 25 years ago. Morphine was synthesized, albeit in very low yield, in 1952 (Barton *et al.*, 1963; Elad and Ginsburg, 1954; Gates and Tschudi, 1952, 1956). The analgesia caused by morphine is know to be both site- and dose-dependent (Jacquet and Lajtha, 1973; Eddy and Jacobson, 1971; Tatum *et al.*, 1929).

Chemical derivatization of morphine began well before its complete structure was known. Evidently, the drawbacks associated with its clinical use were recognized fairly early. Generally, the side effects that chemists attempted to eliminate by modifying the morphine structure were: (1) the marked respiratory and circulatory depression it elicited, (2) gastrointestinal disturbances, (3) its dependence liability and, (4) the tolerance to it that is developed in its chronic use.

One of the first derivatives of morphine, prepared by acetylation of both the phenolic hydroxyl group and allylic alcohol moiety, was heroin, 3,6-diacetylmorphine (Fig. 1: 2) (Wright, 1874). Heroin has a faster onset of action than morphine in man and is two to three times as potent as an analgesic. The mode of action of heroin is still uncertain. Its faster onset of action is, presumably, a result of the increased lipophilic character of the acetylated molecule that enables it to pass through the "blood–brain barrier" more quickly and in greater amount (Oldendorf *et al.*, 1972). However, heroin may be deacetylated enzymatically *in vivo* and may therefore be acting as either morphine or 6-acetylmorphine (Way *et al.*, 1960; Eddy and Howes, 1935). Although heroin appears to interact well with the narcotic receptors in guinea pig ileum (Kosterlitz and Watt, 1968), recent evidence indicates that it binds poorly to the narcotic receptors in rat brain homogenates, when care is exerted to curtail the deacetylation (Pert *et al.*, 1976). Thus, heroin appears to have little affinity for the narcotic receptor under these *in vitro* conditions. The binding that is noted under these conditions is attributable to the hydrolysis products of heroin, 6-acetylmorphine, or morphine. The increase in potency of heroin over morphine, in man, is perhaps ascribable to the larger quantities of heroin that reach the receptor and are metabolized. Most of the morphine that is injected into man never reaches the brain receptors.

Remarkably, though the drawbacks to the use of morphine had been noted, those associated with heroin went unnoticed, at least for a while (Dreser, 1898). Heroin was hailed as the perfect analgesic. The overanxiousness of the chemist and clinician to greet each new analgesic as the final answer to morphine's recognized drawbacks has plagued the field for almost a century.

Heroin, of course, has all the defects of morphine. It is also shorter acting, making it less useful clinically, and it has the fatal flaw of being able to promote a euphoric state, perhaps more so than morphine or most of the other narcotic analgesics (Eddy *et al.*, 1957*a*; Seevers and Pfeiffer, 1936). The euphoria said to be produced by heroin in normal volunteers has been questioned by Beecher (1959). However, Oldendorf *et al.* (1972) have attributed the more intractable dependence caused by heroin to its rapid entry into the brain relative to morphine.

The search for a drug that would have morphine's analgesic effect with none, or fewer, of its side effects began in earnest in the 1920s. The morphine molecule was chemically attacked at all of the more easily attackable sites.

2.1. Substitutions on the Aromatic Ring (Ring A)

One of the best-known, clinically utilized alkaloids from *Papaver somniferum* is codeine (Fig. 1: 3). Because of the small quantities of codeine that are obtainable from the plant and the medical need for very large amounts of the drug (Cochin and Harris, 1975) (207,551 kg was estimated as the world requirement in 1972), most of the morphine obtained from *P. somniferum* is used to prepare codeine. Morphine's phenolic hydroxyl group can be fairly easily converted to a methoxyl substituent to produce codeine. It is more difficult to hydrolyze that aromatic methoxyl group in good yield. Thus, although improved syntheses have been devised lately for codeine, morphine would be produced in much poorer yield (Schwartz and Mami, 1975; Schoenewaldt and Ihnen, 1974). Codeine and other compounds produced by etherification of the C-3 hydroxyl group of morphine-like alkaloids are considerably less potent analgesics than morphine (Kupchan and Casy, 1967; Braenden *et al.*, 1955). However, etherification of, for example, the C-3 hydroxyl group of morphine produces analgesics that are nearly as potent orally as they are on parenteral administration. Generally, phenolic compounds are less potent orally than they are subcutaneously. Thus, codeine has achieved widespread clinical utility for the treatment of moderate pain by oral administration (Eddy *et al.*, 1970). It has also found utility as an antitussive. Other C-3 ethers that have found clinical utility, but are much less popular, are ethylmorphine (Fig. 1: 4), benzylmorphine (Fig. 1: 5), and pholcodine (Fig. 1: 6), the latter as an antitussive (Eddy *et al.*, 1957*a*).

The mode of action of codeine is uncertain. Codeine does not show the binding to the narcotic receptors in rat brain homogenates that it theoretically should display if it is moderately potent (Pert and Snyder, 1974). Its onset of action, peak, and duration of effect are very similar to morphine subcutaneously (3.8, 22.5, and 126.5 min for the onset, peak, and duration of effect, respectively, in mice, as compared with morphine's 3.8, 28.2, and 145.2 min). It is possible that codeine is slowly demethylated to morphine *in vivo* and its effects are, in fact, those of lesser amounts of morphine.

If moieties such as chlorine, bromine, amino, or acetoxy are introduced on codeine's aromatic ring, the potency is decreased substantially (Braenden *et al.*, 1955). These substituents can exert at least two effects. They are bulky and can interfere with the interaction of the drug with a macromolecule (its receptor) *in vivo*. They also exert inductive and resonance effects on the aromatic ring. It is now believed that the loss of potency is not due to their inductive or resonance effect, which would tend to say that there is little electronic influence of the aromatic ring on *in vivo* binding to macromolecules. This was indicated by the observation that the newly synthesized 1-fluorocodeine (Fig. 1: 7) was essentially equipotent with codeine (Lousberg and Weiss, 1974). The fluorine atom is almost equivalent, in bulk effect, to a hydrogen atom. Its inductive effect is vastly different. Codeine, however, may not have been a very good choice as a parent molecule. A comparison of potencies between relatively weak analgesics can be subject to considerable error (95% confidence limits on the potencies usually have a much wider spread than those found with the more potent analgesics). It would be of interest to see whether 1-fluoromorphine is equipotent with morphine for substantiation of this important point.

Comparison of the analgesic potencies of codeine and morphine indicates that the substitution of a phenolic ether group for a phenolic hydroxyl substantially decreases activity. Similarly, substitution of a hydrogen atom for the aromatic hydroxyl decreases potency, usually by an order of magnitude. These effects are noted in the structurally rigid classes of analgesics. There have been at least two theories that have been used to explain the importance of a phenolic group to analgesic potency in structurally rigid molecules. Beckett and Casy (1954; Beckett, 1956) have stated that the macromolecule with which the analgesic interacts has, or attains, a certain conformation into which the phenolic group must fit before the biological effect (of analgesia) can occur. A "three point" attachment of the macromolecule to a substrate's flat aromatic moiety, its basic center, and its hydrocarbon area was postulated. More recently, Portoghese (1965) postulated a multiple uptake theory in which a common anionic center serves as a pivotal point around which binding can occur in various ways. Portoghese postulated that nonphenolic and phenolic analgesics may bind differently.

The affinity of substrates for their receptor can be affected by steric and by electronic changes in the substrate. If the reported potency of 1-fluorocodeine, relative to codeine, holds for the morphine series, an electronic effect can be discounted as a major factor. The steric effect of the phenolic hydroxyl (vs. other moieties in or around that area), then, should have a major influence on the interaction of the rigid analgesics with their receptor. There is also, however, the likelihood that the hydrogen-bonding capability of the phenolic hydroxyl dictates the strength of the binding of the substrate to its receptor. Although either the steric or hydrogen-bonding characteristics of the phenol may be important in these structurally rigid analgesics, it should be recognized that many potent analgesics (usually the less rigid or acyclic varieties) lack the hydroxyl group on the phenyl ring. The pethidines and methadones have one or more phenyl rings without a hydroxyl. Another example would be etonitazine (Fig. 4: 8), a benzylbenzimidazole (Carroll and Coleman, 1975; Hunger *et al.*, 1960), which has a nitrophenyl and an ethoxyphenyl moiety. It is about 1000 times as potent as morphine. Unless the ethoxyl group in etonitazene is cleaved to a phenolic moiety much more easily and quickly than the ether in codeine, one must hesitate to attach much importance to the phenol, except with quite specific classes of analgesics (i.e., the rigid types) (Kandeel and Martin, 1973). Furthermore, the thiambutenes do not have either a phenyl moiety or an aromatic hydroxyl (Eddy and Leimbach, 1953; Adamson *et al.*, 1951; Adamson and Green, 1950). However, thiambutene (Fig. 3: 9) and all other potent analgesics do have some type of aromatic ring. It has been assumed that van der Waals forces are exerted between the flat aromatic moiety and the macromolecule that can serve as one part of the "three point" attachment, according to Beckett and Casy (1954), or at an additional binding area that can presumably swing, in the less rigid molecules, to a "correct" position from a pivotal anionic site (Portoghese, 1965). The importance of the aromatic ring to biological activity has been shown by Pirkle and Gates (1965) using the rigid morphinan and isomorphinan molecules. They hydrogenated these compounds and obtained β,γ-unsaturated ketones (Fig. 3: 10 and 11) and secondary alcohols (Fig. 3: 12) that had little or no analgesic activity. There are no known potent analgesics without some type of aromatic ring in their molecular structure, although at least one weak analgesic (codeine-like in potency), thujone (Fig. 4: 13), has been found that lacks even an aromatic ring (Rice and Wilson, 1976).

The van der Waals forces are, evidently, disruptable by bulky groups on the aromatic nucleus, but either they are not influenced by changes in the electronic character of the aromatic moiety or these electronic changes are compensated by the additional binding force contributed by the aromatic hydroxyl group or its metabolic precursor (an ether or ester). The van der Waals forces involve induced dipoles and decrease rapidly according to the distance between the dipoles. Possibly, any substituent on the aromatic ring that is bulky enough to cause even slightly increased distances between the involved molecules will lessen that attractive force considerably. The electronic distribution in the aromatic ring should be much less important to this dipolar interaction. Because of the inherent weakness of the van der Waals forces it would seem unlikely that they could account for more than a minor amount of the energy involved in the interaction of a substrate and a receptor. Portoghese (1965) has postulated that the interaction may be due to hydrophobic attractive forces rather than van der Waals forces. Hydrophobic forces could account for considerably larger amounts of energy than van der Waals forces and would not be affected as much by small changes in the distance between interacting groups. In the rigid class of analgesic, if the hydroxyl group is replaced by a somewhat less bulky hydrogen atom, the analgesic activity of the molecule is, as has been noted, decreased. It is possible that with these rigid analgesics the aromatic ring is forced into an area that is further from the interacting dipole of the macromolecule than in the less rigid analgesics. The aromatic moiety of the less rigid molecule can, perhaps, reach a site where maximum van der Waals attraction or hydrophobic interaction can be obtained. The rigid molecules may use their phenolic hydroxyl as an additional binding site (e.g., through hydrogen bonding) to compensate for some loss in van der Waals interaction, or they may, in fact, greatly increase their overall biological effect through this additional binding.

2.2. Changes at the Allylic Alcohol Moiety (Ring C)

The C-6 ethyl ether of morphine (Fig. 1: 14) and that of dihydromorphine (Fig. 8: 15), 6-acetylmorphine (Fig. 1: 16), 6-formylmorphine (Fig. 1:

17), and 6-propionylmorphine (Fig. 1: 18), the C-6 methyl ether of codeine (Fig. 1: 19), and dihydrocodeine (Fig. 8: 20) have been prepared (May and Jacobson, 1977; Braenden *et al.*, 1955). Generally, etherification or esterification at the C-6 quasi-equatorial position in the morphine or codeine molecule tends to increase potency two- to sevenfold, depending on the substituent. Similarly, oxidation of the dihydro alcohol to a ketone (dihydromorphinone or Dilaudid) (Fig. 8: 21) and dihydrocodeinone (Fig. 8: 22) tend to increase potency manyfold over the parent compound.

Isomorphine (Fig. 1: 23) and isocodeine (Fig. 1: 24) are compounds that have their C-6 hydroxyl groups quasi-axially oriented (oriented above the plane of the C ring, toward the nitrogen atom). They are slightly less potent analgesics than morphine or codeine, respectively. Etherification of the allylic alcohol in the isomorphine series causes increased *in vivo* potency, as it did in the morphine series.

The bulky α-chloromorphide (Fig. 1: 25) has been synthesized, as has β-bromo (Fig. 2: 26) and iodomorphide (Fig. 2: 27) (Eddy, 1939; Small and Lutz, 1932). At the time the α- and β-halomorphides were prepared there were few good spectroscopic methods for discerning the stereochemistry of the molecules. Stork and Clarke (1956; Stork, 1960) showed that the allylic alcohol moiety in morphine and codeine could undergo S_N2' reactions (substitution, nucleophilic, bimolecular, with rearrangement of the double bond) to form the β-halo compounds. They used infrared spectroscopy to differentiate between the α and β compounds. It had originally been presumed that the β-halo compounds were C-6 iso compounds. That is, they were substituted in the C-6 position differently from the normal C-6 substituents. Stork and Clarke showed that the β compounds were, in fact, C-8, not C-6 substituted, due to the S_N2' rearrangement. The double bond ended up between the C-6 and C-7 carbon atoms, and the halide was at C-8.

Nuclear magnetic resonance spectroscopy can now be utilized to determine the position and configuration of the halide in the C ring. Thus, α-chloromorphide (Fig. 1: 25) has been shown to be the C-6 quasiaxially substituted (iso) compound (Yeh *et al.*, 1976), perhaps better named as 6(β)-chloromorphide (in this nomenclature the "β" notation represents a group above the plane of the ring, in the plane of the nitrogen containing D ring; it should be used only when the absolute configuration of the molecule is known). β-Bromo and iodomorphide have been found through nuclear magnetic resonance studies to be C-8 quasi-equatorially substituted compounds, and these compounds might better be named 8(β)-bromomorphide (Fig. 2: 26) or 8(β)-iodomorphide (Fig. 2: 27) (Yeh *et al.*, 1976).

With the determination of configuration about the C-6 or C-8 positions, it becomes possible to discuss the structure–activity relationships of these morphides. All of these compounds, α-chloromorphide, β-bromo, and β-iodomorphide, are more potent analgesics than morphine. Thus, we can say that the substitution of the bulky C-6 quasi-axially oriented chlorine atom for the hydroxyl group in isomorphine enhances activity, compared with isomorphine (or morphine). Increased steric interactions at the C-8 position in the morphine nucleus also appear to cause increased *in vivo* potency. Attractive steric effects have been previously noted (Liberles *et al.*, 1973).

The recently synthesized 6-formyl-, acetyl-, and propionylmorphines (Fig. 1: 17, 16, and 18) are about three times as potent as morphine (May and Jacobson, 1977). These should show increased steric interactions at the C-6 (quasi-equatorial) position, compared with the C-6 quasi-equatorially oriented hydroxyl group, unless they are rapidly metabolized *in vivo* to the hydroxyl group. They are also more lipophilic molecules than morphine; efficient transport to the receptor might explain their high potencies.

Unfortunately, the receptor binding affinity of very few C-6 substituted morphine-like compounds is known. Thus, we have no way of differentiating between transport to the receptor and receptor affinity for these compounds. We do know that the C-6 quasi-axially oriented chloro compound (α-chloromorphide) has about half the affinity for receptors in the homogenate system compared with morphine (Klee, personal communication, 1975) and is about 20 times as potent as morphine *in vivo*. If this isolated example pertains to other C-6 substituted morphine-like compounds then, apparently, transport to the receptor is being considerably hindered by the C-6 hydroxyl group in morphine. This extra hydroxyl group could serve as an additional moiety for metabolic inactivation by glucuronide formation. The glucuronide would be rapidly excreted. The α-chloromorphide compound should be much more lipophilic than morphine. It might be of interest to attempt to relate partition coefficients (which reflect transport) to *in vivo* potencies for the variously substituted C-6 compounds. 6-Methyl-Δ^6-desoxymorphine (Fig. 2: 28), which has a methyl group oriented between the equatorial and axial position of the normally substituted morphine, is much more potent than morphine and equipotent with α-chloromorphide. Thus, there is agreement with the idea that bulky groups at or near the C-6 axial position in morphine increase potency. The 6-methyl-Δ^6-desoxymorphine is also, however, a relatively lipophilic molecule, compared with morphine, and thus its *in vivo* potency might be explained more simply by its more facile transport to the receptor.

The recently synthesized 6-isoazidodihydromorphine (Fig. 8: 29) (Knoll, 1973) has been found to have about the same analgesic activity as the C-6 quasi-axially substituted α-chloromorphide and a dihydrodesoxymorphine. Hydrogenation of the C-7,8 double bond coupled with removal of the C-6 hydroxyl group produces potent analgesics.

Hydrogenation of the C-7,8 double bond in morphine or codeine generally produces a compound with the C-6 substituent in an axial position, oriented away from the nitrogen and toward the aromatic ring. There is no longer a C-6 equatorial hydroxyl group that can cause detrimental hydrogen bonding or interfere with the substrate–receptor interaction by some other mechanism. Thus, dihydromorphine (Fig. 8: 30) has twice the potency of morphine. Benzyldihydromorphine (Fig. 8: 31) and chlorodihydromorphide

(Fig. 8: 32) are as potent as, or more potent than their unsaturated relatives. However, monoacetyl (Fig. 8: 33) and diacetyl dihydromorphine (Fig. 8: 34) appear to be exceptions to this generalization; they are less potent than their unsaturated relatives.

2.3. Modifications Affecting the Shape of Morphine (B/C Rings)

Morphine is a B/C *cis*-fused compound. The B/C *trans*-fused morphine (Fig. 9: 35) has been prepared and found to have only one-tenth of the activity of morphine (Kugita *et al.*, 1970). Thus, it has been suggested that the receptor is seeking a substrate with a particular shape, and can only accept, or bind with, molecules that have that shape—namely, the T shape of morphine with two broad hydrophobic regions at right angles (Goldstein, 1975). However, it is known that B/C *trans* morphinan (Fig. 9: 36) is more potent as an analgesic than its B/C *cis* relative (Fig. 9: 37) or morphine when comparably substituted on the N atom and aromatic ring. It would appear more likely, then, from the above analysis of the effects of the C-6 hydroxyl group and the double bond in the C ring, that these moieties are being displaced to even less favorable positions, with regard to the receptor, in the B/C *trans* morphine than they already are in the B/C *cis* morphine. That is, it might be the effect of the displaced hydroxyl group and/or the double bond on the macromolecule, rather than the general shape of the substrate that primarily causes the loss in potency of the B/C *trans* morphine. It would be of interest to prepare B/C *trans* halomorphides, etc., to see whether this theory has validity. This type of molecule has not been synthesized as yet.

2.4. Epoxide Ring Opening and the Effect of C-10 and C-14 Hydroxyl Groups (Rings B and D)

The opening of the epoxide ring, to give 3,4-dihydroxylated morphines (Fig. 2: 38), was achieved in the dihydrodesoxymorphine (Fig. 8: 39) series. A loss in potency was noted. Athough this tends to favor the view that the epoxide ring is important to activity, in fact its complete removal in the morphinan (Fig. 9: 37) series has indicated its nonessentiality. The unbroken ring appears to be preferred to the additional free hydroxyl group that would be formed through ring cleavage, but the epoxide appears to do little, by itself, to alter activity.

Similarly, introduction of a hydroxyl group at C-10 appears to decrease analgesic potency. The effect of a C-14 hydroxyl group is equivocal. In the C-14 position, the hydroxyl could hydrogen bond intramolecularly to the tertiary nitrogen atom (or, when in the salt form, the protonated amine's hydrogen could bond to the oxygen of the hydroxyl group). The C-14 hydroxyl, like the C-6 hydroxyl group, can also be solvated in polar media (under *in vivo* conditions) and thus produce a formidable bulk effect.

Solvation of the C-14 hydroxyl could conceivably block the nitrogen atom on what had been its most freely accessible side. The C-14 hydroxyl group appears to considerably alter the pharmacological effect of a compound that has agonist–antagonist activity. The type of N-substituent that causes the change in activity from narcotic analgesic to agonist–antagonist will be discussed below. It should be noted in this context, however, that the only pure narcotic antagonist (a compound devoid of any pharmacological activity of its own) is naloxone (Fig. 10: 40), a C-14 hydroxylated compound based on oxymorphone. The C-14 hydroxyl group in the morphine series as well as the morphinan (Monkovic *et al.*, 1973) and benzomorphan series appears to increase the antagonist activity of molecules that have particular substituents on nitrogen (such as the allyl group). Although no other pure narcotic antagonist has been prepared, the search for such compounds is being focused on this type of hydroxylated, rigid molecule. There are several nearly pure antagonists (which have no agonist activity *in vivo*). However, all of these display some agonist activity in either the adenylate cyclase assay system (Klee, personal communication, 1975), or the guinea pig ileum assay system (Kosterlitz *et al.*, 1972).

Although a large number of man-years of effort went into the synthesis of the many derivatives of morphine mentioned thus far, a dissociation of the side effects associated with morphine from analgesic activity was not achieved, except for the narcotic antagonists. All of the nonantagonist derivatives of morphine contain, at least, the same drawbacks as morphine itself. Nevertheless, more potent analgesics than morphine were prepared, some of which have limited clinical utility, and some orally effective analgesics were discovered with fewer side effects than morphine. It is likely that the lesser incidence of dependence liability observed with the less potent analgesics (e.g., codeine) corresponds with the lessened euphoria associated with them. Individuals have occasionally become dependent on codeine (which, of course, has dependence liability of the opiate type), and others have become dependent on the more potent analgesics (e.g., Dilaudid). Therefore, the search for a "pure" analgesic continued (Eddy, 1956).

2.5. Substituents on the Nitrogen Atom

An attempt was made to eliminate the respiratory depression caused by the opiates by preparing *N*-allylnorcodeine (Fig. 10: 41) (Pohl, 1915). This compound appeared to cause less respiratory depression, but its analgesic activity was also lessened, as compared with codeine. A chain of events, however, was initiated by that preparation which eventually resulted in the synthesis of *N*-allylnormorphine (Fig. 10: 42) (nalorphine) (Weijlard and Erickson, 1942; McCawley *et al.*, 1941) and the discovery that nalorphine was a narcotic antagonist. The fascinating history of the agonist–antagonists has been recently discussed (Jacobson, 1972) and will not be repeated here.

Nalorphine proved to be a useful compound as an antidote to narcotic overdosage. It can precipitate a withdrawal syndrome in nonwithdrawn (NW) monkeys dependent on the opiates. It was subsequently found that nalorphine had analgesic activity comparable with morphine in man (Keats and Telford, 1956; Lasagna and Beecher, 1954). The animal tests that were used initially had failed to uncover this activity. Thus, nalorphine was found to be a strong agonist–antagonist, the first compound that could be shown to have potent analgesic activity and to simultaneously be a strong antagonist to the effects of narcotic analgesics. Nalorphine, without dependence liability of the opiate type, has side effects of the psychotomimetic type that militate against its clinical use as an analgesic. However, the discovery that a compound could have antagonist activity and still display potent analgesia initiated the synthesis of many other types of N-derivatives of morphine and of the other classes of analgesics. These syntheses are still being pursued.

Although the antagonists have been noted to display relatively little analgesic activity in the hot plate assay (Archer *et al.*, 1964), other pharmacological animal screens (Lewis *et al.*, 1971; Fraser and Harris, 1967) and the binding of these compounds to the narcotic receptor in rat brain homogenates (Klee and Streaty, 1974; Terenius, 1973; Pert and Snyder, 1973; Simon *et al.*, 1973) and in guinea pig ileum (Kosterlitz and Waterfield, 1975*a*; Kosterlitz *et al.*, 1972; Kosterlitz and Watt, 1968; Gyang and Kosterlitz, 1966), and their reversal of the morphine inhibition of adenylate cyclase in neuroblastoma × glioma hybrid cells (Sharma *et al.*, 1975) are now utilized to find their analgesic activities.

Thus, the activity of narcotic antagonists can now be effectively measured. The ability of apparently simple N-substituents of many different types to confer narcotic antagonist behavior on perfectly ordinary analgesics (Archer and Harris, 1965) does not have an acceptable theoretical explanation. Even optical resolution of some analgesics can provide enantiomers that exhibit narcotic antagonist behavior (May and Eddy, 1966). Further, it has been observed in a few types of analgesics that, with the proper N substituent, a change in an alkyl side-chain sited relatively far from the nitrogen atom can also change the pharmacological profile of the compound from agonist to antagonist (or agonist–antagonist) (Rice *et al.*, 1977). This will be discussed in the sections Benzomorphans and Complex Morphine Derivatives.

Some *N*-nor compounds have also been examined by these newer techniques. Generally, few secondary amines among the opiates or their derivatives are known to interact with the narcotic receptors in guinea pig ileum as well as their *N*-methyl parents (Kosterlitz and Waterfield, 1975*b*). Their potencies, *in vivo,* generally are less by an order of magnitude than those of their *N*-methyl relatives. The decline in potency can be ascribed to their inability to penetrate the "blood–brain barrier" to any great extent, to their inability to effectively bind with the narcotic receptors if they do arrive at the active site, or to their rapid metabolic inactivation. Two secondary amines that bind as well to the receptors in guinea pig ileum as their *N*-methyl parents, namely normorphine (Fig. 10: 43) and norcodeine (Fig. 10: 44), may be ineffective analgesics *in vivo* because of their decreased lipophilicity, which precludes significant access to the vertebrate brain. Normorphine has been shown to have both weak antagonist action and strong agonist activity (equipotent with morphine) on the ileum. In man it has only one-third of the analgesic activity of morphine. The weak antagonist activity of normorphine (and morphine) that was observed in the ileum preparation has not been seen *in vivo,* possibly because of the overwhelming predominance of agonist activity.

3,6-Diacetylnormorphine (Fig. 10: 45) and 6-acetylnormorphine (Fig. 10: 46) are much more lipophilic molecules than normorphine (Rice and Jacobson, 1975), better suited to traverse the blood-brain barrier. These compounds have been shown to bind very poorly to the narcotic receptors in guinea pig ileum (Kosterlitz, personal communication, 1975) and are also relatively inactive *in vivo.* The question of why normorphine and heroin bind so well to the receptor in guinea pig ileum when their close relatives, 3,6-diacetyl- and 6-acetylnormorphine, bind so poorly remains unresolved. Two benzomorphan secondary amines (Fig. 11: 47, 48) also do not bind well to the narcotic receptor from rat brain homogenates (Rice *et al.*, 1977). It has been noted (Kosterlitz and Waterfield, 1975*b*) that one of them, normetazocine (Fig. 11: 48) has antagonist but not agonist activity in the ileum, although this antagonist activity could not be seen *in vivo*. Normetazocine does, however, display agonist activity in the mouse vas deferens preparation and in the adenylate cyclase assay system (Klee, personal communication, 1975). Perhaps some of the secondary amines examined in the ileum are acetylcholinesterase inhibitors and, thus, their actions may be indirectly antagonized since acetylcholine is known to be involved in the response of the ileum to narcotics (Cowie *et al.*, 1968; Paton and Zar, 1968). Acetylcholine is not involved in the response of the vas deferens. Compounds may show different effects on the ileum and vas deferens owing to their reaction with acetylcholinesterase.

3. PETHIDINES

Pethidine, or meperidine (Fig. 12: 49), initially synthesized in Germany, was the first totally synthetic molecule that could be shown to have good analgesic activity (Eisleb and Schaumann, 1939). It, like heroin, was at first declared to be free from dependence liability of the opiate type. Although it was soon found to have a physical dependence capacity comparable to morphine (and all of morphine's other side effects), this fact was, evidently, not presented too effectively in the medical compendia, or else it was overlooked. In any case, an unreasonable proportion of the population of individuals whose primary physical dependence was to meperidine came, at least at first, from the medical profession.

Thousands of derivatives of meperidine have been prepared. Meperidine has achieved considerable clinical utility, perhaps equal to that of morphine. Of the compounds based on the pethidine structure, only alphaprodine (Fig. 12: 50), anileridine (Fig. 12: 51), phenoperidine (Fig. 12: 52), ketobemidone (Fig. 12: 53), piminodine (Fig. 12: 54), trimeperidine (Fig. 12: 55), and properidine (Fig. 12: 56) have found any clinical utility, and most of these are, comparatively, seldom used.

Many theories have been offered to relate the structure of variously substituted pethidines to their activity. In one theory the pethidine structure was drawn so as to show a resemblance to part of the structure of morphine (Schaumann, 1949). To do so, the phenyl ring must be drawn in an axial orientation on the piperidine ring, as it is oriented in morphine. However, it is known that the pethidine type of analgesic normally exists in a conformation that has an equatorially oriented phenyl group. This has been shown by X-ray crystallography of pethidine analogs (Portoghese *et al.*, 1973; Ahmed and Barnes, 1963; Ahmed *et al.*, 1963; Kartha *et al.*, 1960). It is, of course, possible that during the interaction of these small moleules with their receptor the conformation of the pethidine molecule can be changed to one that has the axial phenyl group (a higher energy state). There are at least two other possibilities that can be considered. The first would be that the macromolecule has considerable flexibility and can be altered by the substrate, almost as well as it can, itself, alter the substrate, to accept the pethidine-type of molecule in pethidine's (more stable) ground state. Small molecules have been previously assumed to do this to macromolecules (Mautner, 1967; Rice, 1967). Alternatively, we could be looking at a different population of receptors from those with which the structurally rigid type of analgesic interact. The multireceptor hypothesis for different types of analgesics, or for analgesics and antagonists, has been suggested by many workers (Bowman *et al.*, 1973*a*; Harris, 1971; Martin, 1967; Portoghese, 1966; Taber *et al.*, 1964). Chemically, it should be noted, it would be easier to explain the differences between the two structurally different classes of analgesic, rigid and less rigid, by multireceptors. However, the multireceptor hypothesis appears to be less probable biochemically. Grumbach and Chernov (1965) and Casy (1970) support the view that the analgesics (and antagonists) interact at a common receptor site (Villarreal, 1970). Biochemical experiments with the narcotic receptor are consistent with a single type of receptor that interacts with narcotic antagonists and that may undergo an allosteric change to interact with the narcotic agonists (analgesic). There is no biochemical evidence to indicate that different types of receptors exist *in vivo* that interact with the structurally different classes of analgesics (or analgesics and antagonists). Unless such evidence is found in the future, we are left with only a few hypotheses:

(1) The substrate can induce a change in the receptor so as to enable the interaction of structurally and stereochemically diverse types of molecules (Mautner, 1967; Archer and Harris, 1965). Fortunately, this is not an overly

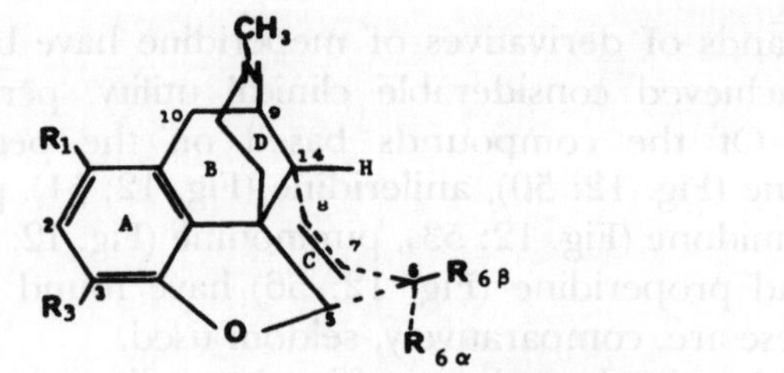

No.	R_1	R_3	$R_{6\alpha}$	$R_{6\beta}$	Compound Name
1	H	OH	OH	H	Morphine
2	H	$OCOCH_3$	$OCOCH_3$	H	Heroin
3	H	OCH_3	OH	H	Codeine
4	H	OC_2H_5	OH	H	Ethylmorphine
5	H	$OCH_2C_6H_5$	OH	H	Benzylmorphine
6	H	$O(CH_2)_2-N$ O	OH	H	Pholcodine
7	F	OCH_3	OH	H	1-Fluorocodeine
14	H	OH	OC_2H_5	H	Morphine ethyl ether
16	H	OH	$OCOCH_3$	H	6-Acetylmorphine
17	H	OH	OCHO	H	6-Formylmorphine
18	H	OH	$OCOC_2H_5$	H	6-Propionylmorphine
19	H	OCH_3	OCH_3	H	Codeine methyl ether
23	H	OH	H	OH	Isomorphine
24	H	OCH_3	H	OH	Isocodeine
25	H	OH	H	Cl	α-Chloromorphide

FIG. 1. Morphine and its derivatives.

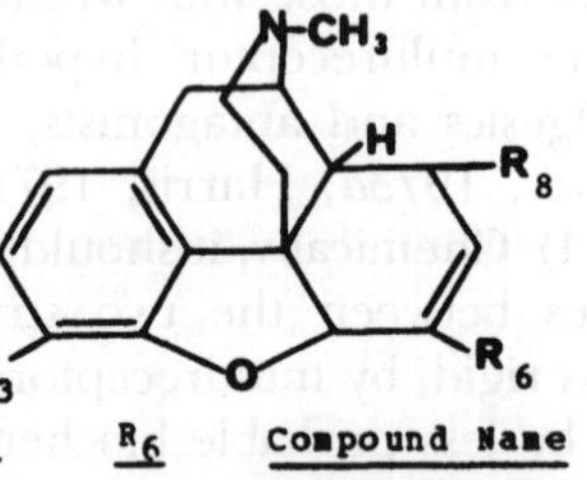

No.	R_3	R_8	R_6	Compound Name
26	OH	Br	H	β-Bromomorphide
27	OH	I	H	β-Iodomorphide
28	OH	H	CH_3	6-Methyl-Δ^6-desoxymorphine

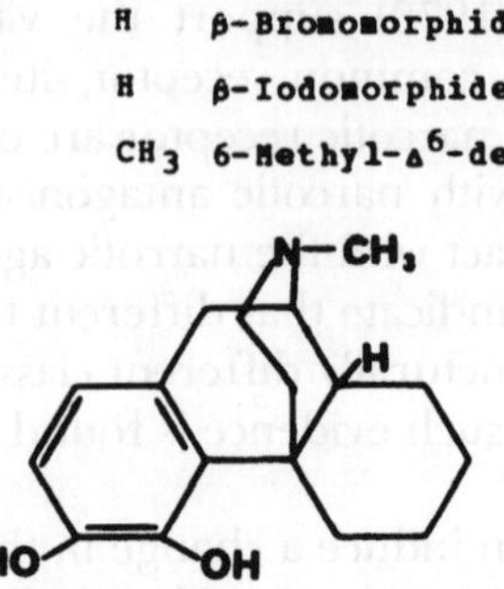

38. 3,4-Dihydroxydesoxydihydromorphine

FIG. 2. Morphine-like structures.

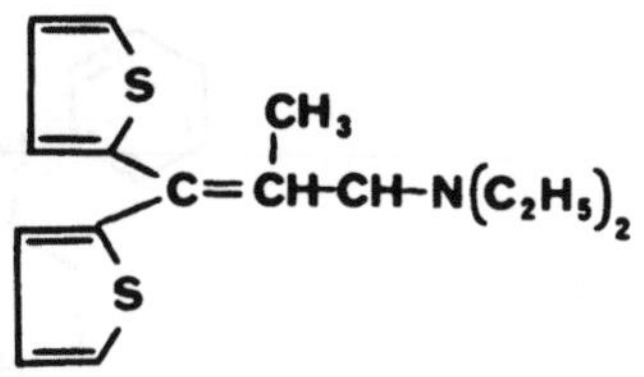

9. Thiambutene

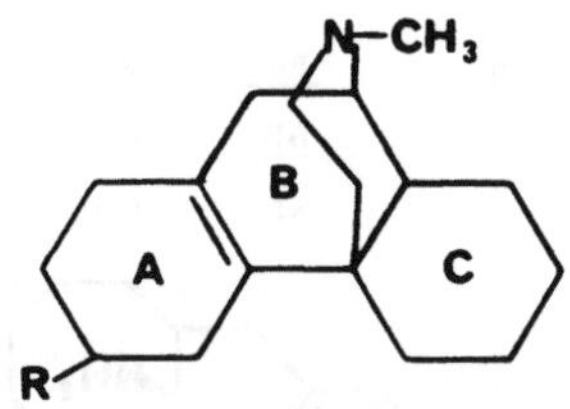

1,2,3,4-Tetrahydro-N-methylmorphinans (B/C cis)

And Isomorphinan (B/C trans)

No.	B/C	R
10	cis	=O
11	trans	=O
12	cis	OH

FIG. 3. Thiambutene and isomeric tetrahydromorphinans.

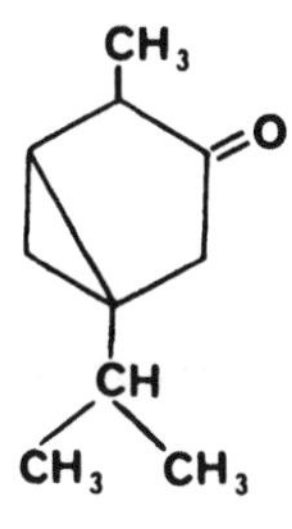

13. Thujone

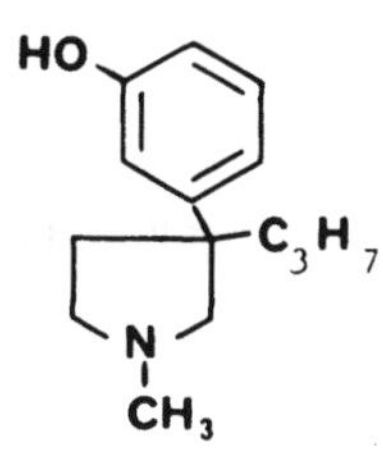

58. Profadol

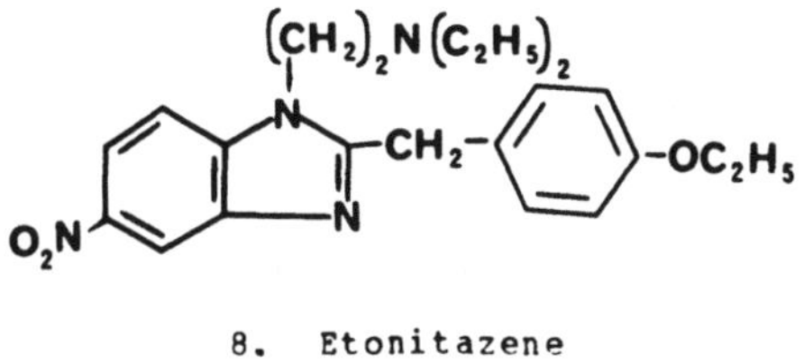

8. Etonitazene

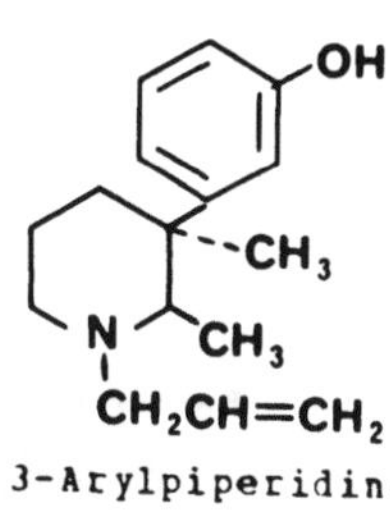

59. 3-Arylpiperidines

(β-Pethidines)

FIG. 4. Thujone, profadol, etonitazene, and β-pethidines.

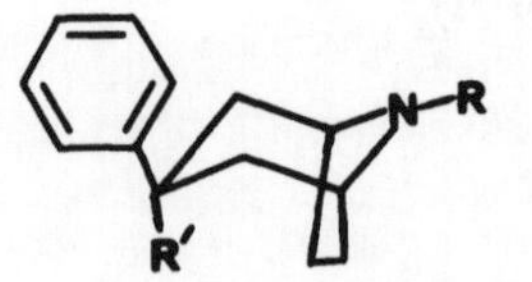

60. Rigid Pethidine Analog

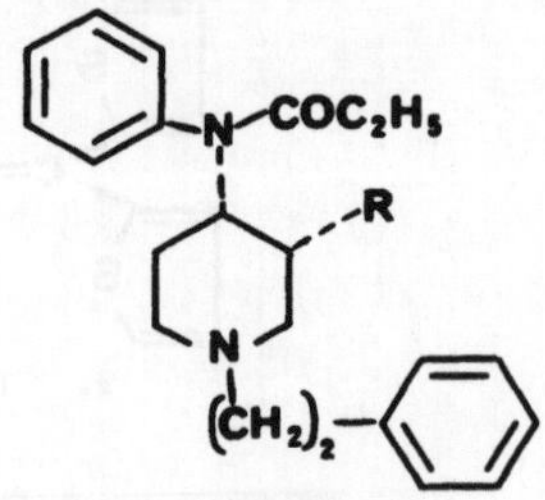

No.	R	Name
65	H	Fentanyl
66	CH_3	Fentanyl Derivative

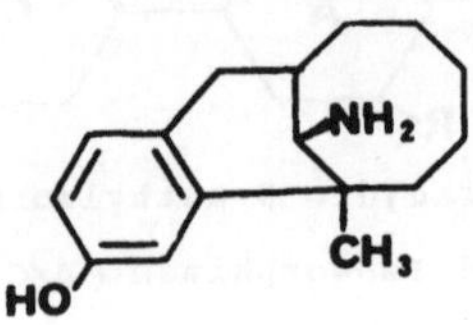

67. Aminotetralin Derivative

FIG. 5. Pethidine analog structure, fentanyl structures, and an aminotetralin derivative.

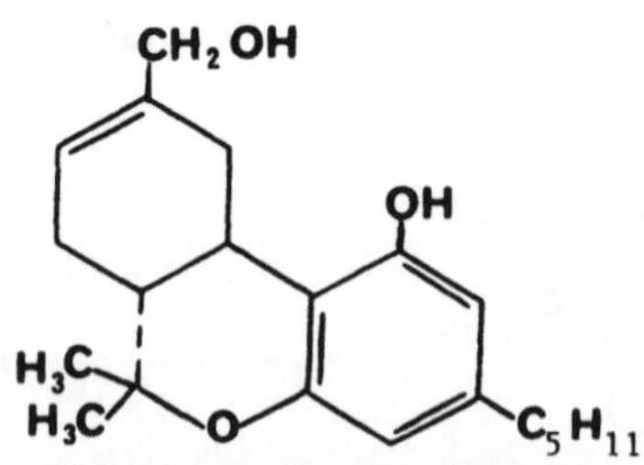

68. 11-Hydroxy-Δ^8-tetrahydrocannabinol

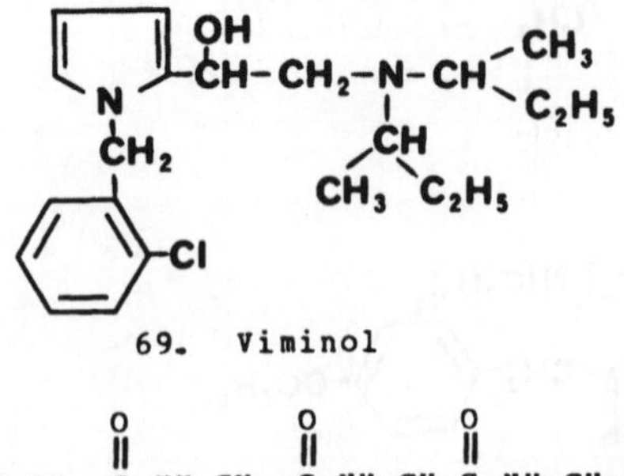

69. Viminol

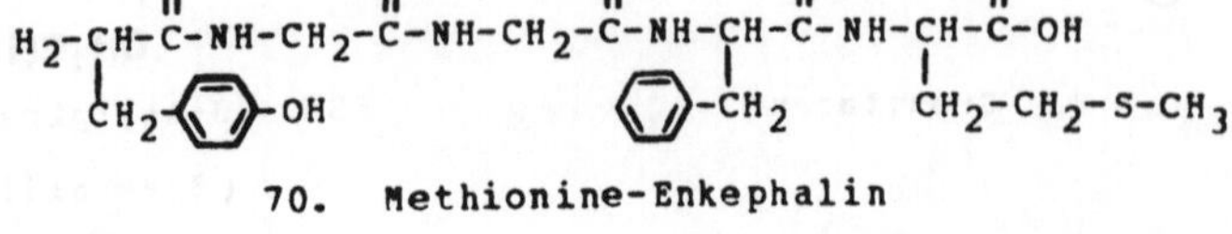

70. Methionine-Enkephalin

FIG. 6. Structure of a tetrahydrocannabinol derivative, viminol, and enkephalin.

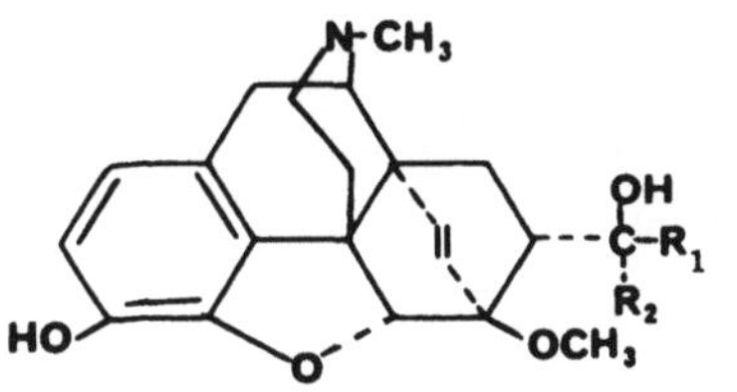

No.	R_1	R_2	Name
71	C_3H_7	CH_3	Etorphine

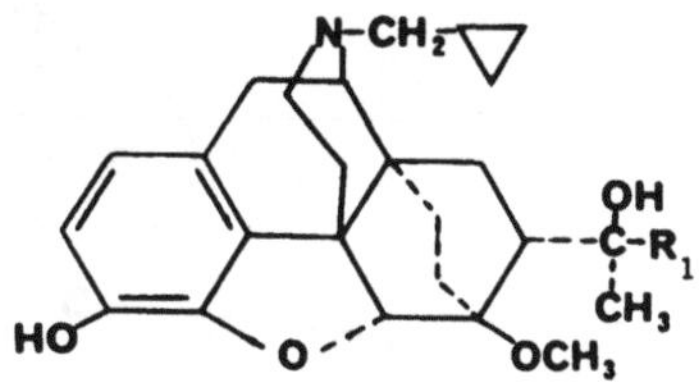

No.	R_1	Name
72	CH_3	Diprenorphine
73	C_4H_9	Buprenorphine

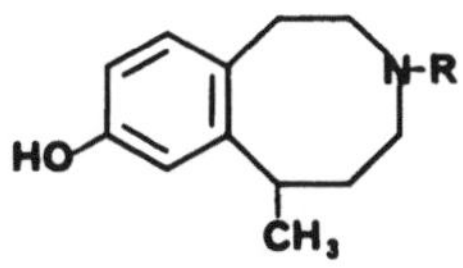

87. N-Substituted (H to Heptyl) Benzazocines

FIG. 7. Oripavine-based endoetheno and endoethano structures, and benzazocine structures.

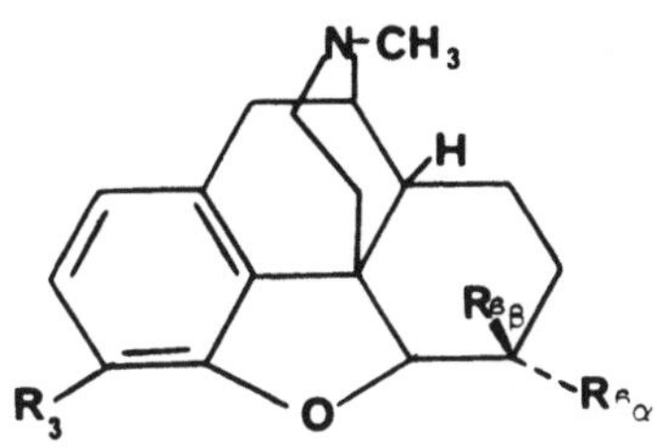

No.	R_3	$R_{6\alpha}$	$R_{6\beta}$	Name
15	OH	H	OC_2H_5	Dihydromorphine ethyl ether
20	OCH_3	H	OCH_3	Dihydrocodeine methyl ether
21	OH	=O	-	Dihydromorphinone
22	OCH_3	=O	-	Dihydrocodeinone
29	OH	H	N_3	6-Isoazidodihydromorphine
30	OH	H	OH	Dihydromorphine
31	$OCH_2C_6H_5$	H	OH	Benzyldihydromorphine
32	OH	H	Cl	Chlorodihydromorphide
33	OH	H	$OCOCH_3$	Monoacetyldihydromorphine
34	$OCOCH_3$	H	$OCOCH_3$	Diacetyldihydromorphine
39	OH	H	H	Dihydrodesoxymorphine

FIG. 8. Dihydromorphine and its derivatives.

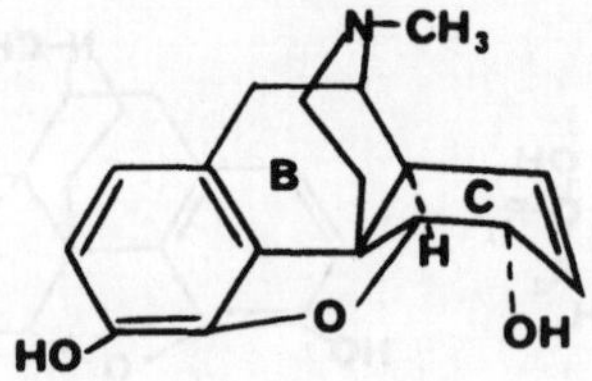

35. B/C trans Morphine

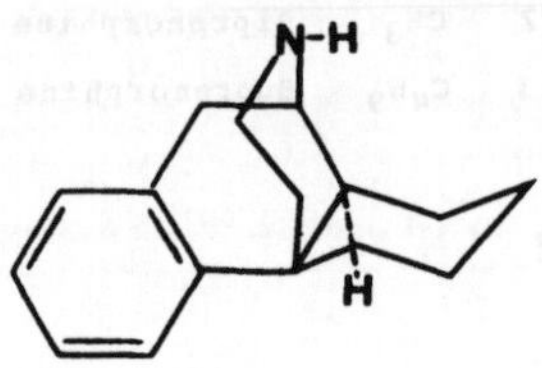

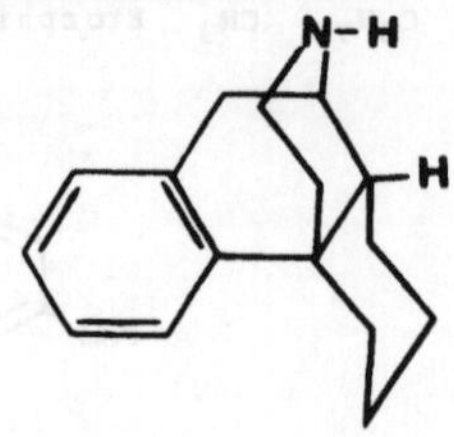

36. B/C trans Morphinan

37. B/C cis Morphinan

FIG. 9. Structures of B/C *cis* and *trans* compounds.

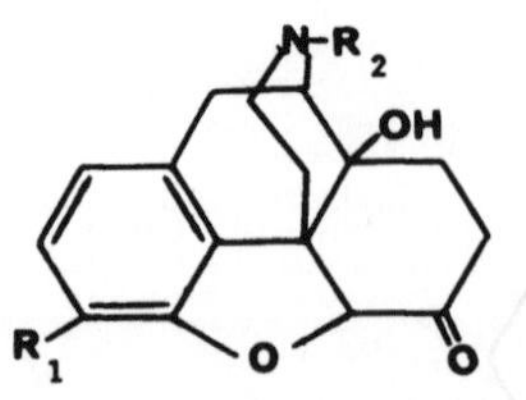

No.	R_1	R_2	Name
40	OH	$CH_2CH{=}CH_2$	Naloxone
86	H	H	Noroxymorphone

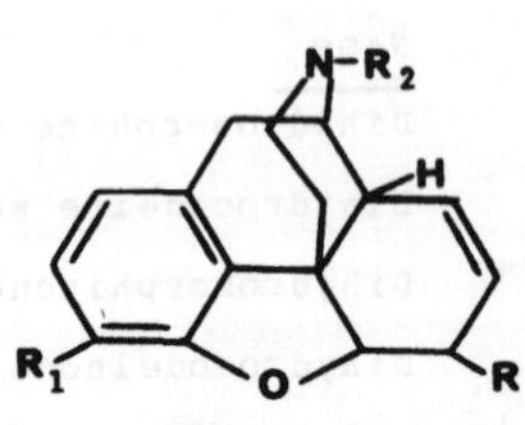

No.	R_1	R_2	R_3	Name
41	OCH_3	$CH_2CH{=}CH_2$	OH	N-Allylnorcodeine
42	OH	$CH_2CH{=}CH_2$	OH	Nalorphine
43	OH	H	OH	Normorphine
44	OCH_3	H	OH	Norcodeine
45	$OCOCH_3$	H	$OCOCH_3$	3,6-Diacetylnormorphine
46	OH	H	$OCOCH_3$	6-Acetylnormorphine

FIG. 10. N-substituted morphine derivatives.

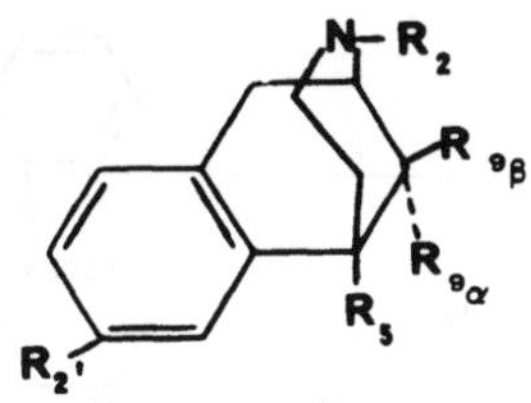

No.	$R_{2'}$	R_2	$R_{9\alpha}$	$R_{9\beta}$	R_5	Name
47	OH	H	C_3H_7	H	CH_3	
48	OH	H	CH_3	H	CH_3	Normetazocine
79	OH	CH_3	H	C_3H_7	CH_3	
80	OH	CH_3	C_3H_7	H	CH_3	
81	H	CH_3	H	H	H	

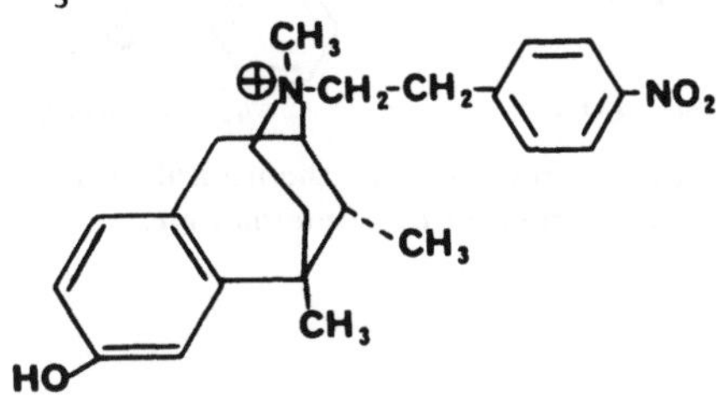

84. Quaternary Ammonium Salt of Metazocine

FIG. 11. 6,7-Benzomorphans.

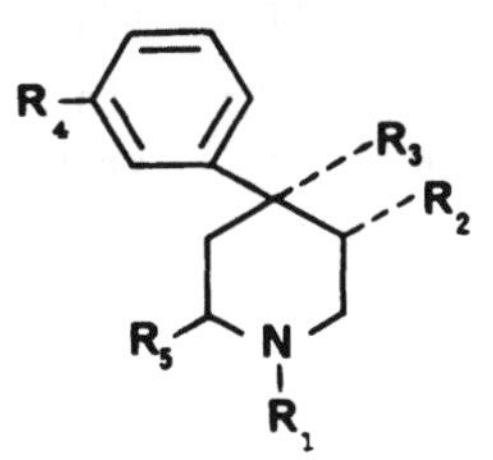

No.	R_1	R_2	R_3	R_4	R_5	Name
49	CH_3	H	$CO_2C_2H_5$	H	H	Meperidine
50	CH_3	CH_3	$OCOC_2H_5$	H	H	Alphaprodine
51	$(CH_2)_2C_6H_4NH_2$	H	$CO_2C_2H_5$	H	H	Anileridine
52	$(CH_2)_2CH(C_6H_5)$-OH	H	$CO_2C_2H_5$	H	H	Phenoperidine
53	CH_3	H	COC_2H_5	OH	H	Ketobemidone
54	$(CH_2)_3NHC_6H_5$	H	$CO_2C_2H_5$	H	H	Piminodine
55	CH_3	CH_3	$OCOC_2H_5$	H	CH_3	Trimeperidine
56	CH_3	H	$CO_2CH(CH_3)_2$	H	H	Properidine
57	H	H	$CO_2C_2H_5$	H	H	Norpethidine
85	H	H	$CO_2C_2H_5$	OH	H	Norbemidone

FIG. 12. 4-Aryl piperidines.

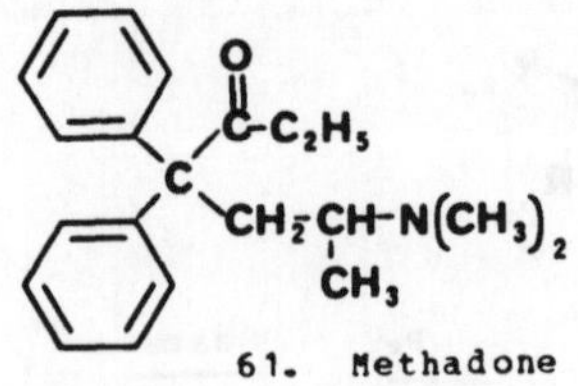

61. Methadone

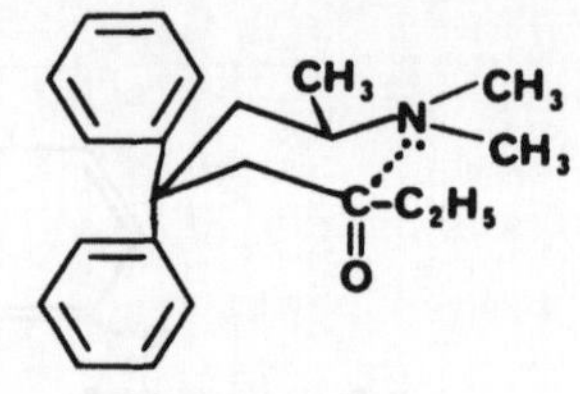

62. Methadone Base

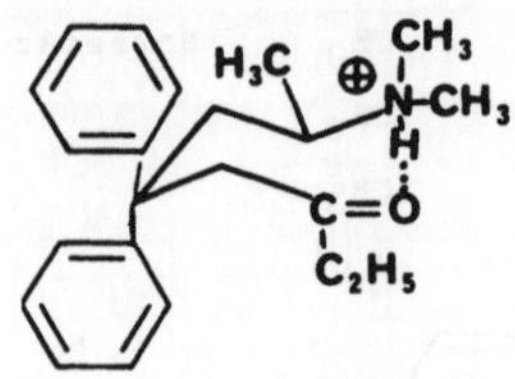

63. Methadone Salt

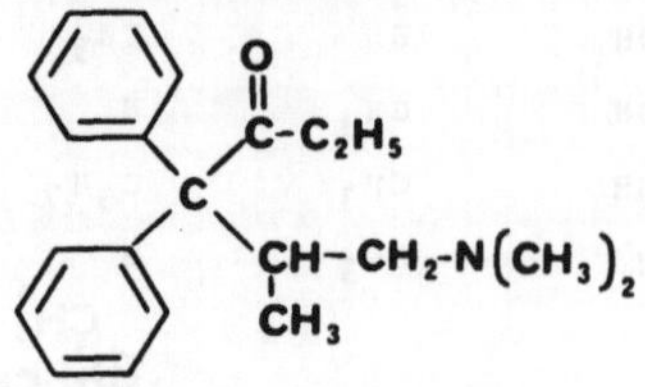

64. Isomethadone

FIG. 13. Structure of methadone, theoretical conformations of methadone, and the structure of isomethadone.

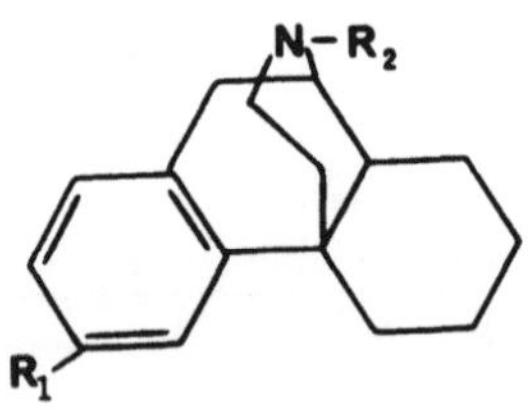

No.	R_1	R_2	Name
74	OH	CH_3	Racemorphan
75	OCH_3	CH_3	Dextromethorphan
76	OH	$CH_2CH{=}CH_2$	Levallorphan
78	OH	CH2–△	Cyclorphan

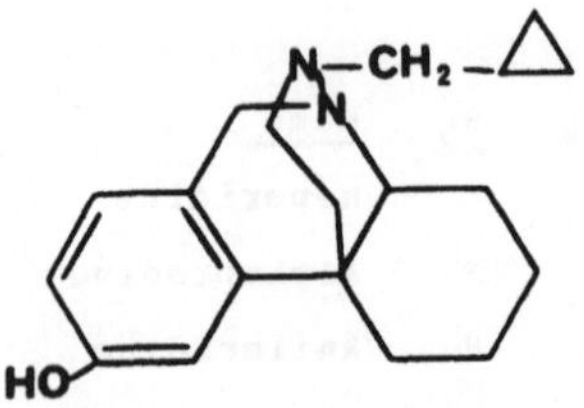

77. 9-Azamorphinan Derivative

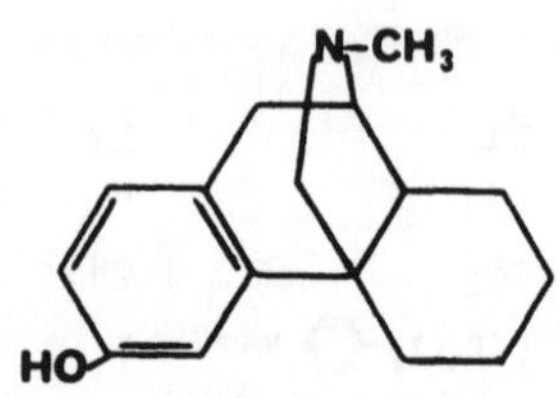

82. D-Normorphinan Derivative

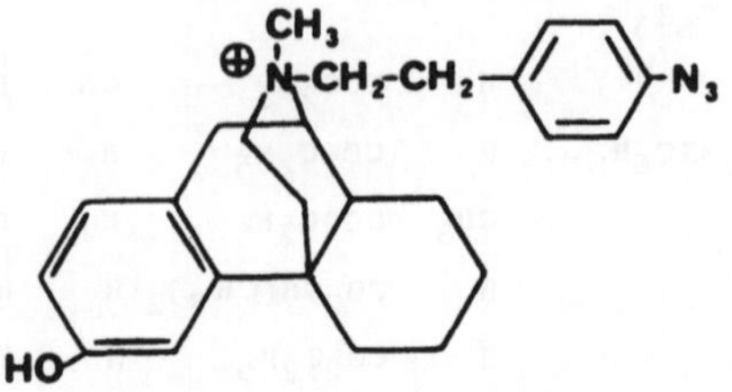

FIG. 14. Structure of racemorphan, substituted morphinans, and morphinan-like compounds.

improbable event, although it tends to make structure–activity correlation among the analgesics more difficult.

(2) The receptor imparts sufficient energy to the less rigid class of substrate to enable it to reach a higher energy state conformation, similar to that which rigid analgesics normally have in their ground state. This latter possibility would not explain why the introduction of a hydroxyl on the phenyl ring does not increase the potency of the pethidines [the carbalkoxy type of compound (Fig. 12: 49)]. Furthermore, introduction of an allyl, propyl, or cyclopropylmethyl group on *N*-norpethidine (Fig. 12: 57) does not convert it to a narcotic antagonist, as such moieties do in the structurally rigid molecules.

In nonrigid pyrrolidines [e.g., profadol (Fig. 4: 58)], replacement of the *N*-methyl group with *N*-cyclopropylmethyl has been asserted to cause weak narcotic antagonist action in mice (Bowman *et al.*, 1973*b*). Profadol, itself, has unusual biological activity. It displays some, but not all, of the characteristics of narcotic antagonists in monkeys and in man. It showed subjective effects similar to those of morphine and very weak antagonist activity in man (Villarreal, 1970). The inability of pethidines to show antagonistic behavior on appropriate substitution has been said by Archer and Harris (1965) to be due to the fact that the pethidines have phenylpropylamine part structures, not the phenethylamine structures of the rigid morphine-like molecules. In fact, when a β-pethidine-like compound was prepared with the phenyl ring in the C-3 position of the piperidine ring (Fig. 4: 59), which would give a phenethylamine part structure, the introduction of an allyl moiety on the nitrogen atom did impart antagonistic properties to the molecule (Iorio and Casy, 1975; Kugita *et al.*, 1965). These 3-phenylpiperidine derivatives appear, in their chemical-structure–biological-activity profile, to be much more closely allied to the rigid analgesics than are the normal 4-phenylpiperidines.

(3) An intermediate situation exists in which the receptor imparts sufficient energy to the pethidine type of molecule to cause it to change from its normal chair conformation to a skew-boat conformation in which the substituents on the piperidine ring are more closely related, stereochemically, to the rigid analgesic structure. The receptor, perhaps, could find it easier to orient its own shape so as to accept this conformer. Casy (1968) has presented spectroscopic evidence to show that some population of pethidine analog skew-boat conformers do exist in polar media. The recent syntheses of more structurally rigid (chair form) pethidine analogs (Fig. 5: 60) (Daum *et al.*, 1975; Portoghese *et al.*, 1968) suggest, however, that the stereochemical configuration of the aromatic ring is not of great importance to the biological activity of this type of analgesic.

The initial hypothesis, that the substrate can modify the receptor, still remains as a possibility due, perhaps, to the difficulty of experimental substantiation.

Substituent changes in the carbalkoxy moiety of the pethidines, from the ethyl ester to other ester moieties, generally reduce potency. Increased potency has been noted by introduction of a phenethyl, and a number of other substituents, on the nitrogen atom, in place of methyl (Hardy and Howell, 1965). The *para*-aminophenethyl analog of pethidine, anileridine (Fig. 12: 51), is two to three times more potent than meperidine. Phenoperidine (Fig. 12: 52), is more potent than meperidine by at least a few orders of magnitude. Piminodine (Fig. 12: 54), also, is more potent than meperidine. Heterocyclic and heteroaromatic moieties have been introduced in that position to give more potent analogs. All of these compounds appear to have the same drawbacks as those associated with meperidine and morphine. They have dependence liability, produce respiratory depression, etc. None of these analogs have achieved the clinical utility of the markedly less potent meperidine. A considerable number of analogs that are based on the pethidine structure have been discussed by Hardy and Howell (1965).

3.1. Prodines and Ketobemidones

There are at least two other series of compounds directly related to the pethidines that are of theoretical interest. These are the prodines (Fig. 12: 50) (4-acyloxy series, in contrast to the 4-carbalkoxypethidines) and the ketobemidones (Fig. 12: 53) (derivatives of 4-keto, 4-metahydroxyphenylpiperidines). The prodines are generally more analgesically potent than the pethidine-like compounds. Although alphaprodine is somewhat less potent than morphine analgesically, its diastereomer (at R_2, see Fig. 12: 50), Betaprodine, has three times the potency of morphine. These are 3-alkyl-substituted prodines. A 2,5-disubstituted prodine, trimeperidine, or promedol (Fig. 12: 55), is about equipotent with morphine. As in the pethidine series, a 1-phenethyl or 2-anilinoethyl substituent in the prodine molecule enhances potency considerably.

Portoghese and co-workers have theorized that a chiral edge of the prodine is of great importance to its biological activity (Larson and Portoghese, 1973; Portoghese *et al.*, 1973). They asserted that the receptor has the ability to differentiate between enantiotopic edges of the prodine molecules and, later, they also found this to be true for trimeperidine (Fries and Portoghese, 1974). Both the configuration and the conformation of substrates were of importance for receptor interaction. An earlier qualitative theory of Beckett and Casy (1954) essentially drew a macromolecular three-point template to which various parts of analgesic molecules were bound. The latter theory relies on the substrate's charged nitrogen atom to fit into an anionic site on a receptor. The bond postulated by Beckett and Casy would depend on the electronic charge on the nitrogen atom. The charge would presumably vary in accord with the effect of the nitrogen atom's substituent. Molecular orbital calculations and the determination of electron density on the nitrogen atom of various analgesics and antagonists by X-ray photoelectron spectroscopy (Saethre *et al.*, 1975) do not support Beckett and Casy's theory.

The ketobemidones are potent analgesics. As with the pethidines, it was thought that it would not be possible to produce antagonists from this class of analgesic, since the ketobemidones were a less rigid type of analgesic with a phenylpropylamine part structure. Recently, however, weak antagonists (in monkey species) have been prepared by substitution of higher alkyl groups on nitrogen (Wilson *et al.*, 1975; Oh-Ishi and May, 1973). This homologous series of N-substituted ketobemidones (where the *N*-alkyl substituents encompass methyl to nonyl) is of theoretical interest. The analgesic potencies of these compounds, as measured by the hot plate assay, have been quantitatively related to receptor binding in rat brain homogenates and guinea pig ileum. This series is one of the few known in which transport, or other pharmacokinetic parameters, evidently play only a minor role, if any, in the analgesic activity of the molecules. Generally, *in vivo* analgesic potencies do not appear to quantitatively correlate with *in vitro* receptor binding. Additional classes of analgesics should be examined to see whether other quantitative relationships can be found.

4. METHADONES

The methadones (Fig. 13: 61) were the second major class of synthetic analgesic to be prepared (Bockmühl and Erhart, 1948). Although several attempts have been made to relate the structure of this class of analgesic to morphine, most of these qualitative theories have defects. Methadones have the general structure: $(Ar)_2—C—(R)—(CH_2)_n—N(R'_2)$, where R represents the ketone, alcohol, etc., and R′ the substituent on nitrogen. The Ar function represents an aromatic ring of some type (there are usually two aromatic rings).

The methadones have a ketone function; the methadols have a corresponding alcohol function. The acetylmethadols are, of course, the acetylated derivatives of the methadols. The methadones have also been chemically modified to amides, nitriles, and sulfones. Howell and Hardy (1965) have listed many of the thousands of individual methadone-like compounds, as has Janssen (1962, 1960). Modified methadone-like compounds have been prepared recently (Regnier *et al.*, 1972).

The methadone family, like the pethidines, include compounds that range from codeine-like in potency to those considerably more potent than morphine. They have side effects essentially identical with those noted for the opiates. Although the methadones and their derivatives do show physical dependence liability of the opiate type in man, the dependence has a somewhat milder withdrawal syndrome with some of them. Perhaps because the withdrawal syndrome occurs over a considerably longer time period with methadone than with morphine, it is easier for an addict to withdraw from physical dependence on methadone. No narcotic antagonist has been prepared from the methadone family's less rigid structures. Interest, after 1960, in the synthesis of new methadone-like compounds was rather limited until long-acting methadone derivatives began to be sought for the treatment of individuals physically dependent on the opiates. Some of the acetylmethadols (Eddy *et al.*, 1952; May and Mosettig, 1948) are being examined in this regard, since they were shown to have a considerably longer duration of action in man.

Gero (1954) and Beckett and Casy (1954) noted that methadone could be drawn (on paper) (Fig. 13: 62, 63) in a conformation that resembles a partial structure of morphine, and they have related the absolute configuration of (—)-methadone (the analgesically active enantiomer) to D-(—)-alanine. Beckett *et al.* (1956*a*) have studied the ionization of methadone-like compounds and found little relationship between analgesic potency and pK_a. Beckett and co-workers (1956*b*), in studying the relationship between steric parameters and biological activity, noted an apparent positive (qualitative) correlation of activity and the effective width of the basic group, measured from molecular models.

More recently, Shefter (1974) determined the crystal structure of α-methadol and (—)-isomethadone (Fig. 13: 64) (a structural isomer of methadone) by X-ray crystallography and compared his results with the previously determined crystal structures of methadone and methadone hydrobromide. He found that these compounds lacked stereochemical similarity. Isomethadone base or salt did not show intramolecular hydrogen bonding. The N···C═O association is more likely to exist in methadone base (Fig. 13: 62) [the N—H···C═O association in the salt (Fig. 13: 63)], but appeared to be weaker in the base than previously assumed. It should be noted, however, that solvent-induced conformational changes are likely. The conformation of a molecule in the solid state is not necessarily the only, or most stable, conformation when it is in aqueous solution. In aqueous solution, for example, the tendency for hydrogen bonding of polar atoms to solvent is enhanced. Intramolecular hydrogen bonding would be favored in nonpolar media. Thus, Henkel *et al.* (1974) used circular dichroism (CD) to show that perturbations in the conformational distribution of methadone were primarily a result of the (polar) solvent's hydrogen bonding to the amine or ketone moiety. The CD study and NMR data (Henkel *et al.*, 1974) indicated that Beckett and Casy's original drawing, which related methadone to morphine, was not very likely (the population of molecules in that conformation was significantly less than in a conformation in which N···C═O association could not occur). The N—H···O═C conformation appeared possible in the methadone salt, but not likely in the isomethadone salt. A possible conclusion from these data would be that it is not at all necessary for a molecule to have the topology of morphine in order for it to bind to narcotic receptors and induce the biochemical events that result in analgesia. Similar conclusions, of course, are noted with the pethidines.

5. MISCELLANEOUS ANALGESICS

Compounds with structures very dissimilar to morphine have been found to bind well to the narcotic receptors and are potent analgesics. Indeed, compounds that do not in the least resemble morphine and that do not even appear to bind to narcotic receptors have been noted to produce analgesia (at least in mice in the hot plate assay). The mechanism of analgesic action of compounds that do not bind to the narcotic receptor may be quite different than that of compounds that have been shown to have good receptor affinity. For example, compounds that lower the body temperature of mice may appear to be analgesics in the hot plate assay. This "analgesia" may not be observable in man, however, nor in other analgesic assays.

Some dissimilar compounds (to morphine) that are known to bind to receptors (*in vitro*) and are highly potent were prepared by Janssen (1962; Janssen *et al.*, 1963). These are phenylpropionamides, such as fentanyl (Fig. 5: 65). Fentanyl, and a recently reported methyl-substituted fentanyl (Fig. 5: 66) (Van Bever *et al.*, 1974), are from five hundred to several thousand times as potent as morphine (Fancher *et al.*, 1964).

Primary amines that are sterically crowded (around the amine) have been found to have good analgesic activity, when present in bridged aminotetralins (Fig. 5: 67) (Freed *et al.*, 1973).

A (—)-11-hydroxy-Δ^8-tetrahydrocannabinol (Fig. 6: 68) has been shown to have good analgesic potency in mice (Wilson and May, 1975). It does not appear to bind to narcotic receptors and it is not structurally similar to morphine, lacking even an amino group.

Thujone, an essential oil constituent, lacks both an amino group and an aromatic ring (Fig. 4: 13). It has been shown to have codeine-like analgesic potency in mice in two pharmacological screens (Rice and Wilson, 1976). Mice show a Straub tail reaction to this compound. Thujone does not bind at all to narcotic receptors *in vitro*.

Viminol (Fig. 6: 69) is a compound that has a tertiary amine function and an aromatic ring two carbon atoms away from it. The aromatic ring, however, is a pyrrole ring. One of the isolated stereoisomers has morphine-like analgesic activity; another stereoisomer will antagonize that activity, but is not a general narcotic antagonist (Della Bella *et al.*, 1973). The analgesically potent compound (*in vivo*) was found to bind only 0.01 times as well as morphine to narcotic receptors in the homogenate system, and had only 0.04 times the activity of morphine in the adenylate cyclase assay (Klee, personal communication, 1975).

Endogeneous morphine-like factors (Terenius and Wahlström, 1974,

1975; Hughes, 1975; Hughes *et al.*, 1975*a,b*; Pasternak *et al.*, 1975; Cox *et al.*, 1975), recently isolated from pig brains and pituitary extracts, are known to be relatively low-molecular-weight peptides and thus do not look at all like morphine. One of the amino acids in the peptide is tyrosine, which does have at least the *para*-hydroxyphenethylamine fragment present in morphine and in most, but certainly not all, potent analgesics. One of the peptides [methionine-enkephalin (Fig. 6: 70)] is 20 times more active than normorphine in the vas deferens preparation and equipotent with normorphine in the guinea pig ileum (Hughes *et al.*, 1975*b*). It is 100 times more potent than morphine as an inhibitor of adenylate cyclase in neuroblastoma × glioma hybrid cells (Klee and Nirenberg, 1976). These peptides have been synthesized and are being extensively investigated. It is, as yet, not certain whether these peptides are acting as analgesics in the brain of vertebrates, or have some other function. Although it has been mentioned (Snyder, 1976) that some analgesic activity can be observed with the endogeneous peptide within the first few minutes after direct intracerebral injection, no analgesic activity was noted after subcutaneous injection, in mice, in the hot plate test (Jacobson and Klee, unpublished results, 1976).

It is fairly clear, from the above examples, that whatever type of molecule initiates the biochemical pathways leading to analgesia, it need not be a molecule that structurally or topologically resembles morphine and the opiates. A few of them may act through rather different biochemical mechanisms than most known centrally acting analgesics, since they do not interact with the narcotic receptors and still appear to produce "analgesia" *in vivo*.

6. COMPLEX MORPHINE DERIVATIVES: THE "M" SERIES

The failure of efforts to obtain an analgesic superior to morphine, and the failure of attempts to eliminate the side effects of the opiates by simplifying the morphine molecule indicated to Bentley and Hardy (1967*a*) that what might be needed were molecules with more highly complicated structures. Presumably, the more rigid and complex compound could fit on some "receptor surface" to give only analgesic action. The more flexible molecules, like the pethidines and the methadones could, as Bentley noted, fit into other receptors as well, and thus cause the noted side effects of the opiates. In a series of papers initiated in 1956 (Bentley and Thomas; Bentley and Hardy, 1963), Bentley and co-workers described a Diels–Alder reaction on thebaine to produce an aromatic methoxy compound and, later, the phenolic hydroxyl compound of the oripavine type (Bentley and Hardy, 1967*b*). They produced endoetheno and endoethano products (Bentley *et al.*, 1967). These molecules appeared to fit the opiate receptor very nicely. One of these compounds, called M-99 or etorphine (Fig. 7: 71), had activity approaching 10,000 times that of morphine in animal species. In man, it is about 100 to 1000 times as potent as morphine. However, the molecule appeared to fit other receptors in the CNS as well as it did the opiate receptor, since its side effects were greater than those from morphine.

In the late 1950s (May and Fry, 1957; Eddy *et al.*, 1957*b*; May and Murphy, 1955), a new type of simplified morphine-like compound was synthesized, a 6,7-benzomorphan, that could reproduce the analgesic activity of morphine and, at least in animals (and, later, in man), showed dissociation of dependence liability of the opiate type from analgesic potency. Thus, the possibility that strong analgesic potency and, presumably, an excellent fit to the receptor were going to inevitably lead to dependence liability as one of the main side effects of analgesics was negated.

About this time, the N-substituted morphine analog, nalorphine, was found to have both agonist and antagonist activity. Thus, soon thereafter, the M series of compounds were similarly derivatized on nitrogen in an attempt to eliminate at least some of the side effects of these compounds and, hopefully, produce powerful narcotic antagonists. Interestingly, substitution of allyl for the methyl on the nitrogen atom of etorphine did not produce a narcotic antagonist. In fact, narcotic antagonists could not be prepared from etorphine by replacing the methyl on the nitrogen atom with any of the usual moieties that were known, by then, to produce antagonists in the morphine series, and in other types of analgesics. In the *N*-cyclopropylmethyl-substituted endoethano series, when the propyl group (R_1) on the side chain at C-7 (see Fig. 7: 71) was changed to methyl or ethyl, or when both R_1 and R_2 (in Fig. 7: 71) were changed to ethyl, potent narcotic antagonists were produced [M-5050, diprenorphine (Fig. 7: 72) (Blane and Dugdall, 1967)]. A longer R_1 alkyl side chain, the *n*-butyl, combined with an *N*-cyclopropylmethyl group on the nitrogen atom, produced a potent agonist–antagonist, buprenorphine (Fig. 7: 73), again in the endoethano series. The possible interaction of the alkyl side chain with the C-6 methoxyl group has been pointed out as a possibility for inducing a different conformational fit of these molecules to a receptor, resulting in the changed pharmacological profile (Lewis, 1974).

The fact that a change in the side chain of the M series combined, of course, with proper N substitution, could alter the pharmacological profile of the compound (from agonist to antagonist or agonist–antagonist) has not been observed in any other series of analgesic until quite recently in the benzomorphans, and this will be discussed later.

Complex molecules, in fact, are not needed to induce potent pharmacological activity, in the sense that these more complex compounds need to be more rigid. Potent narcotic analgesics can obviously be obtained from less rigid or complex molecules (e.g., fentanyl). Etorphine does bind as well as, or better than most of the other analgesics to the narcotic receptor *in vitro*. However, it does not bind to these receptors in accord with its *in vivo* potency in animals. That is, it binds about 10 times as well as morphine does, which is hardly comparable to the difference in potencies of these compounds in animals. Obviously, transport of the more lipophilic etorphine to the receptor site is of great importance in the expression of potency of the compound; the fit to the receptor is only one of many factors that ultimately account for pharmacological potency.

7. MORPHINANS

As we have seen, the pethidines and the methadone-like compounds can be drawn so that they appear somewhat similar to part of the structure of morphine, although crystallographic data do not show these as preferred structures in the solid state and spectroscopic evidence does not show them as preferred in solution. The third large class of totally synthetic analgesics, the morphinans (Fig. 9: 37) (Grewe and Mondon, 1948; Grewe, 1946), are related structurally and stereochemically to morphine. The morphinan rings A to D are structurally identical to those of morphine, but lack morphine's allylic alcohol group and dihydrofuran ring. The phenolic derivative of morphinan, racemorphan (Fig. 14: 74), retains morphine's analgesic potency and essentially all of its side effects.

The analgesic activity of racemorphan lies in its levo isomer, levorphanol. The dextro enantiomer, dextrorphan, and its methoxylated relative, dextromethorphan (Fig. 14: 75), have no analgesic activity but do show cough-reflex suppressant effects. The morphinans have been used in receptor studies. The stereochemically specific binding affinity of levorphanol, and the lack of affinity of its diastereomer, dextrorphan, for narcotic receptors was an essential part of the evidence that was presented to indicate that receptors were present in the CNS of vertebrates through which the centrally acting analgesics exerted their effects.

Structure–activity relationships in the morphinans (Eddy *et al.*, 1958) parallel those in the related morphines. The clinical utility of these analgesics has been limited by their dependence liability and the utility of the derived agonist–antagonists has been limited by their psychotomimetic side effects.

A large number of aralkyl substituents have been introduced on the nitrogen of the normorphinans. The furylethyl and *p*-aminophenethyl derivatives of (—)-3-hydroxynormorphinan were found to have about 100 times the potency of morphine in mice in the hot plate test. The benzyl moiety was among the least potent N substituents (analgesically inactive to 100 mg/kg, subcutaneously).

The structurally rigid morphinans can be converted to agonist–antagonists by appropriate substitution on the *N*-nor base (Gates and Montzka, 1964). The introduction of substituents known to convert analgesics to agonist–antagonists in the morphine series results in a similar change in pharmacological profile in the morphinans. Levallorphan (Fig. 14: 76), *N*-allyl-3-hydroxymorphinan, is a potent agonist–antagonist. It, like nalorphine, exhibits untoward psychotomimetic side effects, which limits its clinical use. The introduction of a C-14 hydroxyl group in a suitably N-substituted morphinan increases narcotic antagonist activity, as it did in the morphine series.

An *N*-cyclopropylmethyl-substituted 9-azamorphinan (Fig. 14: 77) has been found to have twice the potency of pentazocine as an analgesic and antagonist (Kametani *et al.*, 1973). Thus, introduction of a second tertiary amine function in the molecule lowered its potency but did not cause a complete loss of either biological property [compared with cyclorphan (Fig. 14: 78), a very strong agonist–antagonist (Harris *et al.*, 1967)].

The morphinans represented the first instance in which an incomplete, synthetically derived morphine-like structure could be shown to have all of, or more than, the analgesic activity of morphine. They sparked the search for even more simplified morphine-like structures. This effort was culminated by the synthesis of the 6,7-benzomorphans by E. L. May and his coworkers.

8. BENZOMORPHANS

The benzomorphans (Fig. 11) can be viewed as compounds in which the A, B, and D rings of morphine and the morphinans are retained and the C ring is cleaved to form alkyl side chains. The benzomorphans have been the subject of a great deal of contemporary work owing to the observation that analgesia and dependence liability were separable in some of them.

Various substituents have been introduced into the 2′, 2, 5, 9α, and 9β positions, among others (Parfitt and Walters, 1971), of the benzomorphan nucleus (the numbering system has been changed from the morphine skeleton). The 9α and 9β substituents are of special interest. A 9α-substituted benzomorphan stereochemically resembles morphine and the morphinans rather closely. The 9α substituent, when it is a methyl group, for example, can be seen to be affected by the ring current of the aromatic ring when observed spectroscopically by NMR (Fullerton *et al.*, 1962). A 9α substituent is, thus, oriented away from the nitrogen function, allowing the nitrogen to be more rapidly attacked by electrophilic reagents (e.g., methyl iodide) (Fullerton *et al.*, 1962). The 9β substituent is oriented toward the nitrogen atom and effectively blocks it from electrophilic attack; it represents the "wrong" stereochemistry, as compared with morphine. These stereochemical assignments have been confirmed by X-ray crystallographic data (Cochran, 1975; Yokoyama *et al.*, 1970; Karle *et al.*, 1969).

The 9β-substituted benzomorphans are generally more analgesically potent (especially when a 2′-hydroxyl is present in the molecule) and are usually, but not always, more toxic than the comparable 9α-substituted compound. Exceptionally, 2,5-dimethyl-2′-hydroxy-9β-propyl-6,7-benzomorphan (Fig. 11: 79) (9β-propyl group) showed no toxic side effects in monkeys (Rice *et al.*, 1975). The comparable 9α-propyl compound (Fig. 11: 80) did show signs of toxicity. This represents one of the few examples in which the relative toxicities of the 9α- and 9β-substituted benzomorphans appear to be reversed. Although the 5, 9α, or 9β substituents that have been introduced have been predominantly alkyl groups, some other types of substituents have been examined. One of the more interesting 9β substituents that has been examined recently is the hydroxyl group. The 9β position in 6,7-benzomorphan is equivalent to a C-14 on the morphine ring system. It has been found that a C-14 hydroxyl group can enhance antagonist activity in the appropriately substituted morphine; a 9β-hydroxyl group appears to do the same in the benzomorphans. The 9α-hydroxyl group does not have this enhancing effect (Albertson, 1975). It is possible that the 9β-hydroxyl group is conformationally situated so as to enable it to hydrogen-bond to a critical area of the receptor, which could reduce the ability of the macromolecule to shift from its "antagonist" into its "agonist" conformation. The 9β-hydroxyl group, from infrared dilution studies, has been shown to have the ability to intramolecularly hydrogen-bond to the nitrogen atom (May and Kugita, 1961) in the benzomorphan molecule. It has been found to block electrophilic attack on the nitrogen atom, *in vitro*, at least as well as an alkyl group does (Rogers and Jacobson, unpublished results, 1975).

A hydroxyl substituent in the C-8β position on the benzomorphan nucleus should also, theoretically, be able to hydrogen-bond to the nitrogen atom, or to solvent. The C-8α and C-8β hydroxyl-substituted benzomorphans have been prepared recently, and the *N*-nor (secondary amine) C-8β compound had codeine-like activity (Fauley and La Pidus, 1973). Their antagonist behavior has not been investigated, as yet. Introduction of a carbonyl moiety at C-8 reduced narcotic antagonist activity without markedly affecting agonist action (Michne and Albertson, 1972).

2-Methyl-6,7-benzomorphan (Fig. 11: 81), the parent compound in this series, is a relatively weak agonist (Kanematsu *et al.*, 1968, 1969). Generally, the introduction of a 2′-hydroxyl or 2′-acetyl group causes increased potency. The acetyl may well hydrolyze to the hydroxy moiety *in vivo,* after its more efficient transport to the active site. Methoxy, amino, nitro, or halides in the 2′ position reduce analgesic activity (see Table 1). The binding of these compounds to the receptor from rat brain homogenate (Klee, personal communication, 1974) is shown in Table 1. Since these compounds do not have narcotic antagonist activity, their binding constants should be in reasonable accord with their *in vivo* analgesic potencies. Although the correlation is not an excellent one, the trend in *in vivo* potencies is generally reflected in their binding constants. Alkyl groups in the C-5 and C-9 positions in 2′-hydroxy-*N*-methyl-6,7-benzomorphan cause increases in potency until a combined total of about two to four methylene units is reached, at which point potency tends to decrease (see Table 2). It is possible that a parabolic relationship exists between the lipophilicity of these benzomor-

TABLE 1

The Effect of a 2'-Substituent on the Analgesic Activity, Binding Constants, and Physical Dependence Capacity of N-Methyl-6,7-Benzomorphans

NIH number	R_2' [a]	$R_{9\alpha}$	R_5	ED_{50} [b]	EC_{50} [c]	PDC [d]
7389	H	Me [e]	Me	13.7 (11.8–15.8)	—	—
7410	OH	Me	Me	1.2 (1.1–1.3)	9	Very low [f]
7797	OCOMe	Me	Me	0.6 (0.5–0.7)	—	Intermediate [f]
7550	OMe	Me	Me	4.9 (4.1–5.8)	—	Very low [f]
8171	Cl	Me	Me	47.0 (43.1–51.4)	4000	—
8175	F	Me	Me	22.7 (19.6–26.3)	4000	—
8046	H	Et	Et	3.8 (2.9–4.9)	300	None [f]
7856	OH	Et	Et	2.1 (1.9–2.3)	7	Low [g]
8151	NH_2	Et	Et	18.7 (15.6–22.4)	300	—
8104	NO_2	Et	Et	9.4 (8.4–10.6)	—	—
7975	OCOMe	Et	Et	1.5 (1.3–1.7)	—	None [f]

[a] See Fig. 11 for 6,7-benzomorphan numbering system.
[b] Eddy hot plate assay, in mg/kg. Parentheses indicate 95% SE limits on probit analysis, subcutaneous injection, in mice [Eddy and Leimbach, 1953; Jacobson and May, 1965 (see Ref. 9 therein)]. The standard drug, morphine. HCl has an ED_{50} of 1.2 (0.9–1.3) in this test system.
[c] Binding constant, in nmole/liter (Klee and Streaty, 1974).
[d] Physical dependence capacity, in monkeys in comparison with morphine, which has high PDC (Committee on Problems of Drug Dependence, 1973).
[e] Me=CH_3, Et=C_2H_5.
[f] Single-dose suppression studies in monkeys.
[g] Chronic administration to naive monkeys.

TABLE 2
The Effect on Analgesic Potency of Alkyl Substituents at the C-5 and C-9α Positions in 2'-Hydroxy-Substituted N-Methyl-6,7-Benzomorphans

NIH number	R_5[a]	$R_{9\alpha}$	ED_{50}[b]
9124	H[c]	Me	4.3 (3.1–5.9)
7410	Me	Me	1.2 (1.1–1.3)
7938	Et	Me	2.5 (2.0–3.1)
8138	*n*-Pr	Me	2.1 (1.7–2.6)
8505	H	H	4.5 (3.5–6.0)
7327	Me	H	3.3 (2.6–4.2)
7910	Et	H	1.2 (1.0–1.4)
7974	*n*-Pr	H	1.1 (0.9–1.2)
8142	*n*-Bu	H	2.0 (1.7–2.3)
8157	*n*-Am	H	3.4 (3.0–4.0)
8150	*n*-Hex	H	10.8 (9.6–12.1)
7951	Me	Et	0.8 (0.7–0.8)
9092	Me	*n*-Pr	1.6 (1.0–2.5)
7856	Et	Et	2.1 (1.9–2.3)
7993	*n*-Pr	*n*-Pr	35.6 (30.2–41.2)

[a] See Fig. 11 for 6,7-benzomorphan number system.
[b] Eddy hot plate assay, in mg/kg. Parentheses indicate 95% SE limits on probit analysis, subcutaneous injection, in mice [Eddy and Leimbach, 1953; Jacobson and May, 1965 (see Ref. 9 therein)]. The standard drug, morphine. HCl has an ED_{50} of 1.2 (0.9–1.3) in this test system.
[c] H = Hydrogen, Me = Methyl, Et = Ethyl, Pr = Propyl, Bu = Butyl, Am = Amyl, Hex = Hexyl.

phans and their potencies. A substantial decrease in potency can be noted in NIH 7993, the 5,9-dipropyl compound that has a total of six methylene units.

Structure–activity correlations have been made using C-5-substituted 2'-hydroxy-6,7-benzomorphans. The C-5 substituent ranged from hydrogen to hexyl (Table 2). Potency reached a maximum with a C-5 propyl substituent (Inoue *et al.*, 1975). In the 9α- or 9β-substituted 2'-hydroxy-5-methyl-6,7-benzomorphan series, maximum activity is definitely reached with the 9α-ethyl substituent and possibly with the 9β-ethyl substituent (the 9β-propyl substituted compound is practically equipotent with the 9β-ethyl compound). More complex 9β-substituted compounds have not been reported as yet.

The effect of heteroatoms or aromatic rings in the C-5 position can be seen in Table 3, as compared with the C-5 hydrogen (NIH 8420)- or methyl (NIH 6048)-substituted compounds. This comparison was made with the nonphenolic 2-methyl-6,7-benzomorphans and reflects the general decrease in activity upon loss of a phenolic hydroxyl group. Evidently, the carbethoxy ester, or reversed ester (0 Ac), in the 2'-H series caused increased activity. Activity does not appear to be lost when the C-5 substituent becomes phenyl or an amido group. Loss of activity is noted only with the substituted amine

(NIH 7967) and the C-5 hydroxyl (NIH 8500) owing, perhaps, to unfavorable hydrogen-bonding effects or decreased lipophilicity.

The effect of alkyl substituents (from hydrogen to hexyl in Table 4) on the nitrogen atom has been investigated using normetazocine (Rogers *et al.*, 1975; Ager *et al.*, 1963). *N*-Methyl and *N*-amylnormetazocine are both equivalent in potency to morphine: *N*-hexylnormetazocine is a little less potent. The *N*-ethyl, *N*-propyl, and *N*-butyl analogs are rather inactive analgesically in mice on the hot plate. Potencies obtained by the Eddy hot plate procedure have long been known to inadequately reflect the agonist activities of agonist–antagonists. The binding of these homologs to the narcotic receptor from rat brain homogenate, *in vitro*, may be a more realistic approximation to their activity *in vivo*. It can be observed from Table 4 that the N-substituted compounds from methyl to hexyl vary little (fourfold at most) in binding affinity. The *N*-ethyl, *N*-propyl, and *N*-butyl compounds have been found to have narcotic antagonist activity in single-dose suppression (SDS) studies in monkeys and in nonwithdrawn (NW) monkeys. The *N*-propyl analog is 1.5 times as potent as nalorphine in SDS studies. The *N*-ethyl and *N*-butyl compounds have much less narcotic antagonist activity than the propyl. It may be noted that the *N*-isopropyl compound (NIH 9158) in Table 4 has about half the potency of codeine as an analgesic, but it binds to the receptor relatively well (Jacobson and Klee, unpublished results, 1976). Its antagonist activity has not, as yet, been investigated *in vivo*.

As we noted in the discussion of Bentley's M-series, a modification of a side chain coupled with a particular N-substituent produced a change in pharmacological profile in the resultant compounds (e.g., etorphine, or

TABLE 3

The Effect of Analgesic Potency of Heteroatoms or Aromatic Substituents in the C-5 Position of 2′-H, 9-H N-Methyl-6,7-Benzomorphans

NIH number	R_5[a]	ED_{50}[b]
8420	H	11.2 (8.8–14.3)
6048	CH_3	11.0 (9.6–12.6)
8500	OH	42.4 (36.9–48.7)
7964	$CON(CH_3)_2$	9.2 (7.8–10.8)
7967	$CH_2N(CH_3)_2$	Inactive and toxic at 30.0
7962	$CO_2C_2H_5$	5.1 (4.3–6.0)
8501	$OCOCH_3$	5.6 (4.5–7.0)
8502	$OCOC_2H_5$	11.1 (9.1–13.7)
8216	C_6H_5	6.1 (5.3–7.1)

[a] See Fig. 11 for 6,7-benzomorphan number system.

[b] Eddy hot plate assay, in mg/kg. Parentheses indicate 95% SE limits on probit analysis, subcutaneous injection, in mice [Eddy and Leimbach, 1953; Jacobson and May, 1965 (see Ref. 9 therein)]. The standard drug, morphine. HCl has an ED_{50} of 1.2 (0.9–1.3) in this test system.

TABLE 4
The Effect on Analgesic Potency of Acyclic Moieties on the Nitrogen Atom of Normetazocine

NIH number	N substituent	ED_{50}[a]	EC_{50}[b]	PDC[c]
7528	H	Inactive and toxic at 90.0	50	—
7410	Me	1.2 (1.1–1.3)	9	Very low
7527	Et	44.7 (27.8–72.1)	20	None[d]
7549	*n*-Pr	Inactive and toxic at 15.0	5	None[e]
7589	*n*-Bu	Inactive and toxic at 100.0	8	None[f]
7785	*n*-Am[g]	1.1 (0.9–1.3)	10	Very low
8209	*n*-Hex	1.4 (1.3–1.6)	10	
8200	CD_2H	1.0 (0.9–1.2)		
8201	CD_3	1.7 (1.5–2.0)		None
9158	iso-Pr	14.6 (10.0–21.3)	30	
	CH_2CO_2H		3000	
	CH_2CO_2Et		250	
	$CH_2CH(OMe)_2$		8	
8998	$CH_2CH_2(NMe)_2$	Inactive at 20.0 and 50.0	150	

[a] Eddy hot plate assay, in mg/kg. Parentheses indicate 95% SE limits on probit analysis, subcutaneous injection, in mice [Eddy and Leimbach, 1953; Jacobson and May, 1965 (see Ref. 9 therein)]. The standard drug, morphine. HCl has an ED_{50} of 1.2 (0.9–1.3) in this test system.
[b] Binding constant, in nmoles/liter (Klee and Streaty, 1974).
[c] Physical dependence capacity, in monkeys in comparison with morphine, which has high PDC (Committee on Problems of Drug Dependence, 1973).
[d] Narcotic antagonist, longer lasting but much weaker than nalorphine.
[e] Narcotic antagonist, 1.5 times as potent as nalorphine.
[f] Narcotic antagonist, 0.2 times as potent as nalorphine.
[g] H = Hydrogen, Me = Methyl, Et = Ethyl, Pr = Propyl, Bu = Butyl, Am = Amyl, Hex = Hexyl.

comparable analgesics in the endoethano series, as compared with buprenorphine or diprenorphine). An effect of side-chain modification on the pharmacological profile of a compound has recently been observed in the benzomorphan series (Rice *et al.* , 1977). It has been noted above that *N*-pentylnormetazocine, which has a 9α-methyl group, is a potent agonist, with little antagonist activity. The antagonist component of the *N*-pentylnormetazocine has been reinvestigated (Jacobson *et al.*, unpublished results, 1976). Replacement of the 9α-methyl moiety with a 9α-propyl group in the *N*-pentyl-substituted benzomorphan has been found to produce a narcotic antagonist with little agonist activity (Rice *et al.*, 1977). The change in pharmacological profile of a compound caused by a change in the side chain at the 9α position in the benzomorphan (or the C-7 position in the M series) exemplifies the difficulty of attempting to predict the activity of analgesics from their structure. Rather simple modifications in a molecule can produce marked pharmacological changes (Lockhart *et al.*, 1972; Beckett *et al.*, 1956).

The effect of heterocyclics, unsaturated acyclics, aromatics, and cyclic moieties on the nitrogen atom of normetazocine (Archer *et al.*, 1964) can be observed in Tables 5 and 6. Although an *N*-benzyl group lowers the activity of the molecule (Jacobson, unpublished results, 1976), an *N*-phenethyl substantially increases potency (by an order of magnitude over the *N*-methyl). Moving the aromatic ring one carbon atom further away from the nitrogen atom, as in *N*-phenylpropyl, substantially decreases activity. A *p*-nitro or *p*-amino group in the phenethyl moiety tends to increase potency; a *p*-methoxyl group slightly decreases activity, and *p*-fluoro on the aromatic ring causes a further decrease in activity. A thiophene ring in place of the phenyl in the phenethyl moiety increases potency (Gordon *et al.*, 1962). Although the aromatic ethyl analogs on nitrogen show low (thiophenethyl) to high (phenethyl) physical dependence capacity (PDC), none has been shown to be a narcotic antagonist. As we have seen, *N*-benzyl decreases activity, as does an *N*-pyridylmethyl group on nitrogen, but some substituted and unsubstituted furylmethyl analogs are quite potent analgesics and show narcotic antagonist activity (Merz *et al.*, 1974). It is of interest to note that although the *N*-cyclopropylmethyl derivative of normetazocine is a very potent antagonist and has a very high affinity for the receptor, the *N*-cyclobutylmethyl analog, which binds as well as the *N*-cyclopropylmethyl and is also a potent analgesic *in vivo,* has no antagonist activity. The variation in pharmacologic activity with relatively simple changes in structure is quite marked in Table 5. The area of the molecule around the nitrogen atom plays a major part in determining the biological activity of these compounds. Archer and Harris (1965) have noted that strong antagonists are generally obtainable from the more potent *N*-methyl analgesics in the rigid classes of analgesics.

In an *ex post facto* analysis of agonist–antagonists, Archer and Harris (1965) have suggested that the presence of a substituted phenethylamine moiety [preferably by a three-carbon unit (Clark *et al.*, 1953) on the nitrogen atom] is necessary for the molecule to show antagonist activity. No strong antagonist (of the order of magnitude of nalorphine) lacks this part structure (Iorio and Casy, 1975; Iorio *et al.*, 1973). However, the correlation may be fortuitous. As was noted in the section on pethidines, weak antagonists have been prepared in the ketobemidone series that lack this structure. These ketobemidones have a phenylpropylamine moiety, not the phenethylamine moiety. The type of substituent that is likely to confer potent antagonist activity is the allyl-, propyl-, or cyclopropylmethyl group on the nitrogen atom, which is part of a phenethylamine moiety. However, as we have seen, these are not necessarily sufficient, or even necessary. In the ketobemidones, the *N*-hexyl-substituted compound was an agonist–antagonist in the rhesus monkeys, the *N*-cyclopropylmethyl-substituted compound was not an agonist–antagonist.

Quite different types of substituents on the nitrogen atom of the structurally rigid analgesics have been shown to cause this major change in pharmacological profile, from agonist to agonist–antagonist. The data in Tables 5 and 6 indicate that saturated acyclics such as ethyl, propyl, and butyl, unsaturated acyclics such as allyl, dimethylallyl, and pentenyl (Jacobson *et al.*, unpublished results, 1976), and certain cyclic compounds such as

Table 5

The Effect on Analgesic Potency, Binding Constants, and Physical Dependence Capacity of Unsaturated Acyclic, Aromatic, and Cyclic Moieties on the Nitrogen Atom of Normetazocine

NIH number	N substituent	ED_{50}[a]	EC_{50}[b]	PDC[c]
9058	$CH_2C_6H_5$	Inactive at 100.0	90	
7519	$CH_2CH_2C_6H_5$	0.1 (0.08–0.11)	2	High
9144	$CH_2(CH_2)_2C_6H_5$	20.5 (14.0–30.3)		None
7559	$CH_2CH_2COC_6H_5$	1.1 (1.1–1.2)		Very low
	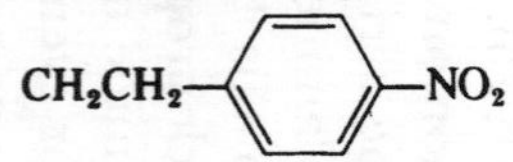		0.4	
7630	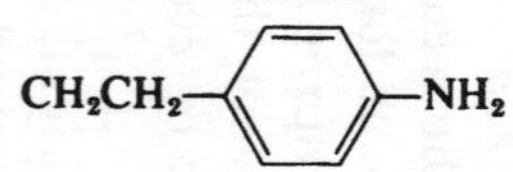	0.06 (0.05–0.06)		Intermediate
7631	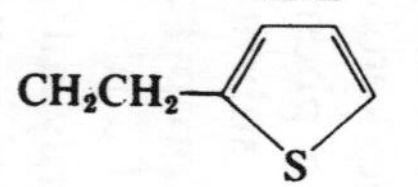	0.03 (0.02–0.03)		Low
7793	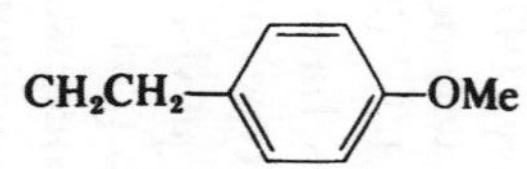	0.2 (0.1—0.2)		Low
	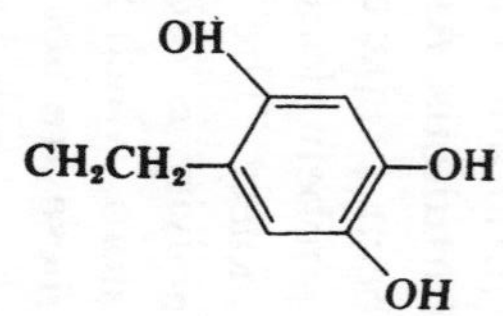		700	

	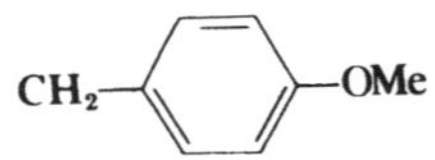		400	
7981	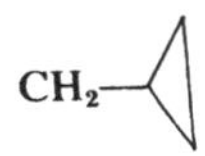	11.5 (8.3–15.9)	0.8	None[d]
8218	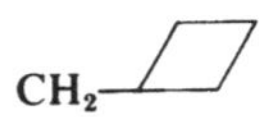	0.3 (0.25–0.31)	0.7	None
8385	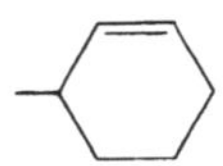	35.0 (27.4–44.6)	5	Low
8455	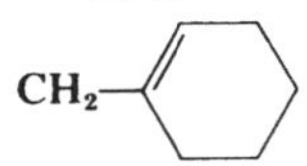	Inactive at 50.0	90	None[e]
7912	$CH_2CH{=}CH_2$	Inactive at 50.0		None[f]
7958	$CH_2CH{=}C(CH_3)_2$	>10.0	10	None[g]
9176	$CH_2CH_2CH{=}CH_2$	4.5 (3.3–6.2)	3	None
9084	$CH_2(CH_2)_2CH{=}CH_2$	6.3 (4.7–8.3)		None[h]

[a] Eddy hot plate assay, in mg/kg. Parentheses indicate 95% SE limits on probit analysis, subcutaneous injection, in mice [Eddy and Leimbach, 1953; Jacobson and May, 1965 (see Ref. 9 therein)]. The standard drug, morphine. HCl has an ED_{50} of 1.2 (0.9–1.3) in this test system.
[b] Binding constant, in nmoles/liter (Klee and Streaty, 1974).
[c] Physical dependence capacity, in monkeys in comparison with morphine, which has high PDC (Committee on Problems of Drug Dependence, 1973).
[d] Narcotic antagonist, 3.5 times as potent as nalorphine.
[e] Exacerbates abstinence in single-dose suppression studies, but does not precipitate abstinence syndrome in nonwithdrawn monkeys.
[f] Narcotic antagonist, twice as potent as nalorphine.
[g] Narcotic antagonist, very much less potent than nalorphine.
[h] Narcotic antagonist, about 0.1 times the potency of nalorphine.

TABLE 6

The Effect on Analgesic Potency, Binding Constants, and Physical Dependence Capacity of Heteroaromatic and Heterocyclic Rings on the Nitrogen Atom of Normetazocine

NIH number	N substituent	ED_{50}[a]	EC_{50}[b]	PDC[c]
8547	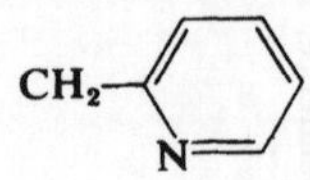	Inactive		None
8753	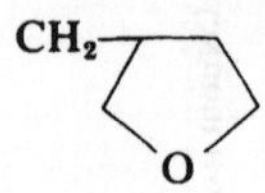	3.0 (2.3–3.9)	4	None
8740	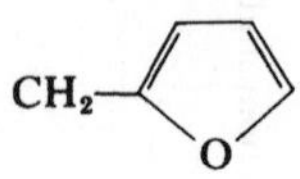	29.5 (20.8–41.8)	2	None[d]
8737	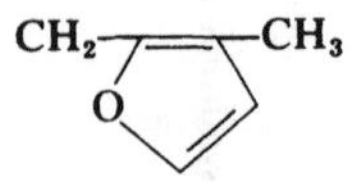	1.8 (1.5–2.3)		None
8738	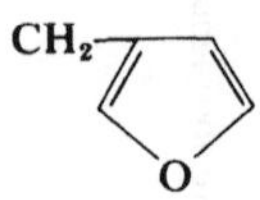	Inactive	2	None[d]
8735	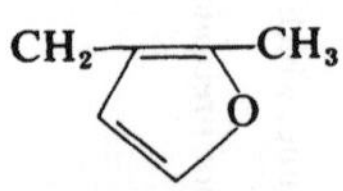	2.2 (1.7–2.8)		None
8965	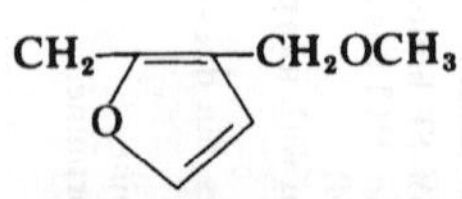	1.9 (1.5–2.5)		None[e]
8958	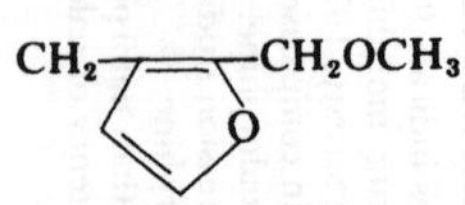	3.2 (2.8–3.7)		None
9098	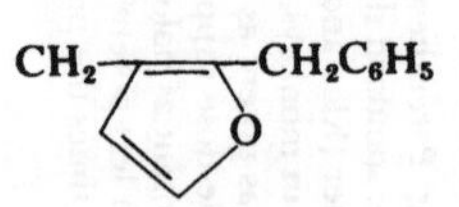	1.5 (1.1–2.1)		
8962	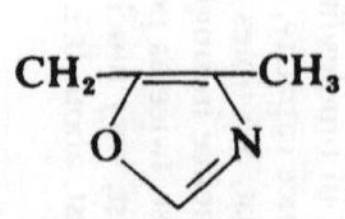	7.6 (6.2–9.4)		

[a] Eddy hot plate assay, in mg/kg. Parentheses indicate 95% SE limits on probit analysis, subcutaneous injection, in mice [Eddy and Leimbach, 1953; Jacobson and May, 1965 (see Ref. 9 therein)]. The standard drug, morphine.HCl has an ED_{50} of 1.2 (0.9–1.3) in this test system.
[b] Binding constant, in nmoles/liter (Klee and Streaty, 1974).
[c] Physical dependence capacity, in monkeys in comparison with morphine, which has high PDC (Committee on Problems of Drug Dependence, 1973).
[d] Narcotic antagonist, 0.5 times as potent as nalorphine.
[e] Narcotic antagonist, 0.1 times as potent as nalorphine.

cyclopropylmethyl and some furylmethyls (Merz *et al.*, 1974) are capable of converting agonists to agonist–antagonists. Others are currently being investigated. Almost all of these compounds show good analgesic activity *in vivo* and will antagonize the activities of narcotic agonists. In monkey species the agonist–antagonists do not have a PDC of the opiate-type but rather of a specific opiate antagonist type (the two types of dependence are said to be qualitatively different) (Eddy and Martin, 1970). The dimethylallyl-substituted normetazocine, pentazocine (Table 5, NIH 7958) (Archer and Harris, 1965; Archer *et al.*, 1964), shows this qualitatively and quantitatively different type of physical dependence. These compounds display dependence of the specific opiate antagonist type to a greater or lesser extent, depending on the particular moiety substituted on nitrogen. Also, those moieties that cause strong agonism and strong antagonism (e.g., the allyl-, propyl-, and cyclopropylmethyl groups) generally display a disconcerting psychotomimetic side effect. The psychotomimetic effect does not, however, appear to be an inevitable concomitant of strong agonist–antagonist behavior. Certain furylmethyl derivatives of the benzomorphans and some agonist–antagonists based on the etorphine structure may not have this effect; this is currently under investigation. Preliminary human studies indicate that buprenorphine does not show signs of dysphoria at dose levels that cause blockade of thermal pain (Lewis, 1974).

The substituents on the nitrogen atom that have been mentioned thus far are not the only ones that can bring about agonist–antagonist behavior. Archer *et al.* (1964; Archer and Harris, 1965) have noted that certain halogenated allyl groups, cyclopentylmethyl and, perhaps, cyclohexylmethyl groups will also have this effect when placed on the nitrogen in normetazocine. There are, no doubt, many other moieties that can produce this effect that remain unexplored. It has also been shown that enantiomers provided by simple optical resolution of some *N*-methyl benzomorphans will produce the shift from agonist to agonist–antagonist behavior in monkey species (May and Takeda, 1970; Ager *et al.*, 1969; May and Eddy, 1966).

In general, the rhesus monkeys used are reasonably good predictors of the physical dependence capacity of analgesics in man. However, it appears that monkeys are more sensitive to pethidine-like compounds and less sensitive to the benzomorphans. Thus, some benzomorphans that appear to be weak agonists and weak antagonists in these monkeys have shown physical dependence of the opiate type in man.

Typical examples of the effect of substituting alkyl substituents on the nitrogen atom of molecules with phenethylamine part structures can be observed with the normetazocine and related 9*β*-propylbenzomorphan compounds. The most potent antagonist activity lies in the *N*-propyl derivative in both series. The *N*-ethyl and *N*-butyl compounds are less potent antagonists. Longer alkyl side chains decrease activity (and binding to the receptors *in vitro*). The binding of some of these compounds to the narcotic receptor, *in vitro*, has been measured and is shown in Table 4. An *N*-allyl group produces potent antagonists. If the double bond is moved further from the nitrogen atom, as in the butenyl and pentenyl groups, the electronic effect due to the π electrons of the double bond should be lessened. The antagonist activity of these molecules does differ (Jacobson *et al.*, unpublished results, 1976). However, the butenyl compound did not substitute for morphine in physically dependent monkeys, nor did it exacerbate abstinence. Thus, it is most likely not an agonist–antagonist. The pentenyl compound, however, does exacerbate the abstinence syndrome in monkeys; it causes severe withdrawal at 8 mg/kg (Jacobson *et al.*, unpublished results, 1976). It would appear that an N substituent does not exert its effect through electronic mechanisms, or some other force counteracts the effect of the double bond in the butenyl substituent.

9. STRUCTURE–ACTIVITY: THEORY

9.1. Qualitative Theory

There are no qualitative or quantitative postulates that are broad enough to satisfactorily relate the activities of all of the compounds listed in Tables 4–6 to their chemical structures, nor is there any theory that can predict the change in pharmacological profile (from narcotic agonist to agonist–antagonist, and from potent analgesic to pharmacological inactivity) due to relatively minor molecular modification. Many qualitative theories have been offered in an attempt to relate structure and activity. One of the early attempts was made by Schaumann (1949). He believed that high analgesic potency was related, in the morphine-like compounds, pethidines and methadones, to (1) a quaternary carbon atom, (2) an aromatic nucleus attached to the quaternary carbon atom, and (3) a tertiary amino group separated from the amino group by two carbon atoms. These postulates, with some addenda, have been oft-repeated. Indeed, this set of rules does appear to describe most of the known potent analgesics, at least those that were known prior to 1949. They do describe those analgesics that are presently available for clinical use in the United States. Some doubt about whether Schaumann's postulates applied to all of the potent morphine-like analgesics was cast by Braenden *et al.* (1955). Eddy (1959) listed specific examples of potent analgesics that violated all of these rules, and some other rules postulated by Braenden *et al.* (1955). It is now known that this set of criteria cannot be said to relate well to many potent analgesics. Further, these criteria would seem to describe naloxone, a presumably pure narcotic antagonist, as well as known agonist–antagonists, and the relatively pure agonists. The postulates are, thus, inadequate even as qualitative generalizations that hope to relate chemical structure to analgesic activity.

A new theory concerning the nature of the interaction of opiate-like compounds with the receptor has been reported by Belleau *et al.* (1974).

They suggested that the relative spatial orientation of the lone pair of electrons on the nitrogen atom of these compounds is of critical importance to their interaction with the receptor. They noted that when these electrons are oriented away from the aromatic ring, as they are in the normal morphinans and benzomorphans, interaction with the receptor is possible. The synthesis of the D-nor morphinan (Fig. 14: 82) in which the electrons on nitrogen were oriented toward the aromatic ring gave them an analgesically inert compound. Since this specific orientation appeared to be required, Belleau and co-workers proposed that a stereospecific electron transfer leading to oxidation of the *N*-methyl substituent occurs after interaction with an electrophilic site on the receptor. This electronic reaction at the receptor level was termed clastic binding (Belleau and Morgan, 1974). They concluded with the suggestion that the introduction of electrons at the receptor level might help create interneuronal connections that allow the observed biological effects of analgesics. Their hypothesis is backed by evidence related to the lesser activity of an N—CD_3-substituted morphine (Elison *et al.*, 1961), as compared with the normal N—CH_3 morphine. Since the N—CD_3 morphine is more basic, it should be more strongly protonated. Thus, if the protonated morphine were the active species, it should be more, not less, active when N—CH_3 is replaced by N—CD_3. This decrease in potency by a factor of about 1.6 was also noted with levorphanol, as compared with its N—CD_3 analog. The effect was reversed with N—CD_2CH_3, as compared with an N—CH_2CH_3-substituted levorphanol owing, presumably, to a decreased rate of degradation at the opiate receptor of the N—CD_2CH_3 analog. Although Belleau noted that the quaternary ammonium salt of morphine (e.g., morphine methiodide), which of course has no free electrons on nitrogen, had been said to have significant analgesic activity, he rationalized that fact by explaining that morphine methiodide was a convulsant. These authors stated that this convulsant activity made the original observation of its analgesic activity unlikely. They concluded that the *N*-methylmorphine (quaternary salt) did not interact with the opiate receptor.

It is likely that Belleau and his co-workers are correct in that morphine methiodide probably does have convulsant activity. Furthermore, in the benzomorphan series, an N—CD_3 compound based on normetazocine has been found to be less active than metazocine (Table 4) (or the N—CD_2H analog of metazocine) in about the same ratio noted for morphine and levorphanol, which would agree with Belleau's argument.

Alternate explanations for the difference in activity between N—CD_3 and N—CH_3 compounds can be cited without invoking "clastic binding." Steric factors and pharmacokinetic differences are two obvious ones. The lack of activity of the five-membered (D-nor) ring morphinan molecule can also be readily rationalized; less major changes in analgesic molecules have caused drastic changes in pharmacological potency *in vivo*. It should be noted that Belleau *et al.* have used *in vivo* activities to create a hypothesis about molecular interactions at the receptor. It would have been preferable to use direct receptor binding in the homogenate, the guinea pig ileum, the vas deferens, or the neuroblastoma × glioma hybrid cells before evolving a general theory on receptor binding. At least two independent studies, based on binding to the opiate receptor in homogenate and on binding to the opiate receptors in guinea pig ileum, appear to directly refute Belleau's conclusions.

(1) It has been noted that quaternary salts, both in the morphinan and in the benzomorphan series, bind very nicely to the narcotic receptor in homogenates. Thus, Schulz and Goldstein (1975) have noted that a quaternary ammonium compound, the *N*-methyl salt of *N*-β(*p*-azidophenyl) ethylnorlevorphanol (Fig. 14: 83), has reasonable affinity for the receptor. An *N*-methyl salt of *p*-nitrophenethylnormetazocine (Fig. 11: 84) has also been noted to have reasonable affinity for the receptor, comparable to that of methadone (Jacobson and Klee, unpublished results, 1976). These results agree with the earlier work of Herz and Teschemacher (1971) and of Kosterlitz *et al.* (1975*b*).

It can, perhaps, be argued that these salts may be dequaternized at the receptor to give the desired free electron pair on nitrogen. This would seem, *a priori*, to be rather doubtful on the time scale required by the *in vitro* experiment.

(2) Kosterlitz and Waterfield (1975*b*) have noted that only a few *N*-nor analgesics have the activity of their *N*-methyl parents when measured on guinea pig ileum. Thus, normorphine and norcodeine are as active as their *N*-methyl parents, morphine and codeine, on the ileum. Dihydronormorphine has 61% of the activity of dihydromorphine. Norbemidone (Fig. 12: 85), norketobemidone, norpethidine, noroxymorphone (Fig. 10: 86), normetazocine, 6-acetylnormorphine, and 3,6-diacetylnormorphine (Rice and Jacobson, 1975) have only about 20% of the activity of their *N*-methyl relatives in the guinea pig ileum. Normetazocine has only one-fifth of the binding affinity of its *N*-methyl parent, metazocine, in rat brain homogenate (Klee, personal communication, 1975). The *N*-nor compounds, of course, have free electrons on their nitrogen atom.

A possible conclusion from these data is that conversion to the *N*-nor compound at the receptor is not only not necessary for binding to opiate receptors, but would appear to be counterproductive.

It is specious to argue that *in vivo* activity must be directly relatable to binding to receptors. As we have seen, even etorphine and fentanyl, which bind quite nicely indeed to the opiate receptor, do not have their *in vivo* activities reflected by that binding. Some quaternary salts that do not pass the blood brain barrier, and thus have little analgesic activity *in vivo* , can display good binding to narcotic receptors *in vitro*. In only three series thus far [with certain ketobemidones, prodines, and benzazocines (Fig. 2: 87)] has receptor binding been demonstrated to directly correlate with analgesic activity (Rice *et al.*, 1977).

9.2. Quantitative Theory

Quantitative structure–activity relationships (QSAR) statistically correlate an experimentally determined biological property, such as analgesic activity, with one, or several, physicochemical parameters. These physicochemical parameters may be determined experimentally for the particular compound or, more usefully perhaps, can be calculated for the entire molecule or individual substituents in the biologically active molecule. The equation that results from the regression analysis of the data may be linear or parabolic. If the equation is statistically satisfactory, it serves to not only relate the biological activity of the molecule to a physiochemical property that the molecule has, but may also indicate the biological importance of various parts, or areas, in the molecule. The equation can then be used, generally within the limits predetermined by the extremes in the variation of the utilized physicochemical parameters, to predict the biological activity of theoretical molecules, or the effects of molecular modifications of the compound.

One of the most widely employed physicochemical parameters has been the partition coefficient. The partition coefficient can be experimentally measured for a molecule or calculated from model compounds. It has been said to reflect the lipophilicity of the molecule, its ability to penetrate to the site at which it acts, and the intrinsic activity of the molecule, the hydrophobic bonding to lipophilic sites on the receptor (Tute, 1971). The usefulness of partition coefficients, and the method of calculating or measuring them, has been demonstrated by Hansch (Hansch, 1971; Leo *et al.*, 1971) and others (Tute, 1971). Lipid solubility has been related to penetration of analgesics through the blood–brain barrier (Kosterlitz *et al.*, 1975*b*). The importance of a partition coefficient parameter to a compound's analgesic activity can be most easily seen with the lipophilic etorphine molecule. Etorphine, with analgesic potency thousands of times greater than morphine in animals, binds to opiate receptors, *in vitro*, merely tenfold better than morphine. Obviously, transport to the receptors *in vivo* must be much more efficient for the less polar (more lipophilic) etorphine than with morphine. As a further example, some monoacyl- and diacylphosphorus analogs of methadone have been prepared (Shelver *et al.*, 1974). Although these compounds had relatively little analgesic activity, the more lipophilic members of the series were somewhat more active. Metabolism of the various molecules can also play a major part in their *in vivo* potencies. It is possible that if a sufficient number of reasonably pure analgesics, like etorphine and morphine, had their partition coefficients experimentally determined, or calculated, and also had their receptor binding affinities (EC_{50}) determined, these could be mathematically combined and regressed against *in vivo* analgesia to obtain an equation that could be helpful in discerning the effect of metabolism. That is, if the molecule's biological activity were statistically adequately expressed by a mathematical combination of transport and binding to the receptor, then the importance of metabolism, or some other pharmacokinetic factors, could be discounted for these molecules. Thus far, sufficient numbers of compounds have not had both their log P and EC_{50} values determined. Generally, a regression equation requires from five to ten compounds for each independent parameter used in the equation. When a larger number of compounds per parameter are used, the probability of obtaining an erroneous, accidental fit to the data is substantially lessened.

There are many other physicochemical parameters that could be used besides partition coefficients (Norrington *et al.*, 1975; Swain and Lupton, 1968). Tute (1971) has discussed a number of these, as have Hansch *et al.* (1973). Molecular orbital calculations have provided other types of usable parameters. Since most of these other parameters have not, as yet, been employed in a quantitative fashion for analgesics we shall not discuss them here. Superdelocalizability and charge density, parameters obtainable from molecular orbital calculations, appear to be correlatable with partition coefficients of aromatic molecules (Rogers and Cammarata, 1969).

The first attempt at quantitation using contemporary QSAR techniques with an assortment of analgesics was made by Kutter *et al.* (1970). These workers attempted to relate log P values (the logarithm of the partition coefficient) for 11 analgesics with "moment of maximal activity" (T_0) at the ED_{10} level, and with analgesic activity after intravenous (iv) and intraventricular (intv) injection. They found that lipophilicity (or log P) could be correlated with T_0 (intv), where T_0 related to the penetration to, and removal from, the receptor site. About 75% of the variance in T_0 (intv) could be explained by linear regression with log P. An even less satisfactory equation was obtained using T_0 values after iv injection. No satisfactory statistical correlation was obtained when the ED_{10} values obtained after iv or intv injection were regressed with log P values. For the regression, the ED_{10} values were converted to log $1/C$, where C represented the molar concentration of the drug. When log $C_{\text{intv}}/C_{\text{iv}}$ was regressed against log P, a statistically good correlation was found. The correlation was improved when a parabolic equation (log P^2 + log P) was used. According to the authors, the $C_{\text{intv}}/C_{\text{iv}}$ ratio reflects the penetration of the drug to the site of action and this should, theoretically, be related to log P. Since log P was positive in the equation, increased lipophilicity would apparently increase the ability of the drug to penetrate to the active site. A conclusion that can be drawn from this work is that, at least with a set of analgesics that were chosen for this study, the biological activity is not directly related to receptor interaction alone, but to receptor interaction combined with "penetration" to the receptor, as reflected by lipophilicity. If the activity of the drugs had been directly related to receptor interaction, one would have expected to see a much better correlation between long $1/C_{\text{intv}}$ and log P than was obtained, since an intraventricular injection, presumably, delivers the drug to, or very near, the receptor. The equation obtained from this work is not very helpful for determining improved (in any sense) analgesics. By dividing C_{intv} by C_{iv} we have removed from the equation the interaction of the drug with the receptor. The statistically derived equation appears to describe only the effect of the blood-brain barrier on biological activity. An interesting quantitative relationship between antinociceptive activity (ED_{50}, in mice, as determined in the hot plate assay), binding to opiate receptors from rat brain homogenates and the lipophilicities (determined by Kutter *et al.*, 1970) of the disparate set of analgesics used by Kutter *et al.* (1970) has been obtained (Jacobson *et al.*, 1977). It was noted that the analgesic activity of these completely different types of molecules can be quantitatively related to a linear combination of lipophilicity and receptor affinity. Neither factor alone would give a reasonable statistical fit to analgesic activity. Thus, although it has been seen that receptor affinity alone can qualitatively, and sometimes quantitatively be related to analgesic activity in a limited subset of closely related molecules, not even qualitative comparisons may be reasonable when the molecules are structurally diverse. It is very important, when attempting to relate the analgesic activities of disparate molecules, to consider both the receptor affinities and the lipophilicities of these molecules. In order to use QSAR predictively, of course, we should be able to calculate something pertaining to the drug–receptor interaction and observe the effect of molecular changes in the drug on this interaction. It is a step forward to be aware that lipophilicity is a factor that must be considered in designing analgesics that must pass through the blood–brain barrier, but we need to combine that with calculable parameters that can reflect the drug–receptor interaction.

A series of quantitative equations have been developed for a much more limited group of analgesics, the 6,7-benzomorphans (Jacobson, unpublished results, 1976). A QSAR determination for 60 *N*-methyl-6,7-benzomorphans (including most of the compounds in Table 1–3) that had predominantly agonist activity was achieved by assigning calculable or literature values of various parameters to four areas in the molecule. These areas were the 2′, 9α, 9β, and C-5 positions on the various rings. The assumption was made that the entire parent molecule, where the 2′, 9α, 9β, and C-5 positions had hydrogen atoms, would have a constant effect. The partition coefficient was, thus, simulated by summing the π values for the four substituents in each of the derivatives of the parent molecule. The independent parameters that were found to be necessary to the equation were the Hammett σ constant for the 2′ substituent, the Taft σ summed for the 5, 9α, and 9β substituents, the four summed π values, and a dummy parameter to relate the 9α and 9β series. About 89% of the variance in the biological activity of the 60 benzomorphans was accounted for by a parabolic equation (in π, σ, and σ^2). Although this equation has been found to be useful for predicting the analgesic activity of theoretical benzomorphans, it fails to relate to the drug–receptor interactions, since the summed parameters are difficult to interpret in regard to the effect of the individual substituents. Also, because it was limited to a particular subset of benzomorphans (the *N*-methyl agonists), it likely has little relevance to other types of analgesics. Nevertheless, the equation suggests that the electronic effects are predominant in these compounds, the lipophilic term (as simulated by π) being less important. QSAR studies in the benzomorphan series are continuing using both the Hansch approach (Jacobson and Dunn, unpublished results, 1976) and the Free–Wilson technique (Katz *et al.*, 1977), and some progress has been made recently.

The electronic density on the nitrogen atom has been studied through the use of quantum chemical calculations and X-ray photoelectron spectroscopy (Saethre *et al.*, 1975). The electronic density appears to be invariant to a substituent change that radically alters pharmacological activity (methyl to allyl, for example). It has been suggested that whereas the nitrogen atom's electronic density (as determined by molecular orbital calculations) does not change, the electronic density of the carbon atoms attached to the nitrogen will change as the substituent is varied. Molecular orbital calculations (e.g., Complete Neglect of Differential Overlap, or CNDO) (Saethre *et al.*, 1975; Kaufman and Koski, 1975; Loew and Jester, 1975; Loew and Berkowitz, 1975; Dinya *et al.*, 1972) or [^{13}C]-NMR analyses (Katz *et al.*, 1976) have not been able to correlate electronic density changes on the carbon atoms in the immediate vicinity of the nitrogen atom, or any other molecular-orbital-derived parameter, with the biological activity of these compounds, except in a very limited way for a few specific compounds (Katz *et al.*, 1976). Also, no quantitative relationship between pK_a and the biological activity of various agonists and antagonists has been found (Kaufman *et al.*, 1975; Beckett, 1956).

The information obtained from these studies could be utilized if the assumption is made that the net electronic density on the nitrogen atom of analgesics and their antagonists, which has been calculated, enables the substrate to be attached to its receptor. The theory of Portoghese (1965) could then serve to rationalize the different effects of agonists and antagonists. It has been suggested (Pert and Snyder, 1975; Simon, 1975) that the macromolecule, or receptor, exists in equilibrium between two interconverting conformations. The conformations have been characterized by their "sodium effect." In the presence of sodium, one receptor conformation has greater affinity for antagonists. In the other conformation, in the absence of sodium, there is a greater affinity for agonists. It is uncertain whether analgesics exist in their salt or base form in the microenvironment of the receptor. In either case, the substrate–receptor complex formed by the binding of the nitrogen atom could then be aided by hydrophobic bonds between the receptor and various areas of the substrate. These hydrophobic forces, combined with van der Waals interactions and hydrogen bonding through the phenolic hydroxyl, if it is present in the molecule, could dictate the strength of the binding of the substrate to the narcotic receptor. It would be essential to hypothesize reasonably precise interactions between an area in the receptor close to the point at which the substrate's nitrogen atom is bound and the substituent on the nitrogen atom. This interaction could either induce a conformational change in the receptor or perturb the equilibrium between conformational states, thus causing the eventual display of agonist and/or antagonist behavior. It should be realized that it is rare to see a "pure" analgesic or a "pure" antagonist. Almost all of these compounds have mixed agonist–antagonist properties that might be rationalized by this shift in an equilibrium between the two conformational states of the receptor.

9.3. Conclusion

Unfortunately, we are without a viable theory that can quantitatively relate molecular structure to biological activity for our multitude of analgesics. Qualitatively, one can still point to the presence of the *para*-hydroxy phenethylamine part structure in all of the structurally rigid analgesics that have attained clinical utility. Levorotatory compounds appear superior to their racemates, and appropriate substitution for the *N*-methyl group in the rigid analgesics can produce agonist–antagonists. Better qualitative theories will, hopefully, evolve in the future from correlations that take receptor binding studies, as well as *in vivo* data, into account. Quantitative work in this area is, of course, still in its infancy. It may be a while before theory can replicate the insight of the medicinal chemist.

Acknowledgments

I would like to thank Dr. N. Albertson (Sterling-Winthrop Co., Inc.) for providing me with samples of N—CH_2CO_2H-, N—CH_2CO_2Et-, and N—$CH_2(OMe)_2$-substituted normetazocine.

I would also like to thank Dr. W. A. Klee (National Institute of Mental Health) for permission to include some of his binding data (EC_{50}).

Lastly, my appreciation goes to Dr. E. L. May and Dr. E. Harrison, Jr. (National Institute of Arthritis, Metabolism, and Digestive Diseases), and to Dr. W. A. Klee (NIMH) for their comments on this manuscript.

10. REFERENCES

Adamson, D. W., and Green, A. F., 1950, A new series of analgesics, *Nature (London)* **165:**122.

Adamson, D. W., Duffin, W. M., and Green, A. F., 1951, Dithienylbutylamines as analgesics, *Nature (London)* **167:**153–154.

Ager, J. H., Fullerton, S. E., and May, E. L., 1963, Structures related to morphine. XXV.

5-Propyl- and 5,9-dipropyl-6,7-benzomorphans and a pharmacologic summary, *J. Med. Chem.* **6**:322–325.

Ager, J. H., Jacobson, A. E., and May, E. L., 1969, Separation of morphine-like effects by optical resolution. Levo isomers as strong analgetics and narcotic antagonists, *J. Med. Chem.* **12**:288–289.

Ahmed, F. R., and Barnes, W. H., 1963, The crystal and molecular structure of *dl*-betaprodine hydrochloride, *Acta Crystallogr.* **16**:1249–1252.

Ahmed, F. R., Barnes, W. H., and Masironi, L. D., 1963, The crystal and molecular structure of *dl*-betaprodine hydrobromide, *Acta Crystallogr.* **16**:237–242.

Albertson, N., 1975, Effect of 9-hydroxylation on benzomorphan antagonist activity, *J Med. Chem.* **18**:619–621.

Archer, S., and Harris, L. S., 1965, *Narcotic Antagonists, Progress in Drug Research,* Vol. 8 (E. Jucker, ed.), pp. 261–320, Birkhauser Verlag, Basel.

Archer, S., Albertson, N. F., Harris, L. S., Pierson, A. K., and Bird, J. G., 1964, Pentazocine. Strong analgesics and analgesic antagonists in the benzomorphan series, *J. Med. Chem.* **7**:123–131.

Barton, D. H. R., Kirby, G. W., Steglich, W., and Thomas, G. M., 1963, The biosynthesis and synthesis of morphine alkaloids, *Proc. Chem. Soc.* **1963**:203–204.

Beckett, A. H., 1956, Analgesics and their antagonists: Some steric and chemical considerations. Part I. The dissociation constants of some tertiary amines and synthetic analgesics the conformations of methadone-type compounds, *Br. Pharm. Conf.* Dublin, **1956**:848–859.

Beckett, A. H., and Casy, A. F., 1954, Synthetic analgesics: Stereochemical considerations, *J. Pharm. Pharmacol.* **6**:986–999.

Beckett, A. H., Casy, A. F., and Harper, N. J., 1956*a*, Analgesics and their antagonists: Some steric and chemical considerations. Part III. The influence of the basic group on the biological response, *Br. Pharm. Conf.* Dublin, **1956**:874–883.

Beckett, A. H., Casy, A. F., Harper, N. J., and Philips, P. M., 1956*b*, Analgesics and their antagonists: Some steric and chemical considerations. Part II. The influence of the basic group on physicochemical properties and the activity of methadone and thiambutene-type compounds, *Br. Pharm. Conf.*, Dublin, **1956**:860–873.

Beecher, H. K., 1959, *Measurement of Subjective Responses,* pp. 321–341, Oxford Univ. Press, New York.

Belleau, B., and Morgan, P., 1974, Clastic binding on the opiate receptor. *J. Med. Chem.* **17**:908–909.

Belleau, B., Conway, T., Ahmed, F. R., and Hardy, A. D., 1974, Importance of the nitrogen lone electron pair orientation in stereospecific opiates, *J. Med. Chem.* **17**: 907–908.

Bentley, K. W., and Cardwell, H. M. E., 1955, The absolute stereochemistry of the morphine, benzylisoquinoline, aporphine, and tetrahydroberberine alkaloids. *J. Chem. Soc.* **1955**:3252–3260.

Bentley, K. W., and Hardy, D. G., 1960, New potent analgesics in the morphine series, *Proc. Chem. Soc.* **1963**:220.

Bentley, K. W., and Hardy, D. G., 1967*a*, Novel analgesics and molecular rearrangements in the morphine-thebaine group. I. Ketones derived from 6,14-endo-ethenotetrahydrothebaine, *J. Am. Chem. Soc.* **89**:3267–3273.

Bentley, K. W., and Hardy, D. G., 1967*b*, Novel analgesics and molecular rearrangements in the morphine-thebaine group. III. Alcohols of the 6,14-endo-ethenotetrahydrooripavine series and derived analogs of *N*-allylnormorphine and norcodeine, *J. Am. Chem. Soc.* **89**:3281–3292.

Bentley, K. W., and Thomas A. F., 1956, The morphine–thebaine group of alkaloids. Part VI. The condensation of thebaine with dienophils, *J. Chem. Soc.* **1956**:1863–1867.

Bentley, K. W., Hardy, D. G., and Meek, B., 1967, Novel analgesics and molecular rearrangements in the morphine-thebaine group. II. Alcohols derived from 6,14-endo-ethanotetrahydrothebaine, *J. Am. Chem. Soc.* **89:**3273–3280.

BLANE, G. F., and DUGDALL, D., 1967, Interactions of narcotic antagonists and antagonist-analgesics, *J. Pharm. Pharmacol.* **20:**547–552.

BOCKMÜHL, M., and EHRHART, G., 1948, Uber eine neue Klasse von spasmolytisch und analgetisch wirkenden Verbindungen, *Ann. Chem. Liebigs* **561:**52–85.

BOWMAN, R. E., COLLIER, H. O. J., HATTERSLEY, P. J., LOCKHART, I. M., PETERS, D. J., SCHNEIDER, C., WEBB, N. E., and WRIGHT, M., 1973*a*, Analgetics based on the pyrrolidine ring. *J. Med. Chem.* **16:**1177–1180.

BOWMAN, R. E., COLLIER, H. O. J., LOCKHART, I. M., SCHNEIDER, C., WEBB, N. E., and WRIGHT, M., 1973*b*, Analgetics based on the pyrrolidine ring, *J. Med. Chem.* **16:**1181–1183.

BRAENDEN, O. J., EDDY, N. B., and HALBACH, H., 1955, Synthetic substances with morphine-like effect, *Bull. WHO* **13:**937–998.

CARROLL, F. I., and COLEMAN, M. C., 1975, Etonitazene. An improved synthesis, *J. Med. Chem.* **18:**318–320.

CASY, A. F., 1968, Probable conformations of some reversed esters of meperidine as solutes in water. Conformational factors in 4-phenylpiperidine analgetics, *J. Med. Chem.* **11:**188–191.

CASY, A. F., 1970, Analgesics and their antagonists: Recent developments, in: *Progress in Medicinal Chemistry,* Vol. 7 (G. P. Ellis and G. B. West, eds.), pp. 229–284, Appleton-Century-Crofts, New York.

CASY, A. F., 1971, The structure of narcotic analgesic drugs, in: *Narcotic Drugs, Biochemical Pharmacology* (D. H. Clouet, ed.), pp. 1–16, Plenum, New York.

CLARK, R. L., PESSOLANO, A. A., WEIJLARD, J., and PFISTER, K., 1953, *N*-Substituted epoxymorphinans, *J. Am. Chem. Soc.* **75:**4963–4967.

COCHIN, J., and HARRIS, L., 1975, *Synthetic Substitutes for Opiate Alkaloids. A Feasibility Study,* p. 5, Drug Abuse Council, Inc., Washington, D. C.

COCHRAN, T. G., and ABOLA, J. E., 1975, 2,9-β-Dimethyl-6,7-benzomorphan hydrochloride, *Acta Crystallogr.* **B31:**919–921.

COMMITTEE ON PROBLEMS OF DRUG DEPENDENCE, 1973, Testing for dependence liability in animals (Revised 1972), *Bull. Narc.* **XXV(2):**25–39.

COWIE, A. L., KOSTERLITZ, H. W., and WATT, A. J., 1968, Mode of action of morphine-like drugs on autonomic neuro-effectors, *Nature (London)* **220:**1040–1042.

COX, B. M., OPHEIM, K. E., TESCHEMACHER, H., and GOLDSTEIN, A., 1975, A peptide-like substance from pituitary that acts like morphine. 2. Purification and properties, *Life Sci.* **16:**1777–1782.

DAUM, S. J., MARTINI, C. M., KULLNIG, R. K., and CLARKE, R. L., 1975, Analgesic activity of the epimeric tropane analogs of meperidine. A physical and pharmacological study, *J. Med. Chem.* **18:**496–501.

DELLA BELLA, D., FERRARI, V., FRIGENI, V., and LUALDI, P., 1973, Agonistic and antagonistic properties of diastereoisomers in a new central analgesic, *Nature New Biol.* **241:**282–284.

DINYA, Z., MAKLEIT, S., BOGNAR, R., and JEKEL, P., 1972, Quantum-chemical calculations for morphine alkaloids, *Acta Chim. Acad. Scientiarum Hungaricae, Tomus* **71(1):**125–126.

DRESER, H., 1898, Pharmakologisches uber einige Morphinderivate, *Deut. Med. Wochenschr.* **24:**185–186.

EDDY, N. B., 1939, The search for more effective morphine-like alkaloids, *Am. J. Med. Sci.* **197(4):**464–479.

EDDY, N. B., 1956, The search for new analgesics, *J. Chron. Dis. (St. Louis)* **4(1):**59–71.

EDDY, N. B., 1959, Chemical structure and action of morphine-like analgesics and related substances, *Chem. Ind.* **47:**1462–1469.

EDDY, N. B., and HOWES, H. A., 1935, Studies of morphine, codeine and their derivatives. VIII. Monoacetyl- and diacetylmorphine and their hydrogenated derivatives, *J. Pharmacol. Exp. Ther.* **53:**430–439.

EDDY, N. B., and JACOBSON, A. E., 1971, Agonists–antagonists, *Curr. Med. Dialog* **38:**330–338.

EDDY, N. B., and LEIMBACH, D., 1953, Synthetic analgesics. II. Dithienylbutenyl- and dithienylbutylamines, *J. Pharmacol. Exp. Ther.* **107:**385–393.

EDDY, N. B., and MARTIN, W. R., 1970, Drug dependence of specific opiate antagonist type, *Pharmakopsych. Neuro-Psychopharmakol.* **3:**73–82.

EDDY, N. B., and MAY, E. L., 1973, The search for a better analgesic, *Science* **181:**407–414.

EDDY, N. B., MAY, E. L., and MOSETTIG, E., 1952, Chemistry and pharmacology of the methadols and acetylmethadols, *J. Org. Chem.* **17:**321–326.

EDDY, N. B., HALBACH, H., and BRAENDEN, O. J., 1956, Synthetic substances with morphine-like effect, *Bull. WHO* **14:**353–402.

EDDY, N. B., HALBACH, H., and BRAENDEN, O. J., 1957*a*, Synthetic substances with morphine-like effect, *Bull. WHO* **17:**569–863.

EDDY, N. B., MURPHY, J. G., and MAY, E. L., 1957*b*, Structures related to morphine. IX. Extension of the Grewe morphinan synthesis in the benzomorphan series and pharmacology of some benzomorphans, *J. Org. Chem.* **22:**1370–1372.

EDDY, N. B., BESENDORF, H., and PELLMONT, B., 1958, *Bull. Narc. U. N.* **10(4):**23–41.

EDDY, N. B., FRIEBEL, H., HAHN, K.-J., and HALBACH, H., 1970, *Codeine and Its Alternates for Pain and Cough Relief*, World Health Organization, Geneva.

EISLEB, O., and SCHAUMANN, O., 1939, Dolantin, ein neuartiges Spasmolytikum and Analgetikum, *Deut. Med. Wochschr.* **65:**967–968.

ELAD, D., and GINSBURG, D., 1954, Synthesis in the morphine series. Part VI. The synthesis of morphine, *J. Chem. Soc.* **1954:**3052–3056.

ELISON, C., RAPOPORT, H., LAURSEN, R., and ELLIOTT, H. W., 1961, Effect of deuteration of N—CH_3 group on potency and enzymatic N-demethylation of morphine, *Science* **134:**1078–1079.

FANCHER, O. E., HAYAO, S., STRYCKER, W. G., and SANCILIO, L. F., 1964, New analgesic N-substituted carboxamides, *J. Med. Chem.* **7:**721–725.

FAULEY, J. J., and LA PIDUS, J. B., 1973, Synthesis and analgetic activity of the diastereomeric 8-hydroxy-6,7-benzomorphans, *J. Med. Chem.* **16:**181–182.

FOLDES, F. F., 1964, Chemistry of narcotics and narcotic antagonists, in: *Narcotics and Narcotic Antagonists* (F. F. Foldes, M. Swerdlow, and E. S. Siker, eds.), pp. 10–26, Charles C Thomas, Springfield, Ill.

FULLERTON, S. E., MAY, E. L., and BECKER, E. D., 1962, Structures related to morphine. XXIII. Stereochemistry of 5,9-dialkyl-6,7-benzomorphans, *J. Org. Chem.* **27:**2144–2147.

FRASER, H. F., and HARRIS, L. S., 1967, Narcotic and narcotic antagonist analgesics, *Ann. Rev. Pharmacol.* **7:**277–300.

FREED, M. E., POTOSKE, J. R., FREED, E. H., and CONKLIN, G. L., 1973, Bridged aminotetralins as novel potent analgesic substances, *J. Med. Chem.* **16:**595–599.

FRIES, D., AND PORTOGHESE, P. S., 1974, Stereochemical studies on medicinal agents. 18. Absolute configuration and analgetic potency of trimeperidine enantiomers, *J. Med. Chem.* **17:**990–993.

GATES, M., and MONTZKA, T. A., 1964, Some potent antagonists possessing high analgesic activity, *J. Med. Chem.* **7:**127–131.

GATES, M., and TSCHUDI, G., 1952, The synthesis of morphine, *J. Am. Chem. Soc.* **74:**1109–1110.

GATES, M., and TSCHUDI, G., 1956, The synthesis of morphine, *J. Am. Chem. Soc.* **78:**1380–1393.

GERO, A., 1954, Steric considerations on the chemical structure and physiological activity of methadone and related compounds, *Science* **119:**112–114.

GOLDSTEIN, A., 1975, Chemistry of opiates, *Neurosci. Res. Prog. Bull.* **13:**11–13.

GORDON, M., LAFFERTY, J. J., TEDESCHI, D. H., SUTTON, B. M., EDDY, N. B., and MAY, E. L., 1962, New benzomorphan analgetics, *J. Med. Pharm. Chem.* **5:**633–635.

GREWE, R., 1946, Das Problem der Morphin-Synthese, *Naturwissenschaften* **33:**333–336.

GREWE, R., and MONDON, A., 1948, Synthesen in der Phenanthren-Reihe, VI. Mitteil.: Synthese des morphinans, *Chem. Ber.* **81:**279–286.

GRUMBACH, L., and CHERNOV, H. I., 1965, The analgesic effect of opiate–opiate antagonist combinations in the rat, *J. Pharmacol. Exp. Ther.* **149:**385–396.

GULLAND, J. M., and ROBINSON, R., 1925, Constitution of codeine and thebaine, *Mem. Proc. Manchester Lit. Phil. Soc.* **69:**79–86.

GYANG, E. A., and KOSTERLITZ, H. W., 1966, Agonist and antagonist actions of morphine-like drugs on the guinea-pig isolated ileum, *Br. J. Pharmacol. Chemother.* **27:**514–527.

HANSCH, C., 1971, Quantitative structure–activity relationships in drug design, in: *Drug Design* (E. J. Ariens, ed.), pp. 271–342, Academic Press, New York.

HANSCH, C., LEO, A., UNGER, S. H., KIM, K. H., NIKAITANI, D., and LIEN, E. J., 1973, "Aromatic" sustituent constants for structure-activity correlations, *J. Med. Chem.* **16:**1207–1216.

HARDY, R. A., JR., and HOWELL, M. G., 1965, Synthetic analgetics with morphine-like action, in: *Analgetics* (G. de Stevens, ed.), pp. 179–279, Academic Press, New York.

HARRIS, L. S., 1971, Structure–activity relationships, in: *Narcotic Drugs: Biochemical Pharmacology* (D. H. Clouet, ed.), pp. 89–98, Plenum, New York.

HARRIS, L. S., PIERSON, A. K., DEMBINSKI, J. R., and DEWEY, W. L., 1967, The pharmacology of (—)-3-hydroxy-*N*-cyclopropylmethylmorphinan (cyclorphan), *Arch. Int. Pharmacodyn.* **165:**112–126.

HENKEL, J. G., BELL, K. H., and PORTOGHESE, P. S., 1974, Stereochemical studies on medicinal agents. 16. Conformational studies of methadone and isomethadone utilizing circular dichroism and proton magnetic resonance, *J. Med. Chem.* **17:**124–129.

HERZ, A., and TESCHEMACHER, H.-J., 1971, Activities and sites of antinociceptive action of morphine-like analgesics, in: *Advances in Drug Research,* Vol. 6 (N. J. Harper and A. B. Simmonds, eds.), pp. 79–119, Academic Press, New York.

HUGHES, J., 1975, Isolation of an endogeneous compound from the brain with pharmacological properties similar to morphine, *Brain Res.* **88:**295–308.

HUGHES, J., SMITH, T., MORGAN, B., and FOTHERGILL, L., 1975*a*, Purification and properties of enkephalin—the possible endogeneous ligand for the morphine receptor, *Life Sci.* **16:**1753–1758.

HUGHES, J., SMITH, T. W., KOSTERLITZ, H. W., FOTHERGILL, L. A., MORGAN, B. A., and MORRIS, H. R., 1975*b*, Identification of two related pentapeptides from the brain with potent opiate agonist activity, *Nature (London)* **258:**577–579.

HUNGER, A., KEBRLE, J., ROSSI, A., and HOFFMANN, K., 1960, Benzimidazol-Derivate und verwandte Heterocyclen. III. Synthese von 1-Aminoalkyl-2-benzyl-nitro-benzimidazolen, *Helv. Chim. Acta* **43:**1032–1046.

INOUE, H., OH-ISHI, T., and MAY, E. L., 1975, Synthesis and pharmacology of 5-noralkyl-9β-methyl-6,7-benzomorphans and stereochemistry of some intermediates, *J. Med. Chem.* **18:**787–791.

IORIO, M. A., and CASY, A. F., 1975, Iosmeric 2,3-dimethyl-3-acylpiperidines with morphine- and nalorphine-like properties, *J. Pharm. Pharmacol.* **27:**140–142.

IORIO, M. A., DAMIA, G., and CASY, A. F., 1973, Synthesis, stereochemistry, and analgesic activities of diastereoisomeric esters of 3-allyl-4-phenyl-4-piperidinol, *J. Med. Chem.* **16:**592–595.

JACOBSON, A. E., 1972, Narcotic analgesics and antagonists, in: *Chemical and Biological Aspects of Drug Dependence* (S. J. Mule and H. Brill, eds.), pp. 101–118, Chemical Rubber Co. Press, Cleveland.

JACOBSON, A. E., and MAY, E. L., 1965, Structures related to morphine. XXXI. 2′-Substituted benzomorphans, *J. Med. Chem.* **8:**563–566.

JACOBSON, A. E., MAY, E. L., and SARGENT, L. J., 1970, Analgetics, in: *Medicinal Chemistry* (A. Burger, ed.), 3rd Ed., Part II, pp. 1327–1349, Wiley-Interscience, New York.

JACOBSON, A. E., KLEE, W. A., and DUNN, W., 1977, A quantitative relationship between antinociceptive activity, opiate receptor affinity and lipophilicity, *Eur. J. Med. Chem.* **12**:49–52.

Jacquet, Y. F., and Lajtha, A., 1973, Morphine action at central nervous system sites in rat: Analgesia or hyperalgesia depending on site and dose, *Science* **182**:490–492.

Janssen, P. A. J., 1960, Diphenylpropylamines, in: *Synthetic Analgesics,* Part I, Pergamon Press, New York.

Janssen, P. A. J., 1962, A review of the chemical features associated with strong morphine-like activity, *Br. J. Anaesth.* **34**:260–268.

Janssen, P. A. J., Niemegeers, C. J. E., and Dony, J. G. H., 1963, The inhibitory effect of fentanyl and other morphine-like analgesics on the warm water induced tail withdrawal reflex in rats, *Arzneimittel-Forsch.* **13**:502–507.

Kalvoda, J., Buchschacher, P., and Jeger, O., 1955, Uber die absolute Konfiguration des Morphins und verwandter Alkaloide, *Helv. Chim. Acta* **38**:1847–1856.

Kametani, T., Kigasawa, K., Hiiraga, M., Wagatsuma, N., Uryu, T., and Araki, K., 1973, Synthesis of analgesics. 34. Synthesis of 3-hydroxy-*N*-cycylpropylmethyl-9-azamorphinan (studies on the syntheses of heterocyclic compounds. 509), *J. Med. Chem.* **16**:301–303.

Kandeel, E. M., and Martin, A. R., 1973, Substituted tetralines. 5. Analgesic properties of some diastereoisometic *N,N*-dimethyl-4-phenyl-1,2,3,4-tetrahydro-2-naphthylamines, *J. Med. Chem.* **16**:947–948.

Kanematsu, K., Parfitt, R. T., Jacobson, A. E., Ager, J. H., and May, E. L., 1968, Synthesis of 6,7-benzomorphan from 4-phenylpiperidine, *J. Am. Chem. Soc.* **90**:1064–1065.

Kanematsu, K., Takeda, M., Jacobson, A. E., and May, E. L., 1969, Synthesis of 6,7-benzomorphan and related nonquaternary carbon structures with marked analgetic activity, *J. Med. Chem.* **12**:405–408.

Karle, I. L., Gilard, R. D., Fratini, A. V., and Karle, J., 1969, The crystal structures of DL-cyclazocine and L-cyclazocine·HBr·H_2O and the absolute configuration of L-cyclazocine·HBr·H_2O (2-cyclopropylmethyl-2′-hydroxy-5,9-dimethyl-6,7-benzomorphan), *Acta Crystallogr.* **B25**:1469–1479.

Kartha, G., Ahmed, F. R., and Barnes, W. H., 1960, The crystal and molecular structure of *dl*-alphaprodine hydrochloride, *Acta Crystallogr.* **13**:525–531.

Katz, R., Jacobson, A. E., and Bates, R. B., 1976, Carbon-13 nmr and biological activity of narcotic antagonists, Tenth Middle Atlantic Regional Meeting in Philadelphia Abstracts, Am. Chem. Soc.

Katz, R., Osborne, S., and Ionescu, F., 1977, Application of the Free-Wilson approach to structurally similar series of homologs: QSAR of narcotic analgesics, *J. Med. Chem.,* in press.

Kaufman, J. J., and Koski, W. S., 1975, Physicochemical, quantum chemical and other theoretical techniques for the understanding of the mechanism of action of CNS agents: Psychoactive drugs, narcotics and narcotic antagonists and anesthetics, in: *Drug Design,* Vol. V (E. J. Ariens, ed.), pp. 252–340, Academic Press, New York.

Kaufman, J. J., Semo, N. M., and Koski, W. S., 1975, Microelectrometric titration measurement of the pK_a's and partition and drug distribution coefficients of narcotics and narcotic antagonists and their pH and temperature dependence, *J. Med. Chem.* **18**:647–655.

Keats, A. S., and Telford, J., 1956, Nalorphine, a potent analgesic in man, *J. Pharmacol. Exp. Ther.* **117**:190–199.

Klee, W. A., and Nirenberg, M., 1976, Mode of action of endogenous opiate peptides, *Nature (London)* **263**:609–612.

Klee, W. A., and Streaty, R. A., 1974, Narcotic receptor sites in morphine-dependent rats, *Nature (London)* **248**:61–63.

Knoll, J., 1973, Azidomorphine and rymazolium (Probon). Approach to the ideal analgesic, *Pharmacol. Res. Commun.* **5**:175–191.

KOSTERLITZ, H. W., and WATERFIELD, A. A., 1975*a*, Analysis of the phenomenon of acute tolerance to morphine in the guinea-pig isolated ileum, *Br. J. Pharmacol.* **53:**131–138.

KOSTERLITZ, H. W., and WATERFIELD, A. A., 1975*b*, *In vitro* models in the study of structure-activity relationships of narcotic analgesics, *Ann. Rev. Pharmacol.* **15:**29–47.

KOSTERLITZ, H. W., and WATT, A. J., 1968, Kinetic parameters of narcotic agonists and antagonists, with particular reference to *N*-allylnoroxymorphone (naloxone), *Br. J. Pharmacol. Chemother.* **33:**266–276.

KOSTERLITZ, H. W., LORD, J. A. H., and WATT, A. J., 1972, Morphine receptor in the myenteric plexus of the guinea-pig ileum, in: *Agonist and Antagonist Actions of Narcotic Analgesic Drugs* (H. W. Kosterlitz, H. O. J. Collier, and J. E. Villarreal, eds.), Macmillan, London.

KOSTERLITZ, H. W., LESLIE, F. M., and WATERFIELD, A. A., 1975*a*, Narcotic agonist and antagonist potencies of a homologous series of *N*-alkylnorketobemidones measured by the guinea-pig ileum and mouse vas deferens methods, *J. Pharm. Pharmacol.* **27:**73–78.

KOSTERLITZ, H. W., LESLIE, F. M., and WATERFIELD, A. A., 1975*b*, Rates of onset and offset of action of narcotic analgesics in isolated preparations, *Eur. J. Pharmacol.* **32:**10–16.

KUGITA, H., OINE, T., INOUE, H., and HAYASHI, G., 1965, 3-Alkyl-3-phenylpiperidine derivatives as analgesics, *J. Med. Chem.* **8:**313–316.

KUGITA, H., TAKEDA, M., and INOUE, H., 1970, Synthesis of B/C *trans*-fused morphine structures. V. Pharmacological summary of *trans*-morphine derivatives and an improved synthesis of *trans*-codeine, *J. Med. Chem.* **13:**973–975.

KUPCHAN, S. M., and CASY, A. F., 1967, Drug latentiation. II. Labile ether derivatives of phenolic analgesics, *J. Med. Chem.* **10:**959–961.

KUTTER, E., HERZ, A., TESCHEMACHER, H.-J., and HESS, R., 1970, Structure–activity correlations of morphine-like analgetics based on efficiencies following intravenous and intraventricular application, *J. Med. Chem.* **13:**801–805.

LARSON, D. L., and PORTOGHESE, P. S., 1973, Stereochemical studies on medicinal agents. 12. The distinction of enantiotopic groups on the interaction of 1-methyl-4-phenyl-4-propionoxypiperidine with analgetic receptors, *J. Med. Chem.* **16:**195–198.

LASAGNA, L., and BEECHER, H. K., 1954, The analgesic effectiveness of nalorphine and nalorphine-morphine combinations in man, *J. Pharmacol. Exp. Ther.* **112:**356–363.

LEO, A., HANSCH, C., and ELKINS, D., 1971, Partition coefficients and their uses, *Chem. Rev.* **71:**525–616.

LEWIS, J. W., 1974, Ring C-bridged derivatives of thebaine and oripavine, in: *Advances in Biochemical Psychopharmacology,* Vol. 8, *Narcotic Antagonists* (M. C. Braude, L. S. Harris, E. L. May, J. P. Smith, and J. E. Villarreal, eds.), pp. 123–136, Raven Press, New York.

LEWIS, J. W., BENTLEY, K. W., and COWAN, A., 1971, Narcotic analgesics and antagonists, *Ann. Rev. Pharmacol.* **11:**241–270.

LIBERLES, A., GREENBERG, A., and EILERS, J. E., 1973, Attractive steric effects, *J. Chem. Ed.* **50:**676–678.

LOCKHART, I. M., WEBB, N. E., WRIGHT, M., WINDER, C. V., and HARE, M. A., 1972, Analgetics based on the pyrrolidine ring, *J. Med. Chem.* **15:**687–690.

LOEW, G. H., and BERKOWITZ, D. S., 1975, Quantum chemical studies of morphine-like opiate narcotics. Effect of N-substituent variations, *J. Med. Chem.* **18:**656–662.

LOEW, G. H., and JESTER, J. R., 1975, Quantum chemical studies of meperidine and prodine, *J. Med. Chem.* **18:**1051–1056.

LOUSBERG, R. J. J. CH., and WEISS, U., 1974, The analgesic action of 1-fluorocodeine, *Experientia* **30:**1440.

MARTIN, W. R., 1967, Opioid antagonists, *Pharmacol. Rev.* **19:**463–521.

MAUTNER, H. G., 1967, The molecular basis of drug action, *Pharmacol. Rev.* **19(2):**107–144.

MAY, E. L., 1960, Analgesics, in: *Encyclopedia of Chemical Technology* (R. E. Kirk, D. F. Othmer, and A. Standen, eds.), 2nd Suppl., pp. 67–80, Interscience Encyclopedia, New York.

MAY, E. L., and EDDY, N. B., 1966, Interesting pharmacological properties of the optical isomers of α-5,9-diethyl-2′-hydroxy-2-methyl-6,7-benzomorphan, *J. Med. Chem.* **9:**851–852.

May, E. L., and Fry, E. M., 1957, Structures related to morphine. VIII. Further syntheses in the benzomorphan series, *J. Org. Chem.* **22:**1366–1369.

May, E. L., and Jacobson, A. E., 1977, Chemistry and pharmacology of homologs of 6-acetyl- and 3,6-diacetylmorphine, *J. Pharm. Sci.* **66:**285–286.

May, E. L., and Kugita, H., 1961, Structures related to morphine. XV. Stereochemical control of methyl-metallo additions to 9-oxobenzomorphans, *J. Org. Chem.* **26:**188–193.

May, E. L., and Mosettig, E., 1948. Some reactions of amidone, *J. Org. Chem.* **13:**459–464.

May, E. L., and Murphy, J. G., 1955, Structures related to morphine. III. Synthesis of an analog of *N*-methylmorphinan, *J. Org. Chem.* **20:**257–263.

May, E. L., and Sargent, L. J., 1965, Morphine and its modifications, in: *Analgetics* (G. deStevens, ed.), pp. 123–177, Academic Press, New York.

May, E. L., and Takeda, M., 1970, Optical isomers of miscellaneous strong analgetics, *J. Med. Chem.* **13:**805–807.

McCawley, E. L., Hart, E. R., and Marsh, D. F., 1941, The preparation of *N*-allylnormorphine, *J. Am. Chem. Soc.* **63:**314.

Merz, H., Langbein, A., Stockhaus, K., Walther, G., and Wick, H., 1974, Structure–activity relationships in narcotic antagonists with *N*-furylmethyl substituents, in: *Advances in Biochemical Psychopharmacology,* Vol. 8, *Narcotic Antagonists* (M. C. Braude, L. S. Harris, E. L. May, J. P. Smith, and J. E. Villarreal, eds.), pp. 91–107, Raven Press, New York.

Michne, W. F., and Albertson, N. F., 1972, Analgetic 1-oxidized 2,6-methano-3-benzazocines, *J. Med. Chem.* **15:**1278–1281.

Monkovic, I., Conway, T. T., Wong, H., Perron, Y. G., Pachter, I. J., and Belleau, B., 1973, Total synthesis and pharmacological activities of N-substituted 3,14-dihydroxymorphinans, *J. Am. Chem. Soc.* **95:**7910–7912.

Norrington, F. E., Hyde, R. M., Williams, S. G., and Wooten, R., 1975, Physicochemical activity relations in practice. 1. A rational and self-consistent data bank, *J. Med. Chem.* **18:**604–613.

Oh-Ishi, T., and May, E. L., 1973, *N*-Alkylnorketobemidones with strong agonist and weak antagonist properties, *J. Med. Chem.* **16:**1376–1378.

Oldendorf, W. H., Hyman, S., Braun, L., and Oldendorf, S. Z., 1972, Blood-brain barrier: Penetration of morphine, codeine, heroin, and methadone after carotid injection, *Science* **178:**984–986.

Parfitt, R. T., and Walters, S. M., 1971, Synthesis and analgetic activity of 3- and 4-methyl-6,7-benzomorphans, *J. Med. Chem.* **14:**565–568.

Pasternak, G. W., Goodman, R., and Snyder, S. H., 1975, An endogenous morphine-like factor in mammalian brain, *Life Sci.* **16:**1765–1769.

Paton, W. D. M., and Zar, M. A., 1968, The origin of acetylcholine released from guinea-pig intestine and longitudinal muscle strips, *J. Physiol. (London)* **194:**13–33.

Pert, C. B., and Snyder, S. H., 1973, Opiate receptor: Demonstration in nervous tissue, *Science* **179:**1011–1014.

Pert, C. B., and Snyder, S. H., 1974, Properties of specific opiate receptor binding in rat brain, *Proc. Nat. Acad. Sci. U.S.A.* **70:**2243–2247.

Pert, C. B., and Snyder, S. H., 1975, Differential interactions of agonists and antagonists with the opiate receptor, *Neurosci. Res. Prog. Bull.* **13:**73–79.

Pert, C. B., Usdin, T., Snyder, S. H., Rice, K. C., May, E. L., and Jacobson, A. E., 1976, Manuscript in preparation.

Pirkle, W. H., and Gates, M., 1965, The derivation of hydroaromatic morphinans and isomorphinans from natural sources, *J. Org. Chem.* **30:**1769–1773.

Pohl, J., 1915, Uber das *N*-allylnorcodein, einen antagonisten des morphins, *Z. Exp. Pathol. Ther.* **17:**370–382.

PORTOGHESE, P. S., 1965, A new concept on the mode of interaction of narcotic analgesics with receptors, *J. Med. Chem.* **8:**609–616.

PORTOGHESE, P. S., 1966, Stereochemical factors and receptor interactions associated with narcotic analgesics, *J. Pharm. Sci.* **55:**865–885.

PORTOGHESE, P. S., MIKHAIL, A. A., and KUPFERBERG, H. J., 1968, Stereochemical studies on medicinal agents. VI. Bicyclic bases. Synthesis and pharmacology of epimeric bridged analogs of meperidine, 2-methyl-5-phenyl-5-carbethoxy-2-azabicyclo[2.2.1]heptane, *J. Med. Chem.* **11:**219–225.

PORTOGHESE, P. S., GOMAA, Z. S. D., LARSON, D. L., and SHEFTER, E., 1973, Stereochemical studies on medicinal agents. 13. Correlation of the solid state conformations of 1,3,5-trimethyl- and 1,3-dimethyl-4-phenyl-4-propionoxypiperidine enantiomers with their absolute stereoselectivity at analgetic receptors, *J. Med. Chem.* **16:**199–203.

RAPOPORT, H., and LAVIGNE, J. B., 1953, Stereochemical studies in the morphine series. The relative configuration at carbons thirteen and fourteen, *J. Am. Chem. Soc.* **75:**5329–5334.

REGNIER, G. L., CANEVARI, R. J., LE DOUAREC, J. C., HOLSTORP, S., and DAUSSY, J., 1972, Triphenylpropylpiperazine derivatives as new potent analgetic substances, *J. Med. Chem.* **15:**295–301.

RICE, K. C., and JACOBSON, A. E., 1975, Preparation and analgesic activity of 3,6-diacetylnormorphine and 6-acetylnormorphine, *J. Med. Chem.* **18:**1033–1035.

RICE, K. C., and WILSON, R. S., 1976, (—)-3-Isothujone: A small non-nitrogeneous molecule with analgesic properties, *J. Med. Chem.* **19:**1054–1057.

RICE, K. C., JACOBSON, A. E., and MAY, E. L., 1975, Synthesis and analgesic activities of 2,5-dimethyl-2′-hydroxy-9α and -β-propyl-6,7-benzomorphans, *J. Med. Chem.* **18:**854–857.

RICE, K. C., KLEE, W. A., ACETO, M. D., SWAIN, H. H., and JACOBSON, A. E., 1977, Potential long acting opiate antagonists: The preparation, pharmacological activity and opiate-receptor binding of N-substituted 2′-hydroxy-5-methyl-9α-propyl-6,7-benzomorphans, *J. Pharm. Sci.* **66:**193–197.

RICE, R. E., 1967, Drug receptors, *J. Chem. Ed.* **10:**565–568.

ROGERS, K. S., and CAMMARATA, A., 1969, Superdelocalizability and charge density. A correlation with partition coefficients, *J. Med. Chem.* **12:**692–693.

ROGERS, M. E., ONG, H. H., MAY, E. L., and KLEE, W. A., 1975, Analgetic activity and in vitro binding constants of some *N*-alkyl-3-benzazocines, *J. Med. Chem.* **18:**1036–1038.

SAETHRE, L. J., CARLSON, T. A., KAUFMAN, J. J., and KOSKI, W. S., 1975, Nitrogen electron densities on narcotics and narcotic antagonists by X-ray photoelectron spectroscopy and comparison with quantum chemical calculations, *Mol. Pharmacol.* **11:**492–500.

SCHAUMANN, O., 1949, The analgiphoric group in morphine, *Pharmazie* **4:**364–365.

SCHOENEWALDT, E. F., and IHNEN, E. D., 1974, Process for converting (−)reticuline to (+)salutaridine, U. S. Patent 3,785,927, Jan. 15, 1974.

SCHULZ, R., and GOLDSTEIN, A., 1975, Irreversible alteration of opiate receptor function by a photoaffinity labelling reagent, *Life Sci.* **16:**1843–1848.

SCHWARTZ, M. A., and MAMI, I. S., 1975, A biogenetically patterned synthesis of the morphine alkaloids, *J. Am. Chem. Soc.* **97:**1239–1240.

SEEVERS, M. H., and PFEIFFER, C. C., 1936, A study of the analgesia, subjective depression, and euphoria produced by morphine, heroin, dilaudid and codeine in the normal human subject, *J. Pharmacol.* **56:**166–187.

SHARMA, S. K., NIRENBERG, M., and KLEE, W. A., 1975, Morphine receptors as regulators of adenylate cyclase activity, *Proc. Nat. Acad. Sci. U.S.A.* **72:**590–594.

SHEFTER, E., 1974, Crystal structures of analgesics. Hydrochlorides of (−)-isomethadone, α-methadol, and α-methadyl acetate, *J. Med. Chem.* **17:**1037–1040.

SHELVER, W. H., SCHREIBMAN, M., TANNER, N. S., and RAO, V. S., 1974, Synthesis of monoaryl- and diarylphosphorus analogs of methadone, *J. Med. Chem.* **17:**120–124.

SIMON, E. J., 1975, Opiate receptor binding with ^{3}H-etorphine, *Neurosci. Res. Progr. Bull.* **13:**43–50.

SIMON, E. J., HILLER, J. M., and EDELMAN, I., 1973, Stereospecific binding of the potent narcotic analgesic [^{3}H]etorphine to rat-brain homogenate, *Proc. Nat. Acad. Sci. U.S.A.* **70:**1947–1949.

SMALL, L. F., and LUTZ, R. E., 1932, *Chemistry of the Opium Alkaloids,* Supplement No. 103 to the Public Health Reports, U. S. Government Printing Office, Washington, D.C.

SNYDER, S. H., 1976, Endorphin: Brain's own "morphine," *Med. World News,* Jan. **12:**55.

STORK, G., 1960, The morphine alkaloids, in: *The Alkaloids,* Vol. VI (R. H. F. Manske, ed.), pp. 226–245, Academic Press, New York.

STORK, G., and CLARKE, F. H., 1956, The S_N2' reaction. III. Structure and S_N2' reactions of the halocodides, *J. Am. Chem. Soc.* **78:**4619–4624.

SWAIN, C. G., and LUPTON, E. C., 1968, Field and resonance components of substituent effects. *J. Am. Chem. Soc.* **90:**4328–4337.

TABER, R. I., GREENHOUSE, D. D., and IRWIN, S., 1964, Inhibition of phenylquinone-induced writhing by narcotic antagonists, *Nature (London)* **204:**189–190.

TATUM, A. L., SEEVERS, M. H., and COLLINS, K. H., 1929, Morphine addiction and its physiological interpretation based on experimental evidence, *J. Pharmacol. Exp. Ther.* **36:**447–475.

TERENIUS, L., 1973, Characteristics of the "receptor" for narcotic analgesics in synaptic plasma membrane fraction from rat brain, *Acta Pharmacol. Toxicol.* **33:**377–384.

TERENIUS, L., and WAHLSTROM, A., 1974, Inhibitor(s) of narcotic receptor binding in brain extracts and cerebrospinal fluid, *Acta Pharmacol. Toxicol.* **35***(Suppl. 1):*55.

TERENIUS, L., and WAHLSTROM, A., 1975, Search for an endogenous ligand for the opiate receptor, *Acta Physiol. Scand.* **94:**74–81.

THULLIER, G., THULLIER, J., LAFOREST, J., and BESSIN, P., 1970, Recherches récentes dans le domaine des analgésiques, *Bull. Chim. Ther.* **1:**79–94.

TUTE, M. S., 1971, Principles and practice of Hansch analysis: A guide to structure–activity correlation for the medicinal chemist, in: *Advances in Drug Research,* Vol. 6 (N. J. Harper and A. B. Simmonds, ed.), pp. 1–77, Academic Press, New York.

VAN BEVER, W. F. M., NIEMEGEERS, C. J. E., JANSSEN, P. A., 1974, Synthetic analgesics. Synthesis and pharmacology of the diastereoisomers of *N*-[3-methyl-1-(2-phenethyl)-4-piperidyl]-*N*-phenylpropanamide and *N*-[3-methyl-1-(1-methyl-2-phenethyl)-4-piperidyl]-*N*-phenylpropanamide, *J. Med. Chem.* **17:**1047–1051.

VILLARREAL, J. E., 1970, Recent advances in the pharmacology of morphine-like drugs, in: *Advances in Mental Science* Vol. 2, *Drug Dependence* (R. T. Harris, C. R. Schuster, and W. Mc Isaac, eds.), pp. 83–116, Univ. of Texas Press, Houston.

WAY, E. L., KEMP, J. W., YOUNG, J. M., and GRASSETTI, D. R., 1960, The pharmacologic effects of heroin in relationship to its rate of biotransformation, *J. Pharmacol. Exp. Ther.* **129:**144–154.

WEIJLARD, J., and ERICKSON, A. E., 1942, *N*-allylnormorphine, *J. Am. Chem. Soc.* **64:**869–870.

WILSON, R. S., and MAY, E. L., 1975, Analgesic properties of the tetrahydrocannabinols, their metabolites, and analogs, *J. Med. Chem.* **18:**700–703.

WILSON, R. S., ROGERS, M. E., PERT, C. B., and SNYDER, S. H., 1975, Homologous *N*-alkylnorketobemidones. Correlation of receptor binding with analgesic potency, *J. Med. Chem.* **18:**240–242.

WRIGHT, C. R. A., 1874, On the action of organic acids and their anhydrides on the natural alkaloids. Part I, *J. Chem. Soc.* **27:**1031–1043.

YEH, H. J. C., WILSON, R. S., KLEE, W. A., and JACOBSON, A. E., 1976, α- and β-halomorphides: Stereochemistry, analgesic potency, toxicity, and their interaction with narcotic receptors *in vitro, J. Pharm. Sci.* **65:**902–904.

YOKOYAMA, N., BLOCK, F. B., and CLARKE, F. H., 1970, 1,2,3,4,5,6-Hexahydro-6-phenyl-2,6-methano-3-benzazocines, *J. Med. Chem.* **13:**488–492.

3

OPIATES: HUMAN PSYCHOPHARMACOLOGY

Peter A. Mansky

1. INTRODUCTION

Although the pharmacology of opiates will be comprehensively reviewed in this chapter, a major emphasis and depth of the discussion will concern the psychopharmacological effects of opiates. Under this rubric the subjectively perceived effects, objective behavioral observations, and correlative influence of physiological function will be emphasized. Underlying mechanisms of action will be discussed if applicable. The reader, however, is referred to Chapter 2 for a thorough discussion of chemical structure–activity relationships. Reference will be made to this area when relevant to the discussion.

In the past the word "opiate" has been used in a restrictive sense to refer to morphine-like drugs derived directly or indirectly from opium. In this chapter, the word "opiate" with the additional labels of "agonist" and "antagonist" will be used to refer to drugs causing effects that closely resemble morphine action in man (opiate agonists) or that antagonize the action of morphine in man (opiate antagonists). Drugs that have mixed agonist and opiate antagonist activity will be discussed as agonist–antagonists. Opiate antagonists then fall into two major categories: (1) opiate agonist–antagonists, and (2) "pure" opiate antagonists.

The word "opioid" is used by some investigators working with morphine-like drugs. Its usage is similar to the broad use of "opiates" in this

Peter A. Mansky • Department of Psychiatry, Albert B. Chandler Medical Center, University of Kentucky, Lexington, Kentucky.

chapter. Additionally, the word "narcotics" has been used in reference to opiates. "Narcotics" has several connotations that might be misleading. The legal use of the word narcotics not only includes opiates but also cocaine and marihuana, which do not produce pharmacological effects similar to the opiates. The word "narcotic" may also be construed to refer to the sedating effects of opiates, ignoring the activating effects described in this chapter.

2. OPIATE METABOLISM

2.1. Introduction

The metabolism of morphine and other opiates is rather involved. The many opiate compounds differ somewhat in their metabolism but several general factors are common to the opiates and will be discussed here along with the specific aspects of metabolism that are relevant to the psychopharmacological effects in man.

2.2. Absorption

Almost every conceivable route of administration has been used for opiates. They have been smoked, snorted, sniffed, and injected subcutaneously, intramuscularly, and intravenously. Opiates are also absorbed through the rectal mucosa and have been administered as rectal suppositories.

Oral administration of opiates reveals marked differences in the rate of absorption among the various opiates. Absorption from the gastrointestinal tract is for the most part passive and is pH dependent, the pH influencing the ratio between the un-ionized and ionized molecule in relationship to the pK_a of the particular opiate compound. The rate of absorption is then ultimately related to both the concentration gradient of the un-ionized fraction and the lipid solubility of the un-ionized opiate. Morphine itself is poorly or irregularly absorbed from the gastrointestinal tract (Way and Adler, 1962; Mulé, 1971). Few controlled studies have compared the relative analgesic potencies of oral versus injectable morphine. Estimates have indicated that oral morphine is approximately one-sixth as potent as parenterally administered morphine compared in single-dose studies measuring analgesia (Houde *et al.*, 1965; Wallenstein *et al.*, 1967; Houde, 1974). In substitution studies involving subjects dependent on 240 mg of parenteral morphine per day, oral morphine was found to be approximately one-third as potent as subcutaneous morphine (Fraser and Isbell, 1961). The relative potency as calculated by comparing single-dose analgesia is confounded by the lower peak action but increased duration of action observed with orally versus parenterally administered morphine. The potency estimate as observed in the substitution studies is concordant with the results of other substitution studies that may show a decrease in the ratio of potency obtained in single-dose comparison studies; i.e., the differing results are related to the operational procedures.

The decrease in potency observed with oral versus parenteral morphine has been attributed to different rates of absorption by the two routes of administration. Some consideration should also be given to the initial passage of orally absorbed morphine through the liver with resulting metabolic alteration (Houde *et al.*, 1965). In contrast to morphine, codeine, meperidine, oxycodone, and methadone are absorbed more predictably through the gastrointestinal mucosa with only slightly lower potency by oral as compared with parenteral routes (Houde, 1974).

2.3. Distribution

Opiates are distributed typically as organic bases, equilibrating rapidly and concentrating in various body tissues (Way and Adler, 1960). Although the distribution of opiates to many body tissues is widespread, the opiates do not accumulate in the tissues, and most of an administered dose is excreted within the first 24 hr. The widespread distribution of opiates avails them for biotransformation at various sites, especially in the liver. The effect of the widespread distribution of opiates upon ultimate brain concentration and resulting observable effects is not clear. Recently it has been found that prior administration of dextromethorphan potentiates the analgesic effects of morphine (Mansky and Jasinski, 1976). Since the distribution of opiates to many body organs may provide nonstereospecific binding sites, the explanation for the potentiating effect of dextromethorphan may be related to interaction of dextromethorphan and morphine at various nonstereospecific binding sites or receptors. Mansky and Jasinski (1976) have postulated that dextromethorphan may displace morphine from nonstereospecific binding sites, increasing the availability of morphine at stereospecific sites in the central nervous system related to analgesic action. More specifically, dextromethorphan may compete with morphine for binding to the nonstereospecific brain stem receptors subserving the cough reflex, thus increasing the availability of morphine to stereospecific central nervous system receptor substances related to analgesia.

Once absorbed into the bloodstream only a fraction of the administered dose of morphine crosses the blood brain barrier. Herz estimates that intraventricularly administered morphine is 500 to 1000 times as potent as intravenously administered morphine (Herz *et al.*, 1970). Indeed, free access to the brain may account for the marked increase in potency estimated for the highly potent opiate agonists such as etionitazine or etorphine, which are considered to be 500 to 1000 times more potent than morphine. Herz's studies can be criticized on the basis of greater drug concentration within the ventricular system, but the effect of the greater concentration is not clear since Herz used lower doses intraventricularly than intravenously and notes additionally that intraventricular morphine has a slow onset of action owing to a slow diffusion of morphine through the paraventricular wall. Herz further indicates that his results are in agreement with those of other investigators addressing a similar question.

2.4. Metabolism and Excretion

The majority of absorbed morphine is metabolized, and only limited amounts of the absorbed compound are excreted unchanged in the urine and in the feces. Morphine and other opiates are postulated to undergo a number of biotransformations that include: (1) conjugation (primarily glucoronide), (2) N-dealkylation (or N-demethylation of appropriate opiates), (3) hydrolysis, and (4) oxidation and reduction reactions. The two biotransformations most relevant to opiate metabolism in man are glucoronide conjugation and N-dealkylation (Mulé, 1971). The conjugation of opiates increases their water solubility leading eventually to more complete renal excretion. Although the conjugated opiate metabolite may or may not retain pharmacological activity (Martin, 1963; Woods, 1954; Scarfani and Clouet, 1971) it is more completely excreted than the unconjugated molecule. Thus, this biotransformation can be considered in either case under the rubric of detoxification.

N-dealkylation has been discussed as a process effecting pharmacological activity (Beckett *et al.*, 1956), tolerance, and physical dependence (Axelrod, 1956*a,b*). Much debate has concerned the role of N-dealkylation as the mechanism underlying the phenomenon of tolerance and dependence. Investigation stimulated by this debate has not supported the hypothesis of biochemical tolerance and dependence related to demethylation in the liver. N-demethylation does effect the pharmacological activity of opiates but norcodeine and normorphine retain the opiate pharmacological properties of morphine and codeine, respectively (Fraser *et al.*, 1958*a,b*).

Since the liver plays a major role in the biotransformation of opiates, caution must be applied in administering opiates to patients with hepatic disease. It is generally considered that some hepatic functions may remain relatively intact until the end stages of liver disease. Additionally, it has been noted that cerebral function may be compromised in severe liver disease (impending hepatic coma) and may thus increase the sensitivity of the brain to many psychotropic medications (Levi, 1965). Laidlow *et al.* (1961) have shown that patients who have a history of hepatic encephalopathy or present with ascites or jaundice are more sensitive to the effects of opiates as measured by EEG changes. Additionally, the EEG changes produced by the opiates occur independently of changes in arterial ammonium and serum electrolytes.

Morphine is excreted in both the urine and the bile, mostly in the conjugated form. Only about 7–10% of an administered dose of morphine appears in the feces. More may actually be excreted in the bile but reabsorbed (Way and Adler, 1960, 1961; Mulé, 1971; Elliot *et al.*, 1954; Martin, 1963). Several studies have been conducted to ascertain the time interval between opiate administration in humans and failure to detect the opiate in the urine, a measurement which is relevant for legal as well as treatment considerations. Heroin and morphine have both been administered in these studies, whereas the assays have measured only morphine in the urine since most of the administered dose of heroin is excreted as morphine glucoronide and morphine with smaller amounts of 6-monoacetylmorphine and heroin (Elliot *et al.*, 1971). Morphine can be detected reliably in the urine by radioimmunoassay about 48 hr after an iv dose of 5 mg/70 kg of heroin, 48 to 56 hr after an iv dose of 10 mg/70 kg of heroin, 48 to 56 hr after an iv dose of 6.0 mg/70 kg of morphine, and about 72 hr after a dose of 12.0 mg/70 kg of morphine (Gorodetzky, 1973, 1975; Gorodetzky *et al.*, 1974).

3. BEHAVIORAL AND GENERAL SUBJECTIVE EFFECTS (ACTIVATING EFFECTS, SEDATING EFFECTS, AND SOMATIC EFFECTS)

3.1. Introduction

Effects of opiate agonists on behavior and mood in man have been described throughout time. In recent years, the effects have been systematically investigated with observations of behavioral responses and related subjective reports. The material discussed in this section will primarily concern opiate agonist effects in non-drug-dependent subjects (both former "addicts" * and nonaddicts) and patients, whereas the behavioral consequences of chronic administration of opiates will be discussed in Section 7. Other sections of the chapter will address the subjective effects and observed behavior related to the mood alteration and analgesia seen with opiate administration.

Behavioral effects of opiate agonist–antagonists will be discussed at the end of this section (Section 3.6). Since many of the behavioral effects of the

* The term "drug-dependent person" or "person with a history of drug dependence" would be preferable to the word "addict" in relation to recent changes in the nomenclature (see Section 7.3.1 and Mansky and Altman, 1977). The word addict is used here for the sake of brevity and because of its use in much of the early literature reviewed in this section. Used in this manner, then, addict carries the same meaning or connotation as drug-dependent person.

agonist–antagonists may result from unique psychopharmacological effects not shared by opiate agonists, it would confuse the discussion of the spectrum of effects due to opiate agonist activity to include the agonist–antagonists in the main discussion. Additionally, the data on the behavioral effects of the agonist–antagonists in man are limited and can be discussed briefly.

3.2. Observations in Former Addict Populations

Behavioral effects of opiates in former addicts have been examined systematically employing questionnaires to be completed by the subjects and by trained observers. One such questionnaire that can be presented as a list of opiate signs and symptoms (see Table 1) has been useful in describing the behavioral and general subjective effects of opiate agonists. All of the signs and symptoms listed can be elicited by opiate administration, whereas selected signs and symptoms have been shown to increase regularly with increasing dose of the opiate agonists. Thus, the symptoms "itchy skin," "drive," "coasting," and "relaxed," along with the signs "scratching," "soap boxing," "coasting," and "nodding" have been noted to be dose responsive (Martin and Fraser, 1961; Martin, 1966). This relationship has been shown repeatedly in studies of opiate agonists given intravenously, subcutaneously, and intramuscularly (Jasinski *et al.*, 1971; Kay *et al.*, 1967).

The above signs and symptoms along with other observations have been noted with single-dose administration of opiate agonists in former addicts. The subjects may exhibit increased activity and arousal. The activity can consist of readily observable increases in movement such as a persistent activity related to cleaning living quarters. As such this activity is often accompanied by a feeling of increased energy or motivation ("drive"). The increase in activity can be recorded accurately by trained observers as well as

TABLE 1
Signs and Symptoms of Opiate Administration

Symptoms	Signs
Itchy skin[a]	Scratching[a]
Drive (active–passive)[a]	Soap boxing[a]
Soap box	Coasting[a]
Coasting[a]	Relaxed
Relaxed[a]	Nodding[a]
Turning of the stomach	Vomiting
Pleasant sick	Red eyes
Sleepy	Sleepy

[a] Dose–response relationships significant.

by instruments calibrated to measure activities such as pedometers (Fraser *et al.*, 1963). Verbal behavior is also increased. Subjects may carry on lengthy conversations identified by former addicts as "soap boxing" or being "on the rap." The increase in both general motor and verbal behavior, decreased pupil size, and scratching of the skin are excellent indicators of opiate intoxication in former addicts.

Some former addicts may not exhibit increased activity but may nonetheless report feelings of "drive," revealing not only a sense of increased potential to act or increased motivation but also a characteristic discussion of plans to start several active projects. The state of increased activity (active "drive") or feelings of increased energy without increased activity (passive "drive") may alternate with periods of decreased activity or energy. Thus, a subject may feel relaxed and at times sit quietly and content with a sense of marked tranquility ("coasting"). "Coasting" in its ultimate form represents a state in which the subject may be awake and relaxed but often unresponsive to environmental stimuli of the particular setting. At other times, increased general motor and verbal activity may supervene. During either the relaxed period of "coasting" or in the middle of activity or conversation, the subject may go "on the nod." This is a unique phenomenon seen with opiate agonist intoxication in which the subject appears to be asleep with eyes closed and neck flexed. Skeletal muscle tension, however, may decrease only in muscles above the shoulder so that the neck and facial muscles relax whereas other skeletal muscles may maintain their tone. While "on the nod," the subject may stand upright with neck flexed and eyes closed appearing to be asleep on his feet. The perception of time in such a state is altered so that a "nod" of several minutes may seem like only a second to an intoxicated subject.

The range of behavioral effects described above include items indicating both arousal and sedation. Thus, "drive" and "soap boxing" indicate increased activity whereas "coasting," "nodding," and "sleepy" are items implying sedation. Additionally, constipation, sweating, difficulty urinating, and dry mouth are common complaints of the former addicts when administered an opiate agonist. Notably, the studies discussed have been conducted with former addicts (drug free for 6 months prior to the study) who are subjects involuntarily confined within the setting of the Addiction Research Center.

3.3. Comparison of Effects in Nonaddict Populations

Measurement of the general subjective effects of single doses of opiate agonists have been studied in patients and experimental subjects, both groups having negative histories of opiate dependency. In these studies general subjective effects or "psychological" and "physical" consequences of opiate administration are noted. No systematic observations quantizing motor behavior are included in these studies.

In a classical study designed to measure drug-induced mood changes a group of Harvard investigators (Lasagna *et al.*, 1955) reported the effect of amphetamine, placebo, and two opiate agonists (heroin and morphine) in three different patient populations in various settings. The first group of subjects contained 20 opiate-naive volunteer male college students. The second group consisted of 22 male and 8 female chronically ill elderly patients. Only a small percentage of the patients had complaints of chronic pain. The third group consisted of 30 postaddict volunteers confined at the U.S. Public Health Service Hospital in Lexington, Kentucky. The subjective effects were measured utilizing structured questionnaires and trained interviewers with all 80 subjects, but the technique of interview, the questionnaires, and the principal investigators differed in the examination of each of the three groups.

The settings of the three studies were quite different and some of the studies employed additional drugs for comparison. The college students were not allowed to smoke but were allowed to read and relax, sitting or lying down, during the observational periods. The postaddict subjects were confined to the hospital grounds but were allowed to smoke and had less restrictions on other activities during the study period. The patients were examined while hospitalized in a chronic disease hospital. Most were hospitalized for a malignant disease or a chronic neurological disorder. Only five complained of constant pain, and the administration of regular medication for pain was not interrupted for the study. All three groups were given amphetamine, morphine, heroin, and placebo utilizing double blind technique. Additionally, the college student group and the patient group were given a sedative–hypnotic (pentobarbital), whereas the postaddicts group was given higher doses of the three standard drugs.

Results of the three groups were compared with comments concerning the drug alteration of mood and other subjective effects related to sedation and arousal. The results pertaining to mood will be discussed later in the chapter, whereas the results cited here will be restricted to the subjective effects emphasizing the spectrum of activation to sedation. The college students responded to amphetamine administration in divided fashion, about one-half indicating arousal or stimulation. The responses indicating stimulation revealed a decrease in frequency following the administration of pentobarbital, heroin, and morphine such that the latter three drugs appeared to be sedating in the college students. In contrast, the chronically hospitalized patients reported few items indicating arousal after all four drugs and placebo. The postaddicts, on the other hand, revealed a tendency to experience stimulating effects under all drug conditions, more with amphetamine than with the two opiate agonists.

The results concerning the three groups are strikingly different and within this context it has been concluded that opiates produce stimulating effects in postaddicts whereas they lead to sedation in opiate-naive volunteers and patients. This is only one of the many conclusions possible from comparing the three groups. It must be remembered that actual motor and verbal activity were not compared but the comparison was restricted to the quality or content of verbal responses. Additionally, it is obvious that the postaddicts responded to more arousal items and less sedation items under all drug conditions. It is possible that the greater relative freedom of movement available to the postaddicts after treatment administration and the exclusion of pentobarbital from the treatment conditions for the postaddicts biased the results in the direction of verbal responses with a greater content of items indicating arousal.

Difference in freedom of movement, the range of drug conditions, and the grossly differing experiences with self-administration of illicit drugs are the most obvious variables in the three differing experimental conditions. Other variables involving set, setting, personality of subjects, instruments of measurement, history of drug self-administration, and systematic alteration of drug dosage could account for the variability in results of the three groups. Unfortunately, it was not possible to control all the variables by either holding them constant or systematically altering them in the three groups of subjects.

Several subsequent studies by the Harvard group of investigators were restricted to the study of healthy male volunteers with double blind administration of opiate agonists and placebo in equally well-designed experiments (Smith and Beecher, 1959; Pearson *et al.*, 1971; Beecher, 1959*a*). Measurement instruments consisted of a multiple adjective checklist and a 12-item questionnaire consisting of opposing subjective effects (e.g., sad. . . .happy). Additionally, voluntary responses from the subjects were elicited during the experiments. In these studies the opiate agonists were found to produce mental clouding and responses indicating inactivity or lack of motivation along with feelings of sleepiness. Responses indicating mental clouding included the feelings of retardation of thought processes such that the subjects reported that their minds were "slower," "duller," and more "sluggish." They felt more "groggy and confused" and had feelings of "dreaminess" in that "things seemed more unusual and unreal" (Beecher, 1959*a*). Questionnaire items such as "sleepy" and "no pep" were elicited more often after opiate administration. Frequently volunteered items included nausea, itching, and feelings of warmth. Occasionally, volunteered responses such as shakiness, sweating, and talkativeness were noted after morphine administration and a "pepped-up feeling" was noted with another opiate agonist (Gravenstein *et al.*, 1956).

Other studies conducted with volunteer subjects have noted a variety of effects with opiates. In a study involving the effects of opiates on pain thresholds, feelings of relaxation, lethargy, apathy, and mental clouding were noted. Additionally, an increase in verbal activity with agreeable conversations has been reported (Wolf *et al.*, 1940). It is interesting that the increase of verbal activity, an indication of arousal, coexists with measurements of sedation.

Other effects such as light-headedness or dizziness have been noted in volunteer subjects (Hewer and Keele, 1948). Clinical studies of opiates in the relief of pain have often included behavioral and general subjective effects in the incidence of side effects. Behavioral activation is rarely reported but sedation and sleepiness commonly accompany the relief of pain. Other effects, such as nausea, vomiting, itchiness, dry mouth, dizziness, light-headedness, constipation, and urinary retention, have been noted as side effects with the administration of morphine or other opiate agonists (Foldes, 1974; Lee, 1942, Kerr and Donald, 1975; Paddock *et al.*, 1969; Beaver *et al.*, 1966; Forrest *et al.*, 1969; Thomas *et al.*, 1965; Bellville *et al.*, 1968*b*, 1971).

In summary, it is clear that physical inactivity, mental clouding, mental inactivity, dizziness, nausea, and itching are noted as opiate effects in healthy non-opiate-dependent volunteers. Additionally shakiness, sweating, talkativeness, and a pepped-up feeling are occasionally noted with opiate agonist administration in this population.

3.4. Effects on Sleep

Since opiate agonists such as morphine are noted throughout medical and lay literature for their ability to induce sleep, the systematic studies of the effects of opiate agonists on sleep will be discussed as part of the behavioral effects of opiates. Observations of sleep after single-dose administration of morphine (Kay *et al.*, 1969) and methadone (Kay, 1975) have been described and discussed. In studies using single-dose administration of 7.5, 15, and 20 mg of morphine in former addicts, increases in the lighter stages of sleep (stages 1 and 2) were seen with concomitant decreases in the deeper states (stages 3 and 4). Thus, REMS and Delta sleep are decreased after single doses of opiate agonists (Kay, 1973). In addition to the shift in sleep stages away from the deeper stages, increased wakefulness and increased muscle tension were noted during the sleep following the opiate administration.

Effects of heroin on sleep (7.5 mg heroin) have been described in non-addicts. Initial insomnia or delay in onset of sleep was observed along with a decrease in REM sleep. Delta sleep was not affected in the subjects by this dose of heroin (Lewis *et al.*, 1970). Bellville *et al.* (1971) investigated the hypnotic effects of 30 and 90 mg of codeine in 43 medical and surgical patients who volunteered for the study. Codeine in this study caused initial and terminal insomnia in painfree patients. This was especially evident with the 90-mg dose.

3.5. Methodological Considerations

3.5.1. Introduction

We have examined findings concerning the effects of single doses of opiates in former addicts, nonaddict volunteers, and patients. Most of the

TABLE 2
Behavioral and General Subjective Effects of Opiates

I. Activating effects
- "Drive"—increased energy
- "Soap boxing," "on the rap"—Talkative

II. Sedating effects
- Relaxed
- "Coasting"
- Sleepy, stupor, and coma
- Nodding
- Mental clouding

III. Somatic effects
- Nausea and vomiting
- Lightheadedness and dizziness
- Itchy skin and scratching
- Warm feeling
- Sweating
- Shakiness or nervous
- Dry mouth
- Constipation
- Difficulty urinating or urinary retention

IV. Sleep effects
- Decrease in deeper stages
- Increased wakefulness
- Increased muscle tension

behavioral and general subjective effects can be observed in any of the three populations noted above and are summarized in Table 2. The rate of occurrence of the many effects does vary from one group to the other in the studies reviewed. Most notably, with the exception of sleep studies, there is a seemingly weighted occurrence of activating effects in the former addicts as opposed to patients and volunteers. We have suggested that this weighted differential may be due to alteration of numerous factors in the various studies, some unrelated to former opiate use. Clearly, the key factor influencing the differential of activating verus sedating effects cannot be identified from the studies discussed in the previous section. Nevertheless, examination of the factors influencing the results can provide some perspective in analyzing various studies and in planning future experiments.

The factors that are postulated to influence the experimental results are presented in Table 3 in terms of variables influencing the observations. Some of the variables can be considered as dependent variables and others as independent variables. Most, however, cannot be categorized neatly into

TABLE 3
Variables Related to the Behavioral and Subjective Effects of Opiates

Psychological factors
Biological profile
Drug factors
Environmental factors
Measurement of drug effects

dependent and independent variables since they interact, so that statistical methods such as factorial analysis may eventually provide a useful tool in investigating the degree of interplay of the several variables.

Certainly, future studies should be constructed considering the factors in the experimental design and, when possible, controlling the various factors. By increasing the size of the population studied the relative statistical variance due to multiple factors may be reduced. Obviously, the most valuable information could be gained by altering, when possible, the variables in a systematic manner. If the measurements studied change in relationship to conditions altering a given variable, the case for the influence of the variable on the results is strengthened. Such is the situation in studies with drug effects showing a graded response with change in drug dose. In analyzing these drug dose–response data the drug dose is altered and certain parameters are measured. The parameters that undergo a clear variation with drug dose can establish a strong relationship between the drug action and the particular effect measured in the study.

3.5.2. Defining the Pertinent Variables

The variables alluded to in the above section deserve further elaboration at this point. The psychological variables influencing the drug effects could include not only indicators of psychological composition such as personality and coping style but also the psychological state of the subject at the time of drug administration. The latter refers to states of arousal or anxiety along with other mood factors that may be determined not only by psychological composition but by both the biological profile and the environmental influences, thus indicating one area of multidependency of the variables. The psychological factors are also related to prior exposure to the class of drugs being studied. The effect of this exposure would be determined by the degree of prior use whether intermittent and occasional or frequent enough to have produced physical and psychological dependence.

The biological profile refers to such factors as individual variation in drug metabolism (absorption, distribution, biotransformation, and excretion) and differences among individuals in the anatomical and functional aspects of the neuronal substrate influenced by the drug. These biological differences may represent variations within healthy individuals or may be the result of diseases such as schizophrenia, bipolar depressive disorder, or other medical illness such as a pain-producing malignancy. Again the biological profile could be influenced by prior exposure to the drug whether casual or intense enough to produce physical dependence.

Drug factors refer to the variation in activity between drugs of the same class, in this case opiate agonists or opiate antagonists. The pharmacological effects of opiate agonists may also be contaminated by agonistic activity not common to other opiates. Additionally, the mixture of opiate agonist and opiate antagonist activity may greatly influence the behavioral effects of a given drug.

Measurement or assay of drug effects can also influence the experimental results. Reports of subjects and observers can be structured or more open ended. Motor activity can be estimated, counted by observers, or measured by instrumentation.

The following sections will discuss studies and observations that indicate the influence of these five factors upon studies of opiates, with particular reference to their alterations of the sedating and activating effects of opiates.

3.5.3. Psychological Variables

Psychological factors in addict and former addict populations have been examined in order to differentiate between the psychological composition or personality of the two groups. Many of the studies conducted to ascertain the personality characteristics of former addicts have included the use of objective tests (such as the MMPI), open interview, and projective tests (Feldstein *et al.*, 1973; Mott, 1972). Most have concluded that sociopathy or psychopathy is a common feature among addicts (Monroe *et al.*, 1971). In spite of this common feature of sociopathy, addicts do not present homogeneous personality constellations, even if one selects a restricted population involving subjects hospitalized for treatment of opiate dependence (Hill *et al.*, 1960). Expanding the studies to include outpatients (Brotman *et al.*, 1965) or opiate users from a population exposed to easily available drugs (Robins *et al.*, 1975) reveals even more diversity in the populations studied.

Descriptions of the addict personality have been for the most part prospective and have involved subjects who have spent some time obtaining personal supplies of opiates by illegal or semilegal activity. Certainly, personality traits can be altered and affected by learning (Rioch, 1972), thus being the result rather than the cause of drug dependence. Alternatively, the personality or personal history (e.g., delinquency) may predispose to a lifestyle conducive to obtaining the drug (Robins and Murphy, 1967).

Even if some personality of psychological traits are recognized as etiologically important in developing drug dependence, they may not be specific factors in predicting the use of a given class of drugs or even drug dependency; i.e., the etiological factors identified may be nonspecific in determining particular drug-seeking behavior as opposed to other behavior associated with sociopathy (Winokur *et al.*, 1970).

The work cited above has provided useful information for clinicians treating drug-dependent patients. In no way, however, do the personality factors cited account for the more frequent arousal effect (or as we shall discuss later, euphoria as opposed to dysphoria) of opiate agonists in former addicts. Speculations as to the relationship of personality traits to opiate effects can be inferred from the work cited, but the speculations raise more questions than they answer. To establish a clear relationship, studies would have to involve the predictive hypothesis relating activation and euphoric effects of opiates to personality traits in opiate-naive subjects measured prior to a controlled experiment ascertaining objective measurements of activity (motor and verbal) and mood after opiate administration. Von Felsinger *et al.* (1955) were able to identify certain characteristics of volunteer subjects (college students) who experienced euphoric responses to opiate administration in a study cited from the Harvard group. The relationship of these traits to both euphoria and arousal is not clearly established but does deserve further investigation.

To predict euphoric responses or activating effects of opiates from personality alone may be possible. The inverse, however, predicting personality from responses to opiates, has lead to many difficulties inherent in this unproven inference. Nonetheless, patients have been labeled sociopathic or abnormal because they respond to opiate analgesia with activation or euphoria. Any reader who has experienced pleasant feelings or increase in activity after receiving opiates for pain (dental procedure, surgery, etc.) would object to this line of reasoning.

In summary, then, personality constellations of the addict population have been described and often differ from the societal norm. Most of the studies have concerned a "core" group of addicts often selected from hospitals that specialize in the treatment of this disorder. The use of larger groups of people taking opiates has often revealed an increased diversity in the personality or coping style of the subjects studied. Nevertheless, the particular personality factor or factors that might be related to arousal or euphoria following opiate administration have not been identified.

3.5.4. Biological Profile

As we shall discuss later, opiate dependency does lead to long-range changes in physiological function that have been detected for up to 6 months after withdrawal (Martin and Jasinski, 1969). Fraser and Isbell (1952) designed a study to detect differences in physiological responses to morphine between former addicts and nonaddicts. The former addicts had been drug free for at least 6 months prior to the study. Each group was given 20 mg of morphine sulfate subcutaneously, after which measurements were obtained periodically of pupil size (photographically), rectal temperature, blood pressure, respiratory rate, pulse rate, and incidence of nausea and vomiting. The only difference in these measurements indicated a higher incidence of nausea and vomiting and a greater drop in rectal temperature in the nonaddicts. The cause of the difference in these two parameters was not identified but the two most likely suggestions of the authors were that the differential was due to prolonged abstinence (longer than 6 months) or, less likely, to an inherent physiological difference.

Certainly, the physical substrate upon which the opiates act or the state of the physiological systems they alter will effect the action of the administered drug. Unfortunately, specific physiological factors have not been well identified as predictors of opiate action. From the above work, it is known only that opiates do produce minor physiological differential effects in addicts and nonaddicts. Again, more studies organized to examine mood and arousal–sedating effects of administered opiates in patients or subjects with alterations of the central nervous system, anatomically or functionally, would be useful.

Two sets of observations, one involving opiate effects in manic–depressive patients and the other involving effects of opiates in chronic psychotic patients, should be mentioned.

Opiates were used (primarily in European countries) to treat depression or manic excitement in patients with unipolar and bipolar depressive disorders (Lindesmith, 1947). Sleep induction has been noted by Berger (1931) who refers to a patient in the manic phase who was able to sleep after the administration of 20 mg of morphine and 1 mg of scoplamine. In contrast, the failure of mania to respond to morphine has been reported (Geoghegan, 1946). These conflicting reports may reflect the individual variations noted in this section concerning the opiate effects of sedation, drowsiness, and dysphoria following opiate administration in some subjects as opposed to behavioral stimulation and euphoria observed in other subjects. Alternatively, the differences cited may be a result of a multiplicity of factors that are not clearly defined due to the anecdotal nature of the reports.

Psychotic and depressed patients have been noted to show a low rate of opiate dependence following treatment of the disorder with opiates (Sceleth and Kuh, 1924). As noted, opiates are rarely used today to treat psychiatric disorders, thus, few systematic observations of the effects of opiates in psychotic patients have been studied recently. Wikler *et al.* (1952), however, did administer opiates to schizophrenic patients to ascertain differential effects of therapeutic frontal lobotomy upon the purposive and nonpurposive symptoms of opiate withdrawal (see Section 7.3.2). Notably, morphine in single doses was noted to have little if any effect upon the behavior of patients prior to or following lobotomy.

The studies cited do not indicate the pharmacological mechanisms at a neuronal level but they do illustrate that observed behavioral effects of drugs are altered in patients with diseases of the brain inherent in a chronic psychosis. Furthermore, the evidence cited in manic–depressive patients reflects either the individual variability referred to above or the difficulty in forming a hypothesis solely from anecdotal reports.

Thus, in summary, it can be seen that differences in effects of opiates in addicts as opposed to nonaddicts and in patients with psychotic or affective disorders have been described. Again, unfortunately, the observations fail to account for or predict a differential of activating–sedating effects in subjects based upon biological factors.

3.5.5. *Drug Factors*

The drug itself and the manner of administration may alter the conclusions inferred from various measurements of drug effects. Martin and

Fraser's (1961) classical study referred to earlier clearly illustrates the ability of the use of dose–response data in identifying selected signs and symptoms of opiate intoxication. Studies comparing newer opiates to standard opiates such as morphine or heroin may differentiate agonistic effects of a nonopiate nature inherent in the new drugs investigated. Nonopiate agonist effects have been noted in various opiate agonists and are of special interest here if the effects lead to either behavioral sedation or activation not common to all opiates.

Unique behavioral arousal with agitation and tremors has been noted with moderate to high doses of meperidine. This opiate may also produce an acute delirium with confusion, disorientation, and a recent memory disturbance (Martin, 1963). Meperidine has specific atropine-like anticholinergic activity in addition to depression of the release of acetylcholine shared by other opiate agonists (Paton, 1957). Thus, the atropine-like action of meperidine could account for the increased arousal and delirium. Marked peripheral anticholinergic effects have not been described in meperidine intoxication, but this does not exclude central anticholinergic intoxication. The syndromes of anticholinergic poisoning seen with tricyclic antidepressants (especially amitriptyline) and with the combined use of phenothiazines and anti-Parkinson medications often show marked evidence of central nervous system toxicity with minimal peripheral signs (Granacher and Baldessarini, 1975). The successful treatment of delirium and agitation seen in meperidine intoxication with physostigmine could identify this syndrome as anticholinergic.

3.5.6. Environmental Factors

The variables discussed to this point do alter the behavioral effects of opiates. Unfortunately, in most of the studies the variables were not altered in a systematic manner such that the full nature of their effect on behavior could be ascertained. In most cases the studies cited were limited to observations primarily designed to measure other aspects of opiate action. Several examples may suffice to illustrate this point. The studies of the Harvard group have been designed to develop the systematic description of the subjective effects of opiates. The descriptions of behavior consequent to opiate intoxication in chronic psychotic patients were part of an investigation designed to ascertain the effects of lobotomy upon purposive and nonpurposive indicators of opiate dependency. The studies of personality traits were constructed to determine common personality traits among addicts.

The aspects of the environment effecting behavior and psychotropic drug actions are legion. Several studies, however, have been constructed to measure systematically the effect of environmentally induced motivation on behavior. Hill *et al.* (1957) related the performance of a task (reaction time) to several conditions differing in the consequent reinforcers. They considered various levels of motivation based upon the nature and schedule of the reinforcers as low, standard I, high, and standard II motivational conditions affected, respectively, by low, standard, and high incentives. The standard I incentive consisted of a fixed amount of morphine received as a consequence of completing the performance task (4 series of 18 reactions with 15 min between each series). In the high incentive group, the amount of reward was contingent upon the quality of the performance, i.e., the ability to react rapidly. In the low incentive condition the reinforcer, a fixed dose of morphine, was administered at least 1 week prior to the study and clearly indicated as advanced payment for participation. The standard II condition involved reinforcement similar to the standard condition with the addition of reinforcement based upon the quality of performance as a consequence of competitive factors, i.e., performance scores were compared to that of other participants or to the subject's previous scores. The participants in the standard II condition had all formerly been subjects in a high incentive group and during their participation in the standard II condition they received continuing feedback concerning their reaction time.

The reinforcing conditions were each compared in subjects receiving saline placebo, 15 mg morphine sulfate, or 250 mg pentobarbital intramuscularly 50 min prior to the test of reaction time. In the subjects receiving placebo (control), the reaction time decreased significantly as a function of the incentive condition so that the reaction time was longest for the low incentive condition and shorter, stepwise, for the standard I, high, and standard II incentive conditions (see Fig. 1). Morphine compared to no-drug control appeared to decrease the reaction time in low incentive condition, have no effect on the reaction time in the standard I and high incentive

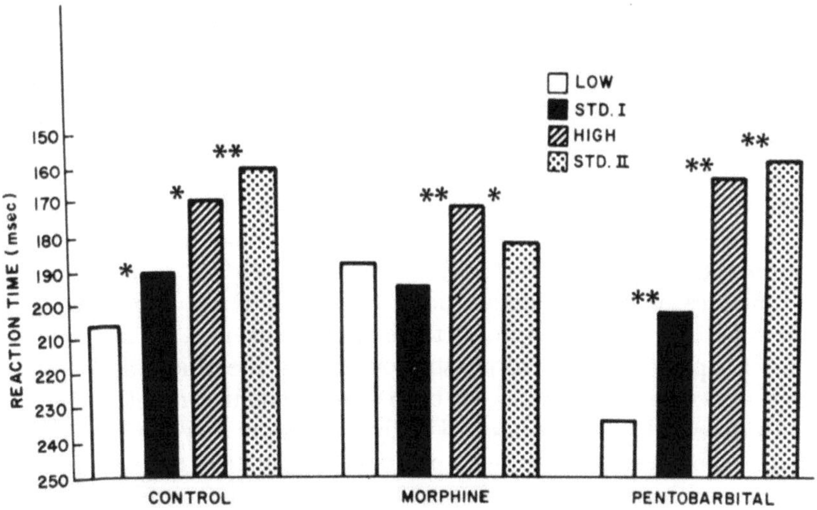

FIG. 1. Task performance related to incentive conditions and altered by morphine and penobarbital. * $P \leq .05$. ** $P \leq .01$.

condition, and increase the reaction time in the standard II incentive condition. Thus, morphine would appear to be a stimulant in the low incentive condition, to be inactive in the standard I and high incentive condition, and to be a depressant in the standard II incentive condition. Additionally, the authors noted that subjects who received morphine were influenced less by the incentives than subjects given either placebo or pentobarbital.

Therefore, it could be concluded that morphine or other opiates could be considered stimulants or sedatives, depending upon the reinforcers related to the performance of the measured activity. Additionally, morphine may decrease the effects of extrinsic positive reinforcers upon behavior. Notably, the various extrinsic positive reinforcers in this particular study appear to effect the performance less in all subjects given morphine. Interestingly, Hill *et al.* (1952*b*, 1955) have also found that morphine decreases the disruption of performance related to pain anticipatory anxiety. Thus, morphine may decrease the effects of selective extrinsic positive and negative reinforcers. Conceivably, this action of morphine could be mediated through brain structures related to reinforcement such as the medial forebrain bundle and the periventricular areas (Olds and Olds, 1965).

It is then clear that opiate agonists can be considered either as agents of arousal or sedation depending upon the subject's motivation as effected by various incentives or reinforcers consequent to the behavior. Therefore, to label opiate agonists solely as sedating or activating agents may be misleading in that alteration of environmental variables may not merely effect the conclusions but actually may appear to support opposing or mutually exclusive hypotheses.

3.5.7. Assessment Variables—Measurement of Drug Effects

Consideration of differing assessment variables indicates that opiates can produce both activating effects and at the same time sedating effects. Additionally, opiates may markedly depress some areas of the brain leaving others intact to react to environmental stimuli.

Several examples serve to illustrate these effects. Observations of sleep in subjects intoxicated with opiates can be deceiving. Unlike the subjects sedated with moderate doses of a barbiturate who may be difficult to arouse, the person intoxicated with moderate doses of morphine or other opiates may appear to be in a sound sleep only to be easily awakened. In fact, the sleep seen after opiate agonist administration, often identified as a calming "narcotic effect," may reveal (as has been stated) a lightening of the stages of sleep. Unexpected areas of arousal and stimulation may remain intact in stupor or coma resulting from intoxication with a high dose of an opiate agonist. A patient in "coma" observed to have pinpoint pupils, minimal or absent reaction to pain, and markedly depressed respirations as a result of ingestion of an opiate agonist may breathe if a loud verbal command to do so is given. At the neuronal level, unlike barbiturates and other sedative-hypnotics, opiates do not produce depression of all neurological activity. To the contrary, intoxication with high doses of opiates can lead to convulsive activity even if anoxia is prevented. More specific examinations have revealed that whereas sedative–hypnotics typically elevate the seizure threshold, opiates have the opposite effect, i.e., they decrease the seizure threshold (Gibbs and Maltby, 1943; Carruyo *et al.*, 1968; Gilbert and Martin, 1975).

3.6. Behavioral Effects of Opiate Agonist–Antagonists

The opiate agonist–antagonists such as nalorphine and cyclazocine in low doses produce subjective and behavioral effects similar to low doses of morphine. As the dose of the agonist–antagonist is increased effects emerge that can be labeled as psychotomimetic and sedative. This will be discussed again in Section 4 concerning the mood effects of opiates and will include a discussion of the ARC Inventory that reflects the above findings. At this point a brief description of the behavioral effects of the agonist–antagonist will be sufficient.

The agonist–antagonists frequently elicit the signs and symptoms of "sleepiness" and "drunkenness" often in a dose-related fashion. The signs and symptoms of "itchy skin," "coasting," and "scratching" are not as prominent as with opiate agonists. The effect of the feelings of sleepiness and drunkenness is rather like being overtired, trying to sleep, but not being able to sleep enough to feel rested. Thus, the subject who attempts to sleep in response to the feelings of sleepiness and drunkenness may fall asleep only to awake quickly feeling nervous and restless. In addition to drunkenness and sleepiness, irritability, racing thoughts, delusions, hallucinations, and drug-induced illusions have been noted with the administration of opiate agonist–antagonists, especially at higher doses. The latter group of effects are generally considered unpleasant or dysphoric by volunteer subjects, patients, and "former" opiate addicts (Martin *et al.*, 1965; Martin and Gorodetzky, 1965; Martin, 1967*a*; Martin and Sloan, 1968; Pennes and Hoch, 1957; Lasagna and Beecher, 1954*a*; Keats and Telford, 1957; Huggens and Moyer, 1955; Freedman *et al.*, 1968; Isbell, 1956).

4. EFFECTS OF OPIATES ON MOOD

4.1. Introduction

Opiate agonists are known for their ability to produce a pleasant mood change identified as euphoria. This is an unfortunate choice of wording for the mood state since euphoria has been used to connote merely a feeling of well-being as well as feelings of marked mood elevation with increased sense of vigor and health as seen in the manic phase of bipolar depressive illness (Winokur *et al.*, 1969). Others have defined the even more dramatic rush or high feeling that occurs simultaneously with the intravenous administration of opiates as euphoria.

Euphoria will be used here to describe the subjective effects of opiates that are identified as pleasurable by former addicts and that lead to mood elevation and a sense of increased well-being. This feeling state follows opiate administration in former addicts and usually lasts for several hours. Although the same mood changes reported by former addicts can be experienced by nonaddict volunteers and patients, appreciation of euphoria in the two latter groups is not universal. In fact, opiates have been found to produce dysphoric or unpleasant mood changes in the majority of nonaddict subjects within particular experimental settings. Some investigators have reported a very low incidence of euphoric feelings consequent to opiate administration in nonaddict populations (Lasagna *et al.*, 1955), whereas others have indicated a higher incidence of euphoria in patients receiving opiates for pain (Batterman, 1943). Nevertheless, the incidence of reported euphoric responses is usually much higher in former addict populations.

Several explanations have been offered for the differential mood effects of opiates in addicts and nonaddicts. Some investigators attribute this differential to learning and others to underlying personality. Certainly nausea, dizziness, vomiting, and smooth muscle spasm are unpleasant somatic symptoms of opiate intoxication. These symptoms are often interpreted as neutral or even pleasant by former addicts who state that the somatic symptoms are not bothersome. In fact, the symptoms signify to the subject that he has received an active opiate or good "dope." As such, the former addict has learned that the somatic symptoms are indicators of drug action and either precede or accompany the subjective mood changes he enjoys so much. In this sense the subject may learn to ignore or even enjoy the usually unpleasant sensations especially with the facilitation of the analgesic effect of the opiates. The nonaddict, on the other hand, may attribute the sensations to harmful somatic effects of the drug or to illness. This may then affect the nonaddict so that he is not able to appreciate the effects of the drug.

Interestingly, volunteer subjects who failed to experience euphoria in the studies conducted by the Harvard group (see Sections 3.3 and 3.5.3) are noted to be high achievers. In addition to the unpleasant somatic symptoms, the subjects experienced sedation and mental clouding. These latter two symptoms may be unpleasant for some high achievers who value alertness and clear mentation. This valuation is reflective of coping style or personality composition which then may be related to the dysphoric mood effects of the opiate agonists in this population. The authors suggested that the subjects who have experienced euphoria can be characterized as self-centered with tendencies to react emotionally, immaturely, and impulsively along with the frequent use of fantasy as a coping mechanism (Von Felsinger *et al.*, 1955). Although these findings reflect studies utilizing open interview and Rorschach technique, the explanation concerning the interaction of achievement style and mental clouding may be sufficient to account for the differential mood effects. Certainly, further studies are needed to make firm conclusions. Consideration can also be given to the discussion of the influence of the variables described in the previous section (Section 3.5) upon euphoric responses. Again, the precise influence of each of the variables upon opiate-induced mood change is far from clear.

Since euphoric mood changes are more universally experienced in former addicts much of the investigation of drug-induced euphoria has been conducted with former opiate addicts. From his work with opiate addicts Kolb (1925) formulated the concepts of euphoria utilizing the terms "positive euphoria" and "negative euphoria." In producing positive euphoria a drug would generate feelings better than normal, or a high, whereas negative euphoria would represent the removal of dysphoric feelings induced by various environmental (extrinsic) or endogenous (intrinsic) factors. As such, the generation of the mood state or euphoria has been considered to be the result of either positive or negative reinforcement paradigms; negative euphoria resulting from the removal of an extrinsic or an endogenous negative reinforcer and positive euphoria resulting from extrinsic or intrinsic positive reinforcement consequent to drug administration (Mansky, 1975). Extrinsic negative reinforcers may result from social or physical factors of the environment, whereas intrinsic negative reinforcers may be related to the pain and discomfort of certain physical illnesses or to other illnesses such as unipolar depression. The intrinsic positive reinforcement may result from the direct pharmacological action of the drug on the brain, whereas extrinsic positive reinforcement is most likely derived from social or interactional factors. Using the above operant paradigms, measurements of subjective effects or mood changes have been postulated to be related to reinforcement paradigms. More specifically, the psychological instrument referred to as the subjective drug-effect questionnaire containing 40 items from the ARC Inventory has been considered to measure euphoria on items from the MBG scale (see Section 4.2). Furthermore, it has been postulated that this measurement of euphoria is the result of intrinsic or direct positive reinforcement as a consequence of opiate action on CNS centers (Mansky and Altman, 1977).

4.2. Measurement of Mood Effects of Opiate Agonists and Agonist–Antagonists

Few instruments have been used extensively in the measurement of subjective and mood effects consequent to opiate administration. The single-dose questionnaire developed at the Addiction Research Center has a graded scale that ascertains the degree of "liking" of the drug by former opiate addicts as a measure of euphoric effects after single-dose administration (Fraser, *et al.*, 1961; Fraser and Isbell, 1960; Martin, 1967*b*). This scale has been found to correlate with other measurements of opiate effects including physiological measurements such as pupil size and other subjective and somatic effects described previously as the signs and symptoms of opiate intoxication (see Table 1).

Another more sophisticated psychological instrument sensitive to drug effects including mood alteration has been developed at the Addiction Research Center and thus has been referred to as the ARC Inventory. This instrument consists of 550 items requiring a true or false response on each item and has been validated utilizing various groups of psychotropic drugs in defined populations (Hill *et al.*, 1963*a,b*; Haertzen *et al.*, 1963; Haertzen, 1974). Three scales derived from the ARC Inventory (MBG, LSD, and PCAG) have been found to be of value in ascertaining the subjective effects of opiate agonists and opiate agonist–antagonists. Each of the three scales has been considered to measure a specific type of drug effect. Thus, the MBG (morphine–benzedrine group) scale is considered to be sensitive to euphoric effects, the PCAG (pentobarbital, chlorpromazine, alcohol group) scale to sedative effects, and the LSD scale to psychotomimetic effects.

Single doses of opiate agonists such as morphine produce dose-related responses on the MBG scale. An occasional significant response has been produced on the other two scales by morphine or other opiate agonists but the latter responses are sporadic and are not usually dose related. Opiate agonist–antagonists such as nalorphine and cyclazocine produce dose-related responses on the PCAG and LSD scales but not on the MBG scale (Haertzen, 1966, 1970, 1974).

The subjective drug effects questionnaire can be considered a brief form of the ARC Inventory (Jasinski *et al.*, 1967). The questionnaire, consisting of 40 items representing the most discriminating items of the MBG, PCAG, and LSD scales, has been used to discriminate between the effects of opiate agonists and agonist–antagonists in single-dose studies. Since the subjective drug effect questionnaire contains only 40 true–false items it permits multiple testing after drug administration. As can be anticipated, morphine and other opiate agonists usually produce dose-related responses on the MBG items, whereas opiate agonist–antagonists produce mixed responses on the three scales. For example codeine, *d*-propoxyphene, and morphine usually produce dose-related elevations of the MBG scale, whereas nalorphine usually produces dose-related responses only on the PCAG and LSD scales (Jasinski *et al.*, 1970, 1971; Jasinski and Mansky, 1972). Occasionally a low dose of nalorphine (15 mg/70 kg) may produce a significant response on the MBG scale (Mansky and Jasinski, 1970). This latter phenomenon is reflective of the morphine-like effects observed with low doses of nalorphine or cyclazocine. Notably, even at doses of 10 mg/70 kg nalorphine can produce significant responses on the LSD and PCAG scales.

The LSD and PCAG responses due to nalorphine are considered to measure the psychotomimetic and sedative effects noted with opiate agonist–antagonists. These effects are generally considered to be dysphoric by both former addicts and nonaddicts (see Section 3.6). Thus, although nalorphine may provide some degree of analgesia at doses of 5 to 15 mg, the dysphoric effects are frequently elicited within this dose range, leading to patient rejection of subsequent use.

In contrast to nalorphine and cyclazocine some agonist–antagonists have been found to be acceptable analgesics in clinical studies. For example, pentazocine and nalbuphine are opiate agonist–antagonists that provide excellent analgesia (Beaver *et al.*, 1966; Forrest *et al.*, 1969; Keats and Telford, 1964; Paddock *et al.*, 1969; Potter and Payne, 1970; Mansky, 1976; Elliot *et al.*, 1970). At lower doses both pentazocine and nalbuphine produce significant responses on the MBG scale, whereas much higher doses are required to produce responses on the LSD and PCAG scales (Jasinski and Mansky, 1972; Jasinski *et al.*, 1970). Thus, pentazocine and nalbuphine can provide analgesia or produce euphoric responses at doses that will usually not elicit the dysphoric sedative and psychotomimetic effects unique to opiate agonist–antagonists.

It is of importance to note at this point that most opiate agonists that produce significant analgesia also, when tested, produce dose-related responses on the MBG scale of the ARC Inventory or on the MBG items contained in the subjective drug effect questionnaire. Additionally, the relative potency of various opiate agonists to morphine are similar when comparing clinical analgesia or when comparing responses on the MBG scale in former addicts. For example, 20 to 30 mg of profadol have been shown to produce analgesia equivalent to 10 mg of morphine (Pearson *et al.*, 1971; Keats and Telford, 1968; Sunshine *et al.*, 1970), whereas the relative potency of profadol to 1 mg of morphine using data from the MBG scale is 1.9 with 95% confidence limits of 0.9–7.5 (Jasinski *et al.*, 1971). In a similar fashion the analgesic potency of intramuscular methadone has been shown to be equal to intramuscular morphine, whereas oral methadone is one-half as potent as both intramuscular morphine and intramuscular methadone (Beaver *et al.*, 1967). The same relative potencies comparing morphine with intramuscular and oral methadone are obtained using the MBG scale of the single-dose drug effects questionnaire given to former addicts after administration of the opiates (Martin *et al.*, 1973*a*).

Thus, there is presently indirect evidence to indicate that euphoric responses to opiates and analgesic effects of opiates may be related to similar mechanisms of drug action. The evidence as presented is descriptive and based on parallel observations alluded to above. Future elucidation of the mechanisms of opiate analgesia and euphoria identifying specific CNS structures involved may confirm or refute this conclusion.

5. PAIN AND ANALGESIA

5.1. Pain Phenomenology

5.1.1. Introduction

Pain is perceived as a subjective experience, a symptom, involving conscious awareness of the pain-producing (nociceptive) stimulus, affective response to the stimulus along with reflexive and nonreflexive behavioral reactions. Although this division of the phenomenology of pain into various components may appear to be an arbitrary construct and does not necessarily reflect introspective data (Merskey, 1974), the various components are useful in understanding the analgesic action of opiates and in describing the phenomenology of various pain experiences in which one or more of the components are altered. The absence or alteration of any one or more components does not negate the subjective experience, but merely adds to the descriptive quality of the particular pain experience. The division may be merely artificial or may reflect the underlying anatomical structures and physiological functions subserving pain. Thus, the conscious awareness of a nociceptive sensation as painful may be akin to other nondistant sensory perceptions such as touch and temperature. The affective and nonreflexive behavioral reactions to pain are often associated with the conscious perception of a nociceptive stimulus as painful, whereas the musculoskeletal and autonomic reflexive reactions to pain are more accurately designated as nociceptive reactions since the reflexive reactions may be observed in situations in which conscious perception of the pain is anatomically impossible; e.g., the withdrawal reflex to a nociceptive stimulus after spinal cord injury (Beecher, 1957; Berlin *et al.*, 1952).

5.1.2. The Components of the Pain Experience

The division of pain into components, one largely perceptual and the other reactive, is agreed upon by many investigators although the phenomonological experience included under each category varies (Beecher, 1956*a*, 1957; Wolfe and Hardy, 1947; Barber, 1959; Mountcastle, 1968). Opiate analgesia often makes this separation more evident in that the analgesia is not universally accompanied by an inability to perceive nociceptive stimuli. Patients may state that they still are aware of the pain but it no longer bothers them. To support the latter statement, the patients may appear to be comfortable and relaxed, they may fall asleep, and observations of several reactive components will support the global observations.

It has been shown under some conditions that morphine may appear to affect the perception or recognition of a stimulus as nociceptive. However, if pain anticipatory anxiety is decreased, morphine has been shown to have little effect upon the perception of an experimentally induced painful stimulus (Hill *et al.*, 1952*a*). In comparison, patients with frontal lobe lesions may be able to recognize a stimulus as nociceptive but may state that the pain-producing stimulus does not bother them (Beecher, 1957). The latter phenomenon can be related to the complex function of the frontal lobe but it is unclear whether or not attentional factors dominate in the altered reaction to pain (Luria, 1973).

The phenomonological division of pain into its various components are represented in Table 4. The cognitive perceptual qualities of pain are often described by its location and similarity to previous pain experiences as well as associated tactile sensations and the temporal quality of the pain. Many descriptive terms have been used to designate qualitatively and quantitatively the parameters describing pain and have recently been reviewed by Melzack and Torgerson (1971). In addition to the multiple terms used to describe pain perception, there has been much discussion of two major qualities of cutaneous pain termed "fast and slow" pain or "first and second" pain. Phenomonologically, they have been noted to occur in sequence. The first or fast pain is faster traveling, described as sharp, epicritic, bright or pricking, and is postulated to be related to the sensory perceptive component of pain. The other is slower traveling, described as dull, aching, and protophatic. It occurs as an aftermath and is often associated with both the reactive and

TABLE 4
Pain

- I. Sensory component (perception of the nociceptive stimulus as pain)
- II. Reactive components
  - A. Reflexive
    - 1. Withdrawal reflex (flexion of the ipsilateral limb, extension of the contralateral limb)
    - 2. Pseudoaffective reflexes
      - a. Autonomic (usually tachycardia, hypertension, hyperpnea, pupillary dilatation, sweating)
      - b. Immediate vocalization (e.g., "ouch!")
      - c. Grimace
      - d. Muscular guarding
      - e. Alerting reaction
  - B. Affective (pain-related discomfort or dysphoria, e.g., fear, anxiety, suffering)
  - C. Behavioral
    - 1. Escape
    - 2. Avoidance

perceptual component. The latter two types of pain have some relevance to opiate analgesia, even though their existence has been debated (Libet, 1957; Jones, 1956).

Reflexive reactions to nociceptive stimuli that include the withdrawal reflex, alerting reaction, immediate vocalization, and autonomic reflexes have been used in clinical and experimental studies of pain. The reflexes represent the common experiences of a quick withdrawal of a limb from a nociceptive stimulus, immediate vocalization or a shout seemingly simultaneous with exposure to the nociceptive stimulus, hyperalertness to other environmental stimuli, and reflexive autonomic changes easily observable such as sweating, respectively.

The autonomic reflex reactions to acute pain are usually sympathetic, although some severe visceral pains have been more frequently associated with parasympathetic reactions (Mountcastle, 1968). The usual sympathetic response to pain includes tachycardia, pupillary dilatation, increase in blood pressure, and sweating. The reflexive reactions occur with the acute application of a nociceptive stimulus and thus are considered primarily to be components of the acute pain experience. The reflexive reactions to an acute nociceptive stimulus may vary with the type of stimulus and the areas of the body stimulated, and this is especially evident if cutaneous pain is compared with visceral pain. The vocalization and autonomic reactions may be accompanied by a reflexive grimace and thus appear to be affective, but they have been observed in decorticate preparations and have, therefore, been termed pseudoaffective (Lim and Guzman, 1968). This reaction may also be similar to the fear reaction or conditioned emotional response associated with a nociceptive stimulus (Maher, 1966).

The affective response to pain mediated through the cortex and associated with perception of the stimulus may be quite varied. A feeling of discomfort accompanied by fear, tension, worry, suffering, and other associated affects may be secondary to the nociceptive stimulus. Conversely, the affective state of the individual at the time of the nociceptive stimulus may influence the entire pain experience including the perceptions and reactions. The nonreflexive behaviors associated with pain are purposeful in limiting the on-going pain experience or in preventing the recurrence of the pain. When the pain-induced activities are not able to eliminate the source of the pain (e.g., lever pressing, fighting, muscular guarding, etc.) they involve attempts to escape the pain situation or to avoid the situations that have produced pain.

5.1.3. Acute and Chronic Pain

In the acute pain experience, escape behavior is observed, whereas in patients with chronic pain, avoidance may be more prominent. Escape and avoidance behaviors have very different implications if one follows the logical conclusions of the operant paradigms. Escape behavior is dependent upon the unconditioned nociceptive stimulus, whereas once the avoidance response is learned it is maintained in the absence of the nociceptive stimulus and is difficult to extinguish (Maher, 1966). If one assumes that escape behavior is related to acute pain and avoidance behavior to chronic pain, it becomes evident that the two types of pain experience present very different dilemmas to the pain patient and to those treating acute and chronic pain. In fact, avoidance behavior in patients with chronic pain may be maintained by the many positive reinforcers consequent to the avoidance behavior as opposed to the unconditioned pain stimulus initiating the avoidance behavior.

Chronic pain has been associated with changes in personality and with the development of associated psychiatric disorders. Woodforde and Merskey (1972) investigated patients with chronic pain referred for psychiatric consultation. The patients were investigated utilizing open-ended interviews along with the Middlesex Hospital Questionnaire (M.H.Q.) and the Eysenck Personality Inventory (E.P.I.). The patients were separated into two groups, the organic group (O), with a known organic basis for the pain, and a psychiatric (P) group, who lacked evidence for an organic disorder related to the pain (idiopathic pain). Both subgroups of pain patients appear to have scores similar to psychoneurotic outpatients, differing from normal controls. Male patients in the O group had higher scores for anxiety- and obsessionality-related items along with a higher L score on the E.P.I. This constellation of effects for the male O patients may reflect mechanisms of coping with a chronic illness and its effect upon the patient's life and self-image. All patients scored low on the E scale of the E.P.I. interpreted by the authors to indicate increased depression in the patients. The authors postulate that their findings may be the result both of the process of subject selection and of the presence of chronic pain.

Other authors have reported the development of a depression syndrome in some patients with chronic pain, consisting of weight loss, sleep disturbance, psychomotor retardation, along with a depressed mood and crying spells (Sternbach, 1974*a*, Merskey, 1974). Although chronic pain does not invariably result in the development of this depression syndrome, it is clear that chronic pain produces alterations in behavior and mood that far exceed the changes seen in acute pain of relatively short duration.

5.2. Psychological Factors Influencing Pain

5.2.1. *Introduction*

Pain may be influenced by numerous factors such as learning and associated cultural milieu, resulting coping style, suggestion, the meaning or significance of the pain, motivation, anxiety, and fear. The multiple psychological factors can be classified under the broad categories of cognition, affect or mood, and attention. Although many studies describing the alteration of pain do not clearly separate the perceptive and reactive components, it appears that the behavioral and affective reactions to pain are more easily and consistently influenced by psychological factors.

As we discussed, pain does differ from other sensory experiences especially considering the multiple involvement of diverse areas of the brain in the processing of the nerve impulse resulting from a nociceptive stimulus. Nevertheless, even the more straightforward sensory processes such as sight can be influenced by psychological factors (Gilchrist and Nesberg, 1952) so that it would be an error to ascribe the alteration of pain by psychological factors solely to influence upon the reactive components.

5.2.2. Cognitive Factors

The many cognitive factors included in the concepts of learning theory, coping style, the meaning or significance of pain, and the resulting influence on motivation are often vaguely defined and frequently inferred from observations or verbal reports. It may be useful, when appropriate, to express the experimental or investigational observations in the more exacting operant and respondent conditioning paradigms. Such attempts will be made throughout this section.

The nonreflexive reactions to pain described as escape and avoidance behavior appear to be influenced by early life experiences. Melzack and Scott (1957) in a classical experiment showed that dogs reared in a painfree environment showed altered reactions to nociceptive stimuli as revealed by a decreased frequency of escape and avoidance behavior. It is probable that early pain experience is also crucial for the development of pain behavior in man. Wikler (1966) has postulated that reactions of adults to nociceptive stimuli may not only represent unconditioned reactions to the unconditioned nociceptive stimulus but may be conditioned reactions to the naturally occurring stimuli preceding the unconditioned stimulus. Thus, the nonnociceptive sensations that precede such naturally occurring phenomena as colic or cramping pain may eventually elicit a conditioned reaction similar to the unconditioned pain reaction to the unconditioned nociceptive stimulus of intestinal distention.

Such a mechanism was postulated by Dorcus and Kirkner (1948) in explaining persistent dysmenhorrhea. They suggested that pain (the unconditioned reaction) is initially experienced as the result of nociceptive visceral stimulation (the unconditioned stimulus) during a particular period of menstruation. This unconditioned nociceptive stimulus is associated with edema, body temperature changes, muscle tone alteration, and other physiological stimuli producing changes occurring during menstruation (conditioned stimuli). The latter conditioned stimuli inherent in normal physiological menstruation may lead to a conditioned pain reaction in spite of the cessation of the initial unconditioned nociceptive stimulus, resulting in chronic dysmenhorrhea.

Learning as reflected by ethnocultural background has been shown to affect reactions of patients to clinical pain. In a study addressed to this question Zborowski (1952) described the different reactions to pain of patients from four diverse ethnic backgrounds: Jewish, Italian, Irish, and "old American." The differences were attributed to cultural attitudes and values acquired from early family experiences. It is of some interest that the observation concerning the cultural influence on pain can also be generalized to cultural influence on the reaction to disease and illness in general (Fabrega and Van Egeren, 1976).

Cognitive style may be the result of ethnic rearing but can be investigated without consideration of social or cultural milieu. Such styles can influence pain. Adler and Lomazzi (1973) found that pain tolerance could be related to perceptual style as measured by the dimensions of field dependence and independence. They also cite the work of Petrie who examined subjects who tend to overestimate external stimulation (augmenters) in opposition to subjects who tend to underestimate (reducers). Pain tolerance was greater in reducers.

The relationship of cognitive style to pain has been postulated from research often employing experimental pain and frequently producing contradictory results. These contradictions may be due to the method of experimental pain produced and the method of ascertaining the subjective pain experience rather than to differences inherent in the hypothesis that perceptual style influences the pain experience.

The cognitive labeling of the meaning or significance of a nociceptive stimulus may greatly influence the perceived pain and suffering. Beecher (1946) noted that soldiers who received serious wounds in battle surprisingly reported less pain than might be expected from the wounds. All of the soldiers interviewed were mentally clear when questioned concerning pain. Of the patients questioned 32.1% indicated "no pain," 25.6% "slight pain," 18.6% "moderate pain," and 23.7% "bad pain." The validity of the verbal responses were supported by a parallel between bad pain reports (23.7%) and desire for pain medication (27.0%). The relative insensitivity to the nociceptive stimulus of the serious wounds was selective in that the soldiers were clearly noted to complain vigorously of other painful procedures such as difficult venipunctures or rough handling of their wounds. Beecher postulated that the pain experienced and the resulting suffering might be related to the significance of meaning of the wound for the soldiers considering that the sustained wound had already removed the soldiers from the height of the front line battle and had the possibility of leading to the soldier being sent home.

Later, Beecher (1956*b*) reported on a comparison group of civilian patients undergoing surgery with wounds in the same body areas as the soldiers. In contrast to the military patients, more of the civilian patients desired pain medication. Comparing abdominal, thoracic, and bone tissue damage, 32% of the soldiers and 83% of the civilians desired pain medication. Beecher postulated that the wound had a much different significance for the civilian patient. Instead of removing them from a dangerous situation the wounds and surgery disrupted the civilian patients' lives, leading to temporary or permanent changes in their life-styles. The striking differences in the two groups of patients can be considered as the difference in the perceived consequence of the nociceptive unconditioned stimulus (the wound). Thus, it appears that the suffering component of pain as ascertained by verbal reports and requests for medication is greatly influenced by the perceived significance of the wound to future behavior. This is a similar process postulated for convert operant conditioning whereby behavior is influenced by imagined or expected consequences (Cautela, 1967, 1970, 1971).

In summary then, learning, memory, significance or consequence of a nociceptive stimulus, and perceptual style all affect the resulting symptom of pain. Certainly, immediate expectations of a person (set) and the place of occurrence of the nociceptive stimulus (setting) may greatly affect the resulting pain. The cognitive factors discussed so far could be included in set and setting as can affectual and attentional factors. The latter factor, attentional, although included in cognitive processes, deserves a special section below.

5.2.3. Influence of Affect on Pain

Pain may be influenced by the affectual state of the individual at the time he or she reports pain. The most systematic studies involving the influence of affect on pain have described the alteration of pain related to anxiety, which may be considered as a symptom either by itself or as a part of a psychiatric disorder such as depression, schizophrenia, or anxiety neurosis. Anxiety as an affectual state can also be influenced by external circumstances and is frequently considered in this sense to be synonymous with fear, especially when the circumstances would produce the symptom of anxiety in the majority of the population. In most of the works cited, anxiety is either described operationally and measured by a psychological instrument or more commonly is inferred from the conditions of the experiment or study. Clearly, the heterogeneity inherent in the different uses of anxiety allows for limited rather than for sweeping conclusions concerning the effects of anxiety on pain.

Additionally, consideration must be given to the causal relationship of anxiety to pain. Anxiety may result as an affectual reaction to a nociceptive stimulus or alternatively to the conditioned stimuli or the discriminative stimuli associated with the nociceptive stimulus. In the latter case, the anxiety may be termed anticipatory anxiety. Alternatively, anxiety may represent an independent variable, i.e., it may exist independent of the nociceptive stimulus. In the latter case, the anxiety may have no influence on the pain experience or may have a marked effect on the perceptions and reactions to the nociceptive stimulus.

To summarize at this point, it is important to realize that anxiety as discussed in relationship to pain represents a multidetermined affect. The anxiety may be the result of a nociceptive stimulus (or related conditioned stimuli) or it may be present prior to the nociceptive stimulus. Anxiety existing prior to the nociceptive stimulus may be such that it alters the pain experience or it may have no effect on the pain experience. Few studies have been designed to separate the various possible relationships described above and even fewer have measured anxiety specifically as an independent variable.

In experiments designed to produce anticipatory anxiety related to a nociceptive stimulus, Hill *et al.* (1952*a*) showed that the estimation of the intensity of a nociceptive stimulus is not affected by opiates in a low anxiety condition but that the tendency of the subjects to overestimate the intensity of a nociceptive stimulus in a high anxiety condition is eliminated by opiates. The authors conclude that opiates specifically decrease pain anticipatory anxiety, which leads to the overestimation of the intensity of the nociceptive stimulus, but that they do not interfere with the actual perception of the stimulus intensity.

Pain-related anxiety is considered as an important aspect of clinical pain as compared to experimentally induced pain. This is evident in the many studies involving an experimental pain stimulus of limited duration. In these studies, inconsistent relief from standard analgesics such as morphine as well as an inconsistent placebo effect is evident. Smith *et al.* (1966, 1968; Smith and Beecher, 1969) have shown that experimental pain of increased severity and duration utilizing ischemic pain induction responds to opiates similarily to clinical pain. The results of subsequent studies (Adler and Lomazzi, 1973) using the method of ischemic pain production suggests that pain-related anxiety may indeed be an important factor in simulating clinical pain experimentally.

Beecher also implicated anxiety in his studies comparing the reactions of soldiers and civilian surgery patients to body wounds. The soldiers were removed from a high-anxiety-producing situation (the front line) to the safety of the hospital. In contrast, the civilians faced increasing anxiety as the result of surgery that interrupted their life pattern, and accompanied disease or injury, which often left them with uncertainty concerning the consequence of the wound producing the nociceptive stimulus. Beecher did not independently measure the level of anxiety in the two groups of patients, but he offers alternative explanations (see above) that may explain the results using cognitive factors such as meaning or significance of the wounds. Nevertheless, Beecher's explanation employing anxiety deserves consideration.

Anxiety reduction has also been implicated as a measure of analgesic effect. Using speed of reaction time as a measurement of performance, Hill *et al.* (1952*b*, 1955) noted that reaction time was increased when poor performance was followed by a nociceptive stimulus (shock). The decrease in performance was attributed to pain anticipatory anxiety and might be expected from the decrease in performance observed with high levels of anxiety. This is represented by an inverted U-shaped curve with performance as the ordinate and anxiety as the abscissa. As anxiety increases, performance increases to a peak and it then decreased as anxiety increases (Yerkes and Dodson, 1908; Hebb, 1955). Hill *et al.* observed that reaction time improved with the administration of morphine in the shock condition, whereas morphine alone in the standard condition did not affect the reaction time. The authors conclude that anxiety reduction can account for the opiate effect on performance.

Anxiety reduction has also been implicated as a major mechanism of hypnotic analgesia (Shor, 1962). In a like fashion, placebo effect has been attributed to anxiety reduction (Sternbach, 1968). It is interesting to note that the hypnotic procedure itself can be shown to have a placebo component and an additional component thought to be due to the hypnotic process itself (Orne, 1974). It would be difficult to account for this latter finding postulating anxiety reduction as the sole mechanism of both the placebo and the "hypnotic" effects of the hypnosis procedure.

Anxiety as a state and as a symptom unrelated directly to a nociceptive stimulus has also been noted to increase sensitivity to pain. Malmo and Shagass (1949) examined a number of patients with conditions characterized by chronic anxiety. This group showed an overreaction to painful stimuli; the greater the presenting anxiety the more intense the reaction to the nociceptive stimulus. It has also been noted that patients diagnosed to have anxiety neurosis by strict research criteria (Feighner *et al.*, 1972) are more sensitive to nociceptive stimuli (Woodruff *et al.*, 1974). Pain sensitivity may also be increased in other psychiatric disorders. Thus, pain symptoms regardless of the etiology of the pain are more common among manic–depressive, anxiety-neurotic, and female hysterical patients than among healthy controls (Sternbach, 1974*b*).

It is evident then that various affective states can alter reactions to nociceptive stimuli and perhaps in the case of the psychiatric disorders mentioned above the individual patients may be more sensitive to the conditioned stimuli related to the nociceptive stimulus if anxiety is high. The mechanism postulated for dysmenorrhea in the previous section may be applicable to the reports of pain in patients with various psychiatric disorders. Just as in the case of dysmenorrhea the nociceptive unconditioned stimulus may no longer be present but a conditioned stimulus not generally thought to be nociceptive may lead to the pain reaction and the reporting of pain symptoms in this group of psychiatric patients.

Thus, it appears that anxiety and other dysphoric affects may alter the perceptions and reactions to nociceptive stimuli. Notably, anxiety appears to increase the intensity or frequency of reported pain and a decrease in anxiety appears to have an effect in producing analgesia. In contrast to these conclusions, it has been noted that soldiers in battle and athletes during competition may fail to react to a nociceptive injury until they are removed from the heat of the battle or the excitement of competition. It has been suggested that the extreme fear present in battle may account for this lack of reaction to a nociceptive stimulus (Merskey, 1974). Although this may be the case, attentional factors and intense motivation focusing attention on the task in combat or competition appear to be a more likely explanation for the lack of pain during the particular event (see below).

If anxiety accentuates the reactive component of pain and if anxiety reduction in part accounts for the analgesic action of opiates, hypnosis, placebo, and other procedures, then medications that primarily affect anxiety should produce analgesia at the dose levels that have been shown to decrease anxiety. This should apply especially to sedative–hypnotics. It is common knowledge that sedative–hypnotics have been used in high doses as anesthetic agents. Sedative–hypnotics, however, in dose levels that relieve anxiety have only limited effects on pain. Indeed, Keats and Beecher (1950) found that pentobarbital in doses of 60 and 90 mg intravenously produced relief of postoperative pain in 50% of patients as compared with a 20% relief rate for saline and an 80% relief rate for morphine. This result was criticized by Hill *et al.* (1955) who noted that the criteria for pain relief and the order of administration biased results in favor of the sedative-hypnotic. Beecher and Keats used both comfort without pain relief and reports of comfort with pain relief in obtaining the 50% figure. If only verbal reports of pain relief are used the rate is reduced to approximately 40%. Furthermore, if reports are restricted to saline versus pentobarbital comparisons, the relief rate drops to 30%. Regardless of this astute critique intravenous pentobarbital does appear to produce some analgesia but much less than would be expected if anxiety reduction in general could account for the pain relief. Additionally, it must be noted that considering the criticism stated above, the sedative–hypnotic did appear to be slightly more effective than placebo but far less effective than morphine in producing analgesia.

In the experiment cited earlier, Hill *et al.* (1955) showed that 15 mg of morphine intramuscularly reduced the deficit of reaction time performance produced by the anticipation of a nociceptive stimulus. In the same study the investigators showed that 250 mg of pentobarbital intramuscularly was not effective in reducing the performance deficit. They concluded that morphine reduces pain anticipatory anxiety whereas pentobarbital does not. Again, it must be remembered that pain anticipatory anxiety was inferred as the mechanism of the increased reaction time. No psychological instrument was used in this case to measure the pain anticipatory anxiety as an independent or dependent variable.

Chapman and Feather (1973), using the ischemic pain method of Smith and Beecher (1969) showed that 10 mg of diazepam orally was effective in reducing anxiety (measured independently) associated with a nociceptive stimulus. The authors found an inverse relationship between the reduction in anxiety by diazepam and pain tolerance such that as the anxiety was decreased pain tolerance increased. The effects of diazepam noted here were shown to be dependent upon prior experience with the nociceptive stimulus. Unfortunately, the authors used placebo and aspirin as comparison treatments. Opiates specifically were not used in the experimental design so that the relative effectiveness of diazepam in comparison with a strong analgesic can not be inferred from this study.

In summary then, anxiety generally increases the reaction to a nociceptive stimulus. Specifically, anxiety, which may be related to anticipation of a nociceptive stimulus (anticipatory anxiety), may be of particular significance in the total reaction to the nociceptive stimulus. Opiates produce pain relief in part by decreasing pain anticipatory anxiety. Additionally, opiates may affect the perception of pain by eliminating the overestimation of the intensity of a nociceptive stimulus as the result of decreasing anticipatory anxiety. Sedative–hypnotics are superior to placebo and inferior to opiates in relieving pain, thus indicating that anxiety as affected by sedative–hypnotics is only one factor influencing the reaction to a nociceptive stimulus. Finally, the various results may be influenced by the lack of measuring anxiety as an independent variable and by the lack of precision in defining anxiety. Other dysphoric affects associated with various psychiatric disorders alter the sensitivity to pain or the reaction to the discriminative or conditioned stimuli associated with a previous pain experience.

5.2.4. *Attentional Factors*

Attention or the ability to focus conscious awareness affects the perceptions and reactions to nociceptive stimuli. The often quoted anecdote of the soldier in battle or the athlete in competition sustaining a nociceptive injury without perceiving the pain associated with the injury is an excellent example of the powerful effect of attention on pain perception and reaction. It has been argued that motivational factors may be of prime importance in these situations. Perhaps this is accurate but it is difficult to describe the lack of conscious appreciation of the nociceptive stimulus to motivation without invoking the extreme concentration of conscious awareness upon the task of the battle or the competition as a mediating process. Less dramatic examples of anecdotal evidence concerns an increased request for pain medication in hospitalized patients during the quiet hours of the evening and night shifts. The same patients may well request less medication during the day when there are many distractions to compete with the nociceptive stimulus.

Distraction from or inattention to a nociceptive stimulus has been invoked as an important aspect of pain reduction (Beecher, 1959*a,b*; Melzack, 1974). This is nicely described by Hackett (1971) who relates a personal account of his experience with a painful corneal laceration. He was able to better cope with the pain utilizing activities that distracted his attention from the nociceptive stimulus.

Patients with frontal lobe syndromes have exhibited a seemingly paradoxical reaction to nociceptive stimuli that may be accounted for in part by attentional factors. The pain perceptual threshold in frontal lobe patients may be unchanged or decreased along with an increase in the skeletal muscle reflex reactions and affective reactions to the nociceptive stimulus (Beecher, 1959*a*). Frontal lobotomy, however, has often decreased the complaints of pain and suffering in cancer patients (Hackett *et al.*, 1966). Furthermore, it is noted that frontal lobe patients may vigorously complain of pain such as that accompanying venipuncture only to be quickly and easily distracted by a simple question involving another activity. These observations may well be related to the attentional deficit described in frontal lobe patients (Luria, 1973).

5.3. Pain Pathways—The Neuroanatomical and Neurophysiological Aspects of the Processing of Nociceptive Stimuli

5.3.1. Introduction

The neuroanatomical substrate and the neurophysiological basis for the conscious appreciation of pain are not precisely defined. The voluminous information arising from the studies of pain and related pathways can best be understood as pieces of a very complex, multidimensional puzzle that has yet to be assembled. It is multidimensional in a consideration of several nerve centers, fibers, and tracts with complex connections originating from nociceptive excitation of peripheral afferent nerve fibers and ending in higher brain centers. This network of neurons and fibers integrates various electrical and chemical information initiated by the nociceptive stimulus. The system is also influenced by other sensory input and by endogenous regulation of neuronal and hormonal activity.

In this section, the structural components of the nervous system implicated as pain pathways will be discussed, followed by theories concerning the functional aspects of this network. The relationship of this incompletely understood system to the phenomenology of pain is far from certain. Some speculations, however, will be entertained and discussed.

5.3.2. Neuroanatomical Aspects (see Fig. 2)

Nociceptive stimulation can result from application of mechanical, thermal, electrical, and chemical energy to cutaneous or visceral structures innervated by afferent nerve terminals. Physical energy stimulation such as heat, cold, pressure, and electricity may affect nerve endings directly or may

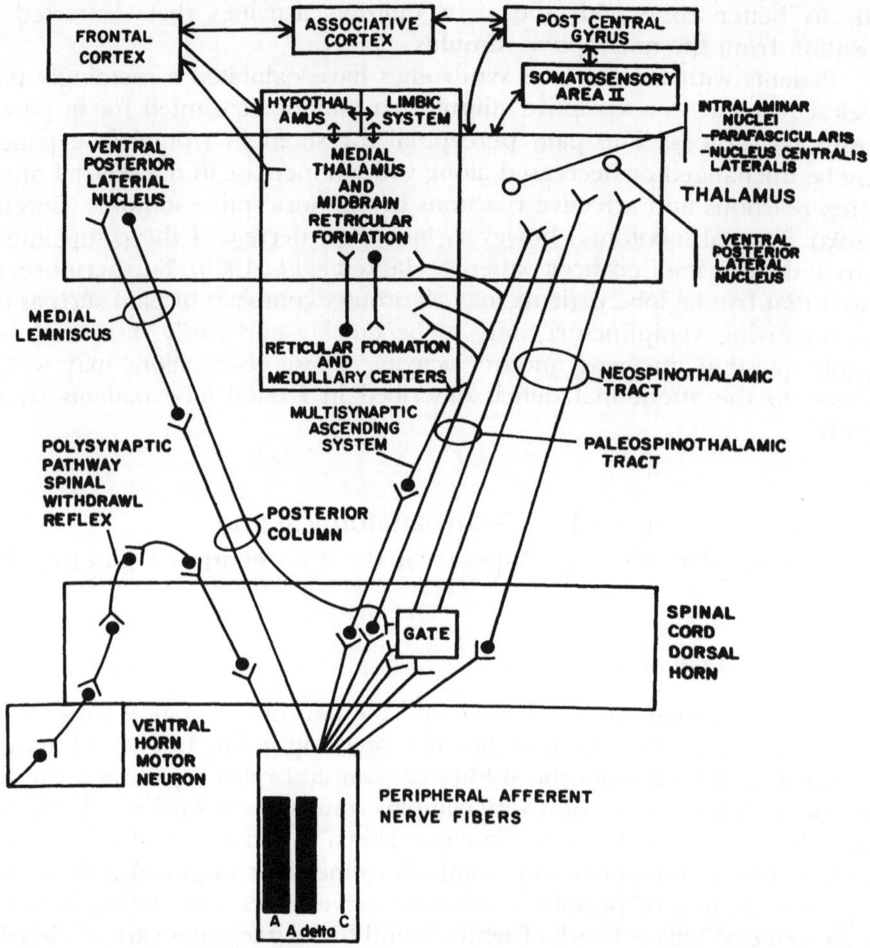

FIG. 2. Theoretical scheme of afferent system related to pain perception and reaction.

at times produce nociceptive stimulation through chemical mediation resulting from tissue damage. The chemical stimuli invoking nociceptive impulses include acetylcholine, serotonin, histamine, acids, bases, excess sodium or potassium, and polypeptides such as bradykinin (Keele and Armstrong, 1964). Cutaneous nociceptive stimuli have been studied most extensively but some experimental studies have involved applied mechanical tension to visceral organs and chemical stimulation of the peritoneum (Lim and Guzman, 1968).

Most evidence indicates that electrical nerve impulses originating from nociceptive stimuli are transmitted by A delta and C nerve fibers. The A delta fibers are 2–5 μm in diamter and occupy the lower range of the larger myelinated nerve fibers. In general, the A delta fibers have a higher threshold of stimulation and are slower conductors (12 to 30 m/sec) than the larger A fibers but faster conductors than the C fibers (0.5 to 2 m/sec). The C fibers occupy the lower range of the peripheral nerve fiber size and are unmyelinated. They are relatively slow conducting and generally have a high threshold of stimulation. Melzack and Wall (1968) have noted that each peripheral nerve fiber may have a profile of thresholds to various stimuli such as touch, heat, cold, or intense stimulation of any type. Conversely, intense nociceptive stimulation may not only stimulate high-threshold receptors and fibers but other fibers throughout the spectrum of cutaneous sensations.

The peripheral fibers, which conduct impulses originating from nociceptive stimuli, synapse in the dorsal horn usually within one or two segments after entering the spinal cord. The synapses involve connections with two very different neuronal systems. One system contains many neurons with short axons and is termed *multisynaptic*, whereas the other system contains fewer neurons with long axons and is labeled *oligosynaptic*. The fibers that belong to the oligosynaptic system ascend in the anteriolateral funiculus usually after crossing to the contralateral side within one or two segments. Due to the length of the axons the oligosynaptic system has been readily identified in studies of neuronal degeneration and labeled the *spinothalamic tract*. Few fibers are contained in the true spinothalamic tract terminating in the thalamus, whereas many terminate in the brain stem reticular formation and in the central gray substance of the midbrain (see below).

The spinothalamic tract described in standard neuroanatomy texts actually represents two ascending systems in the anterior lateral funiculus, one lateral and the other medial. The lateral fibers are relatively few in number and are of recent phylogenetic development, thus being termed the *neospinothalamic tract* (Nauta, 1975; Noordenbos, 1968; Mountcastle, 1968). The neospinothalamic fibers in primates terminate in the nucleus ventralis posterolateralis (VPL) of the thalamus in an archipelago or island-like pattern and lie in close proximity to terminations of the medial lemniscus (Nauta, 1975).

The more medial group of oligosynaptic fibers of the spinothalamic tract may be phylogenetically comparable to the spinodiencephalic system of lower vertebrates and is therefore termed the *paleospinothalamic tract*. Fibers in this tract terminate in the medial or intralaminar thalamic nuclei including the nucleus parafasicularis and the nucleus centralis lateralis (Mehler *et al.*, 1960; Bowsher, 1957; Nauta, 1975).

Many of the oligosynaptic fibers ascending in the lateral funiculus with the paleospinothalamic fibers terminate within the brain stem at the medullary, pontile, or mesencephalic segments. Neurons related to the brain stem terminations of this tract may eventually form connections with the more medial thalamic nuclei. This system has thus been termed the spinoreticulodiencephalic system (Mountcastle, 1968). Some of the medial oligosynaptic fibers also terminate in the central gray mesencephalic area. It is also significant that the input of nociceptive impulses is prominent within the tegmental reticular formation and evidence points to connections with the subcoeruleus nuclei (adjacent to the nucleus coeruleus or nucleus pigmentosa pontis), an area rich in norepinepherine or other adrenergic transmitters.

The group of nociceptive afferent stimuli that are not transmitted by the spinothalamic systems or the spinoreticulodiencephalic system may lead to impulse generation in the chains or networks of the multisynaptic neurons with short interneuronal connections. This multisynaptic network forms the basis for the withdrawal reflex at the spinal cord level. Additionally, this network may well form ascending tracts with multiple synapses that by their nature are difficult to demonstrate by studies of nerve degeneration. This network may ascend more diffusely in the spinal cord in the anteriolateral segments and other areas. The network crosses the midline and sends some fibers that ascend in the posterior columns (Noordenbos, 1968). In the brain stem this system provides much input into the areas of the reticular formations.

Thus, the *oligosynaptic* and *multisynaptic* systems both connect with brainstem centers. The processing of nociceptive stimuli in this area is far from certain but several networks have been implicated. The central gray substance of the midbrain may form a functional system that includes the central gray core of the periaqueductal area, the periventricular area, and the medial thalamus (Nauta, 1975). This functional unit is suggested by studies involving the dorsal longitudinal fasciculus of Schütz that constitutes reciprocal connections with the mesencephalic gray substance and the diencephalic periventricular area. This system may incorporate an ascending tract containing catecholamines (dorsal periventricular bundle), thus indicating connections from the midbrain raphe region and the mesencephalic gray substance to areas of the medial thalamus and hypothalamus (Lindvall *et al.*, 1974; Clark, 1932).

Multiple connections link the mesencephalic gray core and the tegmental reticular formation. Nauta (1958) has described connections of the central gray substance with a large area of the mesencephalic tegmental area that sends impulses in descending tracts into the pons, medulla, and spinal cord. These descending tracts may be related to those described by Melzack and Wall (1968), eventually descending in the posterior columns and providing modulation of the dorsal horn cell gate.

The nociceptive system eventually connects with higher cerebral centers. The VPL nucleus of the thalamus sends postsynaptic fibers to the somatosensory cortex and other cerebral centers. Connections are also evident between the brain stem centers subserving pain, the frontal lobe, and structures of the limbic system.

The conscious appreciation of pain and the nociceptive reactions have implicated multiple higher brain centers. Thus, the frontal lobe, hypothalamus, and structures of the limbic system have been implicated as structures involved in pain perception and reaction as well as related to the analgesic actions of medications or surgery. Many of these structures plus those described in the brain stem and the thalamus have also been implicated in studies involving electrical stimulation and analgesia. Additionally, many of these same structures have a great affinity for morphine and other opiate-like analgesics.

5.3.3. Functional Aspects

The complexity of the processing of nociceptive stimuli is further evident in consideration of functional aspects of the anatomical system described in the previous section. Appreciation of this complexity is enhanced by considering that many neurons within the brain or spinal cord are affected by numerous connections with other neurons; each connection is subserved by a synapse that involves neural transmitter release by the presynaptic fibers and postsynaptic receptor membranes sensitive to the particular neural transmitters. Furthermore, within this system of membranes and transmitter substances some events tend to depolarize the neuron (excitatory events) and others tend to hyperpolarize the neuron (inhibitory events). Summation of excitatory and inhibitory transmitter release over time influences the passage of information over the chain of neurons. Little is known concerning the role of these events in the transmission of nociceptive signals initiated by peripheral stimulation and ultimately perceived as conscious appreciation of pain along with the concomitant reactions to the nociceptive stimulus.

The neuroanatomical pathways described in the previous section, however, have been thought to function in a number of complex manners. Much controversy still surrounds the precise relationship of each aspect of the anatomical system to the observed phenomenology of pain. Nevertheless, information points to some useful hypotheses that indicate putative processing of nociceptive stimuli.

Peripheral nerve impulses resulting from a nociceptive stimulus are processed in some manner at the first synaptic level in the spinal cord. This processing is considered to involve both direct transmission of adequate signals and filtered transmission depending upon the total nature of the cutaneous stimulation. Thus, Melzack and Wall (1965, 1968) have postulated that some peripheral signals may lead to ascending transmission via the posterior column and medial lemniscus to higher centers that then send returning or descending modulating signals to a spinal cord neuronal network. This network then filters incoming cutaneous impulses and has been termed the "gate." The network or gate then may send ascending signals in the spinothalamic tract or other ascending tracts if excitatory nociceptive impulses prevail. Cutaneous sensory stimuli other than nociceptive stimuli tend to close the gate, whereas the lack of cutaneous sensory stimuli as seen in postherpetic neurologias may tend to open the gate. In recent years the gate theory has received much criticism (Schmidt, 1972; Iggo, 1972). Nonetheless, the theory must still be considered and recent evidence has supported some of the major hypotheses (Kerr, 1975).

Signals that ascend in the neospinothalamic tract and terminate in an organized although diffuse pattern in the ventral posterior lateral nucleus of the thalamus may account for both the perceptual component of pain and the localization of the nociceptive stimulus. Although it has been noted that the phenomenology of slow and fast pain is controversial, some investigators postulate that the neospinothalamic oligosynaptic system is responsible for the sharp quality of perceived pain. The slow or aching pain may be due to transmission in the multisynaptic system described in the previous section.

The oligosynaptic paleospinothalamic system and the multisynaptic system may subserve the various reflexive components of pain. At the spinal cord level multisynaptic connections are involved in the ipsilateral withdrawal and contralateral extention seen in the limbs resulting from nociceptive stimulation. The autonomic reflexes and alerting reflex may result from the termination of both systems within the brain stem reticular formation and the resulting hypothalamic connections. The immediate vocalization observed as a reflex to a nociceptive stimulus is also postulated to be processed within the brain stem (Hoffmeister, 1968; Charpentier, 1968; Lim and Guzman, 1968).

The reactive components to pain such as the affective and behavioral are related to the cerebral centers, the limbic system, and their descending connections to the brain stem and spinal cord. The exact pathways involved in the processing of the nociceptive stimuli at the cerebral level are far from clear. As described earlier, implications of structures in the frontal lobe and the limbic system have received much investigative and experimental attention (Charpentier, 1968).

No one of the various putative neurotransmitters in the central nervous system is solely associated with the perception of and reaction to pain. In fact, the involvement of various neurotransmitters is somewhat confusing. For example, dextroamphetamine has been noted to potentiate the analgesic effects of opiates. Likewise, neuroleptic medications are commonly used to provide increased analgesia in combination with an opiate. These observations are rather intriguing since the mechanism of amphetamine activity is associated with an increased release of dopamine, whereas neuroleptics antagonize the activity of dopamine. Similar confusion surrounds the role of each of the central nervous system putative transmitters when considered as the sole neural transmitter involved in pain (Evans, 1962; Forrest *et al.*, 1970; Theobald *et al.*, 1968; Herold and Cahn, 1968). Additionally, no drug that produces analgesia solely by affecting one or another neurotransmitter is as effective an analgesic as are opiate agonists.

5.4. Analgesia

Measurement of the analgesic effects of medications in man have involved two major methodologies, the first employing experimentally induced pain, the second concerned with the relief of clinical pain. The results of studies utilizing experimental pain differ from clinical pain studies in that opiates and placebo appear to show inconsistent analgesic effects with experimental pain, whereas they produce consistent analgesia in patients. Experimental pain investigation does, however, allow for more effective control of variables such as the intensity of the nociceptive stimulus, the subject's set, and the experimental setting.

The inconsistent results utilizing experimental pain in man may be due to several factors defined in more recent investigations. Hill *et al.* (1952*a,b*, 1955) and Kornetsky (1954) have shown that the set and setting can influence the results of analgesic studies. Specifically, they illustrated that pain anticipatory anxiety altered by variation in the subject's set and experimental setting could influence the perception of nociceptive stimuli and the effects of opiate analgesia. Smith and Beecher (1969) and Smith *et al.* (1966, 1968) have shown that changes in the nature of the nociceptive stimulus have an influence in analgesic assays. Smith *et al.* (1966, 1968, 1969) discussed the contrast between experimental and clinical pain. Experimental pain usually involved cutaneous nociceptive stimulation that was relatively mild in intensity, of short duration, and frequently terminated voluntarily by the subjects. In contrast, clinical pain was of uncertain duration and anxiety provoking. This type of anxiety may very well be related to the concern of possible tissue damage and of a possible underlying disease process (Keats *et al.*, 1950; Beecher, 1959*a*, 1960, 1966). Studies using experimentally induced pain that is of uncertain duration with the subjects perceiving the possibility of tissue damage in spite of assurance to the contrary show promise in simulating clinical pain. Examples of this type of experimental pain are found in the studies of the submaximal tourniquet method (Smith and Beecher, 1969; Smith *et al.*, 1966, 1968), other studies of ischemic pain (Hewer and Keele, 1948), and studies involving chemical irritation of the peritoneum (Lim and Guzman, 1968). Interestingly, these latter studies involve a quality of pain described as aching and originating from effects on either the skeletal muscles or the abdominal viscera, whereas studies lacking the uncertainty of possible tissue damage involve mostly cutaneous nociceptive stimulation and are often described as sharp or burning.

More recently, investigators of experimental pain have utilized the technique of signal detection (Goldiamond, 1958), which is thought to differentiate the stimulus-induced perceptive components or *sensitivity* from the psychological influence of perception or *response bias* in reporting pain. In utilizing signal detection, investigators have attempted to differentiate to some extent the perceptual and reactive components resulting from nociceptive stimuli, relating the former component to perceptual sensitivity and the latter to response bias (Chapman and Feather, 1973; Feather *et al.*, 1972; Chapman *et al.*, 1973; Clark, 1969).

The reliability of a well-designed study of clinical pain can be ascertained by its ability to give consistent measurements of analgesia induced by placebo and opiates, whereas the validity of the methodology is illustrated by its ability to obtain relative analgesic potencies of several opiate analgesics with consistent and reproducible results. Further use of the newer methodologies for experimental pain may demonstrate this capability in experimental pain studies utilizing the more sophisticated control of experimental design considering set, setting, the type of stimulus, and the techniques of measuring the perception and reactions to the nociceptive stimulus.

Although studies of clinical pain present many difficulties, most information concerning the effectiveness of opiates as analgesics derives from clinical investigation. Furthermore, clinical study of opiates has provided reliable information concerning the relative potency of various opiates as analgesics. As we have illustrated, pain and analgesia are both affected by multiple biological factors as well as by psychological aspects such as patient set and clinical setting. Most clinical situations involve many of these variables but provide little opportunity to control for them. Therefore, since each clinical situation varies and often includes different subjects, the key to reliable clinical studies is the inclusion of a standard opiate in each population studied and a placebo when possible. Additionally, for a valid bioassay to ascertain relative potency a dose-response curve should be obtained for both the standard opiate and the analgesic being tested by using several doses of the drug to be analyzed and comparable doses of the known opiate. Appropriate doses of the experimental drug can be estimated by preliminary uncontrolled studies with the drug to be analyzed in order to estimate the effective dose range. Excellent reviews of clinical studies of opiates have been published and will not be discussed in detail (see: Wallenstein and Houde, 1975; Houde *et al.*, 1960, 1965; Hewer *et al.*, 1949; Bellville *et al.*, 1968*a,b*; Keats and Beecher, 1952; Beecher, 1957).

It is appropriate at this point to briefly discuss the effectiveness of placebo. Placebo appears to be most effective in clinical situations involving anxiety related to the nociceptives stimulus such as a wound resulting from injury or surgery. Likewise, in those situations in which placebos are most effective, opiates also seem to be more effective as analgesics (Lasagna, *et al.*, 1954). This is not to presume that opiates and placebo act by the same mechanism but they may nonetheless alter similar reactions to pain.

The effectiveness of placebo has been reviewed by Beecher (1955). Summarizing the results of 15 studies (1082 patients) placebo was found to be effective as an analgesic in about 35% of the patients, although the range of effectiveness varied with the individual study. Many investigations of analgesics, however, involved only administration of the active medication or placebo one or at the most two times. With repeated doses, the number of placebo responders decreases. In one study, Lasagna *et al.* (1954) showed that 53% of their subjects responded to a single dose of placebo, 40% to two or three doses, and 15% responded consistently to four or more doses. Thus, the effectiveness of placebo may vary in the same person with repeated administration. In the group of patients investigated by Lasagna *et al.* (1954) 55% of the patients receiving more than two doses of placebo responded inconsistently, having relief from placebo at one time but not at another, 14% received consistent relief with placebo, and 31% consistently did not respond to placebo. Thus, although for single doses placebos can be quite effective in relieving pain, this effectiveness is not usually consistent in any given patient.

The mechanism of placebo action has frequently been discussed in terms of personality structure, coping style, physician–patient relationship, and the symbolic meaning of the medication with little concrete evidence to support the proposed mechanism. Placebo effect has been compared to hypnotism and some have felt that placebo and hypnotism involve similar mechanisms in the relief of pain. Orne (1974), however, has shown that hypnotic analgesia can be differentiated from relief of pain by placebo. Intriguingly Herrnstein (1962) has produced a placebo effect in animals and attributed this effect to classical or Pavlovian conditioning. Pihl and Altman (1971) have also shown evidence that can account for placebo effect in terms of operant or instrumental conditioning.

5.5. Opiate Analgesia

Opiates are certainly recognized as excellent analgesic agents. Notably, they may affect the perceptual and reactive components of pain differentially in that the perception of the nociceptive stimulus as pain is inconsistently affected by opiates, whereas the reactive components of pain are more regularly and consistently diminished by opiates. This phenomenon may often be observed in clinical settings in which a patient may state that he still perceives the pain but may rest comfortably and even sleep easily. Some patients may state that they no longer perceive the pain, others stating that the pain is still present but bothers them less after the opiate administration. In line with this phenomenon, many studies of clinical pain either state the quantitative subjective percentage of relief of pain by the opiate or use a quantal (all or none) measurement such as 50% relief of the pain as a cutoff point. The subjective percentage of relief measured quantitatively may very well reflect more of a decrease in the reactive rather than the perceptive components of pain although both may be diminished in the clinical setting.

Some light may be shed on this clinical phenomenon by the studies of Hill *et al.* (1952*a*,*b*, 1955) and Kornetsky (1954) with experimental pain cited in previous sections. Opiates failed to alter the perception of a nociceptive stimulus unless the setting was conducive to pain anticipatory anxiety. This type of setting actually induced reports of increased pain intensity with the same nociceptive stimulus, whereas opiates tended to decrease this sensitivity to a baseline value. Again, it must be emphasized that these studies involved cutaneous pain. It would be of interest to apply the methodology of increasing pain anticipatory anxiety to studies employing ischemic pain while using subjective reports including, if possible, a modification of the signal detection assay.

Clinically, then, a physician should not expect his patients to report complete relief of pain after opiates. As a practical measure the physician may state to the patient that he or she may still feel "the pain" after the opiate but that usually "the pain" will be more tolerable. Conversely, although physicians should relieve the pain and related suffering of their patients, they should not use the complete lack of the perception of pain as an endpoint in administration of opiate analgesics.

Opiates do consistently alter the reactive components of pain at all levels of the central nervous system. The alteration of the reactive components of pain at the spinal cord level have been clearly demonstrated in animals and man (Wikler, 1958). Wikler and Frank (1948), Martin *et al.* (1964), and McClane and Martin (1967) have shown that the ipsilateral flexor withdrawal reflex to a nociceptive stimulus in spinal animals is exquisitely sensitive to morphine and other opiates. Relatively small doses of the opiates depress this withdrawal reflex with a clear response of increasing depression with increasing dose of the opiates. Doses that depress this multisynaptic reflex do not depress the monosynaptic patellar reflex. Relative potencies of various opiate agonists and agonist–antagonists can be assayed by this method, so that the withdrawal reflex may be a useful animal method for screening drugs for opiate-like action.

Although not as thoroughly studied as the flexor reflex, other multineuronal reflex pathways that have been postulated to subserve the reactive components of pain are depressed by opiates. Hoffmeister (1968) has demonstrated that opiates depressed the immediate vocalization reaction to a nociceptive stimulus postulated to be a medullary reflex. In similar studies, Charpentier (1968) has shown that numerous multisynaptic pathways subserving the reactive components of pain are depressed by morphine.

As discussed earlier in this section, opiates generally diminish the affective and behavioral components of the reactions to a nociceptive stimulus at doses that do not grossly affect other sensory modalities and do not produce marked sensory clouding. Notably, the escape behavior such as muscular guarding is affected by opiates, whereas avoidance behavior established in chronic pain patients often is independent of the nociceptive stimulus and consequently not altered by the opiate administration. This latter aspect of the behavioral reaction has been discussed in Section 5.1.2 and will be elaborated on later in this section. Some of the affective and behavioral reactions to a nociceptive stimulus are decreased by barbiturates and other anesthetic drugs only at dose levels that produce a marked alteration in other sensory modalities along with a dramatic decrease in alertness and cognitive functioning.

A dose of morphine needed to produce analgesia varies with the individual, the clinical setting, and the resulting degree of experienced pain. In studies involving moderate to severe clinical pain doses of morphine lower than 5 mg/70 kg intramuscularly rarely produce sufficient analgesia. More consistent analgesia is observed with doses of 10 mg/70 kg intramuscularly, and occasionally doses as high as 15 mg/70 kg are required for sufficient relief of acute pain. Relative potency of various opiate analgesics are expressed in Table 5, and these drugs can be substituted in non-opiate-dependent subjects for morphine at appropriate doses. Some limitations of dosage may result from the side effects peculiar to a particular opiate.

The various opiates listed in Table 5 and others have been useful in treating pain in various clinical settings. Most of the clinical studies cited have involved treatment of postoperative pain or the treatment of acute episodes of chronic pain in cancer patients. Just as pain itself may be affected by cognitive factors such as learned associations to pain resulting from developmental and ethnocultural background, cognitive style, and cognitive labeling

TABLE 5
Relative Analgesic Potencies[a]

Drug	Route of administration: Intramuscular or subcutaneous	Route of administration: Oral
Morphine	1.0—time action 4–6 hr	0.17
Heroin	2–3	
Methadone	1.0—notably time action similar to morphine	0.5
Mepereridine (Demerol)	0.10–0.13—time action appreciably less than morphine, approximately 3 hr—2–4 hr	0.05–0.07 effectiveness variable
d-Propoxyphene (HCl) (Darvon)		0.03–0.05
Codeine	0.08–0.10	0.05–0.06
Oxycodone (dihydrohydroxycodeinone, Percodan)		0.7–1.0
Hydromorphone (dihydromorphinone, Dilaudid)	6–7	
Oxymorphone (dihydrohydroxymorphinone, numorphan)	7–10	
Pentazocine (Talwin)	0.25–0.40	0.08–0.10

[a] References: Houde *et al.*, 1965; Wallenstein *et al.*, 1967; Lasagna and Beecher, 1954; Murphree, 1962; Beaver *et al.*, 1967; Lasagna, 1964; Reynolds and Randall, 1957; Eddy *et al.*, 1957; Potter and Rayne, 1970; Paddock *et al.*, 1969; Keats and Telford, 1964; Forrest *et al.*, 1969; Beaver *et al.*, 1966; Mansky, 1976; Batterman, 1943.

as to significance (Section 5.2.2); by affectual factors such as anxiety state, pain anticipatory anxiety, and depression (Section 5.2.3); and by attentional factors (Section 5.2.4); analgesia resulting from opiate administration may be expected to be altered by these same factors, resulting in differential effects in various patients and in the same patient in different settings.

The continued or repeated administration of opiates in patients with chronic pain has engendered much debate. That opiates can be useful is clear, but such factors as the method of administration (e.g., on demand or request of patient versus scheduled administration) and the dosage level to be used in treatment are not considered as established procedures at this time (Houde, 1974). The continued and regular opiate use for chronic pain can result in both physical dependence and tolerance to the analgesia. In terminal cancer patients tolerance to the analgesic effect of opiates leads to a major dilemma in obtaining continuing analgesia, whereas physical dependence requires continued scheduled administration of the opiate agonist and caution in substituting agonist–antagonists such as pentazocine for opiate agonists. Tolerance to analgesia as described by Houde (1974) moves the dose–response curve for analgesia further to the right. It is not certain, but much evidence indicates that with the gradual increase in dose needed to surmount tolerance to analgesia there may be a point at which the opiate receptors or potential receptors are completely saturated (see Sections 7 and 8). This would then mean that as the scheduled dose increased to overcome tolerance, the analgesic dose–response curve would not only be shifted to the right but would eventually show a decrease in slope. Houde (1974) indicates that lower relative doses of another opiate agonist might be used at this juncture. Such an alteration would produce mild withdrawal symptomatology similar to that seen in experimental substitution studies (Fraser and Isbell, 1960; Fraser, 1968). If the new drug is to be effective, then a decrease in tolerance must accompany the mild withdrawal symptomatology. Theoretically, then, merely decreasing the dosage of the opiate agonist rather than substitution should lead to the same results (see Section 7.2 for further discussion). Dilemmas such as those just described are faced clinically every day, but further well-designed studies are needed to more clearly examine the aspects of tolerance and physical dependence seen with opiate use and chronic pain.

As alluded to above opiate use with chronic pain has generated much controversy (Houde, 1974; Fordyce, 1974*a,b*; Sternbach, 1974*b*; Greenhoot and Sternbach, 1974) in addition to that generated by the factors involved in tolerance and physical dependence. Some authors of papers on chronic pain go as far as to state that opiates have no role in the treatment of chronic pain.

Perhaps this controversy relates to the very nature of chronic pain alluded to in previous sections (Sections 5.1.2 and 5.1.3). Chronic pain or recurring pain may produce anxiety, depression, and suffering along with both escape and avoidance behavior. In situations where the results of the chronic pain are due to a recurring nociceptive stimulation, the recurring acute reactions to the stimulus such as anxiety, suffering, and escape-related behavior are clearly dependent on the recurring nociceptive stimulation and should respond to opiate analgesia. In contrast, avoidance behavior is not dependent on continued nociceptive stimulation but is reinforced primarily by other environmental contingencies unrelated to the nociceptive stimulation and secondarily or minimally by recurrence of the acute pain. Thus, avoidance behavior seen in chronic pain patients may be expected to respond primarily to behavioral modification and minimally to opiate administration. The mood effects of chronic pain (Section 5.1.3) such as depression and anxiety may respond to opiate administration. Other medications such as tricyclic antidepressants have been effective in altering the mood changes of chronic pain and may be used cautiously along with opiate agonists.

Morphine and other opiates may have some value as anesthetics as well as analgesics. Lowenstein *et al.* (1969) have reported the successful use of high doses of morphine (0.5–3.0 mg/kg) in open heart surgery in over 1000 patients. This use of morphine presents a new area for the investigation of pain, opiate analgesia, and the effects of acute administration of high doses of opiates.

6. OTHER PHARMACOLOGICAL ACTIONS OF OPIATES

6.1. Gastrointestinal Effects

6.1.1. Nausea and Vomiting

Morphine and other opiates produce nausea and vomiting in patients and in both formerly opiate-addicted and opiate-naive subjects. Interestingly, Fraser and Isbell (1952) showed that nausea and vomiting occurred less frequently in former addicts than in naive subjects in a study using a 20-mg dose of morphine administered subcutaneously. This finding may reflect learned behavior of the former addicts since it has been shown that morphine may increase the vestibular response to motion (Guttner *et al.*, 1952) so that physical activity may increase the vestibular input to the medullary centers related to nausea and vomiting. The former addicts may have shown a decreased incidence of vomiting merely by limiting their activity. Additional support for this hypothesis is evident in the studies of Comroe and Dripps (1948) who showed an increased incidence of nausea and vomiting in ambulatory as opposed to bedridden patients given morphine. Opiates, however, do not appear to cause direct vestibular stimulation.

Wang and Galviano (1954) have shown in dogs that morphine stimulates the medullary chemoreceptor trigger zone directly, which then stimulates the emetic center also in the medulla oblongata. Higher doses of morphine appear to depress the emetic center itself. Thus, it has been observed that repeated administration of opiates within the same day leads to a decreased incidence of nausea and vomiting. Further support for this hypothesis in man derives from the reports of high doses of morphine (0.5–3.0 mg/kg body weight) used as anesthetic agents in open heart surgery (Lowenstein *et al.*, 1969). Notably, there are no reports of nausea and vomiting occurring during the surgery.

Apomorphine, which produces nausea and vomiting in doses of 5–10 mg parenterally in man, is also a prominent dopamine agonist. It is then probable that the medullary structures related to nausea and vomiting involve dopamine transmission. This is further supported by evidence that neuroleptics such as chlorpromazine or prochlorparazine are excellent antiemetics as well as exhibiting dopamine antagonism in the central nervous system. Neuroleptics can be used to counteract opiate nausea and vomiting, whereas antihistamines appear to be ineffective. This use of neuroleptics can increase the opiate respiratory depression as well as the orthostatic hypotension seen with opiates and is seldom necessary since bed rest alone may adequately decrease the incidence of vomiting seen with opiates.

6.1.2. Constipating Effects

Opiates in general cause constipation or can be used to treat diarrhea. Several factors contribute to this effect. Opiates decrease gastric and intestinal secretions and also slow the passage of ingested food through the entire gastrointestinal tract. This slowing appears to be due to a decrease in the rhythmic peristaltic contractions and an increase in sphincter tone (Daniel *et al.*, 1959; Paton, 1957). Nonrhythmic contractions of the intestines may occur and may actually be painful. The constipating effect of opiates is further enhanced by decreased central awareness of rectal and colonic distention or fullness.

6.1.3. Biliary Tract Effects

Opiates have been noted to cause an increase in common bile duct pressure with spasm of the sphincter of oddi (Butsch *et al.*, 1936; Bergh and Layne, 1940; Caroli *et al.*, 1960). This spasm may also be related to increase in serum amylase and lipase seen in some patients without pancreatic disease up to 24 hr after a single dose of morphine (Bogoch *et al.*, 1954). Some opiates show a decrease spasmatic effect on the bile duct in equal analgesic doses, and phenazocine has been suggested as the opiate of choice in the treatment of biliary pain (Hopton and Torrance, 1967).

6.1.4. Mechanism of Opiate Action on the Intestines

The mechanism of the effects of morphine on the peripheral innervation of the intestines in man and animals is significant in that this peripheral effect is one of the best studied and may suggest central nervous system analogs of activity of morphine. The latter may be of limited value until studies of the central nervous system confirm the findings with isolated intestinal tissue. It is, however, essential to note that the studies employing guinea pig ileum have been useful in predicting relative potencies of various opiates as analgesics and in investigating the opiate agonist and antagonist action of various opiates as well as indicating possible mechanisms of additional nonopiate agonist activity, e.g., meperidine as described in Section 3.5.5 (Paton, 1957; Gyang and Kosterlitz, 1966; Kosterlitz *et al.*, 1974).

Morphine has a slight anticholinesterase activity that does not account for its effect on the intestines. Most dramatically and specifically morphine decreases the twitch amplitude of the longitudinal smooth muscle of the intestine after coaxial electrical stimulation. At the same time, morphine does not appear to affect other cholinergic transmission at the ganglionic synapses or at neuromuscular junctions using this particular preparation. In contrast to depression of the electrically stimulated contraction related to a diminished release of acetylcholine from the preparation, morphine does not directly antagonize the action of acetylcholine applied directly to the perfused intestine. Paton (1957) noted that morphine diminishes the output of acetylcholine from the electrically stimulated intestines in a quantal manner. This preparation was noted to respond as if there were two types of quantal acetylcholine release upon electrical stimulation, one sensitive to morphine and the other insensitive to morphine. This not only lends some support to Martin's theory of redundancy (see Section 7) but leaves room for further speculation. Paton (1957) suggests that morphine acts specifically to decrease acetylcholine release at the postganglionic cholinergic innervation of the longitudinal smooth muscle of the intestine. He also notes that Kosterlitz has postulated that morphine may act upon the interstitial cells of Cajal. The significance of this is unclear but speculation may assume that it is possible that just as in the innervation of the urinary bladder where acetylcholine has been shown to stimulate an adrenergic inhibitory system affecting the parasympathetic ganglia on the bladder surface (Saum and de Groat, 1972) so morphine may inhibit selectively a similar system in the gut. Indeed, norepinephrine inhibits the electrically stimulated twitch similar to morphine (Ehrenpreis *et al.*, 1975). Thus, the hypothesis of an intervening noradrenergic system inhibiting parasympathetic effects on the gut is a tempting hypothesis for it could explain the resulting smooth muscle spasm seen after opiate administration and the partial response of this spasm to atropine. Unfortunately, there is no further evidence at this time to support the hypothesis. Other explanations of the effects of opiates on the intestines have concerned the antagonism of 5-hydroxytryptamine by opiates and the release of histamine seen after opiate administration.

6.2. Respiratory Effects

6.2.1. General Effects of the Respiratory System

Opiates depress the medullary respiratory center in man in a dose-related fashion eventually causing marked respiratory depression at very high doses. At lower doses this depression is not always evident by measuring either respiratory rate or tidal volume, whereas at higher doses both the rate and rhythm of breathing may be affected with slow (1–4 breaths/min), irregular breathing (Eckenhoff and Oech, 1960). Higher cerebral centers may effect respirations and breathing may be maintained by verbal command, even at doses of opiates that may produce stupor and coma (Lowenstein *et al.*, 1969). Maximal respiratory depression occurs within 7 to 15 min after intraveneous administration of opiates and within 30 min after intramuscular administration (Dripps and Comroe, 1945). Martin *et al.* (1968) have shown that morphine depresses the respiratory response to increasing concentration of carbon dioxide by shifting the response curve of minute volume to P_{CO_2} (ordinate: minute volume; abscissa: P_{CO_2}) to the right and also by decreasing the slope slightly. Martin notes that his results are in general agreement with those of Seed *et al.* (1958).

Most investigators have recognized a great deal of variation in the response of each individual to the respiratory depressant effects of opiates. Factors such as pain and emotional stress may diminish the respiratory depressing effects of morphine (Eckenhoff and Oech, 1960). Opiate addicts have used this fact to treat mild overdoses by producing pain in various manners, e.g., injection of an irritating substance subcutaneously. Caution should be used in giving high doses of opiates to patients who have pain of duration likely to cease prior to the effect of the opiate.

Although reports have appeared indicating that one opiate may be superior to another in terms of decreased effects on the respiratory center, there is no convincing evidence that any opiate may have less respiratory depressing effects at equal analgesic doses. Data must be analyzed carefully considering the relative potency limits and if possible using the same group of subjects to measure both analgesia and depression of the respiratory center.

Opiates also may effect the peripheral respiratory system as part of the generalized decrease in the normal secretory activity of glands in the respiratory tract and may occasionally cause spasm of the bronchial smooth muscle. The drying of secretions, bronchospasm, and release of histamine have convinced many clinicians of the relative contraindication of the frequency of use of opiates in asthma attacks. It is remarkable, however, that some clinicians continue to find opiates useful during asthma attacks and there may be some basis for this practice. It is possible that opiates have differential effects on bronchial musculature depending upon the state of contraction at the time of administration. Evidence also indicates that sputum production may not be adversely affected by opiates in certain patient populations. Sevelius *et al.* (1971) found no decrease in the 24-hr sputum volume in patients with emphysema and chronic bronchitis given codeine in doses as high as 60 mg. Sevelius, however, comments that the measurement of sputum production represents crude measurements. Additionally, opiates depress the cough reflex that can be useful in clearing the tenacious mucus seen in an asthma attack (Sheldon *et al.*, 1967). Obviously this clinical area deserves further investigation and opiates cannot be recommended at this time as treatment for asthma.

6.2.2. *Cough*

Cough represents the end process of a reflex reaction mediated in the brain stem. If compared to similar reflexes such as vomiting and sneezing, cough appears to be under more voluntary control (Bickerman, 1962). Thus, antitussives may act on the afferent component, the processing component in the brain stem, the effector or efferent system, or upon modulation of the medullary cough center from higher cerebral centers. Opiates clearly have been shown to act upon the brain stem centers by Chakravarty *et al.* (1956), who illustrated that opiates depress coughs produced by electrical stimulation of the dorsal portions of the medulla oblongata in cats. The antitussive activity of opiates may also involve direct effects on higher centers modulating the cough reflex or may actually promote more effective inhibition by potentiating the inhibitory effects of the efferent terminations from higher center neurons upon the medullary neurons subserving the processing of the cough reflex. It would be of interest to compare an opiate and placebo in an experiment with instructions that would tend to increase voluntary control over the reflex. In such a study the patients could be requested to attempt to resist the urge to cough, being told that the medicine (opiate or placebo) may help them to accomplish this task. Such a study could ascertain the degree of voluntary control (placebo condition) and the effect of opiates (opiate condition) on this process.

Antitussive activity has been measured by subjective reports and by objective recordings of the frequency of cough. Both methods have shown opiates to be effective antitussive agents (Nicolis and Pasquariello, 1962). Subjective relief, however, might not be as accurate a measure of antitussive activity as actual measurement of cough frequency. Sevelius *et al.* (1971) showed that codeine in single doses from 15 to 60 mg can relieve cough in a dose-related fashion in chronic lung patients measuring the actual frequency of cough. This group of patients, however, reported no relief of the cough or change in sputum on a structured multi-item questionnaire.

Most opiates produce antitussive activity at doses that do not produce significant analgesia in moderate to severe pain (e.g., 15–30 mg codeine). Other opiates such as meperidine require much higher relative doses (50 mg) to produce antitussive activity. It is interesting to note that the time action for meperidine is much shorter than that for codeine. Many clinical studies of antitussive activity examine the effects of low doses of opiates given frequently (Nicolis and Pasquariello, 1962). Codeine may have the opportunity to accumulate and the actual level of the drug needed at the receptors may be higher than that produced by a single dose. Meperidine, on the other hand, has a shorter duration of activity and may not accumulate in repeated doses to give effective antitussive activity. Thus, each dose of meperidine by itself must be sufficient to inhibit the medullary neurons subserving cough.

The antitussive action of opiates does not appear to be related to activity of the drugs on stereosensitive receptors as compared to analgesia, which is stereosensitive. For example, levomethorphan is an effective analgesic and antitussive, whereas dextromethorphan is an effective antitussive but does not have analgesic activity and does not produce subjective effects similar to morphine (Mansky and Jasinski, 1970).

It is also evident that cough is an effective and necessary reflex in combating respiratory irritation or disease and that it is not always desirable to decrease this reflex. Additionally, as previously noted, opiates dry respiratory secretions and may cause bronchial spasms. Opiates also depress the respiratory center and may lead to respiratory failure or respiratory acidosis in patients with chronic lung disease. Potential drug dependence is low with opiate agonists used as antitussives but must also be considered. Therefore, opiates should only be used when cough must be diminished for adequate treatment. Dextromethorphan or other non-morphine-like drugs may be preferred because they represent no potential for opiate-like dependence.

6.3. Cardiovascular Effects

In normal healthy subjects, morphine has little effect upon pulse and blood pressure if measured in the supine position. Any changes that occur are usually slight even when very high doses of morphine are administered intravenously in noncardiac subjects and multiple measures of cardiac function are obtained (Lowenstein *et al.*, 1969). Some investigations, however, have revealed a trend toward a slight increase in blood pressure after opiate administration. This trend has been observed in former addicts studied at the Addiction Research Center and also in normal subjects examined by Drew *et al.* (1946) and may be related to changes in the sympathetic nervous system activity.

Orthostatic hypotension, however, has been well documented after opiate administration. Drew *et al.* (1946) used a tilt board that clearly demonstrated the development of orthostatic hypotension after opiate administration in healthy subjects. Older subjects tended to show a greater tendency to develop orthostatic hypotension and occasionally patients with cardiac and respiratory disease have been noted to show a precipitous drop in blood pressure (Thomas *et al.*, 1965). Although some carefully designed controlled studies have shown little change in blood pressure in recumbent patients with uncomplicated myocardial infarction after both intramuscular (15 mg) and intravenous (7.5 mg) administration of morphine (Grendahl and Hansteen, 1969), orthostatic hypotension should be prevented by restricting postural changes.

Postural hypotension was prevented by Drew *et al.* in 82% of their subjects by wrapping the lower extremity with an elastic bandage prior to tilting. Additionally, hypotension seen occasionally after opiate administration without apparent orthostatic change and definitive orthostatic hypotension can both be treated by elevating the legs and lowering the head and shoulders.

The mechanism of orthostatic hypotension is unclear, although most evidence points to venous pooling in dependent extremities. This pooling may in part be related to histamine release after opiate administration and is partially blocked by antihistamines. Depression of the vasomotor center or direct myocardial depression cannot account for the orthostatic alteration of blood pressure seen with clinical use of opiates (Eckenhoff and Oech, 1960). In contrast, the hypoxia seen late in severe opiate intoxication or overdose may lead to dramatic depression of all central nervous system function including the brain stem centers related to cardiovascular functioning.

6.4. Pupillary Effects

Opiates constrict the pupils in a dose-related manner leading to pinpoint pupils in states of severe opiate intoxication. If anoxia intervenes as a result of opiate depression of the respiratory center, the pupils may then dilate secondary to the anoxia. The only other known cause of bilateral pinpoint pupils is pontine (tegmentum) hemorrhage, which may cause this effect by interrupting sympathetic innervation while at the same time causing irritation of parasympathetic innervation to the pupil (Plum and Posner, 1972). Since the sympathetic nervous system innervates the radial pupillary muscles leading to dilation and the parasympathetic system innervates the sphincter-like smooth muscle, which leads to pupillary constriction, this combined effect of sympathetic blockade and parasympathetic overactivity can produce pin-point pupils. The pupils still react to light in both opiate overdose and pontine hemorrhage, but a magnifying lens may be required to note the small change in pupil size seen after exposure to light (Fisher, 1967, 1969).

Opiates will cause pupillary constriction in the dark but nonetheless require integrity of the optic nerve for their maximum constricting effects in the dog. Morphine appears to exaggerate the light reflex and delay the recovery of the pupil to light exposure (McCrea *et al.*, 1942).

Fraser *et al.* (1954) showed that most opiates lead to pupillary constriction in a dose-related fashion (e.g., morphine given in doses of 10, 20, and 30 mg), measuring pupil size after 15 min accommodation to darkness using a camera and a rapid strobe light (duration of flash 2×10^{-4} sec). The photographic method for measuring pupil size has been further refined and can be used in a lighted room utilizing a Polaroid camera held a fixed distance from the pupil (Marquardt *et al.*, 1967; Jasinski and Martin, 1967; Gorodetzky and Martin, 1965).

Pupillary constricting effects of opiates usually outlast the analgesic effects by two or four times and can sometimes be distinguished from control measurements at up to 24 hr after morphine administration. Some opiate agonists have been noted to have less pupillary constricting effects after equianalgesic doses. Such may be the case with meperidine, which Fraser *et al.* (1954) showed to have constricted the pupils after 160 mg administered both orally and subcutaneously, although the pupillary constriction after meperidine was slight and lasted only about 3 hr. More recently, Jasinski and Nutt (1973) have reported that meperidine in doses of 75, 150, and 300 mg/70 kg constricts the pupils in a dose-related fashion. They also note, however, that meperidine shows a tendency to be about one-half as potent in causing miosis as compared with its ability to produce the subjective effects including euphoria seen after morphine administration. This tendency did not reach statistical significance in the analysis of their data. The decreased effect of meperidine on pupillary constriction, however, has been noted repeatedly and may be a result of the unique anticholinergic activity seen with meperidine and described in Section 3.5.5 of this chapter.

The pupillary constricting effects of opiates not only require the intact optic nerve to exert its full effects but also seem to be mediated by the Edinger–Westphal Nuclei (Martin, 1963). These nuclei lie in the midbrain between the oculomotor nuclei and send fibers that exit from the brain with the oculomotor nerve and provide the major source of preganglionic parasympathetic innervation of the pupils.

6.5. Urinary Tract Effects

Opiates have similar effects on the urinary tract as they do on the gastrointestinal tract in that they cause constriction of the sphincters and spasm of the smooth muscle of both the ureters and the bladder along with decreasing urinary output. Although the discomfort of bladder distention may be decreased by the antinociceptive activity of the opiates, urgency may be present along with difficulty initiating the flow or urine because of sphincter spasm.

The secretion of antidiuretic hormone appears to be increased by morphine possibly as a direct effect of opiates on the hypothalamus.

Increases in urinary antidiuretic hormone have been noted after morphine administration in animals (Martin, 1963).

6.6. Other Effects of Single-Dose Opiate Administration

Single doses of opiates have been noted to lower body temperature in some species including man (Martin, 1963; Fraser and Isbell, 1952; Mansky and Jasinski, 1970). This effect has not been well studied in man but it has been noted that sweating is increased after opiate administration, especially when associated with exercise. Additionally, some investigators have described cutaneous vasodilatation after opiate administration leading not only to a flushed appearance but a slight decrease in body temperature. The latter effect has been postulated to be related to histamine release, which also produces the itchiness and scratching seen with acute opiate administration.

As discussed earlier in this chapter (Section 3.5.7) opiates are generally considered to lower the seizure threshold and to cause seizures at higher dose levels (Gibbs and Maltby, 1943; Carruyo *et al.*, 1968). This is of interest in that opiates are sometimes considered to be central nervous system depressants at higher dose levels. Gilbert and Martin (1975) have shown that the mean quantity of heroin needed to produce seizures in mice was approximately 30 mg/kg. The mean effective dose of *d*-propoxyphene and meperidine was in the same general range, in contrast to the relative analgesic doses of *d*-propoxyphene and meperidine to heroin. Surprisingly, similar doses of naloxone antagonized the ability of all three drugs to produce seizures, indicating a similar pharmacological mechanism of action.

It is important, however, to realize that high doses of opiates (0.5–3.0 mg/kg) have been used in man for anesthesia by Lowenstein *et al.* (1969) without report of increased behavioral excitement or seizure activity. No EEG recordings were made during the surgery and other drugs were used in some of the patients, so that definitive conclusions are difficult to formulate from the observations of Lowenstein *et al.* in relation to seizure thresholds.

The effects of morphine upon pulmonary edema have not been discussed in this chapter and will only be alluded to briefly at this point. Morphine has been useful in treating acute pulmonary edema but the mechanism of this effect is unclear. Some have attributed this to an antianxiety effect of the opiates decreasing the emotional excitement accompanying acute pulmonary edema and to the decrease in hyperpnea due to the depression of the medullary respiratory center. Although these may be strategic factors, it appears that the increase in the capacitance of peripheral vessels may lead to decreased venous return with resulting decrease in pulmonary arterial pressure and pulmonary arterial flow along with a decrease in left atrial pressure and left ventricular end-diastolic pressure (Vasko *et al.*, 1966).

Pulmonary edema has been observed in heroin addicts and in patients with heroin overdose. It is likely that this is due either to contamination, especially if the pulmonary edema occurs during injection long before heroin has a chance to exert its peak pharmacological effect on medullary structures or, if seen long after injection of the opiate, to the hypoxia secondary to respiratory depression.

7. CHRONIC ADMINISTRATION OF OPIATES

7.1. Phenomenology

There have been many anecdotal reports of the chronic use of opiates emphasizing the paucity of physical effects and the abilities of the subjects to function adequately. Martin and Jasinski (1969) refer specifically to a 1930 survey of a report to the Mayor's Committee and reports by physicians working in "narcotic" wards during the same era, both indicating little physical illness among the opiate-dependent populations and little evidence of physical toxicity due to long-term exposure to opiates. Indeed, it is felt by many who treat opiate-dependent patients today that few physical ailments are due to the opiates but many to the mode of administration, i.e., nonsterile intravenous self-administration. Hepatitis, tetanus, bacterial endocarditis, septicemia and thrombophlebitis, the nephrotic syndrome, and other similar ailments are common among opiate-dependent patients who use intravenous self-administration (Sapira, 1968; Cherubin, 1967; Kilcoyne *et al.*, 1972).

This is not to imply that chronic opiate use may not have its toxic effects upon the physical well-being of the subjects. Although not specifically delineated, gastrointestinal ailments do appear more common, and some physical deterioration may be due to the life-style related to drug acquisition and use including the lack of concern for adequate nutrition and hygiene so nicely described in lay literature by Burroughs (1959).

There now exists a large population of opiate-dependent patients maintained chronically on oral methadone. Investigations have already begun concerning the physical, especially endocrine status of this patient population. A comprehensive study of such effects has been discussed by Bloom and Butcher (1970) and several recent studies have defined isolated endocrine abnormalities. Further studies are needed to more thoroughly examine methadone patients and to elucidate the mechanisms of described physical abnormalities, especially in relationship to the pharmacological effects of opiates.

Few systematic studies have been conducted observing subjects prior to, during, and after chronic opiate administration. Those that have been done have observed former addicts for long periods in relatively confined environments. It may be argued that what these studies gain in observation may be lost in the restricted environment. Nonetheless, they represent careful, well-planned investigations and do add to our knowledge of opiate dependency. Some of the findings may indeed be related to a confined environment, others may not. Careful observation of patients in methadone maintenance programs may eventually confirm or refute some of the results and conclusions of these studies.

One of the earlier studies (Wikler, 1952) was confined to one patient and therefore has limited value in drawing general conclusions. This study will not be discussed here but certainly deserves review by the interested reader.

Fraser *et al.* (1963) studied a group of five former addicts for 30 days of placebo administration followed by 60 days of intravenous heroin administration reaching a level of 95 mg heroin per day in four divided doses. The subjects at first exhibited increased activity as measured by observers and pedometers. As the period of heroin maintenance continued activity decreased below control levels. Several subjects stayed in their rooms and exhibited less social interaction. They became hypochondriacal and some complained of feeling depressed although they did not exhibit the vegetative signs and symptoms of depressive illness. One subject stated that he felt more alert and relaxed during the period of heroin administration. Motor performance on the pursuit rotor test was not impaired so that the authors concluded that the decreased activity and decreased sense of "drive" seen after chronic heroin administration as opposed to single-dose administration may be explained by a decreased responsiveness to external stimuli rather than by decreased motor ability. Alternatively, the phenomenon observed by the authors may represent tolerance to the activating and "drive" effects of opiates.

Martin and Jasinski (1969) studied a group of seven subjects (former addicts) for a period of 74 weeks that included a 7-week period of controlled observations followed by a 34-week period during which morphine was given subcutaneously, reaching a stable dose of 240 mg per day in four divided doses by the end of the 3rd week. During the period of chronic morphine administration the investigators observed a decreased respiratory rate, pupillary constriction and a slight increase in mean blood pressure, pulse rate, and body temperature along with an increase in urinary catecholamine excretion (Eisenman *et al.*, 1969).

Haertzen and Hooks (1969) studied 15 subjects, most of whom were included in the group studied by Fraser *et al.* (1963) and by Martin and Jasinski (1969). The subjects were examined while being maintained on 95 mg heroin intravenously per day or 240 mg morphine subcutaneously per day using psychological instruments including the MMPI and the ARC Inventory. Haertzen and Hooks found increases on the hypochondriasis scale of the MMPI and increases on scales of the ARC Inventory related to sedative effects and to social withdrawal. Some of the items are summarized by the authors when they state that "during the chronic phase relative to the acute no-drug phase there is less motivation for physical, mental, social, and sexual activity, plans are less likely to be carried out, requests for activity arouse irritation, which is more apt to be expressed, social affairs become a waste of time, people seem less friendly and too 'nosy,' resentment is felt over being questioned. . .individual pursuits are preferred, and boredom with people increases." These findings were obtained using the structured questionnaires and are similar to the findings reported by Fraser *et al.* (1963) and Martin and Jasinski (1969).

Martin *et al.* (1973*a*) reported a study of six subjects who after a control period were given methadone chronically for 14 weeks, reaching a stabilizing dose of 100 mg methadone given orally once a day. The effects on physiological function were similar to those observed during chronic administration of morphine with the exception of blood pressure and pulse rate, which were slightly depressed rather than elevated as with morphine. The authors suggest that these latter changes differ from the physiological observations during chronic morphine administration and may be related to a greater stimulation of the sympathetic nervous system by morphine as compared to methadone. Additionally, hemodilution in most of the patients and dependent edema in one patient were observed and may be related to a chronic increase in antidiuretic hormone during chronic methadone administration.

The subjects in the methadone study also showed increased social withdrawal, hypochondriasis, and irritability similar to the subjects in the morphine and heroin studies. The subjects in the methadone study did, however, appear to be more sedated or to elicit more items on sedative scales than the subjects maintained on morphine (240 mg per day) or heroin (95 mg per day).

The subjective effects of chronic opiate administration described in the above studies do indicate social withdrawal and decreased psychomotor activity along with an increase in negative feeling states as opposed to positive feeling states. This total mood state, which Martin (1975) has termed hypophoria, may increase slightly during a phase of opiate dependency in that Martin *et al.* (1973*a*) have observed a statistically significant decrease in items signifying positive feelings and an increase in negative feelings during the chronic administration of methadone. Although depression might well describe the objective findings and changes in feeling state, the syndrome may be different from unipolar or bipolar depressive illness and thus should be differentiated at this time as a unique depressive syndrome.

In summary then, the above studies indicate effects upon the psychological profile and physiological function of subjects maintained on opiates. Slight but defined changes in physiological function do occur during chronic opiate administration in former addicts in a confined environment. Furthermore, similar changes in physiological function may occur in nonconfined patients on methadone maintenance. The effects of chronic opiate administration upon psychological function do vary greatly from patient to patient. On the average, however, the effects seem to result in a state of hypophoria characterized by hypochondriasis and social withdrawal. It must be emphasized again that this state of hypophoria may be a result of the confined environment and may not occur in all subjects maintained on chronic opiates.

7.2. Tolerance

7.2.1. *Introduction*

Chronic administration of opiates does lead to the development of tolerance to some of the effects observed after single-dose administration. As commonly understood, tolerance develops to a drug when it takes a larger amount of the drug to produce the same effect or the same amount of the drug produces less effect when administered repeatedly. In a more sophisticated sense, tolerance can be described at the receptor level as a shift of the dose–response curve to the right with or without a change in the slope of the dose–response curve. Several types or degrees of tolerance have been described for differing opiate effects. Some exhibit complete tolerance, some partial tolerance, and others no tolerance. This division in terms of degree of tolerance may be an artifact of the effect measured and will be subsequently discussed with each category of tolerance.

7.2.2. *Complete Tolerance*

Complete tolerance has been described for the euphoric effects of opiates. Haertzen and Hooks (1969) note that in subjects maintained on 240 mg of morphine per day the euphoria scale of the ARC Inventory, the MBG scale, returns to no-drug level or control level early during the period of chronic morphine administration. Furthermore, while stabilized on 240 mg morphine per day or 60 mg four times a day, the subjects were given a single dose of 120 mg, twice their normal dose, without any euphoric effects reported and without any alteration of the MBG scale.

The evidence for complete tolerance to analgesic effects is not as well defined. Houde (1974) and others have noted the occurrence of tolerance to analgesia in cancer patients receiving chronic opiate administration. This tolerance at times is complete and Houde (1974) has found switching to a relative lower dose of another opiate is required at this point. As discussed briefly in Section 5.5 Houde attributes this ability to switch analgesics as an indication of incomplete cross-tolerance.

There is also other evidence that the analgesic effect of opiates eventually leads to complete tolerance. Analgesia and euphoria produced by opiates appear to be closely related phenomena. All opiate analgesics appear to produce euphoria in former addicts. Many of the opiate analgesics have been specifically examined by the ARC Inventory and have been found to produce dose–response effects on the MBG scale. Additionally, it has been noted that the relative potency of opiates needed to produce analgesia as measured by modern clinical assays is similar to their relative ability to produce euphoric responses as measured by objective instruments such as the ARC Inventory MGB Scale (see Section 4.2). If the similarity in terms of relative potency also holds for tolerance then one would expect complete tolerance of the analgesic effects of opiates to develop in the same way that complete tolerance has been described for the euphoric effects. This conclusion is based on descriptive evidence and the assumptions that the described parallel of analgesic and euphoric effects applies to tolerance. More exacting studies involving the nature and location of receptors related to analgesia and euphoria are not available so that this conclusion must be considered tentative until such information is known.

The second observation made by Houde, that a lower relative dose of another opiate may substitute for the original when the original opiate no longer produces analgesia, has a parallel in the substitution studies conducted at the Addiction Research Center. As just noted, 240 mg of morphine per day represents a dose level at which complete tolerance to euphoria has been observed. In the substitution studies it is noted that the total abstinence score for substituting placebo for morphine (240 mg per day) over a 24-hr period is approximately 154, whereas the control value obtained from subjects remaining on the same dose of the opiate, the no-substitution control condition, is approximately 43 (Fraser, 1968). Substituting 10, 20, and 50% of the dose of morphine produces a straight regression of abstinence score upon log dose (Fraser and Isbell, 1960). Fifty percent of the daily dose of morphine gives a score of approximately 60. Thus, decreasing the maximal dose of morphine by 50% does not produce a very dramatic abstinence syndrome in that placebo substitution leads to close to a 400% increase in abstinence score and substitution of one-half the maintenance dose leads to only a 50% increase in abstinence score above control levels. Thus, either a lower dose of morphine or a dose of another opiate equipotent to the lower dose of morphine may produce a similar low intensity of abstinence. Additionally, although not specifically measured, some of the tolerance to euphoria appears to be lost during the 24-hr substitution studies employing lower doses of morphine or relatively lower doses of another opiate in that subjects state that they feel the euphoric effects when returned to their regular dose of morphine at the end of the 24-hr period. It can be seen then that substituting a much lower dose of the same opiate leads to both a mild abstinence syndrome and the loss of tolerance to the euphoric effects in the same way that administration of a lower relative dose of another analgesic may lead to the loss of tolerance to the analgesic effects as described by Houde. Further evidence of alterations in analgesia-utilizing substitution technique will be required to establish a more exacting parallel of tolerance to euphoria and to analgesia resulting from repeated opiate administration. Nevertheless, the above results could explain the phenomena of incomplete cross-tolerance described by Houde (1974).

In addition to euphoria and analgesia, tolerance appears to develop to the activating or "drive"-producing effects of opiates (see Section 7.1). This tolerance appears to be complete.

Complete tolerance to the analgesic, euphoric, and activating effects of opiates may be an artifact in that some opiate activity may continue at the opiate receptor sites related to euphoria and analgesia. It does seem likely that a minimal dose level of opiates at the receptors is required to produce euphoric and analgesic effects, so if tolerance develops to most of the administered dose of an opiate then the remaining active receptors might not be sufficient in number to produce analgesia or euphoria. Again, indirect evidence supports this attractive hypothesis. First, maintenance on a 240 mg per day dose schedule of morphine, during which complete tolerance to euphoria develops, represents a state in which approximately 90% of opiate receptors may be occupied (Martin, 1966), thus leaving little range for increased activity if the subject is tolerant to the activity of 240 mg of morphine. Second, the analgesic and euphoric effects of several opiates may be measurable for only 4–6 hr, whereas the effects on other functions such as pupillary constriction may last up to 24 hr, thus indicating that more opiate receptor occupancy or more opiate activity at the receptors may be needed to produce analgesia and euphoria than to constrict the pupils. Therefore, at the opiate sites related to analgesia or euphoria there may be some active receptor occupancy in subjects dependent on morphine 240 mg per day, which at higher levels of receptor occupancy or activity would produce either analgesia or euphoria.

7.2.3. *Partial Tolerance*

The evidence for the development of partial tolerance is derived from studies of the pupillary constricting and respiratory depressing effects of opiates. These effects are rather sensitive to opiate administration and can be measured quantitatively using a standard technique of photographic pupillography (see Section 6.4) or the rebreathing technique of Eckenhoff *et al.* (1956), respectively.

As can be observed in Fig. 3, single-dose administration of an opiate constricts the pupils markedly but as the dose of morphine is repeatedly given and maintenance dependent levels are reached, the pupils no longer remain markedly constricted by morphine but nonetheless do remain below control size. Furthermore, if the maintenance dose of morphine is doubled little additional pupillary constriction is noted. Thus, although the pupils remain chronically constricted below control levels while receiving 60 mg morphine four times a day, the pupils appear to be resistent to higher doses of morphine. This can then be described as partial tolerance in that although

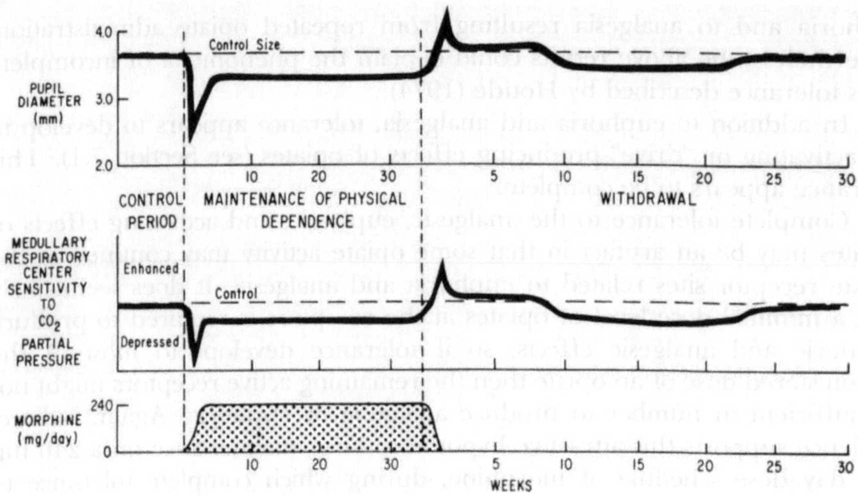

FIG. 3. Cycle of opiate dependency and withdrawal (schematic representation). Based on Martin *et al.* (1968) and Martin and Jasinsky (1969).

the pupils are tolerant to the constricting effects of higher doses of morphine they still are affected by the morphine in that they remain below control size.

Partial tolerance also develops to the effects of morphine on the medullary respiratory center. The center remains chronically depressed during opiate administration (see Fig. 3) but is highly resistent to further depression by larger doses of morphine (Martin *et al.*, 1968). Martin describes this situation as the "persistence of *chronic depression*" of the respiratory center by large doses of opiates but resistence to the "*phasic depression*" by higher doses. The phenomenon of partial tolerance described here is essential in formulating the theoretical basis for the redundancy theory of tolerance and physical dependence, which will be discussed in Section 7.4.

The phenomenon of resistance to phasic depression of the respiratory center in subjects on high-dose opiate maintenance (240 mg per day) implies that the subject is tolerant to the lethal effects of severe respiratory depression. Thus, true opiate overdose leading to death due to respiratory depression in a patient or street addict maintained on high doses of opiates should be exceedingly rare if not impossible.

7.2.4. *Failure to Develop Tolerance*

Tolerance does not appear to develop to some effects of opiates during a cycle of maintenance. The constipating effects of opiates are present throughout a cycle of dependency. In a similar fashion, difficulty in initiating urine flow and acute urinary retention can occur while a patient or experimental subject is taking chronic doses of an opiate. As Haertzen and

Hooks (1969) illustrate little tolerance may be observed in some subjects to the sedating effects of opiates. Indeed, one subject in the chronic methadone study (Martin *et al.*, 1973*a*) continued to exhibit "nodding" throughout the 3 months of methadone administration.

The gastrointestinal autonomic innervation represents a rather complicated interplay of the sympathetic and parasympathetic systems (see Section 6.1.4). The total interactions within the system have not been clearly elucidated. Likewise, the effects of opiates on the gastrointestinal innervation have received much attention but still leave many questions unanswered. Nevertheless, speculation is possible although the conclusions must be tentative. Paton (1957) has described the release of acetylcholine from stimulated gut as having a morphine-sensitive and a morphine-resistant component. Thus, when tolerance of gut to morphine develops as described by Ehrenpreis *et al.* (1975) this may represent a hypertrophy of the morphine-insensitive component described by Paton (1957) and thus represent another system that exhibits partial tolerance at the neuronal level and conforms to the redundancy hypothesis of Martin.

The continued constipation seen in opiate-dependent subjects and patients could be a result of the inability of the opiate-insensitive system to compensate completely for the depression of the morphine-sensitive system. Alternatively, continued slight depression of passage time of digested food through the intestines along with continued suppression of gastrointestinal secretions could account for the chronic constipation. It must be remembered that constipation is usually considered to be a quantal (all or none) phenomenon as opposed to other effects, such as pupillary constriction, that can be expressed as continuous change in given units of diameter. Thus, once the threshold for constipation is reached it will occur as an all-or-none phenomenon, and it is difficult to compare such quantal data with those obtained for pupillary constriction or depression of the medullary respiratory center.

In summary then, some effects of opiates at the level of measured phenomenon appear to be present throughout a cycle of addiction. As such, tolerance does not develop to these effects. Some of the effects such as constipation represent an all-or-none phenomenon, and it is possible that they are the result of partial tolerance at the neuronal level.

7.3. Dependence

7.3.1. Introduction

The use of the term "drug dependence" with a segregation of the components of drug dependence into the categories of physical dependence and psychological dependence has engendered much debate. As a consequence, "drug dependence" was defined by the WHO Expert Committee on

Drug Dependence (1969) as a "compulsion to take a drug on a continuous or periodic basis in order to experience its psychic effects and sometimes to avoid the discomfort of its absence." This state of drug dependence was recognized by the committee to be the result of the "interaction between a living organism and the drug." Thus, the committee recognized that drug dependence may reveal differing patterns of behavior with differing classes of drugs. This also implies that differing individuals may react in various manners to the same class of drugs.

Psychic or psychological dependence was recognized by the WHO Committee at that time as the *sine qua non* of drug dependence. Consequently, physical dependence or the appearance of a withdrawal syndrome upon discontinuation of the drug can be a powerful reinforcer of continued drug use only if the drug produces psychological dependence (Mansky and Altman, 1977). Thus, nalorphine, cyclazocine, and anticholinergic drugs may be observed to produce an abstinence syndrome when abruptly withdrawn but fail to produce drug dependence.

Psychological dependence can be determined by (1) the ability of a drug "to produce pleasure or avoid discomfort" or (2) operationally by the observation of drug-seeking behavior in spite of high personal cost (Isbell and Chruściel, 1970), or, in operant terminology, in spite of a high response cost. Using the above terminology somewhat loosely the ability of a drug to produce pleasure can be inferred from its ability to act as a positive reinforcer and vice versa. Mansky and Altman (1977) note that in both human and animal studies only those opiates that either act as a positive reinforcer in animal studies or indicate their ability to "produce pleasure" by a dose-related response on the MBG of the ARC Inventory have been found to lead to drug-seeking behavior or self-administration upon withdrawal. The ability of an opiate to produce drug dependence or drug-seeking behavior in relationship to its other effects are illustrated in Table 9 describing the various effects of opiate agonists, antagonists, and agonist-antagonists and will be discussed in more detail in Section 8. The present section will elaborate the phenomenon related to the development of physical dependence resulting from the chronic administration of opiates, whereas Section 4.2 serves as an excellent discussion of the ability of various opiates to produce euphorogenic effects intimately related to psychological dependence.

7.3.2. *Primary Abstinence Syndrome*

The primary or acute abstinence syndrome from withdrawal of chronically administered opiates is quite dramatic. It usually starts within hours of discontinuing the drug, reaching a peak within days and ending within one to several weeks, depending upon the particular opiate (see Table 6). The syndrome is unpleasant, often compared to a bad case of "the flu." Fatality is rare in otherwise healthy individuals if left untreated for withdrawal but it is

TABLE 6
Time Course of Primary Abstinence Syndrome[a]

Drug	Start (hr)	Peak (hr)	Duration	Peak intensity (Himmelsbach scores)
Morphine	8–12	48–72	7–10 days	Severe
Meperidine	3–4	8–12	4–5 days	Greater than morphine
Methadone	24–48	72–84	4–7 weeks	Less than morphine

[a] Nonpurposive signs of abstinence used. Data from: Isbell, 1948; Isbell and White, 1953; Martin *et al.*, 1973*a*.

considered ethical and humane to treat the withdrawal from opiate agonists. Many excellent descriptions of the primary abstinence syndrome appear in the literature. The following description is based on the author's personal experience treating patients and the descriptions of Himmelsbach (1941*a*), Martin and Jasinski (1969), and Wikler (1953).

The patient's general appearance is often disheveled. Early during withdrawal the patient may be drowsy with frequent yawning and brief restless sleep. After the first 24 hr the patient becomes more anxious, apprehensive, and restless, finding it difficult to sleep or even rest comfortably. He (she) is frequently anorexic, and weight loss averaging about 7 lb may occur during the first day or so secondary to both decreased intake of calories and fluid loss. Glandular secretion is hyperactive, resulting in or adding to the signs of rhinorrhea, lacrimation, vomiting, diarrhea, perspiration, and salivation described below. The pupils are dilated and the eyes appear moist due to conspicuous lacrimation. The nose is "stuffy" with prominent watery secretions (rhinorrhea). The tongue may appear tremulous and the gag reflex is often hyperactive. The respiratory rate is usually accelerated although it may appear within normal limits. The bronchial mucous glands hypersecrete resulting in clear sputum production and mucous rales that often clear upon coughing. Nausea, vomiting, and diarrhea are common and accompanied by complaints of stomach cramps and diffuse abdominal tenderness. Bowel sounds are usually hyperactive with borborygmus.

Sweating is increased and the patient's skin may feel cold and moist. The patient often complains of hot or cold flashes (usually cold predominates) with the periodic appearance of gooseflesh due to piloerection from which the term "cold turkey" owes its derivation. The muscles, bones, and joints ache and there is often a slight tremor in the extremities with occasional involuntary muscle twitches, especially in the lower extremeties, resulting in an occasional sudden kicking or stepping-like activity from which the term "kicking a habit" is derived. Additionally, involuntary ejaculations in the male and spontaneous climax in the female may occur. Laboratory studies may indicate hyperglycemia, hemoconcentration, and leukocytosis with a sudden decrease in circulting eosinophils (Wikler, 1953).

Prominent drug-seeking behavior accompanies the signs and symptoms described above. Wikler (1953) characterizes the abstinence syndrome into *nonpurposive* and *purposive* changes. The nonpurposive changes include all of the above signs and symptoms with the exception of intense craving and drug-seeking behavior that are characterized as purposive in that they represent attempts of the patient to obtain the drug.

Andrews and Himmelsbach (1944) examined the intensity of the signs of withdrawal in patients who were admitted to the U.S. Public Health Service Hospital in Lexington, Kentucky, stabilized for at least 1 week on a daily dose of morphine needed to prevent abstinence, and then abruptly withdrawn. The average doses of stabilization ranged from 40–407 mg per day for a total of 127 patients, with 5–31 patients at each dose increment. The authors used a scoring system for the signs of abstinence similar to that presented in Table 7. The TAS-7 or Total Abstinence Score for 7 days was compared to the stabilization dose and was clearly illustrated to reveal a relationship of total abstinence score to the level of dependence. If the TAS-7 is plotted against $\log_n$ dose, a curve similar to the classical sigmoid-shaped curve for dose–response is evident (see Fig. 4). Some have speculated that this curve is representative of the saturation of opiate receptors related to physical dependence. This will be discussed further in Section 8.

It is important to notice several aspects of Andrews's and Himmelsbach's results. First, the lowest daily dose of morphine that produced withdrawal symptoms was 40 mg per day. There are more recent unpublished data from

TABLE 7
Source Points for Total Abstinence Score (TAS)[a]

	Withdrawal sign	Point value
Mild	1. Yawning	1
	2. Lacrimation	1
	3. Rhinorrhea	1
	4. Perspiration	1
Moderate	5. Tremor	3
	6. Gooseflesh	3
	7. Anorexia—at least 40% decrease in caloric intake	3
Severe	8. Restlessness	5
	9. Emesis—each episode	5
Measurable signs		
	1. Mydriasis—each 0.1 mm	1
	2. Hyperpnea—each respiration per minute	1
	3. Fever—each 0.1°C	1
	4. Systolic blood pressure (a.m.)—each 2 mm Hg increase	1
	5. Weight loss—each pound	1

[a] Adapted from Martin (1966) and Andrews and Himmesbach (1944).

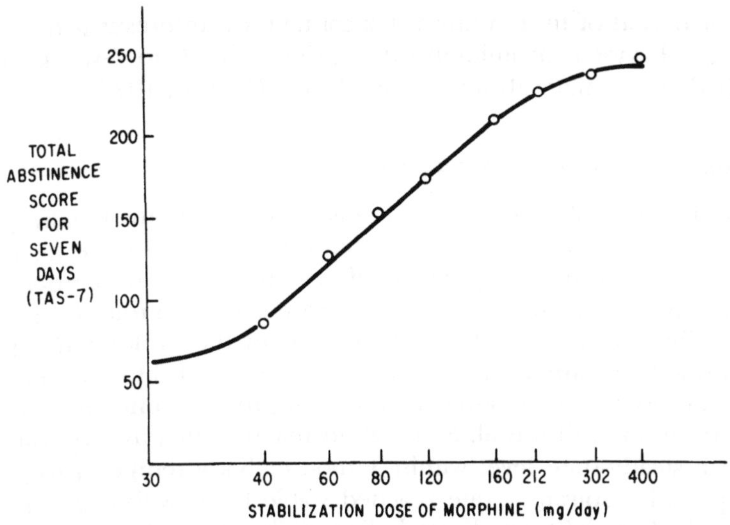

FIG. 4. Abstinence dose-response curve (Himmelsbach abstinence score as a function of $\log_N$ dose). Data from Andrews and Himmelsbach (1944).

opiate studies indicating that measurable abstinence can be obtained from subjects chronically maintained on 30 mg of morphine per day and then abruptly withdrawn. Second, as discussed in Section 7.1 Martin (1966) has indicated that 240 mg of morphine per day will produce an abstinence syndrome that is close to maximal, i.e., 90% of the highest abstinence score obtained by Andrews and Himmelsbach. This maintenance dose of 240 mg morphine per day is well tolerated by subjects and represents the high-dose condition used in substitution studies previously discussed in this chapter. Additionally, it is important to note that all the subjects examined by Andrews and Himmelsbach had a history of prolonged chronic opiate use before they were admitted to the hospital and maintained on their various doses for 10 days.

The time course of the primary abstinence syndrome and the peak intensity of the syndrome varies when different opiates are compared (see Table 6). This variation may depend upon the rapidity with which the particular opiate is eliminated from the body or, more exactly, from the opiate receptors related to dependence. The time course of this elimination during the abstinence period may be related to the relative duration of single-dose effects. Thus, the time course for meperidine is shorter than that for morphine and methadone abstinence is the most prolonged of the three opiates. The peak intensity shows the reverse relationship in that the drug with the shortest duration of action produces the most intense peak withdrawal intensity.

It has been felt by some that drug-seeking behavior is related solely to the peak intensity of the abstinence syndrome as opposed to lower intensity over a longer period of time. Within this context it is interesting to note that drug-seeking behavior is prominent during the entire 4- to 7-week duration of the methadone primary abstinence syndrome (Martin, 1973).

7.3.3. *Secondary Abstinence Syndrome*

During the late 1930s and early 1940s some physicians treating opiate dependency held the clinical impression that 6 to 9 months were needed for adequate recovery from the physical effects of opiate dependency and withdrawal. Stimulated by this clinical impression, Himmelsbach (1942) attempted to find objective evidence in support of the prolonged effects of opiate withdrawal. He studied 21 patients for a period of 6 to 9 months after withdrawal and noted the persistence of several physical abnormalities for at least 6 months after withdrawal. Some abnormalities such as hyperglycemia returned to a steady-state level within 1 month; body temperature, caloric intake, sleep, and respiratory rate reached stable levels within 2–3 months, whereas total body weight, basal metabolic rate, basal systolic blood pressure (taken at 6:00 a.m. in the recumbent position), hematocrit, and sedimentation rate all took 4 to 6 months to become stable. The author noted that body weight was the single most useful parameter indicating physical recovery.

Himmelsbach's studies of opiate withdrawal differ from later studies in animals and man in that he stabilized drug-dependent patients upon admission with a dose of morphine or some other opiate needed to prevent abstinence. He then measured several physiological parameters during the opiate stabilization period after which the measurements were repeated during the acute withdrawal phase and for several months thereafter. Himmelsbach had no measurements of the physiological parameters in the patients prior to opiate dependency so that he could not make pre-drug control comparisons but instead took note of the length of time required for each parameter to return to a stable level. Subsequent studies of opiate dependency have included a pre-drug-administration control period, an opiate-dependence period, and an abstinence or withdrawal interval, so that variation in each parameter measured could be compared to the no-drug control condition.

In order to examine prolonged abstinence changes during a complete addiction cycle in animals, Martin *et al.* (1963) examined several physiological and behavioral measurements during a cycle of opiate dependency in rats. The animals exhibited a primary abstinence syndrome lasting 72 hr consisting of weight loss, "wet dog" shakes, increased activity, along with decreased body temperature and metabolic rate. This was followed by a secondary abstinence syndrome characterized by increases in body weight, body temperature, metabolic rate, and water consumption for 4 to 6 months after initiation of opiate withdrawal.

Martin and Jasinski (1969) later studied a group of seven former addicts throughout a cycle of opiate dependency and withdrawal that included 7 weeks of controlled measurements and 34 weeks of morphine administration stabilized within 4 weeks at 60 mg administered subcutaneously four times a day, followed by observations after withdrawal for 30 weeks. The authors described an acute or primary abstinence syndrome similar to that described in the previous section. Thus, during the primary abstinence phase, blood pressure, pulse rate, pupillary diameter, body temperature, and respiratory rate were all elevated above control preaddiction levels. During the 6th to 9th week after withdrawal, blood pressure, body temperature, pupillary diameter, and pulse rate decreased to levels less than control preaddiction levels and did not return to control levels for up to 30 weeks after withdrawal. This latter period was considered by the authors to be protracted or secondary abstinence.

In a separate report, Martin *et al.* (1968) described the effects of the cycle of morphine dependence on the responsiveness of the respiratory center to the partial pressure of blood carbon dioxide. Figure 3 represents the changes schematically. During the primary abstinence phase the respiratory center is hypersensitive, returning to control levels within 7 weeks of withdrawal and thereafter appearing hyposensitive throughout the period of protracted or secondary abstinence.

This period of protracted or secondary abstinence lasts about 6 months. Since Martin and Jasinski (1969) reported their findings with morphine, Martin *et al.* (1973*a*) have also observed protracted abstinence after methadone dependence. It is of some interest and theoretical importance (see Section 7.3.6) to note that during secondary abstinence some physiological parameters such as pupil size and sensitivity of the medullary respiratory center are depressed below control values in a similar direction observed during opiate dependence (see Fig. 3).

The relationship of secondary or protracted abstinence to relapse to opiate self-administration has not been clearly elucidated. Several findings related to the 6-month period following withdrawal do suggest the tendency to react poorly to stress and possibly to relapse during this period. Himmelsbach (1941*b*) noted that patients showed more physiological reaction to the cold pressor test during opiate dependency and during both primary and secondary abstinence periods. Wikler and Pescor (1967) noted that rats tended to choose to drink an opiate (etonitazene) solution over a control placebo solution during the first 2 months of the rat protracted abstinence period. Furthermore, Valiant (1966) showed that the immediate relapse of patients to opiate use decreased with the length of the drug-free period in the hospital, the most dramatic decrease occurring in the patients who were hospitalized in a drug-free condition for over 6 months.

7.3.4. *Conditioned Abstinence Syndrome*

Anecdotal reports have noted the development of an opiate abstinence syndrome (primary abstinence in quality) in former opiate-dependent subjects who have been drug free for one or more years and experience this syndrome when they return to the neighborhood where they used opiates. Whitehead (1974) has reported an abstinence syndrome occurring in patients while maintained on methadone and has termed this a "pseudowithdrawal syndrome." These two types of occurrences may represent what Wikler (1948, 1968, 1973) has called "conditioned abstinence."

Conditioned abstinence of the primary abstinence syndrome defining specific environmental stimuli associated with its occurrence has not been clearly demonstrated in man. Conditioning to precipitated abstinence with nalorphine, however, has been observed in subjects dependent on morphine, methadone, and heroin (Wikler, 1973) and may have some relationship to both conditioned primary abstinence and Whitehead's pseudowithdrawal syndrome in patients dependent on methadone.

Wikler, however, has developed a very intriguing theory of opiate relapse based upon the theoretical occurrence of conditioned primary abstinence in man. This theory has been shown by Wikler and Pescor (1967) to be supported by animal data that clearly show the occurrence of primary abstinence phenomenon in animals when they are exposed to an environment in which they have previously experienced primary abstinence. Considering these data in animals and the demonstration of conditioned precipitated abstinence in man, Wikler's formulation of conditioned primary abstinence and its relationship to relapse forms a compelling hypothesis.

According to Wikler (1968, 1973), conditioned primary abstinence may occur when a subject formerly dependent on opiates is exposed to stimuli associated with the occurrence of primary abstinence. It is likely that the conditioning events may occur daily in the life of a street opiate-dependent patient who often experiences dysphoric feelings and physiological changes of primary abstinence or withdrawal just prior to obtaining and self-administering his next dose of an opiate. Thus, weeks or months after the patient stops self-administering opiates, the conditioned abstinence phenomenon may still not have been extinguished and may even occur in the mild form. The former opiate-dependent patient has found that opiate administration relieves this dysphoric state of conditioned abstinence just as opiates relieved the dysphoric state of primary abstinence. Therefore, the patient may experience craving and exhibit drug-seeking behavior associated with the occurrence of conditioned abstinence. It is of special interest that this may occur without specific cognitive labeling identifying the process as mild withdrawal and then assuming that opiates will work. Rather, the mild abstinence syndrome may be related to feelings of anxiety or dysphoria unrelated by the patient to opiate withdrawal *per se*. What the patient experiences are the interoceptive cues leading to feelings of dysphoria. The patient knows from his past experience that opiate injection will relieve this feeling or syndrome and related dysphoria from his repeated experience with opiate self-administration (Wikler 1968, 1973; Mansky and Altman, 1976). Treatment may actually lie in teaching the former opiate-dependent patient that feelings that make him want to use opiates may be a conditioned abstinence or related dysphoria and furthermore, by their very nature, may resolve spontaneously with time.

7.3.5. Precipitated Abstinence Syndrome

Opiate antagonists such as nalorphine, cyclazocine, or naloxone can produce a severe abstinence syndrome when administered to subjects or patients dependent on an opiate agonist such as morphine. This abstinence syndrome appears similar to the primary abstinence syndrome and can be quantitatively evaluated using the signs in Table 7 adapted from the original scale used by Andrews and Himmelsbach (1944) to measure the intensity of primary abstinence. The precipitated abstinence syndrome that occurs within minutes of the injection of the antagonist is rather intense but lasts for only 2 to 4 hr (Wikler *et al.*, 1953; Martin *et al.*, 1965; and Jasinski *et al.*, 1967).

Using measurements of the intensity of the precipitated abstinence at 15 and 30 min and at 1, 2, and 3 hr the relative potency of several opiates with antagonist activity can be compared. Table 8 represents the relative antagonist potency of several opiate antagonists compared to nalorphine. Repeated use of the antagonist or agonist–antagonist will eventually lead to a decreased intensity of the abstinence syndrome. If given frequently enough the precipitated abstinence syndrome will cease after administration of the antagonist and abrupt withdrawal of the opiate will not produce primary abstinence (Martin, 1967*a*).

Repeated administration of a narcotic agonist–antagonist such as cyclazocine will lead to tolerance to its agonistic activity but no tolerance to its ability to antagonize the activity of opiate agonists such as morphine

TABLE 8
Relative Opiate Antagonist Activity[a]

Drug	Relative potency (mg equivalent to 1.0 mg nalorphine)
1. "Pure" antagonist	
Naloxone	0.14
Naltrexone	0.06
2. Agonist–antagonist	
a. Unacceptable analgesics	
Nalorphine	1.00
Cyclazocine	0.18
Levallorphan	0.52
b. Acceptable analgesics	
Nalbuphene	3.7
Pentazocine	51.2

[a] Data from: Jasinski *et al.*, 1967, 1970; Martin *et al.*, 1973*a*; Jasinski and Mansky, 1972.

including antagonism of the ability of the opiate agonist to produce physical dependence (Martin *et al.*, 1966). Likewise, chronic administration of "pure" antagonists such as naloxone and naltrexone will prevent the agonist activity of opiate agonists including the development of opiate physical dependence (Martin and Sloan, 1968; Jasinski *et al.*, 1967; Martin *et al.*, 1973*a*).

Precipitated abstinence may also occur when partial agonists are given to subjects dependent on a low opiate habit, e.g., 60 mg morphine per day (Jasinski *et al.*, 1971). This will be discussed further in Section 8.

Intriguing results using opiate antagonists have been produced in elucidating the dose of an opiate agonist and the total time of chronic administration needed to produce both tolerance and dependence. Wikler *et al.*, (1953) were able to precipitate abstinence in subjects who had received morphine, methadone, or heroin in repeated doses for only 2 days. Wikler and Carter (1953) were able to demonstrate signs of precipitated abstinence in the spinal dog after one large dose of morphine followed several hours later by injection of nalorphine. Martin and Eades (1961) were able to demonstrate acute tolerance in the dog to morphine infused over an 8-hr period. Infusion of nalorphine (20 mg/kg) at the end of this period precipitated a severe abstinence syndrome indicating the development of acute physical dependence in addition to acute tolerance, i.e., both tolerance and physical dependence were evident after only 8 hr of morphine administration. Remarkably, Jasinski and Nutt (1974) showed that a single dose of 40 mg of methadone could produce physical dependence evidenced by the precipitation of the abstinence syndrome 1 week later with 4 mg of parenterally administered naloxone.

7.4. Tolerance and Dependence with Opiate Agonist–Antagonists

7.4.1. *Unacceptable Analgesics (Nalorphine and Cyclazocine)*

Tolerance develops to the general subjective effects both of the opiate-agonist-like activity and the unique agonist activity of nalorphine and cyclazocine (Martin *et al.*, 1965; Martin and Gorodetzky, 1965). After chronic administration of nalorphine and cyclazocine the drugs can be abruptly withdrawn with the resulting appearance of an abstinence syndrome which physiologically resembles primary abstinence from opiate agonists such as morphine. Physical examination may reveal lacrimation, rhinorrhea, and gooseflesh along with mydriasis and increases in pulse rate and body temperature above prewithdrawal levels.

The withdrawal syndromes from nalorphine and cyclazocine do differ from the opiate-agonist primary abstinence syndrome in several ways. The abstinence syndrome from cyclazocine does not appear until the 4th or 5th day after withdrawal and reaches peak value on the 7th day with some residual signs up to 6 weeks after withdrawal. The nalorphine abstinence syndrome starts about 8 hr after withdrawal with the appearance of scratching, itching, and shocklike sensations, accompanied at times by myoclonic jerks. Typical opiate primary abstinence phenomenon develops gradually over the first 3 days. Hyperthermia, tachycardia, and anorexia occur during the 1st day while lacrimation, and rhinorrhea appear during the 1st or 2nd day after withdrawal. Hyperpnea and mydriasis appear much later although the abstinence syndrome as measured by modification of the Himmelsbach scoring system (see Table 6, Section 7.3.2) is elevated during the 1st day and remains elevated at the same level for about 3 weeks with a decrease by the 6th week. In rating the intensity of the signs of withdrawal it is evident that hyperpnea and increased blood pressure are relatively more prominent after opiate agonist withdrawal of similar intensity, whereas hyperthermia, mydriasis, and tachycardia are relatively more prominent after withdrawal from cyclazocine and nalorphine. Thus, if one examines the total scores of withdrawal from the agonist–antagonists and from morphine, the rank order of the intensity of the signs of withdrawal are similar for cyclazocine and nalorphine but differ from the rank order for opiate agonists such as morphine. Additionally, shocklike sensations, scratching, itching, and myoclonic jerks are seen only after withdrawal of nalorphine or cyclazocine.

In spite of the moderate intensity of the signs of withdrawal and the very unpleasant shocks and myoclonic jerks, the subjects withdrawn from cyclazocine and nalorphine do not exhibit drug-seeking behavior for the agonist–antagonists or for any other drug (Martin and Gorodetzky, 1965; Martin *et al.*, 1965).

7.4.2. *Acceptable Analgesics (Pentazocine and Nalbuphine)*

Tolerance develops to some of the single-dose effects of pentazocine and nalbuphine with chronic administration. The withdrawal syndromes from both pentazocine and nalbuphine grossly resemble acute opiate abstinence but the intensity is moderate and the rank order of the intensity of the signs resembles completely neither the withdrawal from cyclazocine and nalorphine nor the withdrawal from opiate agonists such as morphine. Specifically, blood pressure increase is less prominent with nalbuphine, pentazocine, and nalorphine withdrawal syndromes compared with morphine withdrawal, whereas hyperpnea is more prominent with pentazocine, nalbuphine, and morphine than in nalorphine withdrawal. Shocks, myoclonic jerks, itching, and scratching were not noted after pentazocine and nalbuphine withdrawal. Notably, however, as with opiate agonists and in contrast to nalorphine and cyclazocine, withdrawal of both nalbuphine and pentazocine led to prominent drug-seeking behavior (Jasinski and Mansky, 1972; Jasinski *et al.*, 1970).

7.5. Theories of Tolerance and Dependence

It is beyond the scope of this chapter to give a complete accounting for the theories of tolerance and dependence seen with chronic opiate administration. Rather, those theories related to the phenomenology of opiate action in man will be emphasized. Other theories, however, deserve mentioning at this point. An altered or more rapid metabolism of opiates has been postulated to account for tolerance and dependence (Axelrod, 1956*a*) and has been rejected in part (Axelrod, 1968). Antagonism of an active enzyme (E) producing a neural transmitter (M) has been invoked proposing that the neural transmitter has a negative feedback on the production of the enzyme. Opiates then may act at the level of E decreasing its activity and thereby decreasing the production of M, which then leads to an increased production of E. Tolerance results from the increase in E and dependence occurs when E in increased amounts is no longer blocked by the opiate (Goldstein and Goldstein, 1968). Another theory postulates that tolerance is accounted for by a decrease in pharmacological receptors for the drug or, conversely, an increase in silent receptors for the drug, whereas an increase in the receptor substance for the blocked neurotransmitter may account for dependence (Collier, 1966). The latter concept is akin to the concept of denervation hypersensitivity proposed by Jaffe and Sharpless (1965) as the mechanism for tolerance and dependence to sedative–hypnotics. Still more intriguing is the theory of tolerance related to substances in the circulation produced by previous exposure to the drug in an analogous fashion to antibody production (Cochin and Kornetsky, 1968).

The more complex theory of redundancy (Martin, 1970) has been proposed to account for much of the phenomenology of opiate tolerance and dependence described in this chapter. This theory applies to functional aspects of the central nervous system and does not necessarily exclude or contradict some of the theories of tolerance and dependence described above. The theory of redundancy postulates dual innervation or redundancy of innervation in the CNS. In the case of morphine, it is proposed that there may be a morphine-sensitive functional system (S) and a morphine-insensitive system (I). Martin (1970) has postulated that morphine inactivates S causing I to hypertrophy from increased use. During normal physiological function either S or I predominate, leading to differing phenomena with acute and chronic opiate administration, depending on the relative ratio of the physiological activity of S to I.

The pupillary diameter and sensitivity of the medullary respiratory center to CO_2 can be considered assuming a relative predominance of S in relationship to I during normal physiologic function. The changes in pupil size and sensitivity of the respiratory center during chronic opiate administration and withdrawal are illustrated schematically in Fig. 3. Initial doses of morphine depress the respiratory center and constrict the pupils. After a few days of morphine administration, the pupils return toward control size and the respiratory center becomes more sensitive to CO_2 or less depressed. With the first one or two doses of morphine, the dose–response curve for minute volume (ordinate) and CO_2 partial pressure (abscissa) shifts to the right (Martin *et al.*, 1968). Remarkably, the slope is also decreased, possibly indicating the influence of dual or secondary innervation. The latter conclusion is speculative but nonetheless attractive.

As repeated morphine administration is continued both the pupils and the respiratory center continue to regain their functional capacity until the respiratory center is depressed slightly below control sensitivity and the pupils return almost to control size. Furthermore, increasing the dose of morphine two times that given in a study of a high degree of physical dependence (240 mg per day) produces very little additional depression of the respiratory center (Martin *et al.*, 1968) and little additional constriction of the pupils. As Martin (1970) pointed out, the systems in effect behave as if a morphine-insensitive system were subserving respiratory function and pupillary constriction during chronic morphine administration. The morphine-insensitive system, however, does not quite compensate completely for the system depressed by morphine so that pupils remain slightly constricted below control size and the respiratory center remains slightly depressed.

Upon abrupt withdrawal of opiates, the morphine-sensitive system again becomes active along with the hypertrophied morphine-insensitive system. The two systems (I and S) acting both at the same time produce the pupillary dilitation and hypersensitivity of the respiratory center seen in primary abstinence. It is furthermore possible that with disuse the morphine-sensitive system becomes slightly atrophied during dependence, to the degree that the hypertrophied morphine-insensitive system and the slightly atrophied morphine-insensitive system acting together during abrupt withdrawal produce hyperactivity such that the pupils dilate and the respiratory center is hyperactive.

It is tempting to postulate the phenomenon of protracted abstinence on the basis of the latter hypothesis. If now, as withdrawal continues, I atrophies toward its usual level of physiological function (preopiate) and the atrophied S continues to slowly recover, then the functioning of the respiratory center and pupil regulation at the predrug control level seen about 2 to 10 weeks after withdrawal may be explained. Furthermore, once I returns to its usual level of physiological functioning S may still be in the state of recovery but not yet completely recovered. This could then explain the depression of the respiratory center sensitivity and decrease in pupil size seen at 8 to 10 weeks. This slight depression of the pupil size and of the respiratory center sensitivity continues for 30 weeks after withdrawal and may well represent the slow return of the morphine-sensitive system to normal preopiate function.

The latter explanation of protracted abstinence is far more tentative than Martin's explanation of tolerance and primary dependence. Martin (1970) does present some compelling evidence referring to neuropharmacological studies of several functional systems exhibiting redundancy. Some additional support for the redundancy theory can also be made from the observations of morphine effects on the intestines. Paton (1957) has noted that the coaxial stimulated intestine behaves as if there is a morphine-sensitive and morphine-insensitive release of acetylcholine (see also Section 6.1.4).

Another theory of tolerance and dependence may involve functional systems in a series rather than in parallel, as with Martin's theory of redundancy. The mechanism for nausea and vomiting as a result of opiate administration (see Section 6.1.1) represents a functional series in that the chemoreceptor trigger zone (CTZ) is stimulated by opiates and in turn stimulates the medullary emetic center. The emetic center itself is inhibited by morphine. Notably, the CTZ is more sensitive to the action of opiate agonists than the emetic center. Thus, a single low dose of an opiate agonist may stimulate the CTZ, leading to stimulation of the emetic center and vomiting. Repeated doses of opiate or a single large dose may confer "tolerance" to the emesis by depressing the emetic center. Vomiting upon withdrawal of the opiate could then be explained by the slow excretion of the opiate with the emetic center recovering from the depressing effects of opiates before the stimulating effects of opiates are terminated at the CTZ. This theory may only be applicable for certain opiate effects such as vomiting that occur through a similar series.

8. CLASSIFICATION OF OPIATES FROM HUMAN STUDIES

This comprehensive review of the psychopharmacology of opiates in human subjects allows for a summary in terms of classification of the various opiate agonists and antagonists solely on the basis of their action in human subjects. Four major categories of the classification are: (1) opiate agonists, (2) opiate partial agonists, (3) "pure" opiate antagonists, and (4) opiate agonist–antagonists. The latter category includes acceptable and unacceptable analgesics. This classification and related data are summarized in Table 9, which forms the basis of the following discussion.

The opiate agonists include all the opiates that resemble morphine and produce none of the effects attributable to opiate antagonists such as precipitation of abstinence in opiate-dependent subjects and the unique constellation of subjective effects (sedative and psychotomimetic) seen with the opiate agonist–antagonists. This group of drugs includes morphine, heroin, codeine, dextropropoxyphene, meperidine, oxycodone, hydromorphone, and oxymorphone.

The opiate partial agonists differ from the opiate agonists phenomenologically in that they precipitate abstinence in subjects dependent upon high doses of morphine (240 mg per day). Unlike the opiate antagonists they do not precipitate abstinence in subjects dependent upon low doses of morphine (60 mg per day). Jasinski *et al.* (1971) has suggested that these opiate drugs behave as if they were partial agonists on the basis of several theoretical assumptions.

TABLE 9
Opiate Agonists, Antagonists, and Agonist–Antagonists

Opiate	Subjective effects (single dose)		Physical dependence		Morphine antagonist		Drug dependence with DSB	PA	
	Mor-phine type	Nalor-phine type	Like M	Like N_1	Low habit (60 mg morphine per day)	High habit (240 mg morphine per day)		N_1	N_2
Agonist									
Morphine	Yes	No	Yes	No	No	No	Yes	Yes	Yes
Heroin	Yes	No	Yes	No	No	No	Yes	Yes	Yes
Codeine	Yes	No	Yes	No	No	No	Yes	Yes	Yes
Dextropro-poxyphene	Yes	No	Yes	No	No	No	Yes	Yes	Yes
"Pure" antagonist									
Naloxone	No	No	No	No	Yes	Yes	No	No	No
Naltrexone	No	No	No	No	Yes	Yes	No	No	No
Partial agonists									
Propiram	Yes	No	Yes	Slight	No	Yes	Yes	Yes	Yes
Profadol	Yes	No	Yes	No	No	Yes	Yes	Yes	Yes
Agonist–Antagonists									
Unacceptable analgesics:									
Nalorphine	Slight	Yes	No	Yes	Yes	Yes	No		
Cyclazocine	Slight	Yes	No	Yes	Yes	Yes	No		
Acceptable analgesics:									
Pentazocine (Talwin)	Yes	Yes	Yes (PT)	Yes (PT)	No data	Yes	Yes	No	Yes
Nalbuphine	Yes	Yes	Yes (PT)	Yes (PT)	Yes	No data	Yes	No	Yes

[a] Key: PA, precipitated abstinence; M, morphine; N_1, nalorphine; N_2, naloxone; DSB, drug-seeking behavior upon withdrawal; PT, partial.

The first assumption concerns Martin's hypothesis of receptor dualism (Martin, 1967*a*) based on evidence supporting the presence of a morphine (M) and a nalorphine (N) receptor to explain the dynamic interaction of morphine and nalorphine on analgesia. The second assumption implies that the subjective and other effects of opiates are due to its agonist activity. It is then possible to assume that the morphine-like subjective effect of euphoria as reflected by a dose response on the MBG scale is due to agonistic activity on the M receptor, whereas the dysphoric subjective effects of the agonist–antagonist are due to activity on the N receptor as reflected by elevation of the PCAG and LSD scales (see Section 4.2 for discussion of the ARC Inventory and the MBG, LSD, and PCAG scales).

Although receptor dualism is not the only explanation for the agonist effects of opiate agonists and opiate agonist–antagonists, there do seem to be several basic differences in the agonist action of the two groups of drugs. The opiate agonists produce euphoric effects in former addicts and lead to physical dependence with a well-defined abstinence syndrome including drug-seeking behavior. The opiate agonists exhibit cross-tolerance and cross-dependence with each other, and the effects of the opiate agonists can be antagonized by both naloxone and nalorphine. The agonist–antagonists, on the other hand, produce some opiate-agonist-like effects at lower doses and dysphoric psychotomimetic and sedative effects at higher doses. In the case of the unacceptable analgesics, the dysphoric effects occur commonly at doses that produce analgesia, whereas in the acceptable analgesics the dysphoric effects usually do not emerge until administration of doses much larger than the standard analgesic dose. The chronic administration of the agonist–antagonist followed by withdrawal produces an abstinence syndrome that has some of the features of primary opiate abstinence but a different rank order of intensity of the various signs and symptoms. Withdrawal of the unacceptable agonist–antagonist analgesics also elicits unique symptoms of withdrawal such as shocklike feelings and myoclonic jerks without drug seeking behavior upon withdrawal, whereas withdrawal of the acceptable agonist–antagonist analgesics produces a withdrawal syndrome with mixed morphine-like and nalorphine-like features without the unique withdrawal symptoms of nalorphine or cyclazocine but with drug-seeking behavior. The occurrence of drug-seeking behavior may be related to the euphoric effects of single-dose administration of low doses of the acceptable agonist–antagonist analgesics without the occurrence of the dysphoric effects at the same dose level. This relationship of the effects of single doses to psychological dependence and drug-seeking behavior was postulated by Mansky and Altman (1977) and is discussed in Section 7 of this chapter. The effects of the agonist–antagonists are not antagonized by nalorphine but are antagonized by naloxone (Jasinski *et al.*, 1968, 1970; Jasinski and Mansky, 1972).

These findings support the first two assumptions underlying the hypothesis presented by Jasinski *et al.* (1971). The other assumptions are that opiate agonists continue to occupy receptors and exert their agonist effects in tolerant subjects and that the degree of physical dependence indicates the percentage of totally available opiate receptors occupied during chronic administration. Martin (1970) has presented evidence indicating that morphine inhibition of certain physiological functions is due to agonistic activity of the opiates. The inhibitory effects then result from stimulation of inhibitory neurons or inhibitory neuronal circuits. The percentage of receptor occupancy is inferred from the studies of Andrews and Himmelsbach (1944) relating the degree of physical dependence to the chronic maintenance dose of morphine (see Section 7.3.2). Figure 4 shows the abstinence dose–response curve, plotting total abstinence score for 7 days (ordinate) against $\log_n$ of the stabilization doses of morphine (abscissa). This graph reveals a sigmoid-shaped curve reminiscent of the classical dose–response curve. This is the only phenomenon seen with opiate administration that reveals both a ceiling effect and a floor effect with a linear function of $\log_n$ dose for effects occurring between the two extremes. Although it is not by any means proof of receptor occupancy, this curve represents evidence in support of maximum receptor occupancy at 400 to 500 mg morphine per day, about 90% or higher receptor occupancy at 240 mg per day, and less than 50% occupancy at 60 mg per day.

Therefore, the opiate partial agonist would be expected to show morphine-like activity in single doses, to produce a morphine-like abstinence syndrome of moderate intensity with chronic administration, and to be sensitive to both nalorphine and naloxone antagonism. The unique feature that separates the partial agonists from the other opiate agonists is the inability of the partial agonists to substitute for morphine in the condition that represents 90% or greater receptor occupancy (240 mg per day), along with their ability to substitute for morphine in the condition of less than 50% receptor occupancy or 60 mg per day. This latter phenomenon is seen with partial agonists and can be explained on the basis of lower intrinsic activity of the opiate partial agonists as compared with the opiate agonists.

A discussion of the "pure" antagonists will complete the discussion of the classification of opiate agonists, antagonists, and agonist–antagonists seen in Table 9. The "pure" antagonists naloxone and naltrexone produce no agonistic activity in low doses administered in man, whereas at the same dose level they antagonize the effects of the opiate and, in the situations referred to above, the effects of the opiate agonist–antagonists.

Thus, the classifications presented in this section appear to separate four major groups according to their human psychopharmacology. The explanation for this classification at the receptor level is tenuous at this point but does provide an acceptable fit to the data.

9. REFERENCES

Adler, R., and Lomazzi, F., 1973, Perceptual style and pain tolerance. I. The influence of certain psychological factors, *J. Psychosom. Res.* **17**:369–379.

ALTMAN, J., and MANSKY, P. A., 1977, A conceptual model of drug dependence, in: *Renewal in Psychiatry: A Critical Rational Perspective* (T. C. Manschreck and A. M. Kleinman, eds.), pp. 139–161, Hemisphere Publishing Corp., Washington, D.C.

ANDREWS, H. L., and HIMMELSBACH, C. K., 1944, Relationship of the intensity of the morphine abstinence syndrome to dosage, *J. Pharmacol. Exp. Ther.* **81:**288–293.

AXELROD, J., 1956*a*, Possible mechanisms of tolerance to narcotic drugs, *Science* **124:**263–264.

AXELROD, J., 1956*b*, The enzymatic *N*-demethylation of narcotic drugs, *J. Pharmacol.* **117:**322–350.

AXELROD, J., 1968, Cellular adaptation in the development of tolerance to drugs, *in: The Addictive States* (A. Wikler, ed.), pp. 247–262, Williams & Wilkins, Baltimore.

BARBER, T. X., 1959, Toward a theory of pain: Relief of chronic pain by prefrontal leucotomy, opiates, placebos, and hypnosis, *Psychol. Bull.* **56:**430–460.

BATTERMAN, R. C., 1943, Clinical effectiveness and safety of a new synthetic analgesic drug, demerol, *Arch. Int. Med.* **71:**345–356.

BEAVER, W. T., WALLENSTEIN, S. L., HOUDE, R. W., ROGERS, A., 1966, A comparison of the analgesic effects of pentazocine and morphine in patients with cancer, *Clin. Pharmacol. Ther.* **7:**740–751.

BEAVER, W. T., WALLENSTEIN, S. L., HOUDE, R. W., and ROGERS, A., 1967, A clinical comparison of the analgesic effects of methadone and morphine administered intramuscularly, and of orally and parenterally administered methadone, *Clin. Pharmacol. Ther.* **8:**415–426.

BECKETT, A. H., CASY, A. F., and HARPER, N. J., 1956, Analgesics and their antagonists: Some steric and chemical considerations. Part III. The influence of the basic group on biological response, *J. Pharm. Pharmacol.* **8:**874–883.

BEECHER, H. K., 1946, Pain in men wounded in battle, *Ann. Surg.* **123:**96–103.

BEECHER, H. K., 1955, The powerful placebo, *JAMA* **159:**1602–1606.

BEECHER, H. K., 1956*a*, The subjective response and reaction to sensation, *Am. J. Med.* **20:**107–113.

BEECHER, H. K., 1956*b*, Relationship of significance of wound to pain experienced, *JAMA* **161:**1609–1613.

BEECHER, H. K., 1957, The measurement of pain, *Pharmacol. Rev.* **9:**59–209.

BEECHER, H. K., 1959*a*, *Measurement of Subjective Responses*, Oxford Univ. Press, New York.

BEECHER, H. K., 1959*b*, Generalizations from pain of various types and diverse origins, *Science* **130:**267–268.

BEECHER, H. K., 1960, Increased stress and effectiveness of placebos and "active" drugs, *Science* **132:**91–92.

BEECHER, H. K., 1966, Pain: One mystery solved, *Science* **151:**840–841.

BELLVILLE, J. W., FORREST, W. H., and BROWN, B. W., 1968*a*, Clinical and statistical methodology for cooperative clinical assays of analgesics, *Clin. Pharmacol. Ther.* **9:**290–302.

BELLVILLE, J. W., FORREST, W. H., ELASHOFF, J., and LASKA, E., 1968*b*, Evaluating side effects of analgesics in a cooperative clinical study, *Clin. Pharmacol. Ther.* **9:**303–313.

BELLVILLE, J. W., FORREST, W. H., SHROFF, P., and BROWN, B. W., 1971, The hypnotic effects of codeine and secobarbital and their interactions in man, *Clin. Pharmacol. Ther.* **12:**607–612.

BERGER, H., 1931, Über das Eliktrencephalogram des Menschen, *Arch. Psychiat. Nervenkr.* **94:**16–60.

BERGH, G. S., and LAYNE, J. A., 1940, A demonstration of the independent contraction of the sphincter of the common bile duct in human subjects, *Am. J. Physiol.* **128:**690–694.

BERLIN, L, GUTHRIE, T., GOODELL, H., and WOLFF, H. G., 1952, Analysis of the reflex function of the isolated human spinal cord using measured stimuli, *Trans. Am. Neurol. Assoc.* **77:**106–110.

BICKERMAN, H. A., 1962, Clinical pharmacology of antitussive agents, *Clin. Pharmacol. Ther.* **3:**353–367.

BLOOM, W. A., and BUTCHER, B. T., 1970, Methadone side effects and related symptoms in 200 methadone maintenance patients, *Proceedings Third National Conference on Methadone Treatment,* pp. 44–49.

BOGOCH, A., ROTH, J. L. A., and BOCKUS, H. L., 1954, The effects of morphine on serum amylase and lipase, *Gastroenterology* **26:**697–708.

BOWSHER, D., 1957, Termination of the central pain pathway in man: The conscious appreciation of pain, *Brain* **80:**606–622.

BROTMAN, R. E., MEYER, A. S., and FREEDMAN, A. M., 1965, An approach to treating narcotic addicts based on a community mental health diagnosis, *Comp. Psychiatry* **6:**104.

BURROUGHS, W. S., 1959, *Naked Lunch,* Castle Books by arrangement with Grove Press, New York.

BUTSCH, W. L., MCGOWAN, J. M., and WALTERS, W., 1936, Clinical studies on the influence of certain drugs in relation to biliary pain and to variations in intrabiliary pressure, *Surg. Gynecol. Obstet.* **63:**451–456.

CAROLI, J., PORCHER, P., PEQUIGNOT, G., and DALATTRE, M., 1960, Contribution of cineradiography to study of the function of the human biliary tract, *Am. J. Dig. Dis.* **5:**677–696.

CARRUYO, L., FLORIO, V., LONGO, V. G., SCOTTI DE CAROLIS, A., 1968, The effect of narcotics and narcotic antagonists on the electrical activity of the brain: Its relationship with their pain-obtunding activity, in: *Pain* (A. Soulairac, J. Cahn, and J. Charpentier, eds.), pp. 425–439, Academic Press, London/New York.

CAUTELA, J., 1967, Covert sensitization, *Psychol. Rep.* **20:**459–468.

CAUTELA, J., 1970, Covert reinforcement, *Behav. Ther.* **1:**33–50.

CAUTELA, J., 1971, Covert extinction, *Behav. Ther.* **2:**192–200.

CHAKRAVARTY, N. K., MATALLANA, A., JENSEN, R., and BORISON, H. L., 1956, Central effects of antitussive drugs on cough and respiration, *J. Pharmacol. Exp. Ther.* **117:**127–135.

CHAPMAN, C. R., and FEATHER, B. W., 1973, Effects of diazepam on human pain tolerance and pain sensitivity, *Psychosom. Med.* **35:**330–340.

CHAPMAN, C. R., MURPHY, T. M., and BUTLER, S. H., 1973, Analgesic strength of 33 per cent nitrous oxide: A signal detection theory evaluation, *Science* **179:**1246–1248.

CHARPENTIER, J., 1968, Analysis and measurement of pain in animals, a new conception of pain, in: *Pain* (A. Soulairac, J. Cahn, and J. Charpentier, eds.), pp. 171–200, Academic Press, London/New York.

CHERUBIN, C. E., 1967. The medical sequelae of narcotic addiction, *Ann. Int. Med.* **67:**23–33.

CLARK, W. C., 1969, Sensory decision theory analysis of the placebo effect on the criterion for pain and thermal sensitivity (d′), *J. Abnorm. Psychol.* **74:**363–371.

CLARK, W. E. LE GROS, 1932, The structure and connections of the thalamus, *Brain* **55:**406–470.

COCHIN, J., and KORNETSKY, C., 1968, Factors in blood of morphine-tolerant animals that attenuate or enhance effects of morphine in nontolerant animals, in: *The Addictive States* (A. Wikler, ed.), pp. 268–277, Williams & Wilkins, Baltimore.

COLLIER, H. O. J., 1966, Tolerance, physical dependence, and receptors, in: *Advances in Drug Research,* Vol. 3 (N. J. Harper and A. B. Simmonds, eds.), pp. 171–188, Academic Press, New York.

COMROE, J. H., and DRIPPS, R. D., 1948, Reactions to morphine in ambulatory and bed patients, *Surg. Gynecol. Obstet.* **87:**221–227.

DANIEL, E. E., SUTHERLAND, W. H., and BOGOCH, A., 1959, Effects of morphine and other drugs on the motility of the terminal ileum, *Gastroenterology* **36:**510–523.

DOLE, V. P., 1970, Biochemistry of addiction, *Annu. Rev. Biochem.* **39:**821–840.

DORCUS, R. M., and KIRKNER, F. J., 1948, The use of hypnosis in the suppression of intractable pain, *J. Abnorm. Soc. Psychol.* **43:**237–239.

DREW, J. H., DRIPPS, R. D., and COMROE, J. H., 1946, Clinical studies on morphine. III. The effect of morphine upon the circulation of man and upon the circulatory and respiratory responses to tilting, *Anesthesiology* **7**:44–61.

DRIPPS, R. D., and COMROE, J. H., 1945, Clinical studies on morphine. I. The immediate effect of morphine administered intravenously and intramuscularly upon respiration in normal man, *Anesthesiology* **6**:462–468.

ECKENHOFF, J. E., and OECH, S. R., 1960, The effects of narcotics and antagonists upon respiration and circulation in man, *Clin. Pharmacol. Ther.* **1**:483–524.

ECKENHOFF, J. E., HELRICH, M., and HEGE, M. J. D., 1956, A method for studying respiratory functions in awake or anesthetized patients, *Anesthesiology* **17**:66–72.

EDDY, N. B., HALBACH, H., and BRAEDEN, O. J., 1957, Synthetic substances with morphine-like effect, clinical experience: Potency, side-effects, addiction liability, *Bull. WHO* **17**:569–863.

EHRENPREIS, S., GREENBERG, J., and COMATY, J. E., 1975, Mechanism of development of tolerance to injected morphine by guinea pig ileum, *Life Sci.* **17**:49–54.

EISENMAN, A. J., SLOAN, J. W., MARTIN, W. R., JASINSKI, D. R., and BROOKS, J. W., 1969, Catecholamine and 17-hydroxycorticosteroid excretion during a cycle of morphine dependence in man, *J. Psychiat. Res.* **7**:19–28.

ELLIOT, H. W., TOLBERT, B. M., ADLER, T. K., and ANDERSON, H. H., 1954, Excretion of carbon-14 by man after administration of morphine-*n*-methyl-C^{14}, *Proc. Soc. Exp. Biol. Med.* **85**:77–81.

ELLIOT, H. W., NAVARRO, G., NOMOF, N., 1970, A double blind controlled study of the pharmacologic effects of nalbuphine (EN-2234A), *J. Med.* **1**:74–89.

ELLIOT, H. W., PARKER, K. D., WRIGHT, J. A., and NOMOF, N., 1971, Actions and metabolism of heroin administered by continuous intravenous infusion to man, *Clin. Pharmacol. Ther.* **12**:806–814.

EVANS, W. G., 1962, The synergism of autonomic drugs on opiate or opioid-induced analgesia. A discussion of its potential utility, *Mil. Med.* **127**:1000–1003.

FABREGA, H., JR., and VAN EGEREN, L., 1976, A behavioral framework for the study of human disease, *Ann. Int. Med.* **84**:200–208.

FEATHER, B. W., CHAPMAN, C. R., and FISHER, S. B., 1972, The effect of a placebo on the perception of painful radiant heat stimuli, *Psychosom. Med.* **34**:290–294.

FEIGHNER, J. P., ROBINS, E., GUZE, S. B., WOODRUFF, R. A., WINOKUR, G., and MUNOZ, R., 1972, Diagnostic criteria for use in psychiatric research, *Arch. Gen. Psychiat.* **26**:57–63.

FELDSTEIN, S., CHESLER, P., and FINK, M., 1973, Psychological differentiation and the response of opiate addicts to pharmacological treatment, *Br. J. Addict.* **68**:151–157.

FISHER, C. M., 1967, Some neuro-ophthalmological observations, *J. Neurol. Neurosurg. Psychiat.* **30**:383–392.

FISHER, C. M., 1969, The neurological examination of the comatose patient, *Acta. Neurol. Scand.* **45**, Suppl. **36**:1–56.

FOLDES, F. F., 1974, The role of drugs in the management of intractable pain, in: *Relief of Intractable Pain* (M. Swerdlow, ed.), Excerpta Medica, New York.

FORDYCE, W. E., 1974*a*, Pain viewed as learned behavior, in: *Advances in Neurology,* Vol. 4, *International Symposium on Pain* (J. J. Bonica, ed.), pp. 415–422, Raven Press, New York.

FORDYCE, W. E., 1974*b*, Treating chronic pain by contingency management, in: *Advances in Neurology,* Vol. 4, *International Symposium on Pain* (J. J. Bonica, ed.), pp. 415–422, Raven Press, New York.

FORREST, W. H., BEER, E. G., BELLVILLE, W. J., CILIBERTI, B. J., and PADDOCK, R., 1969, Analgesic and other effects of the *d*- and *l*-isomers of pentazocine, *Clin. Pharmacol. Ther.* **10**:468–476.

FORREST, W. H., JR., BELLVILLE, J. W., BEER, W. G., and BROWN, B. W., JR., 1970, Interaction of morphine and dextroamphetamine for the treatment of postoperative pain in man, *Pharmacologist* **12**:2 (Abst.).

FRASER, H. F., 1968, Methods for assessing the addiction liability of opioids and opioid antagonists in man, in: *The Addictive States* (A. Wikler, ed.), pp. 176–187, Williams & Wilkins, Baltimore, Maryland.

FRASER, H. F., and ISBELL, H., 1952, Comparative effects of 20 mg. of morphine sulfate in non-addicts and former morphine addicts, *J. Pharmacol. Exp. Ther.* **105:**498–502.

FRASER, H. F., and ISBELL, H., 1960, Human pharmacology and addiction liabilities of phenazocine and levophenacylmorphan, *Bull. Narc.* **12:**15–23.

FRASER, H. F., and ISBELL, H., 1961, Human pharmacology and addictiveness of ethyl 1-(-3-cyano-3,3-phenylpropyl)-4-phenyl-4-piperidine carboxylalate hydrochloride (R-1132, diphenoxylate), *Bull. Narc.* **13:**29–43.

FRASER, H. F., NASH, T. L., VAN HORN, G. D., and ISBELL, H., 1954, Use of miotic effect in evaluating analgesic drugs in man, *Arch. Int. Pharmacodyn.* **98:**443–451.

FRASER, H. F., ISBELL, H., and VAN HORN, G. D., 1958*a*, Norcodeine in man, *Fed. Proc.* **17,** No. 1449.

FRASER, H. F., WIKLER, A., VAN HORN, G. D., EISENMAN, A. J., and ISBELL, H., 1958*b*. Human pharmacology and addiction liability of morphine, *J. Pharmacol. Exp. Ther.* **122:**359–369.

FRASER, H. F., VAN HORN, G. D., MARTIN, W. R., WOLBACK, A. B., ISBELL, H., 1961, Methods for evaluating addiction liability. (a) "Attitude" of opiate addicts toward opiate-like drugs, (b) A short-term "direct" addiction test, *J. Pharmacol. Exp. Ther.* **133:**371–387.

FRASER, H. F., JONES, B. E., ROSENBERG, D. E., and THOMPSON, A. K., 1963, Effects of addiction to intravenous heroin on patterns of physical activity in man, *Clin. Pharmacol. Ther.* **4:**188–196.

FREEDMAN, A. M., FINK, M., SHAROFF, R., and ZAKS, A., 1967, Cyclazocine and methadone in narcotic addiction, *JAMA* **202:**191–194.

FREEDMAN, A. M., FINK, M., SHAROFF, R., and ZAKS, A., 1968, Clinical studies of cyclazocine in the treatment of narcotic addiction, *Am. J. Psychiat.* **124:**1499–1504.

GEOGHEGAN, J. J., 1946, Manic depressive psychosis (manic phase) and electroshock, *Canad. Med. Assn. J.* **55:**54.

GIBBS, F. A., and MALTBY, G. L., 1943, Effect on electrical activity of the cortex of certain depressant and stimulant drugs—barbiturates, morphine, caffeine, benzedrine and adrenalin, *J. Pharmacol. Exp. Ther.* **78:**1–10.

GILBERT, P. E., and MARTIN, W. R., 1975, Antagonism of the convulsant effects of heroin, *d*-propoxyphene, meperidine, normeperidine, and thebaine by naloxone in mice, *J. Pharmacol. Exp. Ther.* **192:**538–541.

GILCHRIST, J. C., and NESBERG, L. S., 1952, Need and perceptual change in need-related objects, *J. Exp. Psychol.* **44:**369–376.

GOLDIAMOND, I., 1958, Indicators of perception: I. Subliminal perception, subception, unconscious perception: An analysis in terms of psychophysical indicator methodology, *Psychol. Bull.* **55:**373–411.

GOLDSTEIN, A., and GOLDSTEIN, D. B., 1968, Enzyme expansion theory of drug tolerance and physical dependence, in: *The Addictive States* (A. Wikler, ed.), pp. 265–267, Williams & Wilkins, Baltimore.

GORODETZKY, C. W., 1973, Time course of morphine (M) detection in human urine after IV morphine, *Fed. Proc.* **32:**764.

GORODETZKY, C. W., 1975, Time course of morphine (M) detection in human urine after IV heroin (H) by EMIT and RIA-I^{125}, *Fed. Proc.* **3:**814.

GORODETZKY, C. W., and MARTIN, W. R., 1965, A comparison of fentanyl, droperidol, and morphine, *Clin. Pharmacol. Ther.* **6:**731–739.

GORODETZKY, C. W., ANGEL, C. R., BEACH, D. J., CATLIN, D. H., and YEH, S. Y., 1974. Validity of screening methods for drugs of abuse in biological fluids. I. Heroin in urine, *Clin. Pharmacol. Ther.* **15:**461–472.

GRANACHER, R. P., and BALDESSARINI, R. J., 1975, Phystostigmine, *Arch. Gen. Psychiat.* **32:**375–380.

GRAVENSTEIN, J. S., SMITH, G. M., SPHIRE, R. D., ISAACS, J. P., and BEECHER, H. K., 1956,

Dihydrocodeine, further development in measurement of analgesic power and appraisal of psychologic side effects of analgesic agents, *N. Engl. J. Med.* **254**:877–885.

Greenhoot, J. H., and Sternbach, R. A., 1974, Conjoint treatment of chronic pain, in: *Advances in Neurology,* Vol. 4, *International Symposium on Pain* (J. J. Bonica, ed.), Raven Press, New York.

Grendahl, H., and Hansteen, V., 1969, The effect of morphine on blood pressure and cardiac output in patients with acute myocardial infarction, *Acta Med. Scand.* **186**:515–517.

Guttner, L. B., Gould, W. J., and Batterman, R. C., 1952, The effects of potent analgesics upon vestibular function, *J. Clin. Invest.* **31**:259–266.

Gyang, E. A., and Kosterlitz, H. W., 1966, Agonist and antagonist actions of morphine-like drugs on the guinea-pig isolated ileum. *Br. J. Pharmacol. Chemother.* **27**:514–527.

Hackett, T. P., 1971, Pain and prejudice, *Med. Times* **99**:130–138.

Hackett, T. P., White, J. C., and Sweet, W. H., 1966, Leukotomy for the relief of pain: The selection of cases and psychological hazards, in: *Pain* (R. S. Knighton and P. R. Dumke, eds.), Little, Brown, Boston.

Haertzen, C. A., 1966, Development of scales based on patterns of drug effects, using the addiction research center inventory (ARCI), *Psychol. Rep.* **18**:163–194.

Haertzen, C. A., 1970, Subjective effects of narcotic antagonists cyclazocine and nalorphine on the addiction research center inventory (ARCI), *Psychopharmacologia* **18**:366–377.

Haertzen, C. A., 1974, Subjective effects of narcotic antagonists, in: *Narcotic Antagonists* (M. C. Braude, L. S. Harris, E. L. May, J. P. Smith, and J. E. Villarreal, eds.), pp. 383–398, Raven Press, New York.

Haertzen, C. A., and Hooks, N. T., 1969, Changes in personality and subjective experience associated with the chronic administration and withdrawal of opiates, *J. Nerv. Ment. Dis.* **148**:606–614.

Haertzen, C. A., Hill, H. E., and Bellville, J. W., 1963, Development of the addiction research center inventory (ARCI): Selection of items that are sensitive to the effects of various drugs, *Psychopharmacologia* **4**:155–166.

Hebb, D. O., 1955, Drives and the cns (conceptual nervous system), *Psychol. Rev.* **62**:243–254.

Herold, M., and Cahn, J., 1968, The possible role of serotonin in pain, in: *Pain* (A. Soulairac, J. Cahn, and J. Charpentier, eds.), pp. 251–280, Academic Press, London/New York.

Herrnstein, R. J., 1962, Placebo effect in the rat, *Science* **138**:677–678.

Herz, A., Albus, K., Metys, J., Schubert, P., and Teschemacher, H. J., 1970, On the central sites for the antinociceptive action of morphine and fentanyl, *Neuropharmacology* **9**:539–551.

Hewer, A. J. H., and Keele, C. A., 1948, A method of testing analgesics in man, *Lancet* **ii**:683–688.

Hewer, A. J. H., Keele, C. A., Keele, K. D., and Nathan, P. W., 1949, A clinical method of assessing analgesics, *Lancet* **i**:431–435.

Hill, H. E., Kornetsky, C. H., Flanary, H. G., and Wikler, A., 1952*a*, Effects of anxiety and morphine on discrimination of intensities of painful stimuli, *J. Clin. Invest.* **3**:473–480.

Hill, H. E., Kornetsky, C. H., Flanary, H. G., and Wikler, A., 1952*b*, Studies on anxiety associated with anticipation of pain, I. Effects of morphine, *Arch. Neurol. Psychiat.* **67**:612–619.

Hill, H. E., Bellville, R. E., and Wikler, A., 1955, Studies on anxiety associated with anticipation of pain. II. Comparative effects of pentobarbitol and morphine, *Arch. Neurol. Psychiat.* **73**:602–608.

Hill, H. E., Belleville, R. E., and Wikler, A., 1957, Motivational determinants in modification of behavior by morphine and pentobarbital, *A.M.A. Arch. Neurol. Psychiat.* **77**:28–35.

Hill, H. E., Haertzen, C. A., and Glaser, R., 1960, Personality characteristics of narcotic addicts as indicated by the MMPI, *J. Gen. Psychol.* **62:**127–139.

Hill, H. E., Haertzen, C. A., Wolback, A. B., and Miner, E. J., 1963*a*, The addiction research center inventory: Standardization of scales which evaluate subjective effects of morphine, amphetamine, pentobarbitol, alcohol, LSD-25, pyrahexyl and chlorpromazine, *Psychopharmacologia* **4:**167–183.

Hill, H. E., Haertzen, C. A., Wolback, A. B., and Miner, E. J., 1963*b*, The addiction research center inventory: Appendix, *Psychopharmacologia* **4:**184–205.

Himmelsbach, C. K., 1941*a*, The morphine abstinence syndrome, its nature and treatment, *Ann. Int. Med.* **15:**829–839.

Himmelsbach, C. K., 1941*b*, Studies on the relation of drug addiction to the autonomic nervous system: Result of cold pressor tests, *J. Pharmacol. Exp. Ther.* **73:**91–98.

Himmelsbach, C. K., 1942, Clinical studies of drug addiction, physical dependence, withdrawal and recovery, *Arch. Int. Med.* **69:**766–772.

Hoffmeister, F., 1968, Effects of psychotropic drugs on pain, in: *Pain* (A. Soulairac, J. Cahn, and J. Charpentier, eds.), pp. 309–319, Academic Press, London/New York.

Hopton, D. S., and Torrance, H. B., 1967, Action of various new analgesic drugs on the human common bile duct, *Gut* **8:**296–300.

Houde, R. W., 1974, The use and misuse of narcotics in the treatment of chronic pain, in: *Advances in Neurology*, Vol. 4, *International Symposium on Pain* (J. J. Bonica, ed.), pp. 527–536, Raven Press, New York.

Houde, R. W., Wallenstein, S. L., and Rogers, A., 1960, Clinical pharmacology of analgesics: 1. A method of assaying analgesic effect, *Clin. Pharmacol. Ther.* **1:**163–174.

Houde, R. W., Wallenstein, S. L., and Beaver, W. T., 1965, Clinical measurement of pain, in: *Analgetics* (G. de Stevens, ed.), pp. 75–122, Academic Press, New York/London.

Huggins, R. A., and Moyer, J. H., 1955, Some effects of *n*-allylnormorphine on normal subjects in a review of the literature, *Anesthesiology* **16:**82–90.

Iggo, A., 1972, Critical remarks on the gate control theory, in: *Pain* (R. Jansen, W. D. Keidel, A. Herz, and C. Steichele, eds.) (English Ed., J. P. Payne, and R. A. P. Burt, eds.), pp. 127–128, Williams & Wilkins, Baltimore.

Isbell, H., 1948, The newer analgesic drugs; their use and abuse, *Ann. Int. Med.* **29:**1003–1013.

Isbell, H., 1956, Attempted addiction to nalorphine, *Fed. Proc.* **15:**442.

Isbell, H., and Chruściel, T. L., 1970, Dependence liability of "nonnarcotic" drugs. *Bull. WHO* **43** (Suppl.):1–111.

Isbell, H., and White, W. M., 1953, Clinical characteristics of addictions, *Am. J. Med.* **14:**558–565.

Jaffe, J. H., and Sharpless, S. K., 1965, The rapid development of physical dependence on barbiturates, *J. Pharmacol. Exp. Ther.* **150:**140–145.

Jasinski, D. R., and Mansky, P. A., 1972, Evaluation of nalbuphine for abuse potential, *Clin. Pharmacol. Ther.* **13:**78–90.

Jasinski, D. R., and Martin, W. R., 1967, Evaluation of a new photographic method for assessing pupil diameters, *Clin. Pharmacol. Ther.* **8:**271–272.

Jasinski, D. R., and Nutt, J. G., 1973, Progress report on the clinical assessment program at the addiction research center. Report of the thirty-fifth annual scientific meeting, Committee on Problems of Drug Dependence, NAS-NRC, p. 108–130.

Jasinski, D. R., Martin, W. R., and Haertzen, C. A., 1967, The human pharmacology and abuse potential of *n*-allylnoroxymorphine (naloxone), *J. Pharmacol. Exp. Ther.* **157:**420–426.

Jasinski, D. R., Martin, W. R., and Sapira, J. D., 1968, Antagonism of the subjective, behavioral, pupillary, and respiratory depressant effects of cyclazocine by naloxone, *Clin. Pharmacol. Ther.* **9:**215–222.

Jasinski, D. R., Martin, W. R., and Hoeldtke, R. D., 1970, Effects of short- and long-term administration of pentazocine in man, *Clin. Pharmacol. Ther.* **11:**385–403.

JASINSKI, D. R., MARTIN, W. R., and HOELDTKE, R., 1971, Studies of the dependence producing properties of GPA-1657, profadol, and propiram in man, *Clin. Pharmacol. Ther.* **12**:613–649.

JONES, M. H., 1956, Second pain: Fact or artifact, *Science* **124**:442–443.

KAY, D. C., 1973, Sleep and some psychoactive drugs, *Psychosomatics* **14**:108–118.

KAY, D. C., 1975, Human sleep and EEG through a cycle of methadone dependence. *Electroencephalogr. Clin. Neurophysiol.* **38**:35–43.

KAY, D. C., GORODETSKY, C. W., and MARTIN, W. R., 1967, Comparative effects of codeine and morphine in man, *J. Pharmacol. Exp. Ther.* **156**:101–106.

KAY, D. C., EISENSTEIN, R. B., JASINSKI, D. R., 1969, Morphine effects on human REM state, waking state and NREM sleep, *Psychopharmacologia (Berlin)* **14**:404–416.

KEATS, A. S., and BEECHER, H. K., 1950, Pain relief with hypnotic doses of barbiturates and a hypothesis, *J. Pharmacol.* **100**:1–13.

KEATS, A. S., and BEECHER, H. K., 1952, Analgesic potency and side action liability in man of heptazone, win 1161-2, 6-methyl dihydromorphine, metopan, levo-isomethadone and pentobarbital sodium as a further effort to refine methods of evaluation of analgesic drugs, *J. Pharmacol.* **105**:109–129.

KEATS, A. S., and TELFORD, J., 1957, Subjective effects of nalorphine in hospitalized patients, *J. Pharmacol. Exp. Ther.* **119**:370–375.

KEATS, A. S., and TELFORD, J., 1964, Studies of analgesic drugs. VIII. A narcotic antagonist analgesic without pschotomimetic effects, *J. Pharmacol. Exp. Ther.* **143**:157–164.

KEATS, A. S., and TELFORD, J., 1968, Annual report, continuing study of narcotic antagonists as analgesics. Report of thirtieth scientific meeting of the Committee of Problems of Drug Dependence, NAS-NRC, pp. 5514–5530.

KEATS, A. S., BEECHER, H. K., and MOSTELLER, F. C., 1950, Measurement of pathological pain in distribution to experimental pain, *J. Appl. Physiol.* **3**:35–44.

KEELE, C. A., and ARMSTRONG, D., 1964, *Substances Producing Pain and Itch,* Williams & Wilkins, Baltimore.

KERR, F. W. L., 1975, Pain, a central inhibitory balance theory, *Mayo Clin. Proc.* **50**:685–690.

KERR, F., and DONALD, K. W., 1974, Analgesia in myocardial infarction, *Br. Heart J.* **36**:117–121.

KILCOYNE, M. M., DALY, J. J., GOCKE, D. J., THOMSON, G. E., MELTZER, J., HSU, K. C., and TANNENBAUM, M., 1972, Nephrotic syndrome in heroin addicts, *Lancet* **i**:17–20.

KOLB, L., 1925, Pleasure and deterioration from narcotic addiction, *Ment. Hyg.* **9**:699–724.

KORNETSKY, C., 1954, Effects of anxiety and morphine on the anticipation and perception of painful thermal stimuli, *J. Comp. Physiol. Psychol.* **47**:130–132.

KOSTERLITZ, H. W., WATERFIELD, A. A., and BERTHOUD, V., 1974, Assessment of the agonist and antagonist properties of narcotic analgesic drugs by their actions on the morphine receptor in the guinea pig ileum, in: *Narcotic Antagonists (Advances in Biochemical Psychopharmacology)* (M. C. Braude, L. S. Harris, E. L. May, J. P. Smith, and J. E. Villarreal, eds.), Raven Press, New York.

LAIDLOW, J., READ, A. E., and SHERLOCK, S., 1961, Morphine tolerance in hepatic cirrhosis, *Gastroenterology* **40**:389–396.

LASAGNA, L., 1964, The clinical evaluation of morphine and its substitutes as analgesics, *Pharmacol. Rev.* **16**:47–83.

LASAGNA, L., 1965, Drug interaction in the field of analgesic drugs, *Proc. Roy. Soc. Med.* **58**:978–983.

LASAGNA, L., and BEECHER, H. K., 1954*a*, The analgesic effectiveness of nalorphine and nalorphine–morphine combinations in man. *J. Pharmacol. Exp. Ther.* **112**:356–363.

LASAGNA, L., and BEECHER, H. K., 1954*b*, The analgesic effectiveness of codeine and meperidine (demerol), *J. Pharmacol. Exp. Ther.* **112**:306–311.

LASAGNA, L., MOSTELLER, F., VON FELSINGER, J. M., and BEECHER, H. K., 1954, A study of the placebo response, *Am. J. Med.* **16**:770–779.

LASAGNA, L., VON FELSINGER, J. M., and BEECHER, H. K., 1955, Drug induced mood changes in man, I. Observations of healthy subjects, chronically ill patients and "post addicts," *JAMA* **157:**1006–1020.

LEE, L. E., 1942, Studies of morphine, codeine and their derivatives. XVI. Clinical studies of morphine, methyldihydromorphinone (metopan) and dihydrodesoxymorphine-d (desmorphine), *J. Pharmacol. Exp. Ther.* **75:**161–173.

LEVI, A. J., 1965, Some aspects of drug metabolism in liver disease, in: *Therapeutic Agents and the Liver* (N. McIntyre, and S. Sherlock, eds.), F. A. Davis, Philadelphia.

LEWIS, S. A., OSWALD, I., EVANS, J. I., AKINDELE, M. O., and TOMPSET, S. L., 1970, Heroin and human sleep, *Electroencephalogr. Clin. Neurophysiol.* **28:**374–381.

LIBET, B., 1957, Delayed pain as a peripheral sensory pathway, *Science* **126:**256–258.

LIM, R. K. S., and GUZMAN, F., 1968, Manifestations of pain in analgesic evaluation in animals and man, in: *Pain* (A. Soulairac, J. Cahn, and J. Charpentier, eds.), pp. 119–152, Academic Press, London/New York.

LINDESMITH, A. R., 1947, *Opiate Addiction*, Principia Press, Bloomington, Indiana.

LINDVALL, O., BJÖRKLUND, A., NOBIN, A., and STENEVI, U., 1974, The adrenergic innervation of the rat thalamus as revealed by glyoxylic acid flourescence method, *J. Comp. Neurol.* **154:**317–348.

LOWENSTEIN, E., HALLOWELL, P., LEVINE, F. H., DAGGETT, W. M., AUSTEN, W. G., and LAVER, M. B., 1969, Cardiovascular response to large doses of intravenous morphine in man, *N. Engl. J. Med.* **281:**1389–1393.

LURIA, R. A., 1973, *The Working Brain* (Trans. by B. Haigh), Basic Books, New York.

MAHER, B. A., 1966, *Principles of Psychopathology, an Experimental Approach,* McGraw-Hill, New York.

MALMO, R. B., and SHAGASS, C., 1949, Physiologic studies of reaction to stress in anxiety and early schizophrenia, *Psychosom. Med.* **2:**9–24.

MANSKY, P. A., 1975, Opiate action, in: *Opiate Receptor Mechanisms* (S. H. Snyder, and S. Matthysse, eds.), *Neurosci. Res. Progr. Bull.* **13:**13–17.

MANSKY, P. A., 1976, Pentazocine (Talwin): A review to be published.

MANSKY, P. A., and ALTMAN, J., 1977, A conceptual model of drug dependence, in: *Renewal in Psychiatry: A Critical Rational Perspective* (T. Manschreck and A. Kleinman, eds.), pp. 139–161, Hemisphere Publishing Corp., Washington/London.

MANSKY, P. A., and JASINSKI, D. R., 1970, Effects of dextromethorphan in man, *Pharmacologist* **12:**231.

MANSKY, P. A., and JASINSKI, D. R., 1976, Potentiation of the antinociceptive action of morphine by prior administration of dextromethorphan, in preparation.

MARQUARDT, W. G., MARTIN, W. R., and JASINSKI, D. R., 1967, The use of the Polaroid CU camera in pupillography, *Int. J. Addict.* **2:**301–304.

MARTIN, W. R., 1963, Analgesic and antipyretic drugs. 1. Strong analgesics, in: *Physiological Pharmacology* (W. S. Root and E. G. Hofman, eds.), pp. 275–312, Academic Press, New York.

MARTIN, W. R., 1966, Assessment of the dependence producing potentiality of narcotic analgesics, in: *International Encyclopedia of Pharmacology and Therapeutics,* Vol. 1 (C. Radauco-Thomas and L. Lasagna, eds.), pp. 155–180, Pergamon Press, Glasgow.

MARTIN, W. R., 1967*a*, Opioid antagonists, *Pharmacol. Rev.* **19:**463–521.

MARTIN, W. R., 1967*b*, Clinical evaluation for narcotic dependence, in: *New Concepts in Pain and Its Clinical Management* (E. L. Way, ed.), pp. 121–132, F. A. Davis, Philadelphia.

MARTIN, W. R., 1970, Pharmacological redundancy as an adaptive mechanism in the central nervous system, *Fed. Proc.* **29:**13–18.

MARTIN, W. R., 1975, Clinical phenomenology of addiction, in: *Opiate Receptor Mechanisms* (S. H. Snyder and S. Matthysse, eds.), *Neurosci. Res. Progr. Bull.* **13:**126–134.

MARTIN, W. R., and EADES, C. G., 1961, Demonstration of tolerance and physical dependence in the dog following short-term infusion of morphine, *J. Pharmacol. Exp. Ther.* **133:**262–270.

MARTIN, W. R., and FRASER, H. F., 1961, A comparative study of physiological and subjective effects of heroin and morphine administered intravenously in post addicts, *J. Pharmacol. Exp. Ther.* **133:**388–399.

Martin, W. R., and Gorodetzky, C. W., 1965, Demonstration of tolerance to and physical dependence on *n*-allylnormorphine (nalorphine), *J. Pharmacol. Exp. Ther.* **150:**432–442.

Martin, W. R., and Jasinski, D. R., 1969, Physiological parameters of morphine dependence in man—tolerance, early abstinence, protracted abstinence, *J. Psychiat. Res.* **7:**9–17.

Martin, W. R., and Sloan, J. W., 1968, The pathophysiology of morphine dependence and its treatment with opioid antagonists, *Pharmakopsych. Neuro-Psychopharmakol.* **1:**260–270.

Martin, W. R., Wikler, A., Eades, C. G., and Pescor, F. T., 1963, Tolerance to and physical dependence on morphine in rats, *Psychopharmacologia* **4:**247–260.

Martin, W. R., Eades, C. G., Fraser, H. F., and Wikler, A., 1964, Use of hindlimb reflexes in the chronic spinal dog for comparing analgesics, *J. Pharmacol. Exp. Ther.* **144:**8–11.

Martin, W. R., Fraser, H. F., Gorodetzky, C. W., and Rosenberg, D. E., 1965, Studies of the dependence-producing potential of the narcotic antagonist 2-cyclopropylmethyl-2′-hydroxy-5,9-dimethyl-6,7-benzomorphan (cyclazocine, win-20, 740, ARC II-C-3), *J. Pharmacol. Exp. Ther.* **150:**426–436.

Martin, W. R., Gorodetzky, C. W., and McClane, T. K., 1966, An experimental study in the treatment of narcotic addicts with cyclazocine, *Clin. Pharmacol. Ther.* **7:**455–465.

Martin, W. R., Jasinski, D. R., Sapira, J. D., Flanary, H. G., Kelly, O. A., Thompson, A. K., and Logan, C. R., 1968, The respiratory effects of morphine during a cycle of dependence, *J. Pharmacol. Exp. Ther.* **162:**182–189.

Martin, W. R., Jasinski, D. R., Haertzen, C. A., Kay, D. C., Jones, B. E., Mansky, P. A., and Carpenter, R. W., 1973*a*, Methadone—a re-evaluation, *Arch. Gen. Psychiat.* **28:**286–295.

Martin, W. R., Jasinski, D. R., and Mansky, P. A., 1973*b*, Naltrexone, an antagonist for the treatment of heroin dependence, effects in man, *Arch. Gen. Psychiat.* **28:**784–791.

McClane, T. K., and Martin, W. R., 1967, Effects of morphine, nalorphine, cyclazocine, and naloxone on the flexor reflex, *Int. J. Neuropharmacol.* **6:**89–98.

McCrea, F. D., Eadie, G. S., and Morgan, J. E., 1942, The mechanism of morphine miosis, *J. Pharmacol. Exp. Ther.* **74:**239–246.

Mehler, W. R., Freeman, M. E., and Nauta, W. J., 1960, Ascending axonal degeneration following contralateral cordotomy, *Brain* **83:**718–750.

Melzack, R., 1974, Psychological concepts and methods for the control of pain, in: *Advances in Neurology, International Symposium on Pain*, Vol. 4 (J. J. Bonica, ed.), pp. 275–288, Raven Press, New York.

Melzack, R., and Scott, T. H., 1957, The effects of early experience on the response to pain, *J. Comp. Physiol. Psychol.* **50:**155–161.

Melzack, R., and Torgerson, W. S., 1971, On the language of pain, *Anesthesiology* **34:**50–59.

Melzack, R., and Wall, P. D., 1965, Pain mechanisms: A new theory, *Science* **150:**971–979.

Melzack, R., and Wall, P. D., 1968, Gate control theory of pain, in: *Pain* (A. Soulairac, J. Cahn, and J. Charpentier, eds.), Academic Press, New York/London.

Merskey, H., 1974, Psychological aspects of pain relief; hypnotherapy, psychotropic drugs, in: *Relief of Intractable Pain* (M. Swerdlow, ed.), Excerpta Medica, New York.

Monroe, J. J., Ross, W. F., and Berzins, J., 1971, The decline of the addict as "psychopath": Implications for community care, *Int. J. Addict.* **6:**601–608.

Mott, J., 1972, The psychological basis of drug dependence: The intellectual and personality characteristics of opiate users, *Br. J. Addict.* **67:**89–99.

Mountcastle, V. B., 1968, Pain and temperature sensibilities, in: *Medical Physiology*, Vol. 2, 12th Ed. (V. B. Mountcastle, ed.), pp. 1424–1464, C. V. Mosby, St. Louis.

Mulé, S. J., 1971, Physiological disposition of narcotic agonists and antagonists, in: *Narcotic Drugs: Biochemical Pharmacology* (D. H. Clouet, ed.), pp. 99–121, Plenum Publishing Corp., New York.

Murphree, H. B., 1962, Clinical pharmacology of potent analgesics, *Clin. Pharmacol. Ther.* **3:**473–504.

NAUTA, W. J. H., 1958, Hippocampal projections and related neural pathways to the midbrain in the cat, *Brain* **81:**319–340.

NAUTA, W. J. H., 1975, Anatomical organization of pain pathways in the central nervous system, in: *Opiate Receptor Mechanisms* (S. H. Snyder and S. Matthysse, eds.), *Neurosci. Res. Progr. Bull.* **13:**84–87.

NICOLIS, F. B., and PASQUARIELLO, G., 1962, Controlled clinical trials of antitussive agents: An experimental evaluation of different methods *J. Pharmacol. Exp. Ther.* **136:**183–189.

NOORDENBOS, W., 1968, Physiological correlates of clinical pain syndromes, in: *Pain* (A. Soulairac, J. Cahn, and J. Charpentier, eds.), Academic Press, New York/London.

OLDENDORF, W. H., HYMAN, S., BRAUN, L., and OLDENDORF, S. Z., 1972, Blood-brain barrier penetration of morphine, codeine, heroin and methadone after carotid injection, *Science* **178:**984–986.

OLDS, J. S., and OLDS, M. E., 1965, Drives, rewards, and the brain, in: *New Directions in Psychology II,* pp. 329–410, Holt, Rhinehart & Winston, New York.

ORNE, M. T., 1974, Pain suppression by hypnosis and related phenomena, in: *Advances in Neurology,* Vol. 4, *International Symposium on Pain* (J. J. Bonica, ed.), **4:**563–582, Raven Press, New York.

PADDOCK, R., BEER, G. E., BELLVILLE, J. W., CILIBERTI, B. J., FORREST, W. H., and MILLER, E., 1964, Analgesic and side effects of pentazocine and morphine in a large population of postoperative patients, *Clin. Pharmacol. Ther.* **143:**157–164.

PADDOCK, R., BEER, E. G., BELLVILLE, J. W., CILIBERTI, B. J., FORREST, W. H., and MILLER, E. V., 1969, Analgesic and side effects of pentazocine and morphine in a large population of postoperative patients, *Clin. Pharmacol. Ther.* **10:**355–365.

PATON, W. D. M., 1957, The action of morphine and related substances on contraction and on acetylcholine output of coaxially stimulated guinea-pig ileum, *Br. J. Pharmacol.* **12:**119–127.

PEARSON, J. W., LASAGNA, L., and LAIRD, R. D., 1971, Analgesic activity of oral and intramuscular profadol, *Clin. Pharmacol. Ther.* **12:**683–690.

PENNES, H. H., and HOCH, P. H., 1957, Psychotomimetics, clinical and theoretical considerations, Harmine, win-2292 and nalline, *Am. J. Psychiat.* **113:**887–892.

PIHL, R. O., and ALTMAN, J., 1971, An experimental analysis of the placebo effect, *J. Clin. Pharmacol.* **11:**91–95.

PLUM, F., and POSNER, J. B., 1972, *The Diagnosis of Stupor and Coma,* F. A. Davis, Philadelphia.

POTTER, D. R., and PAYNE, J. P., 1970, Newer analgesics: With special reference to pentazocine, *Br. J. Anesth.* **42:**186–193.

REYNOLDS, A. K., and RANDALL, L. O., 1957, *Morphine and Allied Drugs,* Univ. of Toronto Press, Toronto.

RIOCH, D. MCK., 1972, Personality, *Arch. Gen. Psych.* **27:**575–580.

ROBINS, L. N., and MURPHY, G. E., 1967, Drug use in a normal population of young Negro men, *Am. J. Public Health* **57:**1580–1596.

ROBINS, L. N., HELZER, J. E., and DAVIS, D. H., 1975, Narcotic use in southeast Asia and afterward, an interview of 898 Vietnam returnees, *Arch. Gen. Psychiat.* **32:**955–961.

SAPIRA, J. D., 1968, The narcotic addict as a medical patient, *Am. J. Med.* **45:**555–588.

SAUM, W. R., and DE GROAT, W. C., 1972, Parasympathetic ganglia: Activation of an adrenergic inhibitory mechanism by cholinomimetic agents, *Science* **175:**659–661.

SCARFANI, J. T., and CLOUET, D. H., 1971, Biotransformations, in: *Narcotic Drugs: Biochemical Pharmacology* (D. H. Clouet, ed.), pp. 137–158, Plenum Publishing Corp., New York.

SCELETH, C. E., AND KUH, S., 1924, Drug addiction, *JAMA* **82:**679–682.

SCHMIDT, R. F., 1972, The gate control theory of pain: An unlikely hypothesis, in: *Pain* (R. Jansen, W. D. Keidel, A. Herz, and C. Stichele, eds.) (English Ed.: J. P. Payne and R. A. P. Burt, eds.), pp. 124–127, Williams & Wilkins, Baltimore.

SEED, J. C., WALLENSTEIN, S. L., HOUDE, R. W., and BELLVILLE, J. W., 1958, A comparison of the analgesic and respiratory effects of dihydrocodeine and morphine in man, *Arch. Int. Pharmacodyn. Ther.* **116:**293–339.

SEVELIUS, H., McCOY, J. F., and COLMORE, J. P., 1971, Dose response to codeine in patients with chronic cough. *Clin. Pharmacol. Ther.* **12:**449–455.

SHELDON, J. M., LOVELL, R. G., and MATHEWS, K. P., 1967, *A Manual of Clinical Allergy,* W. B. Saunders, Philadelphia/London.

SHOR, R. E., 1962, Physiological effects of painful stimulation during hypnotic analgesia under conditions designed to minimize anxiety, *Int. J. Clin. Exp. Hypn.* **10:**183–202.

SMITH, G. M., and BEECHER, H. K., 1959, Measurement of "mental clouding" and other subjective effects of morphine, *J. Pharmacol.* **126:**50–62.

SMITH, G. M., and BEECHER, H. K., 1969, Experimental production of pain in man: Sensitivity of a new method to 600 mg. of aspirin, *Clin. Pharmacol. Ther.* **10:**213–216.

SMITH, G. M., EGBERT, L. D., MARKOWITZ, R. A., MOSTELLER, F., and BEECHER, H. K., 1966, An experimental pain method sensitive to morphine in man: The submaximum effort tourniquet technique, *J. Pharmacol. Exp. Ther.* **154:**324–332.

SMITH, G. M., LOWENSTEIN, E., HUBBARD, J. H., and BEECHER, H. K., 1968, Experimental pain produced by the submaximum effort tourniquet technique: Further evidence of validity, *J. Pharmacol. Exp. Ther.* **163:** 468–474.

STERNBACH, R. A., 1968, Hypnotic and placebo effects, in: *Pain, A Psychophysiological Analysis,* pp. 133–146, Academic Press, New York/London.

STERNBACH, R. A., 1974*a*, Pain and depression, in: *Somatic Manifestations of Depressive Disorders* (A. Kiev, ed.), Excerpta Medica, Princeton.

STERNBACH, R. A., 1974*b*, Varieties of pain games, in: *Advances in Neurology,* Vol. 4, *International Symposium on Pain* (J. J. Bonica, ed.), pp. 423–430, Raven Press, New York.

SUNSHINE, A., LASKA, E., and SLAFTA, J., 1970, A comparison of the analgesic effects of profadol (Parke-Davis CI-572) and morphine, Report of thirty-second scientific meeting of The Committee on Problems of Drug Dependence, NAS-NRC, pp. 6899–6901.

THEOBALD, W., WILHELMI, G., and KRUPP, P., 1968, Analgesic and anticonvalesant activity of derivatives of dibenz (b,f) azepine, in: *Pain* (A. Soulairac, J. Cahn, and J. Charpentier, eds.), pp. 239–249, Academic Press, New York /London.

THOMAS, M., MALMCRONA, R., FILLMORE, S., and SHILLINGFORD, J., 1965, Haemodynamic effects of morphine in patients with acute myocardial infarction, *Br. Heart J.* **27:**863–875.

VALLIANT, G. E., 1966, A twelve-year follow-up of New York narcotic addicts: I. The relationship of treatment to outcome, *Am. J. Psychiat.* **122:**727–737.

VASKO, J. S., HENNEY, R. P., OLDHAM, H. N., BRAWLEY, R. K., and MORROW, A. G., 1966, Mechanism of action of morphine in the treatment of experimental pulmonary edema, *Am. J. Cardiol.* **18:**876–883.

VON FELSINGER, J. M., LASAGNA, L., and BEECHER, H. K., 1955, Drug-induced mood changes in man. 2. Personality and reactions to drugs, *JAMA* **157:**1113–1119.

WALLENSTEIN, S. L., and HOUDE, R. W., 1975, The clinical evaluation of analgesic effectiveness, in: *Methods in Narcotics Research* (S. Ehrenpreis and A. Neidle, eds.), pp. 127–145, Marcel Dekker, New York.

WALLENSTEIN, S. L., HOUDE, R. W., and BEAVER, W. T., 1967, Analgesic studies of orally and parenterally administered morphine and codeine in patients with cancer, *Fed. Proc.* **26:**742.

WANG, S. C., and GALVIANO, V. V., 1954, Locus of emetic action of morphine and hydergine in dogs, *J. Pharmacol. Exp. Ther.* **111:**329–334.

WAY, E. L., and ADLER, T. K., 1960, The pharmacologic implications of the fate of morphine and its surrogates, *Pharmacol. Rev.* **12:**383–446.

WAY, E. L., and ADLER, T. K., 1961, The biological disposition of morphine and its surrogates—1, *Bull. WHO* **25:**227–262.

WAY, E. L., and ADLER, T. K., 1962, The biological disposition of morphine and its surrogates—4, *Bull. WHO* **27:**359–394.

WHITEHEAD, C. C., 1974, Methadone psuedowithdrawal syndrome: Paradigm for a psychopharmacological model of opiate addiction, *Psychosom. Med.* **36:**189–198.

WHO Expert Committee on Drug Dependence, Sixteenth Report (1969), *WHO Techn. Rep.*, Ser. 407.

WIKLER, A., 1944, Studies on the action of morphine on the central nervous system of the cat, *J. Pharmacol. Exp. Ther.* **80:**176–197.

WIKLER, A., 1948, Recent progress in research on the neurophysiological basis of morphine addiction, *Am. J. Psychiat.* **105:**329–338.

WIKLER, A., 1952, A psychodynamic study of a patient during experimental self-regulated re-addiction to morphine, *Psychiat. Quart.* **26:**270–293.

WIKLER, A., 1953, *Opiate Addiction*, Charles C Thomas, Springfield, Ill.

WIKLER, A., 1958, *Mechanisms of Action of Opiates and Opiate Antagonists: A Review of Their Mechanisms of Action in Relation to Clinical Problems*, Public Health Monograph No. 52, U.S. Government Printing Office, Washington, D.C.

WIKLER, A., 1966, Designated discussion, in: *Pain* (R. S. Knighton and P. R. Dumke, eds.), Little, Brown, Boston.

WIKLER, A., 1968, Interaction of physical dependence and classical and operant conditioning in the genesis of relapse, in: *The Addictive States* (A. Wikler, ed.), pp. 280–287, Williams & Wilkins, Baltimore.

WIKLER, A., 1973, Dynamics of drug dependence, implications of a conditioning theory for research and treatment, *Arch. Gen. Psychiat.* **28:**611–616.

WIKLER, A., and CARTER, R. L., 1953, Effects of single doses of *n*-allylnormorphine on hindlimb reflexes of chronic spinal dogs during a cycle of morphine addiction, *J. Pharmacol. Exp. Ther.* **109:**92–101.

WIKLER, A., and FRANK, K., 1948, Hindlimb reflexes of chronic spinal dogs during cycles of addiction to morphine and methadone, *J. Pharmacol. Exp. Ther.* **94:**382–400.

WIKLER, A., and PESCOR, F. T., 1967, Classical conditioning of a morphine abstinence phenomenon, reinforcement of opioid-drinking behavior and "relapse" in morphine-addicted rats, *Psychopharmacologia* **10:**255–284.

WIKLER, A., PESCOR, M. J., KALBAUGH, E. P., and ANGELLUCI, R. J., 1952, Effects of frontal lobotomy on the morphine abstinence syndrome in man, *AMA Arch. Neurol. Psychiatry* **67:**510–521.

WIKLER, A., FRASER, H. F., and ISBELL, H., 1953, *N*-allylnormorphine: Effects of single doses and precipitation of acute "abstinence syndromes" during addiction to morphine, methadone or heroin in man (post-addicts), *J. Pharmacol. Exp. Ther.* **109:**8–20.

WINOKUR, G., CLAYTON, P. J., and REICH, T., 1969, *Manic Depressive Illness*, C. V. Mosby, St. Louis.

WINOKUR, G., REICH, T., RIMMER, J., and PITTS, F. N., 1970, Alcoholism. III. Diagnosis and familial psychiatric illness in 259 alcoholic probands, *Arch. Gen. Psychiat.* **23:**104–111.

WOLF, H. G., and HARDY, J. D., 1947, On the nature of pain, *Physiol. Rev.* **27:**167–199.

WOLF, H. G., HARDY, J. D., and GOODELL, H., 1940, Studies on pain, measurement of the effect of morphine, codeine, and other opiates on pain threshold and an analysis of their relation to the pain experience, *J. Clin. Invest.* **9:**659–680.

WOODFORDE, J. M., and MERSKEY, H., 1972, Personality traits of patients with chronic pain, *J. Psychosom. Res.* **16:**167–172.

WOODRUFF, R. A., GOODWIN, D. W., and GUZE, S. B., 1974, *Psychiatric Diagnosis*, Oxford Univ. Press, New York.

WOODS, L. A., 1954, Distribution and fate of morphine in non-tolerant and tolerant dogs and rats, *J. Pharmacol. Exp. Ther.* **112:**158.

YERKES, R. M., and DODSON, J. D., 1908, The relationship of strength of stimulus to rapidity of habit formation, *J. Comp. Neurol. Psychol.* **18:**459–482.

ZBOROWSKI, M., 1952, Cultural components in responses to pain, *J. Social Issues* **8:**16–30.

4

SEDATIVE–HYPNOTICS: ANIMAL PHARMACOLOGY

Roger A. Nicoll

1. INTRODUCTION

1.1. Definition

The separate classification of CNS depressants into general anesthetics and sedative–hypnotics is based primarily on clinical usage, which in turn is determined largely by pharmacokinetic factors. Thus, volatile anesthetics are not used as sedative–hypnotics because of difficulties with administration and short duration of action, and the sedative–hypnotics, although anesthetics in higher doses, are not routinely used as anesthetics in humans, except for induction, because there is less control over the level of anesthesia. The progressive dose-related effects of all CNS depressants may be indicated as follows: sedation→hypnosis→anesthesia→coma→death. These different states lie on a continuum and, except for an early excitatory phase that is often seen with many agents, there is no convincing evidence that the drug actions that produce sedation are qualitatively any different from those that produce anesthesia for a particular agent. Therefore, much of the research on CNS depressants has focused on their anesthetic action with the belief that such results will also apply to their sedative–hypnotic action.

Placement of drugs in the sedative–hypnotic category implies that their major therapeutic applications are in producing drowsiness and a state of CNS depression resembling normal sleep. Included in this class are such

Roger A. Nicoll • Department of Pharmacology and Physiology, University of California, San Francisco, San Francisco, California 94143.

drugs as the barbiturates, piperidinediones, carbamates, alcohols, quinazolones, and cyclic ethers. There have been a number of excellent articles and symposia covering the general properties of sedative–hypnotics and anesthetics (Way and Trevor, 1971; Goth, 1974; Halsey *et al.*, 1974; Fink, 1975; Harvey, 1975; Mori, 1975). Two chapters in Section III of this *Handbook* deal specifically with alcohol, and another is devoted to the clinical aspects of sedative–hypnotics. The antianxiety drugs, such as the benzodiazepines, which are often included in the sedative–hypnotic group (Way and Trevor 1971), are considered separately in this volume. In this chapter I will concentrate mainly on the cellular mechanism of action of the barbiturates. This restricted scope seems justified for three reasons: First, the barbiturates are one of the oldest and still one of the most effective group of sedative–hypnotics. Second, an enormous body of literature exists on the action of barbiturates. Third, by concentrating on one class, a rather complete account of our present knowledge can be given.

1.2. Nature of the Problem

The discovery that certain agents can reversibly disrupt consciousness has been one of the most intriguing and mysterious puzzles in all of medicine. Aside from the enormous practical benefits derived from the discovery of such agents, e.g., painless surgery, sedation, etc., the mechanism by which these agents produce unconsciousness provides a constant stimulus to the study not only of the site of action of these drugs but also of the more philosophical questions concerning the basis of consciousness. It has often been said in the past that the action of these drugs will not be understood until the basis of consciousness is elucidated. While this may be true, it is quite clear that irrespective of the numerous unanswered questions related to consciousness, consciousness depends on the activity of nerve cells. Silencing neurons or withdrawing their oxygen supply will invariably lead to a loss of consciousness. This fact, although not fully appreciated, was known to the Greeks; the word "carotid," which in Greek means "to stupefy," indicates that they were aware of the consequence of occlusion of these arteries. While it is accepted that some areas of the CNS are more important than others in maintaining wakefulness and consciousness, e.g., the reticular activating system, it is equally well established that CNS depressant agents are rather evenly distributed throughout the CNS and affect all neuronal systems. Thus, it seems reasonable to postulate that the unconsciousness that results from these agents may merely be one obvious and dramatic expression of a generalized action on all parts of the CNS and, indeed, possibly on all cells in an organism (cf. Seeman, 1972). If the reticular activating system is more vulnerable than specific sensory pathways, the difference is presumably a quantitative one owing to the polysynaptic and diffuse nature of the reticular activating system, rather than to some unique property found only in this system. Our ultimate goal, then, is to explain the cellular and molecular mechanism of this generalized neuronal depression. To answer these broad questions we are forced to go to simpler systems and models where such problems can be solved.

1.3. General Properties of CNS Depressants

A remarkable feature of CNS depressants is that there is no structural similarity shared by this group of chemicals. Furthermore, many of these agents are essentially chemically inert. With these facts in mind it is clear that we are not dealing primarily with specific receptor mechanisms, but rather with some physiochemical property that these compounds have in common. The classic observations by Meyer (1899) and Overton (1896, 1901) demonstrated that the ability of a particular agent to produce anesthesia is directly correlated to its lipid solubility. Since all membranes are rich in lipids it was concluded that anesthesia commences when a critical concentration of an agent is present in cell membranes. This concept, based on the lipid solubility or, more precisely, on the hydrophobic properties of anesthetics, with later modifications (cf. Mullins, 1975), has remained the only satisfactory theory for linking this diverse group of chemicals together.

However, it is quite clear that other factors must also play a role, especially in the case of the agents commonly used as sedative–hypnotics. For instance, Richards and Hesketh (1975) have shown that the depressant action of an anesthetic steroid on synaptic transmission can be antagonized by a nonanesthetic steroid, a finding not predicted by current theories of anesthesia. Slight changes in the structure of the barbiturate molecule convert a predominantly depressant agent into a predominantly excitant agent (Ariens, 1964; Downes and Williams, 1969; Downes *et al.*, 1970). Even more surprising is the finding that isomers of the same barbiturate molecule have strikingly different anesthetic potencies, and may even have opposite CNS effects, although they are present in the brain in similar concentrations (Gibson *et al.*, 1959; Wahlstrom, 1968; Downes *et al.*, 1970; Buch *et al.*, 1973; Christensen and Lee, 1973; Grossmann *et al.*, 1974; Daves *et al.*, 1975; Freudenthal and Martin, 1975). All of these findings suggest that specific receptor mechanisms may also play an important role in determining the action of many of these drugs.

It is often assumed that all agents that produce anesthesia do so by a common mechanism. However, the stereospecificity seen within certain groups of CNS depressants suggests that this may not be the case. Also, as Quastel and Linder (1975) have pointed out, the common mode of action implied by the Meyer–Overton rule of anesthesia does not seem to hold at the neuromuscular junction, since there is no single common action of CNS depressants in this system. For instance, barbiturates dramatically shorten the decay of miniature end plate potentials, while ethanol prolongs their decay.

1.4. Site of Action

Until recently, research on the mechanism of CNS depressants has proceeded along two rather independent lines of inquiry. Chemists have concentrated on the properties of the agents and on their molecular site of action, i.e., where in the membrane these agents act. Often, little distinction has been made between different membrane preparations. On the other hand, neurophysiologists have been concerned with the cellular site of action, i.e., what step in the neuronal chain of events is attacked by CNS depressants. This separation is becoming less apparent as the studies in these two areas become more sophisticated. A common goal of the two disciplines is to explain CNS depression and anesthesia as alterations of specific neurophysiological events secondary to a particular molecular perturbation caused by the agent.

A fundamental dilemma in anesthesia research is to determine whether a particular pharmacological property of a depressent is related to its anesthetic action. Since these depressants, especially in high concentrations, will affect all biological processes, the question of possible relevance to the mechanism of anesthesia assumes critical importance. The elucidation of such relevance is generally approached in two ways. First, it is important to determine the concentration that is necessary for an agent to produce its effect. If the concentration is many times higher than that which is normally found in the brain during anesthesia, it is unlikely that this action is of prime importance in the production of anesthesia. However, this approach does not ensure that those effects produced by appropriate concentrations of anesthetics are related to their depressant action. Second, a comparison can be made with a series of agents of the concentrations needed to produce a given effect and to produce anesthesia. A good correlation should exist if the effect studied is important in causing anesthesia. However, as mentioned above, the possibility must be kept in mind that overall gross effects of different groups of agents on the CNS may not necessarily be produced by a common mechanism.

2. AXONS

Studies of the action of CNS depressants on the physiology of axons have often been extrapolated in order to explain the actions of depressants in the CNS. This approach emphasizes the common blocking action of a wide variety of agents, including local and general anesthetics, on the axonal action potential. Indeed, this blocking action, which occurs without any appreciable change in membrane potential, has even been used as the sole criterion for defining an anesthetic agent (cf. Seeman, 1972). In particular, barbiturates are known to block excitation in peripheral nerve (Heinbecker and Bartley, 1940; Schoepfle, 1957). Voltage clamp studies on lobster giant axons (Blaustein, 1968) and squid giant axons (Narahashi *et al.*, 1969) indicate that barbiturates decrease and prolong the early transient (sodium) current. The late steady-state (potassium) current is also decreased to a similar extent. The barbiturates are more potent and act more quickly when applied internally than when applied externally, suggesting an internal site of action (Narahashi *et al.*, 1971; Frazier *et al.*, 1975). It is also generally believed that the uncharged molecular form is responsible for the blocking action (Krupp *et al.*, 1969; Narahashi *et al.*, 1971; but see Blaustein, 1968). No difference in the time course of the blocking action has been found between short and long acting barbiturates (Frazier *et al.*, 1975). Thus, differences in the ability to penetrate nerve membranes does not appear to be important in explaining the differential effects of these barbiturates in the CNS.

A major problem in attempting to relate these findings to the CNS effects of barbiturates is that the concentrations necessary for general anesthesia are about 5% of the concentrations used in the above experiments and, indeed, there is no functional change in peripheral nerves or spinal afferent volleys during anesthesia (Thornton *et al.*, 1963; Løyning *et al.*, 1964). Since these experiments have been conducted on large fibers, one explanation is that the smaller fibers and nerve terminals in the CNS are more vulnerable (Frank and Sanders, 1963; Frank, 1968; Seeman, 1972). Indeed, it is a general and well-documented finding that for local anesthetics small fibers are more susceptible to blockade than large fibers (cf. Seeman, 1972). Recently, Staiman and Seeman (1974) have analyzed this differential effect with a variety of agents and found that phrenic nerves (mean diameter of 11 μm) are more susceptible than sciatic nerves (mean diameter of 16 μm). In particular, the concentration of pentobarbital causing a 50% block was 0.8 mM for the sciatic nerve and 0.4 mM for the phrenic nerve, the latter value approaching the concentrations generally considered to exist during pentobarbital anesthesia (approximately 0.1 to 0.2 mM) (Fisher *et al.*, 1948; Jori *et al.*, 1970; Richards, 1972; Saubermann *et al.*, 1974). Thus, it could be postulated that the size of the action potential in fine presynaptic terminals is reduced by the barbiturates and, since the amount of transmitter released from a synapse is governed by the size of the action potential, less transmitter would be released in the presence of barbiturates.

3. SYNAPSES

3.1. General Effects on Transmission

It has long been recognized that barbiturates have a very selective action on synaptic transmission. The most detailed studies have been performed on the spinal monosynaptic reflex (Eccles, 1946; Brooks and Eccles, 1947; Somjen, 1963; Somjen and Gill, 1963; Løyning, *et al.*, 1964; Shapovalov, 1963; Weakly, 1969) and it has been shown that the reduction of the monosynaptic reflex (Fig. 1A) and excitatory postsynaptic potential (EPSP) (Fig. 1B,C) occur without any changes in the conduction of nerve impulses along sensory or motor axons. A reduction of excitatory synaptic transmission has been demonstrated at a number of other sites in the CNS, including the cuneate nucleus (Galindo, 1969), olfactory bulb (Nicoll, 1972), olfactory cortex (Richards, 1972; Scholfield and Harvey, 1975), and cerebellum (Gordon *et al.*, 1973). Larrabee and Posternak (1952) have shown that concentrations of pentobarbital that completely block transmission through sympathetic ganglia have no effect on the nerve compound action potential. Figure 2A shows this selective action in the cat stellate ganglion, while the records in Fig. 2C are from a rat superior cervical ganglion. Since the pre-

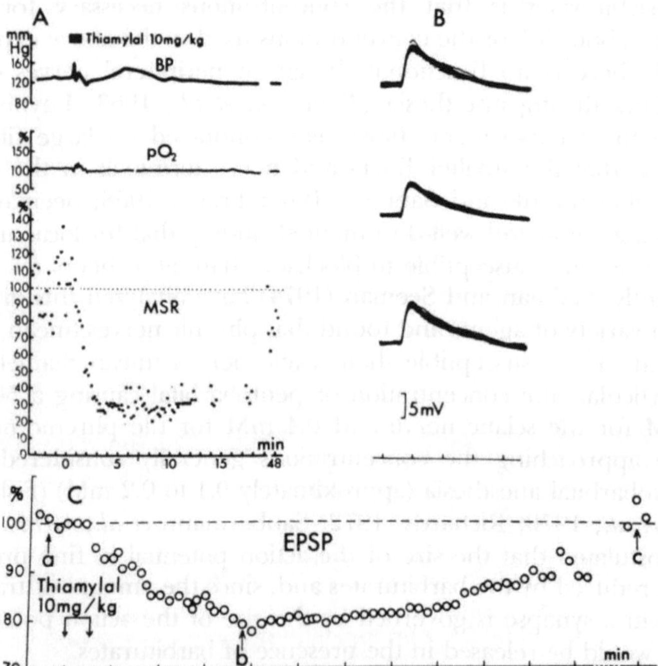

FIG. 1. Effects of thiamylal on the spinal monosynaptic reflex and EPSP. (A) The effect on blood pressure, oxygen tension in the spinal cord, and the monosynaptic reflex. The monosynaptic reflex was evoked by a single volley to the posterior-biceps-semitendinosus nerve and recorded from the L_7 ventral root. (B and C) The effect on the monosynaptic EPSP in the flexor hallucis and digitorum longus motoneuron. In C the EPSP sizes are plotted before and after an injection of 10 mg/kg thiamylal. The top record in B was recorded before the injection (arrow "a" in C), the middle and bottom records were recorded after the injection at the times indicated by arrows "b" and "c" in C. The time scale in B is in msec. (Løyning *et al.*, 1964.)

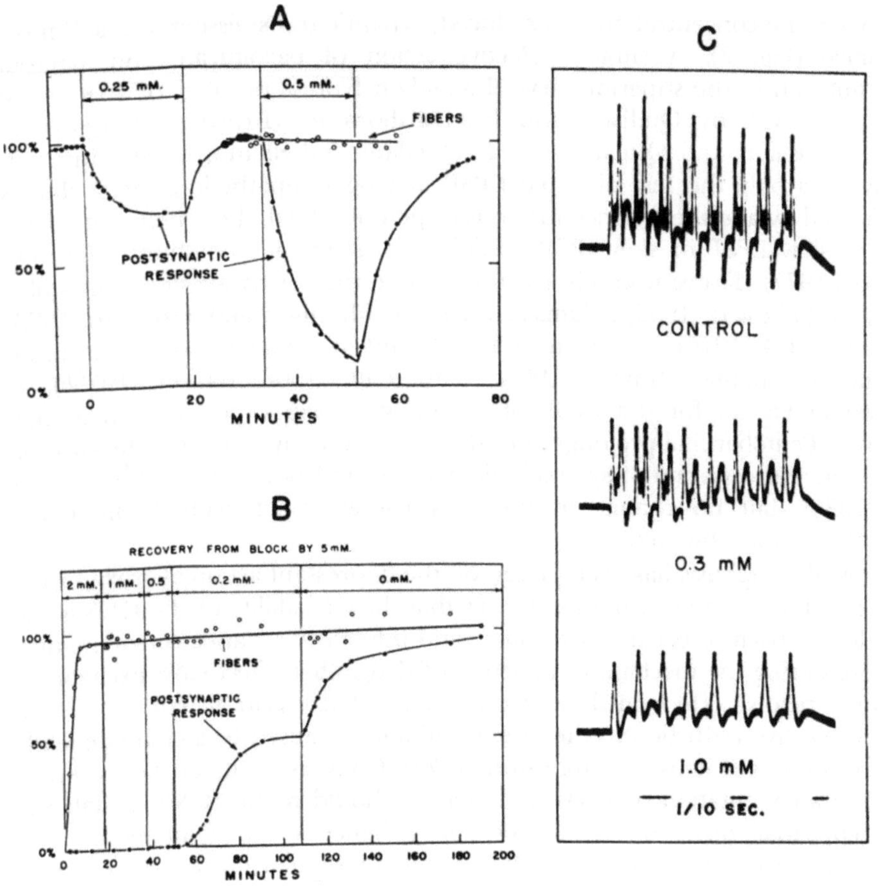

FIG. 2. Selective action of sodium pentobarbital (Nembutal) on synapses in sympathetic ganglia. Stimulation applied to preganglionic nerve. (A and B) Experiments on perfused stellate ganglia of cats. Ordinates represent heights of action potentials of impulses discharged from ganglion cells over postsynaptic fibers ("fibers"). (A) Application and removal of two concentrations of pentobarbital. (B) Stepwise reductions in concentration after application of pentobarbital in a concentration sufficient to block conduction over direct fibers as well as the postsynaptic response. (C) Records from excised superior cervical ganglion of rat. Presynaptic and postsynaptic nerve action potentials in response to repetitive stimulation of the presynaptic nerve, in the absence of anesthetic ("control") and in the presence of two concentrations of pentobarbital. The action potentials normally recur in pairs, the first being the presynaptic nerve action potential and the second the postsynaptic action potential. (The latter is the highest in the control records.) Only the postsynaptic potential was greatly reduced by the anesthetic. (Larrabee and Posternak, 1952.)

and postsynaptic fibers in the rat are both unmyelinated, the selective action cannot be explained by a block of conduction in the postsynaptic fibers. Furthermore, the differential effect cannot be attributed only to differences in time for the effects to develop, because in Fig. 2B the ganglion was initially exposed to a concentration of pentobarbital that blocked both responses and yet when the concentration was reduced, synaptic transmission was still more sensitive (Fig. 2). A similar selective action of barbiturates on synaptic transmission in the superior cervical ganglion from a number of species has been observed by Quilliam and his collaborators (Brown and Quilliam, 1964*a,b*; Elliott and Quilliam, 1964; Quilliam and Shand, 1964). Interestingly, it is only the fast nicotinic EPSP in frog sympathetic ganglia that is depressed by anesthetic concentrations of pentobarbital, there being no effect on the slow EPSP or slow IPSP (inhibitory postsynaptic potential) (Fig. 3A) (Nicoll, 1977). Transmission is also impaired at the vertebrate neuromuscular junction (Thesleff, 1956; Adams *et al.*, 1970; Thomson and Turkanis, 1973; Adams, 1974, 1976), as shown in Fig. 4, and at a number of invertebrate excitatory synapses (Iravani, 1965*b*; Sato *et al.*, 1968; Barker, 1975*b*), as shown in Fig. 5, for the EPSP of a biphasic synaptic potential in a snail neuron. Pentobarbital prolongs both the rise and decay of heart rate with the initiation and cessation of sympathetic nerve stimulation in the cat (Cowan *et al.*, 1975), but no change in the maximal effect of sympathetic nerve stimulation was observed.

While emphasis has been placed on the depressant action of barbiturates on excitatory synaptic action, it is clear that the excitability of the CNS is the result of a balance between excitatory and inhibitory synaptic activity. Thus, in considering the mechanism of action of drugs that affect CNS excitability, it is the relative effect on these two processes that is critical. For instance, a slight selective reduction in the level of inhibition caused by strychnine leads to convulsions (Curtis and Johnston, 1974). Conversely, it can be expected that an augmentation of synaptic inhibition should reduce CNS excitability. Indeed, small doses of barbiturates do enhance synaptic inhibition at a number of sites. The recurrent IPSP in spinal motoneurons is prolonged by

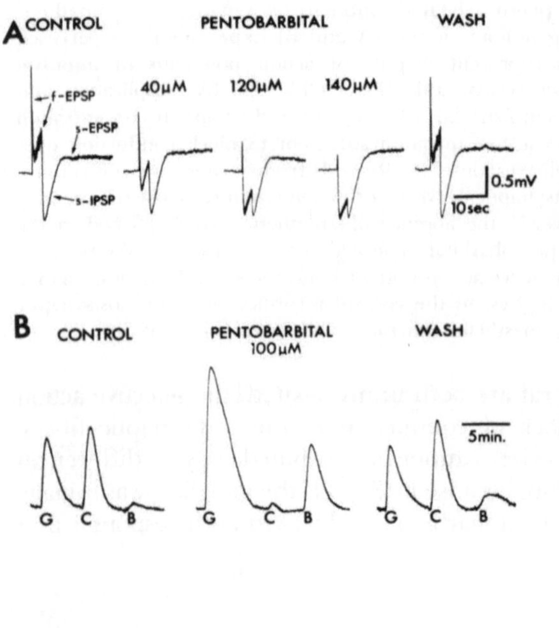

FIG. 3. Differential postsynaptic effects of pentobarbital on frog sympathetic ganglion. (A) Increasing concentrations of pentobarbital markedly depress the fast EPSP, but have no effect on the slow EPSP or slow IPSP. (B) Brief applications of carbachol (C), GABA (G), and β-alanine (B) depolarize the ganglion. Pentobarbital (10^{-4} M) blocks the carbachol response, but augments the GABA and β-alanine responses. Carbachol (2×10^{-5} M) was applied for 15 sec, GABA (4×10^{-5} M) for 10 sec, and β-alanine (2×10^{-4} M) for 30 sec. The voltage calibration in B is the same as in A. (Nicoll, unpublished.)

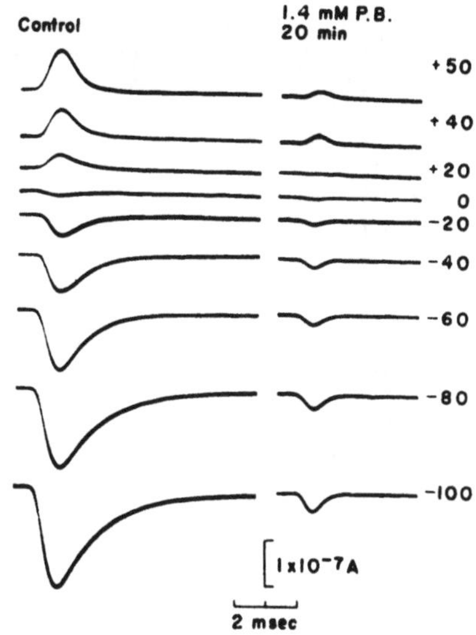

FIG. 4. Effect of pentobarbital on the end plate current of the frog neuromuscular junction. Families of end plate currents recorded at various membrane potentials are shown on the right (millivolts) before and after application of 1.4 mM pentobarbital (PB). Downward deflection shows inward current. Excitation-contraction coupling was blocked after treatment with ethylene glycol. Ringer's solution containing 10 mM Mg was used as the bathing medium. (Seyama and Narahashi, 1975.)

hexobarbital (Larson and Major, 1970). In the olfactory bulb, doses of barbiturate that are without effect on the EPSP in this structure markedly prolong postsynaptic inhibition, anesthetic doses causing a four- to fivefold lengthening of this inhibition (Nicoll, 1972). An important observation was that the enhancement of synaptic inhibition could be demonstrated even when synaptic excitation was severely depressed. As shown in Fig. 6, pentobarbital has a similar action on the IPSP in hippocampal neurons

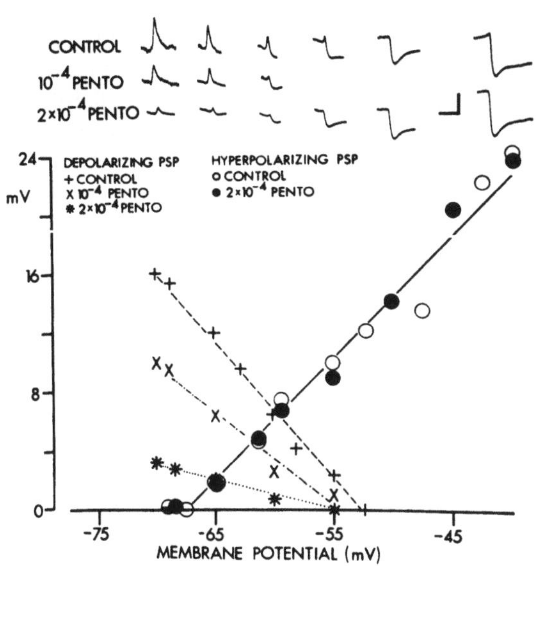

FIG. 5. Pentobarbital selectively depresses the depolarizing phase of a biphasic PSP in a snail neuron. The amplitudes of the de- and hyperpolarizing phases of the biphasic PSP recorded in cell 11 are graphed as a function of the membrane potential for control and 0.1 and 0.2 mM pentobarbital. Specimen records of the PSPs above the potentials at which they were recorded. Calibration: 10 mV, 5 sec. (Barker, 1975*b*.)

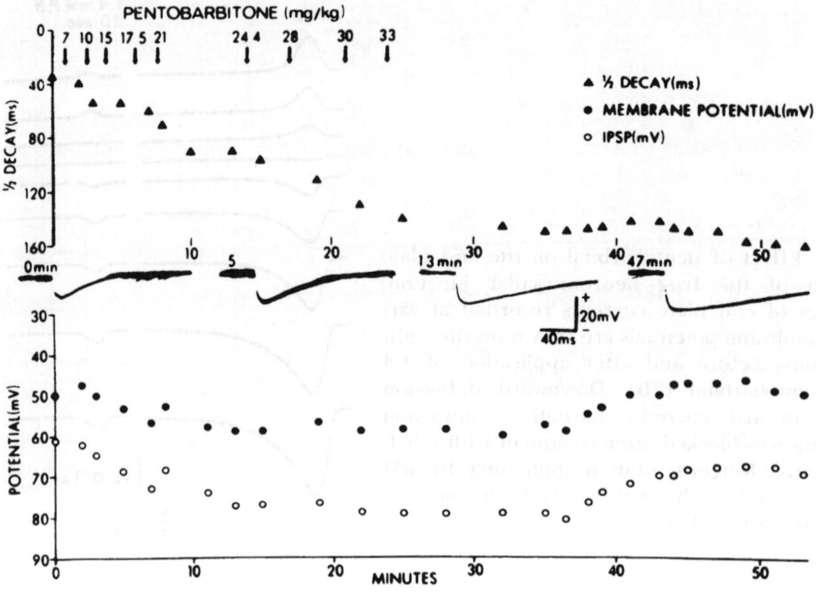

FIG. 6. Prolongation of IPSP in a hippocampal pyramidal cell by pentobarbital. The top graph plots the ½ decay of the IPSP (▲), while the bottom graph plots the membrane potential (●) and peak of the IPSP (○) The time scale applies to both graphs. Sample film records, taken at the indicated times, are shown between the graphs. The cumulative dose (mg/kg) of pentobarbital after each injection is shown at top of figure. (Nicoll *et al.,* 1975.)

(Nicoll *et al.*, 1975). Postsynaptic inhibition at a number of other sites in the CNS may also be increased. These pathways include the recurrent inhibition of cortical pyramidal tract neurons (Veselyunene *et al.*, 1971; Steriade *et al.*, 1974), the recurrent inhibition of thalamic relay neurons (Andersen *et al.*, 1964; Bremer, 1970), the basket cell inhibition of cerebellar Purkinje cells (Bloedal and Roberts, 1969; Eccles *et al.*, 1971), and the olfactory cortex (Scholfield, 1977). However, the inhibition of cortical neurons following direct cortical stimulation is not apparently consistently changed by pentobarbital (Krnjević *et al.*, 1966). Except for the recurrent inhibition of spinal motoneurons, which is mediated by the inhibitory transmitter, glycine, all of the other inhibitory pathways referred to above are thought to release GABA (Curtis and Johnston, 1974; Krnjević, 1974).

Eccles and Malcolm (1946), using the isolated frog spinal cord, were the first to demonstrate that pentobarbital greatly prolongs the decay of the dorsal root potential. This finding has been confirmed in numerous studies, both in the frog (Schmidt, 1963, 1964; Grinnell, 1966; Richens, 1969*a*; Nicoll, 1975*a*) and in the cat (Lloyd, 1952; Eccles *et al.*, 1963). It is now well established that the synaptic depolarization of primary afferents that produces the dorsal root potential results in a presynaptic inhibition of the primary afferents (Eccles, 1964), and GABA is thought to be the transmitter acting on the primary afferent terminals (Davidson and Southwick, 1971; Davidoff, 1972; Barker and Nicoll, 1972, 1973; Barker *et al.*, 1975*b*). Thus, presynaptic inhibition in the spinal cord is prolonged to the same extent as the dorsal root potential in the presence of pentobarbital (Eccles *et al.*, 1963; Miyahara *et al.*, 1966; Nicoll, 1975*a*). Presynaptic inhibition in the cuneate nucleus (Banna and Jabbur, 1969) and the primary afferent depolarization in the solitary tract nucleus (Rudomin, 1966) are also enhanced by pentobarbital.

This action of pentobarbital on presynaptic inhibition in the frog spinal cord is shown in Fig. 7. In the frog, stimulation of the ventral root activates a pathway that synaptically depolarizes the primary afferent terminals. This depolarization, as recorded from the dorsal root, is shown in the top trace of Fig. 7. A microelectrode carefully placed near the primary afferent terminals will also record this depolarizing action (second trace). The synaptic action of the primary afferents is depressed during this depolarization. This is shown in the third trace where the focally recorded EPSP is reduced when it is elicited during the dorsal root potential. In the presence of pentobarbital the depolarization of the primary afferents and the presynaptic inhibition of the EPSP are increased *pari passu*.

On the other hand, as shown in Fig. 5, concentrations of pentobarbital that severely depress EPSPs apparently have no effect on IPSPs at a number of invertebrate synapses (Barker, 1975*b*), and Iravani (1965*b*) reported that the IPSP of crustacean muscle was actually reduced by barbiturates. Weakly *et al.* (1967), using monosynaptic testing, were unable to detect a specific change in the direct inhibition of cat spinal motoneurons. However, their test monosynaptic response was elicited at an interval of only 0.4 to 0.7 msec after

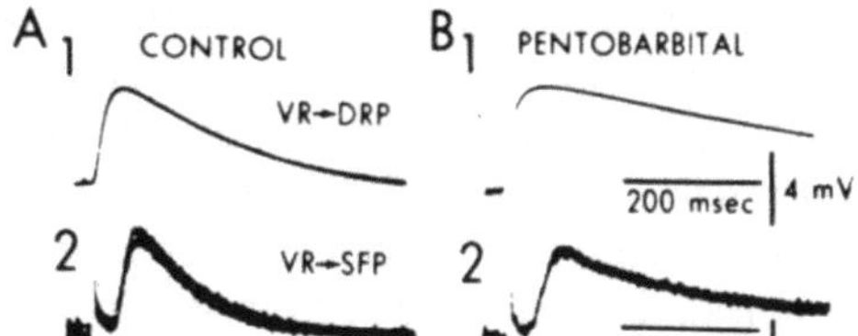

FIG. 7. Effect of pentobarbital on presynaptic inhibition. (A) Top trace (A_1) is the dorsal root potential elicited by ventral root stimulation (VR-DRP), the middle trace (A_2) is the accompanying field potential recorded in the dorsal horn with an extracellular microelectrode (SFP, slow field potential), and lower trace (A_3) shows the focally recorded pre- and postsynaptic responses, obtained from the same site, to stimulation of the dorsal root. Superimposed on the control response ("DR alone") is the response obtained 100 msec after a conditioning ventral root stimulus. The calibration pulse is 0.5 mV and 1 msec. (B) The same responses elicited 20 min after addition of 50 μM pentobarbital. In all traces negativity is up, signifying depolarization. (Nicoll, 1975*a*.)

the inhibitory volley and would arrive prior to the peak of the IPSP. Therefore, any change in the duration of the inhibition would have been missed. The effect of barbiturates on reticulospinal inhibition of motoneurons is not entirely clear. Frank and Ohta (1971) report that this pathway is particularly sensitive to depressant action of barbiturates, while other investigators have seen depression of this pathway only with relatively large doses of barbiturate (Ricci and Zanchetti, 1953; Brooks *et al.*, 1956; Valdman and Arushanyan, 1967). It has been speculated that the prime effect of small doses of thiopental on the electroretinogram is a result of a selective depression of inhibitory cells (Knave and Persson, 1974), but inhibitory processes were not directly examined in these studies.

The above-mentioned studies suggest that, in general, excitatory synaptic transmission is depressed by barbiturates, while inhibitory synaptic transmission is usually preserved or enhanced depending on the synapse examined. An important question concerns the mechanism by which barbiturates produce these changes in synaptic transmission. The processes that could be modified include (1) release of transmitter, (2) postsynaptic sensitivity of transmitter, and (3) excitability of the postsynaptic membrane. It will be shown that, depending on the concentration and site, barbiturates can alter all three of these parameters.

3.2. Presynaptic Effects

3.2.1. Spinal Monosynaptic Reflex

Since the spinal monosynaptic reflex has received the most rigorous analysis, it will be considered in detail and these results will be compared with results obtained at other synapses. In the original studies on barbiturate action in the spinal cord it was shown that the focally recorded presynaptic volley is depressed by pentobarbital (Brooks and Eccles, 1947). This was not considered to be the primary site of action because it was seen only with high doses. However, in later, more detailed studies with small doses of barbiturate, this action on the primary afferent terminals, as illustrated in Fig. 8A, was found to be the only effect that could adequately account for the depression of the EPSP (Løyning, *et al.*, 1964; Richens, 1969*b*; but see Somjen, 1963). A selective presynaptic action in this pathway was clearly established by Weakly (1969). By analyzing quantal synaptic transmission, he showed that with small subanesthetic doses (10 mg/kg) of thiopental and pentobarbital the mean quantum content of the unitary EPSP is reduced by about 25%, while there is no change in the average amplitude of the unitary EPSP. Furthermore, there is no change in the input resistance of the motoneuron membrane or the strength–duration relation. Thus, with this dose of barbiturate the effect is entirely confined to the presynaptic terminals, resulting in a reduction in the amount of transmitter released. The antagonism of the depressant action of pentobarbital on the monosynaptic

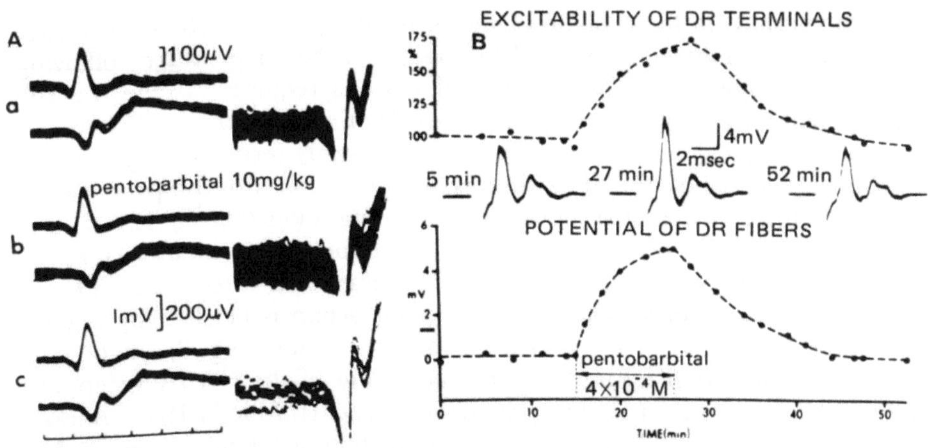

FIG. 8. Effects of barbiturates on the motor nucleus focal potentials and the excitability of primary afferents. (A) The focal potential in the cat spinal cord was evoked by a maximum group Ia afferent volley from the gastrocnemius-soleus nerve and recorded with a low resistance (2 MΩ) NaCl-filled microelectrode placed in the gastrocnemius-soleus motor nucleus at L_7 level. In the left-hand column the upper trace shows the potential recorded on the cord surface and the lower trace is the focal potential. The initial negative spike component is shown with a higher amplification on the right: (b) About 5 min and (c) 2 hr after the injection of 10 mg/kg pentobarbital. Time scale: 0.5 msec. Voltage calibration: 100 μV for trace at right. (Løyning *et al.*, 1964.) (B) The effect of pentobarbital on the membrane potential and the excitability of primary afferents in the frog. Addition of 4×10^{-4} M pentobarbital reversibly increases the excitability of dorsal root terminals (B), the excitability increase having the same time course as the depolarization of the neighboring dorsal root recorded simultaneously across the sucrose gap (B_2). The inserts show samples of the antidromic volley elicited by a stimulating microelectrode located in the dorsal horn. (Nicoll, 1975*a*.)

reflex by catechol (Banna, 1970), a substance that is considered to increase release of transmitter (Otsuka and Nonomura, 1963; Banna and Jabbur, 1972), supports this conclusion.

There are two mechanisms by which the barbiturates could exert their presynaptic action. First, they could decrease the size and/or block terminal invasion of the action potential or second, they could interfere directly with the release mechanism, possibly by blocking calcium influx and/or action. There is no information available at this site for the second alternative. However, the data of Løyning *et al.* (1964) strongly suggest that, although the action potential invades the terminals, its size is reduced. They suggested that barbiturates could be acting like local anesthetics (see Section 2). However, if this were the case, the excitability of the terminals should have been depressed (see Curtis and Ryall, 1966*a*) and yet no change in excitability was detected. On the other hand, Galindo (1969) has reported a decrease in the excitability of primary afferent terminals in the cuneate nucleus. It should be mentioned that stability is a problem in assessing possible presynaptic membrane effects *in vivo* with excitability testing (Wall,

1958). Small shifts in the position of the stimulating microelectrode will alter the size of the antidromic volley. The changes in blood pressure following barbiturate injections and the prolonged periods required to see the full action of barbiturates limit the usefulness of this technique *in vivo*. However, in the isolated spinal cord of the frog one can directly record changes in the membrane potential of primary afferents, and the stability of the preparation is superior to *in vivo* preparations. In this preparation (Nicoll, 1975*a*) low concentrations of pentobarbital (2×10^{-5} M) depolarize primary afferents, possibly by a direct action, and this depolarization is associated with an increase in terminal excitability (Fig. 8B). This action is blocked by GABA antagonists, but not by the glycine antagonist, strychnine (Fig. 9), suggesting that the depolarization results from the activation of the GABA receptors, which are known to exist on the primary afferents (Davidoff, 1972; Barker and Nicoll, 1972, 1973). Interestingly, the depletion of GABA by semicarbazide treatment has no effect on the depressant action of barbiturates on the monosynaptic reflex (Banna, 1973), indicating that the release of endogenous GABA cannot account for the depressant action of barbiturates. Since the barbiturates activate the same receptors as does the presynaptic inhibitory transmitter, it is to be expected that the barbiturate-induced depolarization would decrease the size of the presynaptic action potential and the amount of transmitter released from the primary afferents. These results do not exclude a local anesthetic action that might be masked by the GABA-like action of pentobarbital and, indeed, with high concentrations the local anesthetic property of pentobarbital predominates (Nicoll, 1975*a*). To what extent can these findings at the spinal monosynaptic reflex be applied to other synapses? First, the changes in the presynaptic action potential will be

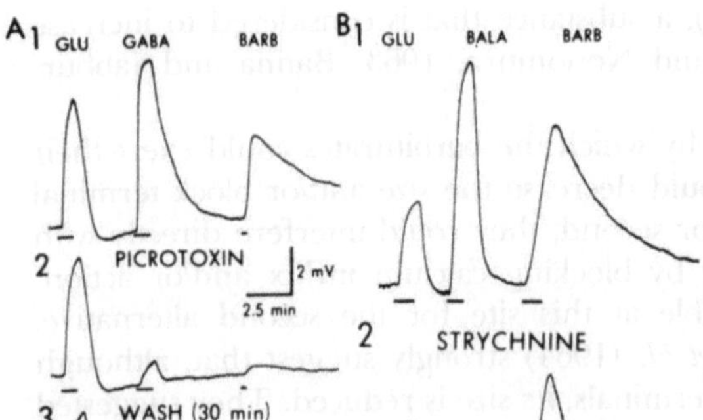

FIG. 9. Pharmacological characterization of the pentobarbital depolarization of primary afferents. (A_1) The control responses to glutamate (GLU) (1 mM), GABA (1 mM), and pentobarbital (BARB) (4 mM). (A_2) Addition of picrotoxin (0.5 mM) for 7 min markedly reduces the GABA and pentobarbital response but not the glutamate response. Washing the preparation (A_3 and A_4) progressively restores the antagonized responses. (B) The addition of strychnine (0.2 mM) for 12 min abolishes the β-alanine response (BALA) but not the glutamate or pentobarbital response. The calibration is the same as in A. (Nicoll, 1975*a*.)

considered, followed by the reduced release of transmitter, since, as will become apparent, these two actions need not invariably be linked.

3.2.2. Other Synapses

a. Changes in Presynaptic Action Potential. GABA-mediated presynaptic inhibition in the CNS is probably restricted to primary afferents in the spinal cord and brain stem (Schmidt, 1971). It remains to be established whether nerve terminals in the CNS, which do not receive presynaptic inhibition, have GABA receptors. However, presynaptic terminals in sympathetic ganglia have GABA receptors (Koketsu *et al.*, 1974; Suria and Costa, 1975), and no presynaptic inhibitory pathway exists in this structure. Moreover, GABA, but not glutamate or glycine, has been reported to increase chloride permeability in synaptosomes isolated from cerebral cortex (Tan, 1975). On the other hand, it appears that motor axon terminals in crab that do not receive presynaptic inhibition do not have GABA receptors (Parnas *et al.*, 1975). Richards (1972) has found no change in the size of the presynaptic spike (Fig. 10A) or in the excitability of presynaptic fibers accompanying the pentobarbital-induced depression of excitatory transmission in the olfactory cortex, while Scholfield and Harvey (1975) found that the presynaptic fibers were only slightly less sensitive than the synaptic potential to depression by barbiturates. There is also no change in the size of the presynaptic mossy fiber response in the cerebellum to small doses (4 to 8 mg/kg) of thiopental (Gordon *et al.*, 1973). In contrast, the lateral column terminals in the frog spinal cord are depressed by methohexital, but the simultaneously recorded postsynaptic response is actually increased in size, despite the reduced presynaptic volley (Richens, 1968). The dendrodendritic pathway in the olfactory bulb provides an unusual case in which the presynaptic element is dendritic, i.e., the mitral cell dendrite. In this pathway (Fig. 10B) the depression of the EPSP is invariably associated with a reduction in the size of the presynaptic dendritic response (Nicoll, 1972), suggesting that the reduction of the EPSP is, at least in part, a presynaptic action. The action of barbiturates on soma and dendritic excitability will be considered in detail later (Section 4). At the vertebrate neuromuscular junction (Fig. 10C) there is a small reduction in amplitude and an increase in duration of the presynaptic spike in the presence of phenobarbital (Thomson and Turkanis, 1973), but, at this site, release has actually been shown to increase during these changes in the presynaptic spike (see below). At the crustacean neuromuscular junction (Iravani, 1965*b*) pentobarbital produces a rather large decrease in the amplitude of the terminal action potential, not unlike the effect of GABA (Dudel, 1965), and also increases its duration. The thiobarbiturates also cause orthodromic repetitive firing of both the excitatory and inhibitory axon (Iravani, 1965*b*), and thus it was concluded that these axons are depolarized by thiobarbiturates.

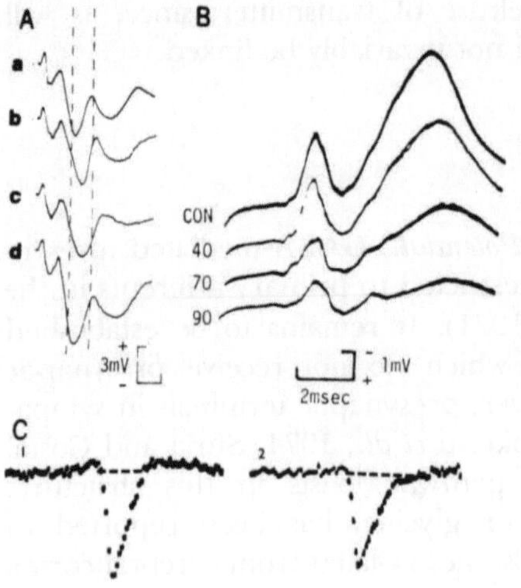

FIG. 10. Presynaptic action of barbiturates at a variety of synapses. (A) The effects of 0.25 mM pentobarbital on the evoked potentials of the guinea pig prepiriform cortex. A: (a) control, (b) after 6 min exposure to 0.25 mM pentobarbital, (c) after 18 min exposure to 0.25 mM pentobarbital, (d) recovery 45 min after removing pentobarbital from the incubation fluid. The first vertical interrupted line is drawn to indicate the (fixed) latency at which the EPSP was measured; the second is drawn 1 msec later and runs approximately through the peak of the first population spike of the control response a. The EPSP slope was reduced by pentobarbital and the first population spike decreased in magnitude and increased in latency. (Calibration: horizontal bar, 1 msec (Richards 1972). (B) The effect of increasing doses of hexobarbital on the mitral-to-granule dendritic EPSP in the olfactory bulb. The first deflection signifies the antidromic invasion of mitral cell dendrites, while the second negativity is due to the synaptic excitation of the granule cell dendrites in the external plexiform layer. Note that as the synaptic potential is depressed the antidromic invasion of the mitral cell dendrites is also depressed. Note also that negativity is up, in contrast to A. (Nicoll, 1972.) (C) The effect of phenobarbital (200 μm) on the nerve terminal action potential at the frog neuromuscular junction. Potentials recorded extracellularly with glass microelectrodes. Each trace represents the sum of 300 action potentials. The dashed line indicates the width of the negative phase of the action potential measured at the level of the baseline. (C_2) 120 min after phenobarbital. (Thomson and Turkanis, 1973.)

b. Release from Peripheral Synapses. The vertebrate neuromuscular junction provides the only site, other than the spinal monosynaptic pathway, where release has been examined neurophysiologically. In response to nerve stimulation the quantal content of the end plate potential increases in the presence of barbiturates (Quastel *et al.*, 1972; Thomson and Turkanis, 1973; Seyama and Narahashi, 1975; Proctor and Weakly, 1976). This increase in release, at a time when the amplitude of the presynaptic spike is somewhat reduced, has been attributed to the prolongation of the presynaptic action potential (Thomson and Turkanis, 1973). The frequency of spontaneous miniature end plate potentials also tends to increase in the presence of barbiturates at the vertebrate neuromuscular junction (Quastel *et al.*, 1971, 1972; Westmoreland *et al.*, 1971; Thomson and Turkanis, 1973) but decreases at the crustacean neuromuscular junction (Iravani, 1965*b*). The increase in spontaneous release might be related to the membrane fluidization produced by CNS depressants, which would favor fusion of the vesicular membrane to the nerve terminal membrane (Seeman, 1972). In this context it has been suggested that barbiturates and other CNS depressants can induce release of acetylcholine by a calcium-independent mechanism (Quastel *et al.*, 1971). Alternatively, the increase in frequency of miniature end plate potentials and in evoked release might be the result of a block in the uptake of calcium by mitochondria, since blockers of mitochondrial uptake produce a similar action (Almaes and Rahamimoff, 1975). Release of acetylcholine at the vertebrate neuromuscular junction by presynaptic nerve stimulation has, in addition, been measured chemically, and no significant change in release in the presence of barbiturates has been detected (Gergis *et al.*, 1972). Presumably, the small increase in release detected neurophysiologically is too subtle to be detected chemically with repetitive presynaptic stimulation.

Quastel *et al.* (1972) have examined the effects of barbiturates on graded release at the neuromuscular junction. Graded release, either by focal electrical polarization or by elevated potassium concentration, was monitored by the frequency of miniature end plate potentials. Barbiturates were found to depress the graded release of transmitter, but not that released by an action potential. It was proposed that the barbiturates and other CNS depressants interfered with depolarization secretion coupling, possibly by altering calcium influx. A possible explanation for this discrepancy between action-potential-evoked release and graded release may be found in the steep relationship that exists between presynaptic polarization and transmitter release (Quastel *et al.*, 1972). Thus, the effect of depolarization on the release process tends to become saturated with depolarization considerably below that which occurs with the presynaptic action potential. Whatever the explanation for this paradox, the findings suggest that results obtained with graded release, as with potassium, may not be directly applicable to action-potential-induced release of transmitter.

There are numerous studies in which release of transmitter has been measured chemically or by bioassay and the effect of barbiturates on this release has been determined. In the peripheral nervous system, release has been examined at the neuromuscular junction, the superior cervical ganglion, and the adrenal medulla. As mentioned above, barbiturates have little effect on action-potential-induced release of acetylcholine at the neuromuscular junction (Gergis *et al.*, 1972). At the superior cervical ganglion one study reported no reduction in acetylcholine release induced by presynaptic electrical stimulation in the presence of anesthetic concentrations of amylobarbital (Exley, 1954), while another study detected a halving of acetylcholine output in the presence of approximately 0.4 mM amylobarbital (Matthews and Quilliam, 1964). The explanation for these conflicting results is not clear. However, even if release is decreased, Brown and Quilliam (1964*b*) concluded that the block of transmission is largely a postsynaptic event. The fact that the depression of the fast nicotinic EPSP by anesthetic concentrations of pentobarbital is not associated with any change in the slow EPSP or slow IPSP (Fig. 3A), which are both dependent on the presynaptic release of acetylcholine suggests that there is no decrease in release (Nicoll, 1977).

Blaustein (1976) has found that 0.4 mM or greater pentobarbital blocks the preganglionic stimulation-induced uptake of ^{45}Ca by rat superior cervical ganglia but not the action-potential conduction in the preganglionic axons, suggesting that pentobarbital may block excitation–secretion coupling. Although this may be occurring at drug concentrations above the anesthetic level, the physiological evidence suggests that there is little effect on release with anesthetic concentrations of pentobarbital.

The effect of pentobarbital on catecholamine secretion from the adrenal gland has been examined in detail (Homes and Schneider, 1973). Concentrations of pentobarbital as low as 0.1 mM reduce the spontaneous release. Both acetylcholine- and potassium-induced release were inhibited by pentobarbital, 50% inhibition of the potassium-induced release occurring at a concentration of 0.15 mM. Acetylcholine receptor blockade cannot explain the inhibitory effect, since potassium-induced release was also blocked. Furthermore, it is unlikely that the pentobarbital inhibition is caused by a block in calcium flux, since pentobarbital had no effect on calcium-induced catecholamine release. It was therefore concluded that pentobarbital prevents a stimulus-induced alteration in the cell membrane, presumably by its membrane-stabilizing action. While these results clearly demonstrate that pentobarbital can inhibit secretory processes, it is unclear how closely secretion from the adrenal gland elicited by depolarizing agents parallels release from synaptic terminals. Release of inhibitory transmitter at a number of inhibitory synapses in invertebrates is presumably affected very little by pentobarbital, since there is no change in IPSPs in the presence of pentobarbital (Barker, 1975*b*; but see Iravani 1965*b*).

c. Release from Central Synapses. Most of the studies on barbiturate effects on transmitter release in the vertebrate CNS have been performed on tissue slices or synaptosomal preparations. These studies have usually examined the release of radioactive substances that have been accumulated by the tissue during a prior incubation. Since amino acids are known to be accumulated and released both by presynaptic nerve terminals and glial cells (cf. Minchin and Iversen, 1974; Roberts, 1974; Schon and Kelly, 1975), it cannot be assumed that the release is occurring solely from nerve terminals. Thus, caution must be exercised in interpreting these results. The effects observed depend both on the transmitter and on the stimulus used to release the transmitter. Electrically induced release of norepinephrine from cortical slices is unaffected by 0.1 mM pentobarbital (Lidbrink and Farnebo, 1973; Carmichael and Israel, 1975) but is reduced to 50% by a concentration of approximately 0.9 mM (Carmichael and Israel, 1975). The simultaneous release of acetylcholine in this study was more sensitive to pentobarbital, 50% inhibition being produced by approximately 0.5 mM. Phenobarbital was also shown to reduce the release of these two transmitters but was less potent than pentobarbital. The effects of barbiturates on the release of GABA and glutamate have been examined in detail by Cutler and his collaborators (Cutler and Dudzinski 1974, 1975; Cutler *et al.*, 1974). While pentobarbital has little effect on the spontaneous efflux of glutamate, the efflux of GABA is depressed by concentrations as slow as 0.01 mM. The electrically induced release of glutamate is unaffected by pentobarbital (5 mM), but GABA release was actually increased, at least in the presence of high pentobarbital concentrations (5 mM). On the other hand, quite different results were obtained when release was induced by the depolarizing agents, potassium and ouabain. Pentobarbital (5 mM) completely blocks potassium-induced release of glutamate and GABA. Amobarbital also blocks GABA release, with concentrations as low as 0.05 mM being effective. The release of GABA produced by ouabain was blocked by both pentobarbital and amobarbital, but not by pentobarbital. Although these results on potassium- and ouabain-stimulated efflux were interpreted as resulting from barbiturate blocking of a carrier-mediated membrane transport of GABA, it is possible that barbiturates block release by interfering with depolarization–secretion coupling. Such a conclusion was reached by Haycock *et al.* (1977) who found that the calcium-dependent release of [^{3}H]-NE and [^{14}C]-GABA was antagonized by pentobarbital. In this context, it has recently been shown that pentobarbital, but not phenobarbital, blocks the entry of labeled calcium ions into synaptosomes induced by depolarizing agents (Blaustein and Ector, 1975). Regardless of the mechanism whereby barbiturates block the release of amino acids by depolarizing agents, these results are in striking contrast to the effect of barbiturates on release provoked by electrical stimulation. This paradoxical situation is remarkably similar to that observed by Quastel *et al.* (1972) at the neuromuscular junction where action-potential-induced release of acetylcholine is increased, while potassium-induced release is decreased by pentobarbital. The explanation for this difference at the neuromuscular junction may also apply for the results from cortical slices.

Akert and his collaborators (1974) have compared synaptic morphology, as revealed by freeze-etched replicas, of barbiturate anesthetized and unanesthetized rat and cat. They have found that the relative number of vesicular attachment sites is strongly enhanced in the waking as compared with the anesthetized state. This presumed decrease in the release of transmitter during anesthesia undoubtedly results from the overall neuronal depression seen with anesthesia (see Section 5) and is not necessarily the result of a direct effect of barbiturates on the nerve terminals.

3.2.3. *Summary*

The variety of effects produced by barbiturates on the release of transmitter makes it difficult to reach any solid generalizations. This variability results both from differences in the techniques used to elicit release as well as from the tissue preparation used. However, it seems clear that the presynaptic effects of barbiturates differ both quantitatively and qualitatively at different presynaptic sites. The reason for these differences is not entirely clear but may be related to the size of the terminals and presence of GABA receptors. It is, perhaps, not surprising that different types of presynaptic terminals might respond differently to barbiturates. For instance, there is evidence that tetanus toxin can block the release of glycine and GABA, but not the release of excitatory transmitter (Curtis and DeGroat, 1968; Curtis *et al.*, 1973). There are also anatomical differences in the presynaptic membranes of excitatory and inhibitory terminals (Landis *et al.*, 1974; Landis and Reese, 1974). It has often been assumed, based largely on the results of Weakly (1969), obtained at the spinal monosynaptic reflex, that a decrease in transmitter release can be expected at all synapses. However, the spinal monosynaptic reflex pathway is not typical, and these results may not be applicable to other synapses that do not receive presynaptic inhibition. Indeed, if we assume that the electrically induced release of transmitter from brain slices most closely approximates the physicological release of transmitter, then there is little evidence that barbiturates in anesthetic concentrations depress the release of any putative transmitters in the CNS, and the release of GABA may even be increased. Furthermore, the preservation of inhibitory synaptic potentials in the presence of barbiturate both in the vertebrate and in invertebrate systems would suggest that there is not a decrease in the release of inhibitory transmitter. Results from the vertebrate neuromuscular junction also support the generalization that barbiturates do not decrease the release of transmitter.

3.3. Effects on Transmitter Action

3.3.1. Peripheral and Invertebrate Synapses

At the vertebrate neuromuscular junction barbiturates depress the size of the end plate potential (Thesleff, 1956; Galindo, 1971; Adams, 1974, 1976; Seyama and Narahashi, 1975), the miniature end plate potentials (Galindo, 1971; Westmoreland *et al.*, 1971; Thomson and Turkanis, 1973; Adams, 1974, 1976; Quastel and Linder, 1975), and the depolarization produced by exogenous cholinergic agonists (Quilliam, 1955; Thesleff, 1956; Adams *et al.*, 1970; Lee Son *et al.*, 1975; Adams, 1974, 1976; Seyama and Narahashi, 1975). The voltage clamp experiments of Seyama and Narahashi (1975) indicate that the reversal potential of the end plate current is unchanged by pentobarbital. An interesting observation is that barbiturates drastically accelerate the falling phase of end plate potentials and miniature end plate potentials (Adams, 1974, 1976; Quastel and Linder, 1975; Seyama and Narahashi, 1975). This effect is illustrated in Fig. 11A and B for the

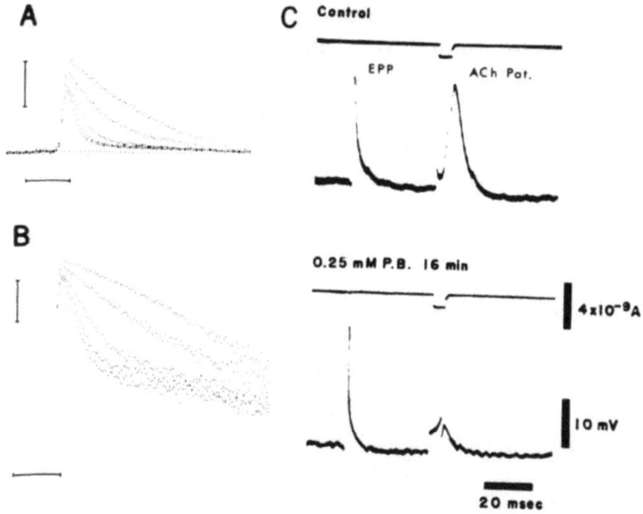

FIG. 11. The postsynaptic action of pentobarbital at the vertebrate neuromuscular junction. (A) Effect of pentobarbital on averaged miniature end plate currents in a mouse diaphragm muscle fiber. 0, 0.05, 0.2, 0.4, 0.8 mM pentobarbital; linear plot; different fibers; 60 mV. Calibration: 2 msec, 2 nA. (B) Semilogarithmic plot of data in A. Calibration: 2 msec, one natural logarithmic unit (Quastel and Linder, 1975). (C) Simultaneous recording of end-plate potential (EPP) and acetylcholine potential (ACh Pot.) before and after application of 0.25 mM pentobarbital (PB) to an end plate in frog sartorius muscle. The upper tracing of each set gives the current applied to the ACh pipet. Ringer's solution containing 10 mM Mg was used as the bathing medium. (Seyama and Narahashi, 1975.)

miniature end plate currents. Another surprising finding (Fig. 11C) is that the response to exogenous acetylcholine at the vertebrate neuromuscular junction is considerably more sensitive to barbiturates than is the end plate potential (Adams *et al.*, 1970; Adams, 1976; Seyama and Narahashi, 1975). This difference in sensitivity can be explained only in small part by the increased quantal content of the end plate potential which would counteract the decreased sensitivity of the end plate to acetylcholine.

A detailed analysis of barbiturate action on the neuromuscular junction has been made by Adams (1974, 1976), who proposed that barbiturates have a very high selectivity for binding to and blocking open-receptor-channel complexes. This attractive model explains why the decay of the end plate current is accelerated and why the much slower response to exogenously applied acetylcholine is more sensitive to barbiturates than the end plate current. Because the opening of channels during the end plate current is very fast, barbiturate molecules do not have time to enter and block during the rising phase, but are able to act during the falling phase. The rising phase of the response to exogenous acetylcholine is always much slower and therefore the barbiturate is able to block channels during the rising phase resulting in a diminished response. This model is also supported by the finding that barbiturates depress the dose–conductance curve to cholinergic agonists much more near the top than near the foot and that the conductance change elicited by a brief iontophoretic carbachol pulse is depressed by a prepulse of carbachol (Fig. 12).

From his study on the superior cervical ganglion, Exley (1954) concluded that amylobarbital blocked ganglionic transmission by an anticholinergic action, since this barbiturate blocked the excitatory actions of acetylcholine, but not potassium, and in anesthetic concentrations had no effect on the presynaptic release of acetylcholine. A similar more detailed study was done by Brown and Quilliam (1964*a,b*), who compared the depressant effects of amylobarbital and pentobarbital on the excitation of the superior cervical ganglion by presynaptic electrical stimulation, stimulation by cholinergic agonists, and stimulation by potassium ions. They found that these barbiturates had a highly selective anticholinergic action. In the frog sympathetic ganglion, the response to carbachol is reduced to a greater extent than the fast EPSP (Fig. 3B) (Nicoll, 1977), a finding similar to that observed at the frog neuromuscular junction (Adams, 1976). Downing (1972) has found that the peak of the dose–response curve to carbachol at the superior cervical ganglion is depressed by amylobarbital, 0.64 mM depressing the maximum value by 65.4%. Thus, it was concluded that amylobarbital does not compete for the nicotinic receptors. The selectivity of barbiturates for the nicotinic response, which is generated by a conductance increase to sodium and potassium ions, is emphasized by the fact that the slow muscarinic EPSP and slow IPSP (which is thought to be generated by an adrenergic interneuron) are unaffected by anesthetic concentrations of pentobarbital (Fig. 3A). Although the ionic mechanism of these slow potentials is controversial, they are clearly not due to an increase in ionic conductance.

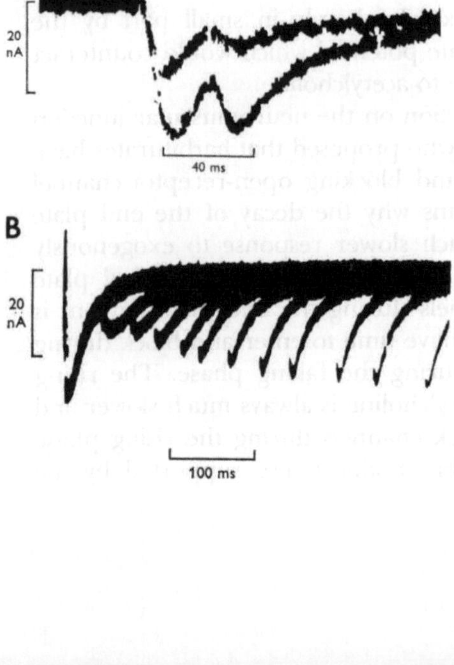

FIG. 12. Effect of amylobarbital on interpulse interaction between carbachol pulses. (A) Two closely spaced equiactive carbachol pulses were applied to a voltage-clamped end plate from separate barrels of a twin pipette. Superimposed on the control responses are the responses to the same pulses in the presence of amylobarbital (80 μM). Note that amylobarbital depressed the second response more than the first. (B) Decay of interpulse interaction. The records were obtained by superimposing responses to a variably delayed carbachol pulse following a carbachol prepulse in the presence of 120 μM amylobarbital. (Adams, 1976.)

The GABA depolarization of sympathetic ganglia which appears to be mediated by an increased conductance to chloride ions (Adams and Brown, 1975) has often been used as a model system for elucidating mechanisms of synaptic inhibition in the central nervous system. Bowery and Dray (1976) found that equilibrated responses to GABA were not effected or slightly reduced by pentobarbital. However, when the response had been blocked by picrotoxin or bicuculline, pentobarbital was found to restore the depressed response. They proposed that barbiturates and GABA antagonists act on a common site that in turn affects GABA receptors. While these findings could be confirmed on frog sympathetic ganglia using equilibrated responses, it was found that responses to brief applications of GABA were increased in amplitude at least twofold and prolonged by pentobarbital (Fig. 3B) (Nicoll, 1977).

Barker (1975*a*) has examined the effects of pentobarbital at a number of invertebrate synapses. Both the glutamate depolarization of crustacean muscle and the acetylcholine depolarization of snail neurons are antagonized in a noncompetitive manner by concentrations of pentobarbital that are considered to exist during anesthesia in vertebrates. Pentobarbital (0.1 mM) also inhibits the excitatory action of glutamate on the crayfish vas deferens (Heavner and Haschke, 1975). Since the glutamate and acetylcholine depolarizations are both due primarily to an increase in sodium conductance, but are elicited by different receptors, the antagonism is presumably occurring at the sodium channel or on the mechanism that couples the receptor to the sodium conductance. Pentobarbital in the same concentrations has no effect on responses generated by mechanisms other than an increase in sodium conductance. Thus, the chloride-mediated GABA response of crustacean muscle is unaffected, although Iravani (1965*a*) observed a competitive antagonism of the action of GABA with similar concentrations of pentobarbital. In snail neurons, chloride-dependent acetylcholine responses, potassium-dependent dopamine and glutamate responses, and 5-HT and acetylcholine responses, which are associated with a decrease in conductance, were all unaffected by concentrations of pentobarbital that markedly depressed sodium-dependent processes. These findings emphasize the fact that there is some property associated with the sodium conductance mechanism in these preparations that is uniquely sensitive to pentobarbital. It should be mentioned that this selectivity is not absolute and that in higher concentrations of pentobarbital, chloride-dependent responses are blocked (Iravani, 1965*a*; Sato *et al.*, 1967, 1968).

3.3.2. *Vertebrate Central Neurons*

a. Excitatory Responses. There are numerous studies on the interaction of barbiturates with putative transmitters in the CNS. Most of these studies have relied on iontophoretic techniques and have monitored the firing rate of neurons extracellularly. A limitation in these studies is that the depression of a response can either result from a direct antagonism of the response or it can be secondary to changes in the excitability of the neuronal membrane. Furthermore, there must also be a level of background activity upon which to observe an inhibitory effect, and this requirement limits the dose of barbiturate that can be given. Virtually all of the studies have shown that the excitatory action of putative transmitters on a wide variety of central neurons is depressed by barbiturates. These studies have examined the excitatory action of acetylcholine (Krnjević and Phillis, 1963; Bloom *et al.*, 1965; Curtis and Ryall, 1966*b*; Crawford and Curtis, 1966; Salmoiraghi and Stefanis, 1967; Phillis and Tebecis, 1967; Salmoiraghi and Weight, 1967; Crawford, 1969, 1970; Tebecis and DiMaria, 1972; Catchlove *et al.*, 1972; Bradley and Dray, 1973; Duggan *et al.*, 1974; Smaje, 1976), acidic amino acids (Crawford and Curtis, 1966; Phillis and Tebecis, 1967; Galindo, 1969; Bradley and Dray, 1973; Nicoll, 1975*b*; Ransom and Barker, 1975; Richards and Smaje, 1976), serotonin (Roberts and Straughan, 1967; Johnson *et al.*, 1969; Sampson and Jaffe, 1975), norepinephrine (Johnson *et al.*, 1969), and tryptamine (Marley and Vane, 1963). Considerable disagreement exists in the literature concerning whether barbiturates affect one type of excitation more than another. On the one hand, no difference in the effect of barbiturates on the excitation of cortical neurons by acetylcholine and acidic amino acids was detected (Curtis and Crawford, 1966; Johnson *et al.*, 1969; Crawford, 1969, 1970), while, on the other hand, Krnjević and collaborators (Krnjević and Phillis, 1963; Catchlove *et al.*, 1972) claimed that acetylcholine responses are considerably more sensitive to barbiturates than are acidic amino acid responses and that the glutamate response may actually be transiently increased (Fig. 13). Krnjević offers the following explanation for this selective action (Catchlove *et al.*, 1972; Krnjević, 1974*b*, 1975). Previous studies suggested that the muscarinic action of acetylcholine on cortical neurons is caused by a decrease in potassium conductance (Krnjević *et al.*, 1971). 2,4-Dinitrophenol (DNP), a metabolic inhibitor, selectively blocks acetylcholine responses (Fig. 13) by causing the opposite membrane effect, i.e., an increase in potassium conductance (Godfraind *et al.*, 1971), by releasing calcium from mitochondria (Krnjević and Lisiewicz, 1972). Barbiturates are proposed to act in a manner similar to DNP. It should be pointed out that the slow muscarinic response in olfactory cortical neurons (Smaje, 1976) and in sympathetic ganglion cells (Nicoll, 1977) is resistant to pentobarbital.

Acetylcholine responses in other areas of the CNS, which have properties intermediate between nicotinic and muscarinic responses, have also been reported to be considerably more sensitive to barbiturates than are glutamate responses (Bloom *et al.*, 1965; Phillis and Tebecis, 1967; Tebecis and DiMaria, 1972; Bradley and Dray, 1973; but see Andersen and Curtis, 1964). In the brain stem of the rat two types of acetylcholine response have been characterized on different neurons; a fast nicotinic response and a slow muscarinic response, and it has been suggested that the former is more sensitive to barbiturates than the latter (Bradley and Dray, 1973; Duggan *et al.*, 1974), findings in accord with results from the sympathetic ganglion

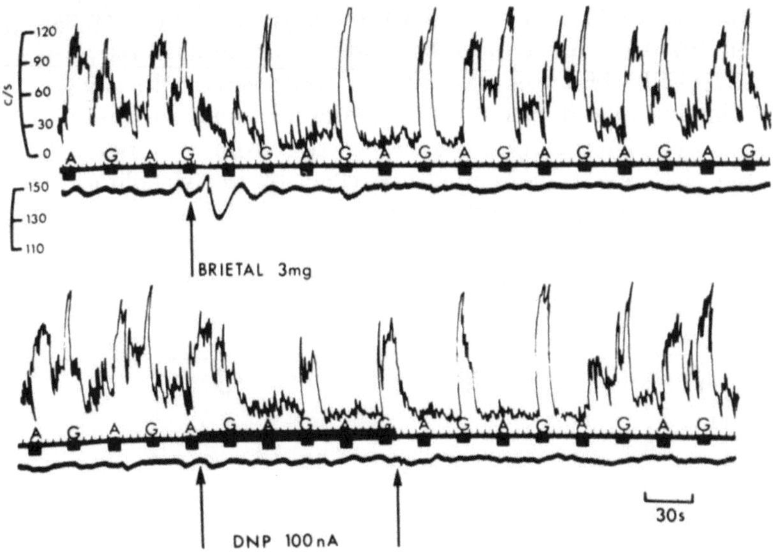

FIG. 13. Effect of methohexital (Brietal) and DNP on the excitatory responses of a cortical unit to glutamate and acetylcholine. Firing frequency (in counts per second) of postcruciate unit in cortex of cat, under light N_2O anesthesia. Black signals on time trace indicate regularly alternating microiontophoretic applications of ACh (A) and L-glutamate (G) by currents of 70 and 56 nA, respectively. The mean femoral arterial pressure is recorded below each trace; it is calibrated by millimeters of Hg. Arrows below lower trace mark the period of iontophoretic release of DNP by a current of 100 nA. Arrow below upper trace signals intravenous injection of methohexital (Brietal). (Catchlove *et al.*, 1972.)

(Nicoll, 1977). However, on Renshaw cells pentobarbital indiscriminately reduces the excitation produced by acidic amino acids, nicotinic agonists, and muscarinic agonists (Curtis and Ryall, 1966*b*).

The variability in the relative sensitivity of excitatory agents to barbiturates reported above is presumably due, in part, to different control conditions upon which the action of barbiturates was examined and to differing populations of neurons sampled in different studies. However, it seems possible that in certain areas, acetylcholine responses, both of the muscarinic and nicotinic type, are more sensitive to barbiturates than are the responses to acidic amino acids. It is unclear whether all of the differences reported can be explained in terms of different ionic mechanisms.

b. Inhibitory Responses. Inhibitory responses have been examined in much less detail than excitatory responses. With one exception, all studies failed to detect any appreciable depression of inhibitory responses to a number of different putative transmitters. The inhibitory effects of serotonin (Roberts and Straughan, 1967; Johnson *et al.*, 1969; Tebecis and DiMaria, 1972), norepinephrine (Bloom *et al.*, 1965; Johnson *et al.*, 1969; but see Phillis and Tebecis, 1967), dopamine (Bloom *et al.*, 1965; Tebecis and DiMaria, 1972), acetylcholine (Bloom *et al.*, 1965), and GABA (Galindo,

1969; Crawford, 1970; Tebecis and DiMaria, 1972; Nicoll, 1975*b*; Ransom and Barker, 1975) are not reduced by moderate amounts of barbiturate. The selective effect of barbiturates on excitatory responses can be clearly appreciated when inhibitory and excitatory responses are simultaneously compared. Bloom *et al.* (1965) recorded simultaneously from two neurons in the caudate nucleus, one of which was excited by acetylcholine, the other inhibited by the same application of acetylcholine. The intravenous injection of hexobarbital abolished the excitatory response but had little effect on the inhibitory response (Fig. 14A–C). On frog motoneurons (Fig. 14D and E),

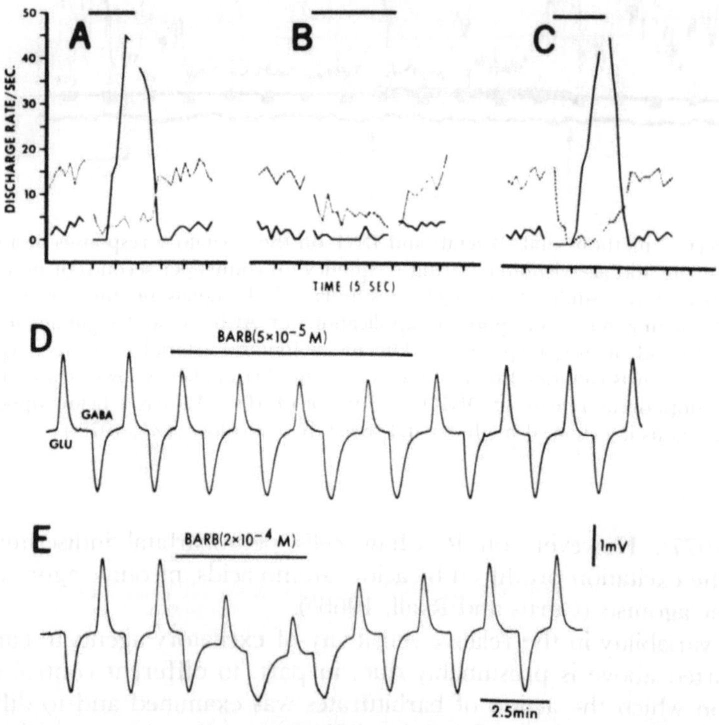

FIG. 14. Differential action of barbiturates on excitatory and inhibitory responses to putative transmitters. (A–C) Effect of hexobarbital on acetylcholine responses of neurons in the caudate nucleus of the cat. Plots from filmed records of two caudate nucleus neurons recorded simultaneously. The electrophoretic administration of acetylcholine by 20 nA of current is indicated by horizontal bars. (A) control; (B) after the intravenous administration of hexobarbital (1.5 mg/kg); (C) 10 min later. (Bloom *et al.*, 1965.) (C and D) The action of pentobarbital on GABA and glutamate responses of frog motoneurons recorded with sucrose gap from a ventral root. In C a concentration of pentobarbital that had no direct hyperpolarizing action reversibly increases the size of the GABA response and decreases the size of the glutamate responses. In D, obtained 20 min after record C, a concentration of pentobarbital was selected that induced a hyperpolarization. In this case the amplitude of the GABA response is reduced but the duration is prolonged to a greater extent than that seen with 5×10^{-4} M. In C and D, GABA was applied for 7 sec and glutamate for 12 sec. (Nicoll, 1975*b*.)

concentrations of barbiturate that depress the depolarization to glutamate actually enhance (D) and prolong (E) the response to GABA (Nicoll, 1975*b*). This enhancement is best seen on responses elicited by very brief pulses of GABA, there being little effect on equilibrated GABA responses. However, as reported by Bowery and Dray (1976), GABA responses that have been blocked by GABA antagonists are restored in the presence of barbiturates (Nicoll, unpublished observations). GABA responses on mouse neurons grown in tissue culture are also prolonged (Ransom and Barker, 1975). The basis for the enhancement of the GABA response is not entirely clear. It could result from a direct effect on the receptor and/or conductance mechanism, or the removal of GABA might be retarded by the barbiturates. The effect of barbiturates on amino acid uptake is controversial. Harris *et al.* (1973) reported that amylobarbital and phenobarbital had no effect on GABA uptake into cortical slices, while Weinberger *et al.* (1975) observed a twofold increase in GABA uptake into synaptosomes in the presence of pentobarbital. The detailed studies of Cutler and collaborators on cortical slices have found that pentobarbital competitively blocks GABA uptake but has no effect on glutamate uptake (Cutler and Dudzinski, 1974; Cutler *et al.*, 1974). The basis for the conflicting results on GABA uptake is not readily apparent. Glycine uptake also has been reported to be blocked by pentobarbital (Johnston and Iversen, 1971), and yet the action of glycine on frog motoneurons is not enhanced by pentobarbital (Nicoll, unpublished observations). The depolarizing action of GABA on primary afferents is enhanced with low concentrations of pentobarbital, but at concentrations that markedly prolong presynaptic inhibition (0.1–0.2 mM) the enhancement gives way to a depression (Nicoll, 1976*a*), which is presumably caused partly by the direct depolarizing action of pentobarbital on primary afferents (Nicoll, 1975*a*). Although earlier studies suggested the involvement of sodium in the GABA depolarizations of primary afferents (Barker and Nicoll, 1973), recent findings suggested that chloride is the major ion involved in this response (Nishi *et al.*, 1974; Gallagher *et al.*, 1975).

3.3.3. Summary

The results reviewed in this section suggest that changes in the postsynaptic sensitivity to neurotransmitters produced by barbiturates play a major role in altering synaptic transmission. While the identification of excitatory transmitters in the CNS has lagged far behind the identification of inhibitory transmitters, the action of all putative excitatory transmitters that are presumed to increase membrane conductance to sodium ions at a variety of sites is depressed by low concentrations of barbiturate. This generalized action on receptor-coupled sodium-conductance mechanisms is consistent with the model of Adams (1976) at the vertebrate neuromuscular junction, in which barbiturate molecules enter and block receptor–channel complexes. However, the sensitivity of excitatory synapses to barbiturates varies considerably, depending on the pathway examined. Thus, the climbing-fiber–Purkinje cell synapse in the cerebellum (Van Gilder and O'Leary, 1971; Gordon *et al.*, 1973; Hackett, personal communication) and the mitral–granule-cell synapse in the olfactory bulb (Nicoll, 1972) are quite resistant to the action of barbiturates, while the mossy-fiber–granule-cell synapse in the cerebellum (Gordon *et al.*, 1973), the excitatory synapses in the prepiriform cortex (Richards, 1972) and the monosynaptic excitation of motoneurons (Weakly, 1969) are quite sensitive to barbiturates. These differences in barbiturate sensitivity might be a result of differences in the kinetics of transmitter release, slower EPSPs being more sensitive, as well as of differences in the sensitivity of the presynaptic terminal. However, until we know the identity of the transmitter at a particular excitatory synapse and the ionic mechanism, the interpretation of results obtained from analyzing the postsynaptic action of suspected transmitters must remain tentative.

The fact that the action of all putative excitatory transmitters is reduced in the presence of barbiturates does not minimize the importance of presynaptic actions. Unfortunately, precise analysis of presynaptic effects requires intracellular recording and fractionation of the EPSP into quantal components, as has been done so elegantly at the neuromuscular junction. The small size of most CNS neurons and the predominantly dendritic location of excitatory synapses virtually exclude this type of analysis in the CNS, except for a few large neurons, e.g., motoneurons. The work of Weakly (1969), showing that the quantal content of the primary afferent EPSP is reduced by barbiturates, witnesses the power of this technique. However, as mentioned in Section 3.2.3, application of results obtained at this synapse to other synapses in the CNS is questionable. Therefore, at present we must rely on less precise data, such as the release of putative excitatory transmitters from brain slices (see Section 3.2.2c).

The situation is considerably better for inhibitory synaptic transmission in the CNS. There is good evidence to indicate that GABA is a transmitter, not only at many supraspinal sites, but also at presynaptic inhibitory synapses, and that glycine is the major transmitter mediating postsynaptic inhibition onto spinal motoneurons (Krnjević, 1974*a*; Curtis and Johnston, 1974; Barker and Nicoll, 1973; Miyata and Otsuka, 1975; Ryall, 1975; Kelly and Beart, 1975). Dopamine is likely to be an inhibitory transmitter in the caudate nucleus and other sites (York, 1975; Snyder and Bennet, 1976) and much evidence indicates that norepinephrine (Bloom, 1975) and serotonin (Bloom *et al.*, 1972) are inhibitory transmitters at a number of sites. The fact that postsynaptic inhibition and the action of the inhibitory substances are, in general, preserved or augmented in the presence of barbiturates strongly suggests that a decrease in release is not occurring at these inhibitory synapses. The enhancement of the postsynaptic action of GABA by barbiturates helps explain the prolongation of GABA-mediated postsynaptic inhibition. However, the observation that the action of exogenously applied glycine, at least on frog motoneurons, is unaltered by concentrations of barbiturates that prolong spinal postsynaptic inhibition, suggests that the release of glycine may actually be prolonged. A similar argument would also apply for GABA and presynaptic inhibition (Nicoll, 1976*a*).

4. POSTSYNAPTIC MEMBRANES

4.1. Muscle and Invertebrate Neurons

In addition to the effects of barbiturates on synaptic transmission per se, many studies have suggested that the barbiturates can also exert direct effects on membrane excitability of the postsynaptic cell. In anesthetic concentrations barbiturates have only minor effects on the membrane properties of vertebrate and crustacean muscle fibers, including a small and variable depolarization and increase in resistance (Thesleff, 1957; Iravani, 1965*a,b*; Westmoreland *et al.*, 1971; Thomson and Turkanis, 1973; Seyama and Narahashi, 1975). Thesleff (1957) also observed a slight lowering of threshold and increase in spike duration in the presence of similar barbiturate concentrations (0.2 mM). In concentrations of 0.4 mM or more pentobarbital has a negative inotropic effect on heart muscle, prolongs relaxation, and diminishes the amount of calcium displaced by lanthanum ions. Higher concentrations interfere with microsomal uptake of calcium, and it was suggested that the pentobarbital-induced increase in the time required for relaxation may be associated with an impaired removal of calcium by the sarcoplasmic reticulum (Nayler and Szelo, 1972).

Goldring and Blaustein (1976) have examined the effects of pentobarbital on sodium and calcium spikes in an identified neuron of aplysia. Both sodium and calcium carry inward current during the rising phase of the action potential in this cell. Pentobarbital (0.05–0.2 mM) had no effect on the resting input resistance or the sodium spike elicited in a calcium-free sea water. However, the calcium spike elicited in a sodium-free sea water was marked attenuated. These findings support Blaustein's proposal that barbiturates block the calcium conductance increase at presynaptic terminals and thereby reduce transmitter release. However, as reviewed before (Section 3.2) there is very little evidence that action-potential-induced release of transmitter is reduced by anesthetic concentrations of barbiturates.

In concentrations above 0.5 mM, barbiturates have been shown to hyperpolarize a number of invertebrate neurons (Sato *et al.*, 1967, 1968; Prichard, 1972; Prichard and Kleinhaus, 1974). This hyperpolarization is shown in Fig. 15. It is associated with a fall in membrane resistance and is dependent on the membrane potential, being reversed by membrane hyperpolarization. These properties indicate that pentobarbital increases membrane conductance to potassium ions in these neurons.

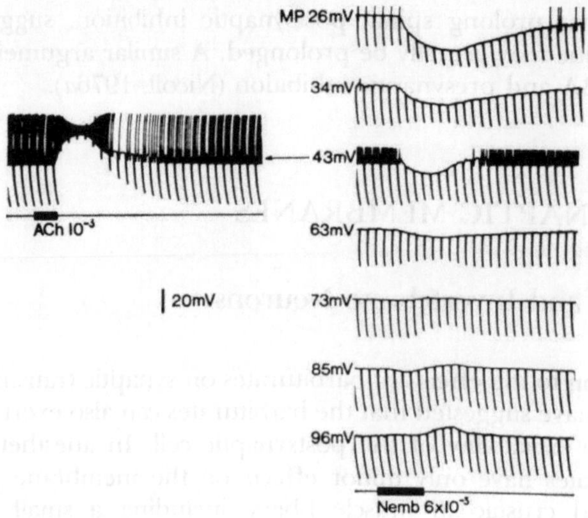

FIG. 15. Determination of reversal potential of "Nembutal"-induced hyperpolarization. The cell was of a D-type with a resting potential of 43 mV. The membrane potential was artificially shifted to various levels described in millivolts by passing inward or outward current through a microelectrode during the recording of the response to "Nembutal." Concentrations are shown in g/ml. Interval of resistance monitoring pulse is 5 sec. (Sato *et al.*, 1967.)

4.2. Vertebrate CNS

The action of barbiturates on neuronal membrane properties in the vertebrate CNS has been studied most extensively on spinal motoneurons. Eccles (1946) and Brooks and Eccles (1947) observed a decreased excitability of motoneurons, as determined by the size of the antidromic field potential, and this decreased excitability was proposed as the basis for the depression of the monosynaptic reflex (see Section 3.1). A similar decrease in excitability has been seen with intracellular recording (Sasaki and Otani, 1962; Somjen, 1963; Somjen and Gill, 1963; and Shapovalov, 1964). In these investigations little change in the membrane potential was found, but a decrease in membrane excitability, measured either by depolarizing current pulses or ramps of depolarizing current was detected. On the other hand, Løyning *et al.* (1964) and Weakly (1969) found no change in the membrane excitability or current–voltage relation. Thus, the decrease in the EPSP in Fig. 1B and C was not associated with any change in the membrane potential or excitability of the motoneuron (Løyning *et al.*, 1964). The difference in these results is undoubtedly related to the dose of barbiturate used, the latter two studies using subanesthetic doses.

There are limitations to these *in vivo* studies such as lack of stability and confusion as to whether a change in membrane excitability is due to a direct effect or to changes in tonic synaptic input. In the isolated frog spinal cord, indirect synaptic effects can be eliminated with magnesium ions and a stable record of membrane potential can be obtained with sucrose gap recording from the spinal roots (Barker *et al.*, 1975*a*). In this preparation, as shown in Fig. 14 and 16, pentobarbital (0.1 mM) hyperpolarizes frog motoneurons (Nicoll, 1975*b*). This hyperpolarizing action has the same pharmacological properties as the GABA hyperpolarization, being blocked by picrotoxin (Fig. 16B) and bicuculline, but not by strychnine, suggesting that pentobarbital activates GABA receptors, as has been proposed for the primary afferents (Nicoll, 1975*a*). The saturable binding of GABA to neuronal membranes, however, is not displaced by 10^{-4} M pentobarbital (Zukin *et al.*, 1974), indicating that barbiturates may not directly activate GABA receptors. It is unlikely that the pentobarbital-induced hyperpolarization of frog motoneurons is due to inhibition of mitochondrial metabolism as suggested by Krnjević (1974*b*, 1975), as DNP, which inhibits mitochondrial metabolism, depolarizes frog motoneurons (Fig. 16A). The hyperpolarization induced by pentobarbital is associated with a fall in motoneuron excitability as measured by the size of the focally recorded antidromic potential (Nicoll, unpublished observations), contrary to the findings of Richens (1969*b*). Possibly the transient increase in excitability seen by Richens resulted from indirect synaptic effects since synaptic transmission in his experiments had not been blocked with magnesium ions. As shown in Fig. 6, a hyperpolarizing action of barbiturates has been observed in hippocampal pyramidal cells (Nicoll *et al.*, 1976) and cortical neurons (Krnjević, 1974). However, the basis for this action is unknown, and a withdrawal of background excitation presumably contributes to the effect. The iontophoretic application of pentobarbital to

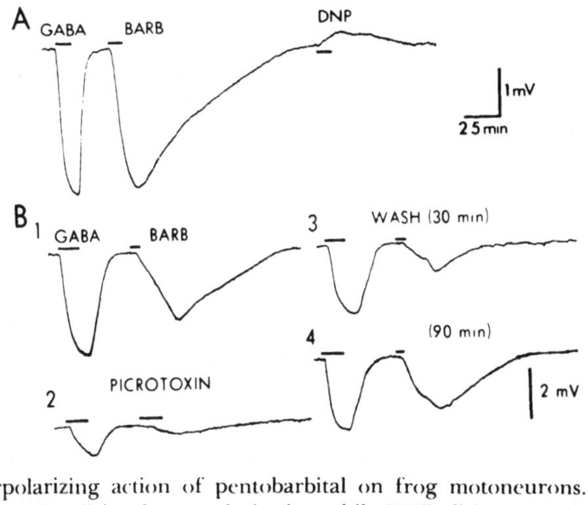

FIG. 16. Hyperpolarizing action of pentobarbital on frog motoneurons. (A) GABA and pentobarbital (BARB) elicit a hyperpolarization while DNP elicits a depolarization. (B) The GABA and pentobarbital responses are reversibly antagonized by picrotoxin (2×10^{-4} M). The concentration of GABA was 5×10^{-4} M, pentobarbital was 4×10^{-3} M, and DNP was 5×10^{-4} M. Positivity is downward, signifying a hyperpolarization. (Nicoll, 1975*b*.)

mouse spinal cord neurons grown in tissue culture causes a hyperpolarization and a fall in membrane resistance (Ransom and Barker, 1975). Gordon *et al.* (1973) found that small doses of thiopental (4–8 mg/kg) had no effect on the mossy-fiber-induced postsynaptic excitatory potentials in cerebellar granule cells, but they abolished the axon discharge of these cells. These authors proposed that there is a hyperpolarization of the granule cell, possibly due to the withdrawal of excitatory input from the reticulocerebellar pathway. Relatively high doses of barbiturate have been shown to depress antidromic invasion of dendrites in both cerebellar Purkinje cells (Eccles *et al.*, 1971) and olfactory bulb mitral cells (Nicoll, 1972). The action of mitral cell dendrites is shown in Fig. 10B. This effect cannot be explained solely on the basis of a removal of excitatory input to the mitral cells, because local iontophoresis of pentobarbital to the soma of mitral cells, which receive no excitatory synapses (Price and Powell, 1970), decreases the excitability of these cells (Nicoll, unpublished observations). In the cuneate nucleus (Galindo, 1969) larger iontophoretic doses of pentobarbital were needed to suppress antidromic spikes compared to orthodromic spikes, and 20 mg/kg given intravenously had no effect on antidromic spikes, but it depressed orthodromic action potentials. In the olfactory cortex, pentobarbital (0.2–0.3 mM) does not impair the coupling between the EPSP and the discharge of cortical neurons, since the relationship between the size of the EPSP and the area of the population spike did not change (Richards, 1972). Thus, it was concluded that there was no change in the firing threshold of the cortical neurons. However, a variable increase in latency of the population spike did occur.

The results in this section suggest that with small amounts of barbiturate, which would be comparable to light anesthesia, little or no change in the properties of soma and dendritic membrane occurs, while with higher amounts the excitability is often depressed. At present it is unclear how much of the change in excitability is due to a stabilizing action on the membrane, the release of mitochondrial calcium, and the activation of GABA receptors. With regard to the last possibility, it has been reported that barbiturates and GABA have a synergistic action (Lingwood and Chiesa, 1967).

A model which might help to explain the variety of interactions which occur between the barbiturates and GABA responses is derived from a proposal made by Bowery and Dray (1976). They proposed that barbiturates might compete with the GABA antagonists, bicuculline and picrotoxin, for sites adjacent to the GABA receptor. The combination of GABA antagonists to this site leads to the block of the GABA receptor. Barbiturates prevent the action of the GABA antagonists by competing for the same sites. It could also be envisaged that barbiturate interaction with these same sites in addition causes the duration of the chloride conductance generated by GABA receptor activation to increase. With higher concentrations of barbiturates this chloride conductance is directly activated. Such a model would explain why the pharmacology of the barbiturate and GABA response are the same even though the barbiturates do not appear to bind directly to the GABA receptors (Zukin *et al.*, 1974).

5. CORRELATION OF BARBITURATE ANESTHESIA WITH SLOW-WAVE SLEEP

The similarities between barbiturate anesthesia and certain phases of slow-wave sleep, as judged by the EEG and unit activity, are so striking that barbiturate anesthesia has often served as a model to explain the changes in neuronal activity during slow-wave sleep (cf. Steriade *et al.*, 1974; Noda and Iwama, 1975) and the alpha rhythm (cf. Andersen and Anderson, 1968). In both slow-wave sleep and barbiturate anesthesia, the spontaneous discharge rate of cortical neurons and other neurons is decreased, the decrease being greater for barbiturate anesthesia (Steriade *et al.*, 1974; Noda and Iwama, 1975). Another feature common to these two states is the presence of spindles (cf. Andersen and Anderson, 1968; Steriade *et al.*, 1974; Noda and Iwama, 1975). Spindles can be recorded from the surface of all areas of the neocortex and from all thalamic nuclei. They consist of a sequence of slow waves varying in size in a typical way. The size of the initial few waves increases gradually, only to decrease after a short while. During barbiturate and sleep spindles, neurons tend to fire synchronously at the same frequency as the slow waves. As reviewed by Andersen and Anderson (1968) the thalamus appears to be the prime mover or pacemaker of spindle activity. These oscillations are transmitted from the thalamus to the cerebral cortex.

From detailed studies Andersen and his collaborators (cf. Andersen and Anderson, 1968) proposed that the rhythmic activity generated in the thalamus is dependent upon a powerful recurrent inhibitory process followed by a postinhibitory rebound. The level of background excitatory input to the thalamus is also important, but based on the construction of models of rhythmic activity, the degree of background activity was less important than the inhibition and rebound present in thalamic neurons. Thus, the occurrence of spindle activity during barbiturate anesthesia and possibly during slow-wave sleep could result from an augmentation of recurrent inhibition in this system, as well as from a decrease in ascending excitatory drive, especially from the reticular formation. Indeed, barbiturates do prolong the p-wave, which is the extracellular correlate of the recurrent IPSP (Bremer, 1970), and increasing the dose of barbiturates decreases the frequency of the spindle (Andersen and Anderson, 1968). In addition, Steriade *et al.* (1974) have shown that during slow-wave sleep, postsynaptic inhibition, both in the thalamus and cortex, is prolonged. Therefore, these results suggest that, as has been documented for other sites in the CNS (see Section 3.1), barbiturates enhance postsynaptic inhibition in the thalamus and that a similar enhancement is seen during slow-wave sleep. Given the crucial role of synaptic inhibition in generating spindle activity, it is not unreasonable to suppose that this effect might provide a basis for the induction of spindle activity by barbiturates in addition to the withdrawal of excitatory input.

Interestingly, there is evidence (cf. Nicoll, 1975*c*) that a sleep-promoting substance(s) is released into the cerebral blood and cerebrospinal fluid of animals deprived of sleep (Fencl *et al.*, 1971; Pappenheimer *et al.*, 1975) or of animals induced to sleep by electrical stimulation of "sleep centers" in the intralaminary thalamus (Monnier and Hosli, 1965). In both studies this factor has been found to be a peptide (Schoenenberger *et al.*, 1972; Pappenheimer *et al.*, 1975). The injection of sleep-promoting factors into the ventricles, but not into the subarachnoid space, increases slow-wave activity in the EEG and decreases motor activity. An intriguing possibility, then, is that certain areas of the CNS may release a sleep-promoting factor that mimics the effects of barbiturates. However, if such a factor is involved in slow-wave sleep, it either does not gain access to the spinal cord or its action differs from barbiturates, since presynaptic inhibition has been reported to be unaltered during slow-wave sleep (Baldissera *et al.*, 1966).

6. EXCITATORY ACTIONS OF BARBITURATES

While early studies failed to demonstrate any appreciable difference in the hypnotic and toxic activity of barbiturate isomers (cf. Hsueh and Marvel, 1928), a number of studies have subsequently shown that enantiomers differ considerably in their hypnotic potency (Wahlstrom, 1966, 1968; Downes *et al.*, 1970; Buch *et al.*, 1970, 1973; Christensen and Lee, 1973). This difference in hypnotic potency, at least for the enantiomers of pentobarbital and secobarbital, cannot be adequately explained by differences in metabolism or entry into the brain, since the brain levels of these enantiomers are similar (Freudenthal and Martin, 1975). In addition, it is well established that some isomers and analogs are frankly convulsant (Knoefel, 1945; Domino, 1956; Downes and Williams, 1969; Downes *et al.*, 1970; Downes and Franz, 1971; Buch *et al.*, 1970, 1973; Grossmann *et al.*, 1974; Daves *et al.*, 1975). The degree of excitation varies considerably with different analogs, and many of the barbiturates used for their sedative–hypnotic properties produce mild preanesthetic excitatory effects.

On the assumption that the barbiturates as a group possess a common excitatory mechanism, Downes and his collaborators have done detailed studies on the mechanism of action of convulsant barbiturates, so that the excitatory effects could be studied in comparative isolation. They have found that 5-(2-cyclohexylideneethyl)-5-ethyl barbituric acid (CHEB) increases the size of the spinal monosynaptic reflex with little consistent change in pre- and postsynaptic inhibition (Downes and Williams, 1969). This effect was antagonized by pentobarbital. Further studies (Downes, 1969; Downes and Franz, 1971) showed that CHEB depolarized motoneurons, but since it was impossible to exclude indirect synaptic effects secondary to the convulsant activity, dorsal root ganglion cells, which receive no synaptic input, were used to analyze the membrane effects of this convulsant. It was found that CHEB depolarizes dorsal root ganglion cells and increases their excitability. The depolarization is associated with a fall in membrane resistance. This action is similar to that observed with pentobarbital at all sites along primary afferents (Nicoll, 1975*a*). This depolarizing action would be expected to reduce the amount of transmitter released by impulses in primary afferent terminals, but if the depolarization were sufficiently large, the spontaneous release of transmitter would increase. Unlike the depolarization by pentobarbital, the CHEB depolarization is not blocked by GABA antagonists (Nicoll, unpublished observations), suggesting that the depolarizing action of CHEB may be a general phenomenon on all excitable membranes. Hupka *et al.* (1969) and Edney and Downes (1975) have found that CHEB causes contractions of a number of smooth muscle preparations by a direct effect, while pentobarbital lacks any contractor effect. Pentobarbital does, however, block the effects of CHEB. In the isolated frog spinal cord CHEB also depolarizes motoneurons, in contrast to the hyperpolarizing action of pentobarbital (Nicoll, unpublished observations). This effect, which could explain the increase in the size of the spinal monosynaptic reflex (Downes and Williams, 1969), is presumably a direct action, since it can be demonstrated in the presence of magnesium ions that block synaptic transmission. These results support the hypothesis of Downes, that the convulsant activity of CHEB and possibly other barbiturates is due, in part, to a generalized increase in membrane excitability.

On the other hand, the postsynaptic action of CHEB and phenobarbital and their action of evoked release of transmitter are similar at the vertebrate neuromuscular junction (Thomson and Turkanis, 1973). The only major difference between the effects of these two compounds at this site is that CHEB markedly increases the frequency of miniature end plate potentials. Thomson and Turkanis (1973) thus suggested that increased release of transmitter could contribute to the excitatory properties of barbiturates.

Crawford (1969) has found that the iontophoretic application of the convulsant 5-ethyl-5-(1,3-dimethylbutyl) barbiturate to cortical neurons depresses the excitatory effects of acetylcholine and DL-homocysteic acid, similar to the results obtained with depressant barbiturates (see Section 3.3.2a). The action of glutamate on frog motoneurons is also depressed by the convulsant barbiturate CHEB (Nicoll, unpublished observations), similar to the findings of Thomson and Turkanis (1973) with acetylcholine at the vertebrate neuromuscular junction. These findings suggest that both the depressant and convulsant barbiturates have a common depressant effect on the postsynaptic action of excitatory transmitters.

Grossmann *et al.* (1974) have compared the action of the optical isomers of 1-methyl-5-phenyl-5-propyl barbituric acid (MPPB) on the cat spinal cord. Similar to the action of CHEB, the convulsant isomer (+)-MPPB increased the spinal monosynaptic reflex, while the depressant isomer (−)-MPPB reduced this reflex. In addition, intracellular recording revealed that (+)-MPPB increased the excitability, but had no effect on the resting potential. However, the additional observation that the membrane resistance was also reduced is difficult to reconcile with the above effects.

By analogy with the action of strychnine, it has been proposed that the excitatory effects of barbiturate might arise from a selective block in synaptic inhibition (Esplin, 1963; Frank and Ohta, 1971). However, as reviewed in Section 3 synaptic inhibition is generally not reduced in the presence of barbiturates. Even with the convulsant barbiturate CHEB (Downes and Williams, 1969), a block in synaptic inhibition could not account for its excitatory action. A more likely possibility is that barbiturates block disfacilitation, rather than synaptic inhibition. Disfacilitation is dependent upon a background activity in excitatory relay neurons upon which an inhibitory input acts. As reviewed in Section 5, barbiturates generally decrease the spontaneous firing rate of neurons. Garrison *et al.* (1974) have examined the effects of lidocaine on cerebellar disfacilitation. In this system Purkinje cells inhibit the background activity of fastigial neurons. Since fastigial neurons have an excitatory action on neurons in Deiters nucleus, a removal of this excitatory action, i.e., disfacilitation, occurs in Deiters neurons when Purkinje cells are activated. It has been found that lidocaine blocks disfacilitation in this pathway by depressing the spontaneous activity of fastigial neurons. Interestingly, the spontaneous activity of fastigial neurons is particularly sensitive to barbiturates (Eccles *et al.*, 1974), which suggests that a similar action on disfacilitation may occur with barbiturates.

In summary, the excitatory effects of barbiturates could arise from a number of actions including (1) an increased sensitivity of the postsynaptic membrane to excitatory transmitter, (2) a selective block of synaptic inhibition, (3) a direct excitatory action on neuronal membranes, and (4) an increased release of transmitter. The first possibility is unlikely, since excitatory transmitter action is depressed by both convulsant and depressant barbiturates. Although a selective block in synaptic inhibition is unlikely to play a major role in the excitatory properties of barbiturates, a block in disfacilitation could contribute to some of the excitatory effects observed. A direct excitatory action on neuronal membranes may well contribute to the excitatory properties, at least for some of the convulsant analogs. Finally, the enhanced release of transmitter, including evoked and spontaneous release, may also play a role in the excitatory action of both depressant and convulsant barbiturates.

7. CONCLUSIONS

Since only fragmentary and sometimes conflicting results are available at many regions of the CNS, the generalizations presented below should be regarded only as a framework. At virtually all sites examined excitatory synaptic transmission is reduced by barbiturates, but the sensitivity varies at different sites. The depression of the monosynaptic EPSP generated by spinal primary afferents on motoneurons by subanesthetic doses of barbiturate is caused solely by the decreased release of excitatory transmitter. This presynaptic action may be related to the interaction of barbiturates with the GABA receptors that exist on these terminals. It is unclear whether anesthetic doses, in addition, decrease the sensitivity of the postsynaptic membrane to the excitatory transmitter. If glutamate is a transmitter released from primary afferents (cf. Curtis and Johnston, 1974), this is likely to be the case, since barbiturates in anesthetic concentrations severely depress the action of glutamate on motoneurons. It would be interesting to know the effect of barbiturates on the action of substance P, a peptide considered to be a strong candidate as a transmitter released from primary afferents (Otsuka *et al.*, 1975; Nicoll, 1976*b*).

In general, there is little evidence to suggest that barbiturates in anesthetic concentrations decrease action-potential-evoked release of excitatory transmitter at other synapses. For instance, pentobarbital depresses the EPSP in the olfactory cortex without any change in the presynaptic action potential, and these same concentrations of barbiturate markedly depress the excitatory action of glutamate, a putative excitatory transmitter in this system. Anesthetic concentrations of barbiturate have little or no effect on the [^{14}C]glutamate or acetylcholine release evoked by electrical stimulation of cortical slices. This generalization is supported by results obtained at the vertebrate neuromuscular junction where transmitter release is actually increased by barbiturates. On the other hand there is good evidence to suggest that barbiturates may impair excitatory transmission by depressing the action of the transmitter in the CNS, since the action of all putative excitatory transmitters at a variety of sites is markedly depressed by barbiturates. These findings are in accord with the large volume of literature on peripheral and invertebrate synapses where the depression of transmission can be attributed in large part, or entirely, to a block in the action of the excitatory transmitter. However, it must be borne in mind that there are very few excitatory synapses in the vertebrate CNS where the identity of the transmitter has been established.

In general, synaptic inhibition in the CNS is preserved and greatly prolonged by barbiturates, including that in pathways that are considered to use both glycine and GABA as transmitters. The prolongation of the inhibitory action of exogenously applied GABA can account for much of the effect seen on GABA-mediated postsynaptic inhibition. However, the weak enhancement of the depolarizing action of GABA on primary afferents suggests that the release of GABA may also be prolonged at presynaptic inhibitory synapses in the presence of barbiturate. A similar argument would apply for inhibitory synapses that release glycine, since the action of glycine is not enhanced by barbiturates. If barbiturates were to impair calcium removal by mitochondria in the synaptic terminal, as they do with calcium uptake into sarcoplasmic reticulum (Nayler and Szelo, 1972) and mitochondria (Dransfeld, *et al.*, 1969) in the heart, a prolonged release of transmitter, especially following the repetitive activity that is seen with inhibitory interneurons, would be expected (Almaes and Rahamimoff, 1975).

With concentrations of barbiturate that would correspond to deep anesthesia, the excitability of the soma and dendrites of many types of neurons in the CNS is depressed. This depression, at least on frog motoneurons, is associated with membrane hyperpolarization that is pharmacologically similar to the action of GABA. The membrane-stabilizing action of barbiturates could also contribute to this decreased excitability.

The actions of barbiturates discussed above would have an overall depressant effect on neuronal systems and, therefore, would be expected to contribute in varying degrees to the sedative–hypnotic and anesthetic properties of these agents. The basis for the early excitatory phase of barbiturate anesthesia is unclear, but it is more likely to represent a block in disfacilitation than a selective block in postsynaptic inhibition. It is also possible that an initial enhancement in the release of excitatory transmitter, as has been demonstrated at the vertebrate neuromuscular junction, could contribute to this excitatory phase (cf. Thomson and Turkanis, 1973).

The present review has considered only the mechanism of action of barbiturates. Although considerable work has been done on this group of depressant agents, we are still at a very rudimentary level in our understanding of their action on the CNS. We have virtually no knowledge as to the cellular mechanism of action of other groups of sedative–hypnotics, and it will be of interest to determine if the homogeneity found clinically for this class of drugs is also seen at the cellular level.

8. REFERENCES

Adams, P. R., 1974, The mechanism by which amylobarbitone and thiopentone block the end-plate response to nicotinic agonists, *J. Physiol. (Lond.)* **236**:41–43P.

Adams, P. R., 1976, Drug blockade of open end-plate channels, *J. Physiol. (Lond.)* **260**:531–552.

Adams, P. R., and Brown, D. A., 1975, Actions of γ-aminobutyric acid on sympathetic ganglion cells, *J. Physiol. (Lond.)* **250**:85–120.

Adams, P. R., Cash, H. C., and Quilliam, J. P., 1970, Extrinsic and intrinsic acetylcholine and barbiturate effects on frog skeletal muscle, *Br. J. Pharmacol.* **40**:552–553P.

AKERT, K., LIVINGSTON, R. B., MOOR, H., and STREIT, P., 1974, Ultrastructure of synapses in the waking state, *J. Neurol. Trans. Suppl.* **XI:**1–11.

ALMAES, E., and RAHAMIMOFF, R., 1975, On the role of mitochondria in transmitter release from motor nerves terminals, *J. Physiol. (Lond.)* **248:**285–306.

ANDERSEN, P., and ANDERSON, J. A., 1968, *Physiological Basis of the Alpha Rhythm,* Appleton-Century-Crofts, New York.

ANDERSEN, P., and CURTIS, D. R., 1964, The excitation of thalamic neurones by acetylcholine, *Acta Physiol. Scand.* **61:**85–99.

ANDERSEN, P., ECCLES, J. C., and SEARS, T. A., 1964, The ventro-basal complex of the thalamus: Types of cells, their responses and their functional organization, *J. Physiol. (Lond.)* **174:**370–399.

ARIENS, E. J., 1964, *Molecular Pharmacology,* Academic Press, New York.

BALDISSERA, F., CESA-BIANCHI, M. G., and MANCIA, M., 1966, Phasic events indicating presynaptic inhibition of primary afferents to the spinal cord during desynchronized sleep, *J. Neurophysiol.* **29:**871–887.

BANNA, N. R., 1970, Antagonism of barbiturate depression of spinal transmission by catechol, *Experientia* **26:**1330–1331.

BANNA, N. R., 1973, The effect of semicarbazide pretreatment on the depressant action of barbiturates, *Experientia* **29:**819–820.

BANNA, N. R., and JABBUR, S. J., 1969, Pharmacological studies on inhibition in the cuneate nucleus of the cat, *Int. J. Neuropharmacol.* **8:**299–307.

BANNA, N. R., and JABBUR, S. J., 1972, Facilitation of spinal synaptic transmission by catechol, *Neuropharmacol.* **11:**565–571.

BARKER, J. L., 1975*a*, CNS depressants: Effects on post-synaptic pharmacology, *Brain Res.* **92:**35–55.

BARKER, J. L., 1975*b*, Inhibitory and excitatory effects of CNS depressants on invertebrate synapses, *Brain Res.* **93:**77–90.

BARKER, J. L., and NICOLL, R. A., 1972, GABA: Role in primary afferent depolarization, *Science (N.Y.)* **176:**1043–1045.

BARKER, J. L., and NICOLL, R. A., 1973, The pharmacology and ionic dependency of amino acid responses in the frog spinal cord, *J. Physiol. (Lond.)* **228:**259–277.

BARKER, J. L., NICOLL, R. A., and PADJEN, A., 1975*a*, Studies on convulsants in the isolated frog spinal cord. I. Antagonism of amino acid responses, *J. Physiol. (Lond.)* **245:**521–536.

BARKER, J. L., NICOLL, R. A., and PADJEN, A., 1975*b*, Studies on convulsants in the isolated frog spinal cord. II. Effects on root potentials. *J. Physiol. (Lond.)* **245:**537–548.

BLAUSTEIN, M. P., 1968, Barbiturates block sodium and potassium conductance increases in voltage-clamped lobster axons, *J. Gen. Physiol.* **51:**293–307.

BLAUSTEIN, M. P., 1976, Barbiturates block calcium uptake by stimulated and potassium-depolarized rat sympathetic ganglia, *J. Pharmacol. Exp. Ther.* **196:**80–86.

BLAUSTEIN, M. P., and ECTOR, A. C., 1975, Barbiturate inhibition of calcium uptake by depolarized nerve terminals *in vitro, Molec. Pharmacol.* **11:**369–378.

BLOEDEL, J. R., and ROBERTS, W. J., 1969, Functional relationship among neurons of the cerebellar cortex in the absence of anesthesia, *J. Neurophysiol.* **32:**75–84.

BLOOM, F. E., 1975, Amine receptors in CNS. I. Norepinephrine, in: *Handbook of Psychopharmacology,* Vol. 6 (L. L. Iversen, S. D. Iversen, and S. H. Snyder, eds.), Plenum, New York.

BLOOM, F. E., COSTA, E., and SALMOIRAGHI, G. C., 1965, Anesthesia and the responsiveness of individual neurons of the caudate nucleus of the cat to acetylcholine, norepinephrine and dopamine administered by microelectrophoresis, *J. Pharmacol. Exp. Ther.* **150:**244–252.

BLOOM, F. E., HOFFER, B. J., SIGGINS, G. R., BARKER, J. L., and NICOLL, R. A., 1972, Effects of serotonin on central neurons: Microiontophoretic administration, *Fed. Proc.* **31:**97–106.

Bowery, N. G., and Dray, A., 1976, Barbiturate reversal of amino acid antagonism produced by convulsant agents, *Nature* **264**:276–278.

Bradley, P. B., and Dray, A., 1973, Modification of the responses of brain stem neurones to transmitter substances by anaesthetic agents, *Br. J. Pharmacol.* **48**:212–224.

Bremer, F., 1970, Inhibitions intrathalamiques recurrentielles et physiologie du sommeil, *Electroenceph. Clin. Neurophysiol.* **28**:1–16.

Brooks, C. McC., and Eccles, J. C., 1947, A study of the effects of anaesthesia and asphyxia on the mono-synaptic pathway through the spinal cord, *J. Neurophysiol.* **5**:349–360.

Brooks, C. McC., Koizumi, K., and Siebens, A. A., 1956, Inhibitory action of bulbar and suprabulbar reticular formation on spinal reflex pathway, *Am. J. Physiol.* **184**:497–504.

Brown, D. A., and Quilliam, J. P., 1964*a*, The effects of some centrally acting drugs on ganglionic transmission in the cat, *Br. J. Pharmacol.* **23**:241–256.

Brown, D. A., and Quilliam, J. P., 1964*b*, Observations on the mode of action of some central depressant drugs on transmission through the cat superior cervical ganglion, *Br. J. Pharmacol.* **23**:257–272.

Buch, H., Knabe, J., Buzello, W., and Rummel, W., 1970, Stereospecificity of anesthetic activity, distribution, inactivation and protein binding of the optical antipodes of two *N*-methylated barbiturates, *J. Pharmacol. Exp. Ther.* **175**:709–716.

Buch, H. P., Schneider-Affeld, F., Rummel, W., and Knabe, J., 1973, Stereochemical dependence of pharmacological activity in a series of optically active *N*-methylated barbiturates, *Naunyn-Schmiedeberg's Arch. Pharmacol.* **277**:191–198.

Carmichael, F. J., and Israel, M., 1975, Effects of ethanol on neurotransmitter release by rat brain cortical slices, *J. Pharmacol. Exp. Ther.* **193**:824–834.

Catchlove, R. F. H., Krnjević, K., and Maretic, H., 1972, Similarity between effects of general anesthetics and dinitrophenol on cortical neurones, *Canad. J. Physiol. Pharmacol.* **50**:1111–1114.

Christensen, H. D., and Lee, I. S., 1973, Anesthetic potency and acute toxicity of optically active disubstituted barbituric acids, *Toxicol. Appl. Pharmacol.* **26**:495–503.

Cowan, M. J., Scher, A. M., and Hildebrandt, J., 1975, Heart rate response to sympathetic stimulation before and after sodium pentobarbital, *Am. J. Physiol.* **228**:1568–1574.

Crawford, J. M., 1969, Effects of convulsant barbiturates on cortical neurons, *Brain Res.* **12**:485–489.

Crawford, J. M., 1970, Anaesthetic agents and the chemical sensitivity of cortical neurones, *Neuropharmacology* **9**:31–46.

Crawford, J. M., and Curtis, D. R., 1966, Pharmacological studies on feline Betz cells, *J. Physiol. (Lond.)* **186**:121–138.

Curtis, D. R., and DeGroat, W. C., 1968, Tetanus toxin and spinal inhibition, *Brain Res.* **10**:208–212.

Curtis, D. R., and Johnston, G. A. R., 1974, Amino acid transmitters in the mammalian central nervous system, *Ergeb. Physiol.* **69**:97–188.

Curtis, D. R., and Ryall, R. W., 1966*a*, Pharmacological studies upon spinal presynaptic fibres, *Exp. Brain Res.* **1**:195–204.

Curtis, D. R., and Ryall, R. W., 1966*b*, The excitation of Renshaw cells by cholinomimetics, *Exp. Brain Res.* **2**:49–65.

Curtis, D. R., Felix, D., Game, C. J. A., and McCulloch, 1973, Tetanus toxin and the synaptic release of GABA, *Brain Res.* **51**:358–362.

Cutler, R. W. P., and Dudzinski, D. S., 1974, Effect of pentobarbital on uptake and release of [^{3}H]-GABA and [^{14}C]glutamate by brain slices, *Brain Res.* **67**:546–548.

Cutler, R. W. P., and Dudzinski, D. S., 1975, Release of ^{3}H-GABA and C-glutamic acid from rat cortex slices: The relationship between the tissue pool size and rates of spontaneously and electrically induced release, *Brain Res.* **88**:415–423.

Cutler, R. W. P., Markowitz, D., and Dudzinski, D. S., 1974, The effect of barbiturates on ^{3}H-GABA transport in rat cerebral cortex slices, *Brain Res.* **81**:189–197.

Daves, G. D., Belshee, R. B., Anderson, W. R., and Downes, H., 1975, Solution conformations of ethyl-1-methylbutylbarbituric acids: Implications for drug–receptor interactions, *Mol. Pharmacol.* **11:**470–477.

DAVIDOFF, R. A., 1972, Gamma-aminobutyric acid antagonism and presynaptic inhibition in the frog spinal cord, *Science (N.Y.)* **175:**331–333.

DAVIDSON, N., and SOUTHWICK, C. A. P., 1971, Amino acids and presynaptic inhibition in the rat cuneate nucleus, *J. Physiol. (Lond.)* **219:**689–708.

DOMINO, E. F., 1956, Pharmacological actions of a convulsant barbiturate. II. Effects compared with pentobarbital on cerebral cortex and some brain stem systems of the cat, *J. Pharmacol. Exp. Ther.* **119:**272–283.

DOWNES, H., 1969, as quoted by Esplin, D. W., and Zablocka-Esplin, B., Mechanisms of action of convulsants, in *Basic Mechanisms of the Epilepsies* (H. H. Jasper, A. A. Ward, and A. Pope, eds.) Little, Brown, Boston.

DOWNES, H., and FRANZ, D. N., 1971, Effects of a convulsant barbiturate on dorsal root ganglion cells and dorsal root discharges, *J. Pharmacol. Exp. Ther.* **179:**660–670.

DOWNES, H., and WILLIAMS, J. K., 1969, Effects of a convulsant barbiturate on the spinal monosynaptic pathway, *J. Pharmacol. Exp. Ther.* **168:**283–289.

DOWNES, H., PERRY, R. S., OSTLUND, R. E., and KARLER, R., 1970, A study of the excitatory effects of barbiturates, *J. Pharmacol. Exp. Ther.* **175:**692–699.

DOWNING, D. A., 1972, The effects of procaine, amylobarbitone on drug induced changes in the surface potentials of an isolated sympathetic ganglion, *Br. J. Pharmacol.* **45:**159–160P.

DRANSFELD, H., GREEFF, K., SCHORN, A., and TING, B. T., 1969, Calcium uptake in mitochondria and vesicles of heart and skeletal muscle in presence of potassium, sodium, *K*-strophanthin and pentobarbital, *Biochem. Pharmacol.* **18:**1335–1345.

DUDEL, J., 1965, The action of inhibitory drugs on nerve terminals in crayfish muscle, *Pflugers Arch.* **284:**81–94.

DUGGAN, A. W., HEADLEY, P. M., and LODGE, D., 1974, Acetylcholine-sensitive cells in the caudal medulla of the rat: Distribution, pharmacology and effects of pentobarbitone, *Br. J. Pharmacol.* **54:**23–31.

ECCLES, J. C., 1946, Synaptic potentials of motoneurones, *J. Neurophysiol.* **9:**87–120.

ECCLES, J. C., 1964, *The Physiology of Synapses,* Springer, Berlin.

ECCLES, J. C., and MALCOLM, J. L., 1946, Dorsal root potentials of the spinal cord, *J. Neurophysiol.* **9:**139–160.

ECCLES, J. C., SCHMIDT, R., and WILLIS, W. D., 1963, Pharmacological studies on presynaptic inhibition, *J. Physiol. (Lond.)* **168:**500–530.

ECCLES, J. C., FABER, D. S., and TABORIKOVA, H., 1971, The action of a parallel fiber volley on the antidromic invasion of Purkinje cells of cat cerebellum, *Brain Res.* **25:**335–356.

ECCLES, J. C., SABAH, N. H., and TABORIKOVA, H., 1974, Excitatory and inhibitory responses of neurones of the cerebellar fastigial nucleus, *Exp. Brain Res.* **19:**61–77.

EDNEY, S. M., and DOWNES, H., 1975, Contractor effect of barbiturates on smooth muscle, *Arch. Int. Pharmacolodyn.* **217:**180–196.

ELLIOTT, R. C., and QUILLIAM, J. P., 1964, Some actions of centrally active and other drugs on the transmission of single nerve impulses through the isolated superior cervical ganglion preparation of the rabbit, *Br. J. Pharmacol.* **23:**222–240.

ESPLIN, D. W., 1963, Criteria for assessing effects of depressant drugs on spinal synaptic transmission with examples of drug selectivity, *Arch. Int. Pharmacodyn. Ther.* **143:**479–497.

EXLEY, K. A., 1954, Depression of autonomic ganglia by barbiturates, *Br. J. Pharmacol.* **9:**170–181.

FENCL, V., KOSKI, G., and PAPPENHEIMER, J. R., 1971, Factors in cerebrospinal fluid from goats that affect sleep and activity in rats, *J. Physiol. (Lond.)* **216:**565–589.

FINK, B. R., ed., 1975, Molecular mechanisms of anesthesia, in: *Progress in Anesthesiology* (R. L. Katz, ed.), Raven Press, New York.

FISHER, R. S., WALKER, J. T., and PLUMMER, C. W., 1948, Quantitative estimation of barbiturates in blood by ultra-violet spectrophotometry, *Am. J. Clin. Pathol.* **18:**462–469.

FRANK, G. B., 1968, Drugs which modify membrane excitability, *Fed. Proc.* **27:**132–136.

FRANK, G. B., and OHTA, M., 1971, Blockade of the reticulospinal inhibitory pathway by anaesthetic agents, *Br. J. Pharmacol.* **42:**328–342.

FRANK, G. B., and SANDERS, H. D., 1963, A proposed common mechanism of action for general and local anesthetics in the central nervous system, *Br. J. Pharmacol. Chemother.* **21:**1–9.

FRAZIER, D. T., MURAYAMA, K., ABBOTT, N. J., and NARAHASHI, T., 1975, Comparison of the action of different barbiturates on squid axon membranes, *Eur. J. Pharmacol.* **32:**102–107.

FREUDENTHAL, R. I., and MARTIN, J., 1975, Correlation of brain levels of barbiturate enantiomers with reported differences in duration of sleep, *J. Pharmacol. Exp. Ther.* **184:**664–668.

GALINDO, A., 1969, Effects of procaine, pentobarbital, and halothane on synaptic transmission in the central nervous system, *J. Pharmacol. Exp. Ther.* **169:**185–195.

GALINDO, A., 1971, Procaine, pentobarbital, and halothane: Effects on the mammalian myoneural junction, *J. Pharmacol. Exp. Ther.* **177:**360–368.

GALLAGHER, J. P., HIGASHI, H., and NISHI, S., 1975, The ionic requirements for the production of the GABA depolarization at cat primary afferent neurons, *Fed. Proc.* **34:**418.

GARRISON, D. L., SINCLAIR, J. G., KEE, R. D., and YIM, G. K. W., 1974, The differential action of intravenous lidocaine on cerebellar inhibition and cerebellar disfacilitation, *Brain Res.* **77:**443–450.

GERGIS, S. D., DRETCHEN, K. L., SOKOLL, M. D., and LONG, J. P., 1972, Effect of anesthetics on acetylcholine release from the myoneural junction, *Proc. Soc. Exp. Biol. Med.* **141:**629–631.

GIBSON, W. R., DORAN, W. J., WOOD, W. C., and SWANSON, E. E., 1959, Pharmacology of stereoisomers of 1-methyl-5-(1-methyl-2-pentynyl)-5-allyl-barbituric acid, *J. Pharmacol. Exp. Ther.* **125:**23–27.

GODFRAIND, J. M., KAWAMURA, H., KRNJEVIĆ, K., and PUMAIN, R., 1971, Actions of dinitrophenol and some other metabolic inhibitors on cortical neurones, *J. Physiol. (Lond.)* **215:**199–222.

GOLDRING, J. M., and BLAUSTEIN, M. P., 1976, Barbiturates block Ca spikes but not Na spikes in Aplysia neurons, *Neurosci. Abst.* **2:**411.

GORDON, M., RUBIA, F. J., and STRATA, P., 1973, The effect of Pentothal on the activity evoked in the cerebellar cortex, *Exp. Brain Res.* **17:**50–62.

GOTH, A., 1974, *Medical Pharmacology*, C. V. Mosby, St. Louis.

GRINNELL, A. D., 1966, A study of the interaction between motoneurones in the frog spinal cord, *J. Physiol. (Lond.)* **182:**612–648.

GROSSMANN, W., JURNA, I., and THERES, C., 1974, The site of action of the optical isomers of 1-methyl-5-phenyl-5-propyl barbituric acid, *Naunyn-Schmiedeberg's Arch. Pharmacol.* **282:**367–377.

HALSEY, M. J., MILLAR, R., and SUTTON, J. A., ed., 1974, *Molecular Mechanisms in General Anaesthesia*, Churchill Livingston, New York.

HARRIS, M., HOPKIN, J. M., and NEAL, M. J., 1973, Effect of centrally acting drugs on uptake of γ-aminobutyric acid (GABA) by slices of rat cerebral cortex, *Br. J. Pharmacol.* **47:**229–239.

HARVEY, S. C., 1975, Hypnotics and sedatives, in: *The Pharmacological Basis of Therapeutics* (L. S. Goodman and A. Gilman, eds.) pp. 102–136, MacMillan, New York.

HAYCOCK, J. W., LEVY, W. B., and COTMAN, C. W., 1977, Pentobarbital depression of stimulus-secretion coupling in brain-selective inhibition of depolarization-induced calcium-dependent release, *Biochem. Pharmacol.* **26:**159–161.

Heavner, J. E., and Haschke, R. H., 1975, Interaction of glutamate and neurotropic compounds with an excitable membrane, *Neurosci. Abst.* **1:**368.

Heinbecker, P., and Bartley, S. H., 1940, Action of ether and nembutal on the nervous system, *J. Neurophysiol.* **3:**210–236.

Holmes, J. C., and Schneider, F. H., 1973, Pentobarbitone inhibition of catecholamine secretion, *Br. J. Pharmacol.* **49:**205–213.

Hsueh, C., and Marvel, C. S., 1928, Optically active hypnotics, *JAMA* **50:**855–859.

Hupka, A. L., Williams, J. K., and Karler, R., 1969, Effects of convulsant barbiturates on vascular smooth muscle, *J. Pharm. Pharmacol.* **21:**838–844.

Iravani, J., 1965*a*, Wechselbeziehung von Barbituraten und Piperazin mit GABA an der Membrane des Krebsmuskels, *Arch. Exp. Pathol. Pharmakol.* **251:**265–274.

Iravani, J., 1965*b*, Die Wirkung einiger zentral wirksamer Pharmaka auf die synaptische Ubertragung im Krebsmuskel, *Arch. Exp. Pathol. Pharmakol.* **251:**375–395.

Johnson, E. S., Roberts, M. H. T., and Straughan, D. W., 1969, The responses of cortical neurones to monoamines under differing anaesthetic conditions, *J. Physiol. (Lond.).* **203:**261–280.

Johnston, G. A. R., and Iversen, L. L., 1971, Glycine uptake in rat central nervous system slices and homogenates: Evidence for different uptake systems in spinal cord and cerebral cortex, *J. Neurochem.* **18:**1951–1961.

Jori, A., Bianchetti, A., and Prestini, P. E., 1970, Relations between barbiturate brain levels and sleeping time in various experimental conditions, *Biochem. Pharmacol.* **19:**2687–2694.

Kelly, J. S., and Beart, P. M., 1975, Amino acid receptors in the CNS. II. GABA in supraspinal regions, in: *Handbook of Psychopharmacology,* Vol. 4 (L. L. Iversen, S. D. Iversen, and S. H. Snyder, eds.), Plenum, New York.

Knave, B., and Persson, H. E., 1974, The effect of barbiturate on retinal functions. III. Effects on the isolated receptor responses and the inner nuclear layer components in the low-intensity electroretinogram of the sheep eye, *Acta Physiol. Scand.* **91:**187–195.

Knoefel, P. L., 1945, Stimulation and depression of the central nervous system by derivatives of barbituric and thiobarbituric acids, *J. Pharmacol. Exp. Ther.* **84:**26–33.

Koketsu, K., Shoji, T., and Yamamoto, K., 1974, Effects of GABA on presynaptic nerve terminals in bullfrog (*Rana catesbiana*) sympathetic ganglia, *Experientia* **30:**382–383.

Krnjević, K., 1974*a*, Chemical nature of synaptic transmission in vertebrates, *Physiol. Rev.* **54:**418–540.

Krnjević, K., 1974*b*, Central action of general anaesthetics, in: *Molecular Mechanisms in General Anaesthesia,* Glaxo Symposium, October 1973, Middlesex, England. Churchill-Livingston, London.

Krnjević, K., 1975, Is general anesthesia induced by neuronal asphyxia? in: *Molecular Mechanisms of Anesthesia* (B. R. Fink, ed.), Raven Press, New York.

Krnjević, K., and Lisiewicz, A., 1972, Injections of calcium ions into spinal motoneurones, *J. Physiol. (Lond.)* **225:**363–390.

Krnjević, K., and Phillis, J. W., 1963, Acetylcholine-sensitive cells in the cerebral cortex, *J. Physiol. (Lond.)* **166:**296–327.

Krnjević, K., Randic, M., and Straughan, D. W., 1966, Pharmacology of cortical inhibition, *J. Physiol.* **184:**78–105.

Krnjević, K., Pumain, R., and Renaud, L., 1971, The mechanism of excitation by acetylcholine in the cerebral cortex, *J. Physiol.* **215:**247–268.

Krupp, P., Bianchi, C. P., and Suarez-Kurtz, G., 1969, On the local anaesthetic effect of barbiturates, *J. Pharm. Pharmacol.* **21:**763–768.

Landis, D. M. D., and Reese, T. S., 1974, Differences in membrane structure between excitatory and inhibitory synapses in the cerebellar cortex, *J. Comp. Neurol.* **155:**93–126.

Landis, D. M. D., Reese, T. S., and Raviola, E., 1974, Differences in membrane structure between excitatory and inhibitory components of the reciprocal synapse in the olfactory bulb, *J. Comp. Neurol.* **155:**67–92.

LARRABEE, M. G., and POSTERNAK, J. M., 1952, Selective action of anesthetics on synapses and axons in mammalian sympathetic ganglia, *J. Neurophysiol.* **15**:91–114.

LARSON, M. D., and MAJOR, M. A., 1970, The effect of hexobarbital on the duration of the recurrent IPSP in cat motoneurons, *Brain Res.* **21**:309–311.

LEE SON, S., WAND, B. E., and WAND, D. R., 1975, A comparison of the potencies of a series of barbiturates at the neuromuscular junction and on the central nervous system, *J. Pharmacol. Exp. Ther.* **195**:251–256.

LIDBRINK, P., and FARNEBO, L. O., 1973, Uptake and release of noradrenaline in rat cerebral cortex *in vitro*: No effect of benzodiazepimes and barbiturates, *Neuropharmacology* **12**:1087–1095.

LINGWOOD, R. N. G., and CHIESA, F., 1967, Barbiturate/γ-aminobutyric acid compositions, British Patent: Brit. 1,085,786.

LLOYD, D. P. C., 1952, Electrotonics in dorsal nerve roots, *Cold Spr. Harb. Symp. Quant. Biol.* **17**:203–219.

LØYNING, Y., OSHIMA, T., and YOKOTA, T., 1964, Site of action of thiamylal sodium on the monosynaptic spinal reflex pathway in CNS, *J. Neurophysiol.* **27**:408–428.

MARLEY, E., and VANE, J. R., 1963, Tryptamine receptors in the central nervous system: Effects of anaesthetics, *Nature (London)* **198**:441–444.

MATTHEWS, E. K., and QUILLIAM, J. P., 1964, Effects of central depressant drugs upon acetycholine release, *Br. J. Pharmacol.* **22**:415–440.

MEYER, H., 1899, Welche Eigenschaft der Anästhetica bedingt ihre narkitische Wirkung? *Arch. Exp. Path. Pharmakol.* (Naunyn-Schmiedelbergs) **42**:109–118.

MINCHIN, M. C. W., and IVERSEN, L. L., 1974, Release of [^{3}H]gamma-aminobutyric acid from glial cells in rat dorsal root ganglia, *J. Neurochem.* **25**:239–244.

MIYAHARA, J. T., ESPLIN, D. W., and ZABLOCKA, B., 1966, Differential effects of depressant drugs on presynaptic inhibition, *J. Pharmacol. Exp. Ther.* **154**:118–127.

MIYATA, Y., and OTSUKA, M., 1975, Quantitative histochemistry of γ-aminobutyric acid in cat spinal cord with special reference to presynaptic inhibition, *J. Neurochem.* **25**:239–244.

MONNIER, M., and HOSLI, L., 1965, Humoral transmission of sleep and wakefulness: II. Hemodialysis of a sleep-inducing humour during stimulation of the thalamic somnogenic area, *Pflugers Arch. Ges. Physiol.* **282**:60–75.

MORI, K., ed., 1975, Neurophysiological basis of anesthesia, in: *International Anesthesiology Clinics*, Vol. 13, Little, Brown, Boston.

MULLINS, L. J., 1975, Anesthesia: An overview, in: *Molecular Mechanisms of Anesthesia* (B. R. Fink, ed.), Raven Press, New York.

NARAHASHI, T., MOORE, J. W., and POSTON, R. N., 1969, Anesthetic blocking of nerve membrane conductances by internal and external applications, *J. Neurobiol.* **1**:3–22.

NARAHASHI, T., FRAZIER, D. T., DEGUCHIK, T., CLEAVES, C. A., and ERNAN, M. C., 1971, The active form of pentobarbital in squid giant axons, *J. Pharmacol. Exp. Ther.* **177**: 25–33.

NAYLER, W. G., and SZELO, J., 1972, Effect of sodium pentobarbital on calcium in mammalian heart muscle, *Am. J. Physiol.* **222**:339–344.

NICOLL, R. A., 1972, The effects of anaesthetics on synaptic excitation and inhibition in the olfactory bulb, *J. Physiol. (Lond.)* **223**:803–814.

NICOLL, R. A., 1975*a*, Presynaptic action of barbiturates in the frog spinal cord, *Proc. Nat. Acad. Sci.* **72**:1460–1463.

NICOLL, R. A., 1975*b*, Pentobarbital: Action on frog motoneurons, *Brain Res.* **96**:119–123.

NICOLL, R. A., 1975*c*, Peptide receptors in CNS, in: *Handbook of Psychopharmacology*, Vol. 4 (L. L. Iversen, S. D. Iversen, and S. H. Snyder, eds.), Plenum, New York.

NICOLL, R. A., 1976*a*, The action of pentobarbital on the amino acid induced depolarization of primary afferents in the frog, *Proc. West. Pharmacol. Soc.* **19**:421–423.

NICOLL, R. A., 1976*b*, Promising peptides, in: *Neurotransmitters, Hormones, and Receptors: Novel Approaches* (J. A. Ferrendelli, B. S. McEwen, and S. H. Snyder, eds.) *Neurosc. Symp.* **1**:99–122.

NICOLL, R. A., 1977, Differential effects of pentobarbital on synaptic potentials in the sympathetic ganglion, (in preparation).

NICOLL, R. A., ECCLES, J. C., OSHIMA, T., and RUBIA, F., 1975, Prolongation of hippocampal inhibitory postsynaptic potentials by barbiturates, *Nature (London)* **258:**625–627.

NISHI, S., MINOTA, S., and KARCZMAR, A. G., 1974, Primary afferent neurons: The ionic mechanism of GABA-mediated depolarization, *Neuropharmacology,* **13:**215–219.

NODA, H., and IWAMA, K., 1975, Behavior of cortical neurons during both sleep and barbiturate anesthesia, *Internat. Anesth. Clin.* **13:**37–66.

OTSUKA, M., and NONOMURA, Y., 1963, The action of phenolic substances on motor nerve endings, *J. Pharmacol. Exp. Ther.* **140:**41–45.

OTSUKA, M., KONISHI, S., and TAKAHASHI, T., 1975, Hypothalamic substance P as a candidate for transmitter of primary afferent neurons, *Fed. Proc.* **34:**1922–1928.

OVERTON, E., 1896, Ueber die osmotischen Eigenschaften der Zelle in ihrer Bedentung fur die Toxikologie und Pharmakologie, *Z. Phys. Chem.* **22:**189–209.

OVERTON, E., 1901, *Studien über die Narkose zugleich sin Beitrag zur allgemeinen Pharmakologie,* Verlag von Gustav Fischer, Jena.

PAPPENHEIMER, J. R., KOSKI, G., FENCL, V., KARNOVSKY, M. L., and KRUEGER, J., 1975, Extraction of sleep-promoting factor S from cerebrospinal fluid and from brains of sleep deprived animals, *J. Neurophysiol.* **38:**1299–1311.

PARNAS, I., RAHAMIMOFF, R., and SARNE, Y., 1975, Tonic release of transmitter at the neuromuscular junction of the crab, *J. Physiol. (Lond.)* **250:**275–286.

PHILLIS, J. W., and TEBECIS, A. K., 1967, The effects of pentobarbitone sodium on acetylcholine excitation and noradrenaline inhibition of thalamic neurones, *Life Sci.* **6:**1621–1625.

PRICE, J. L., and POWELL, T. P. S., 1970, The mitral and short-axon cells of the olfactory bulb, *J. Cell Sci.* **7:**631–651.

PRICHARD, J. W., 1972, Effect of phenobarbital on a leech neuron, *Neuropharmacol.* **11:**585–590.

PRICHARD, J. W., and KLEINHAUS, A. L., 1974, Dual action of phenobarbital on leech ganglia, *Comp. Gen. Pharmacol.* **5:**239–249.

PROCTOR, W. R., and WEAKLY, J. N., 1976, A comparison of the presynaptic and postsynaptic actions of pentobarbitone and phenobarbitone in the neuromuscular junction of the frog, *J. Physiol. (Lond.)* **258:**257–268.

QUASTEL, D. M. J., and LINDER, T. M., 1975, Pre- and postsynaptic actions of central depressants at the neuromuscular junction, in: *Molecular Mechanisms of Anesthesia* (B. R. Fink, ed.), pp. 157–168, Raven Press, New York.

QUASTEL, D. M. J., HACKETT, J. T., and COOK, J. D., 1971, Calcium: Is it required for transmitter secretion? *Science* **172:**1034–1036.

QUASTEL, D. M. J., HACKETT, J. T., and OKAMOTO, K., 1972, Presynaptic action of central depressant drugs: Inhibition of depolarization-secretion coupling, *Canad. J. Physiol. Pharmacol.* **50:**279–284.

QUILLIAM, J.P., 1955, The action of hyptonic drugs on frog skeletal muscle, *Br. J. Pharmacol.* **10:**133–140.

QUILLIAM, J. P., and SHAND, D. G., 1964, The selectivity of drugs blocking ganglionic transmission in the rat, *Br. J. Pharmacol.* **23:**273–284.

RANSOM, B. R., and BARKER, J. L., 1975, Pentobarbital modulates transmitter effects on mouse spinal neurones grown in tissue culture, *Nature (London)* **254:**703–705.

RICCI, G., and ZANCHETTI, A., 1953, Rapporti tra le azioni inhibitrici del cerveletto e della sostanza reticolare mediale del bulbo, *Arch. Fisiol.* **53:**162–177.

RICHARDS, C. D., 1972, On the mechanism of barbiturate anaesthesia, *J. Physiol. (Lond.)* **227:**749–767.

RICHARDS, C. D., and HESKETH, T. R., 1975, Implications for theories of anaesthesia of antagonism between anaesthetic and non-anaesthetic steroids, *Nature (London)* **256:**179–182.

RICHARDS, C. D., and SMAJE, J. C., 1976, Anaesthetics depress the sensitivity of cortical neurones to L-glutamate, *Br. J. Pharmacol.* **58:**347–357.

RICHENS, A., 1969*a*, The action of general anaesthetic agents on root responses of the frog isolated spinal cord. *Br. J. Pharmacol.* **36:**294–311.

RICHENS, A., 1969*b*, Microelectrode studies in the frog isolated spinal cord during depression by general anaesthetic agents, *Br. J. Pharmacol.* **36:**312–328.

ROBERTS, P. J., 1974, Amino acid release from isolated rat dorsal root ganglia, *Brain Res.* **74:**327–332.

ROBERTS, M. H. T., and STRAUGHAN, D. W., 1967, Excitation and depression of cortical neurones by 5-hydroxytryptamine, *J. Physiol. (Lond.)* **193:**269–294.

RUDOMIN, P., 1966, Pharmacological evidence for the existence of interneurons mediating primary afferent depolarization in the solitary tract nucleus of the cat, *Brain Res.* **2:**181–183.

RYALL, R. W., 1975, Amino acid receptors in CNS. I. GABA and glycine in spinal cord, in: *Handbook of Psychopharmacology,* Vol. 4 (L. L. Iversen, S. D. Iversen, and S. H. Snyder, eds.), Plenum, New York.

SALMOIRAGHI, G. C., and STEFANIS, C. N., 1967, A critique of iontophoretic studies of central nervous system neurons, *Int. Rev. Neurobiol.* **10:**1–30.

SALMOIRAGHI, G. C., and WEIGHT, F., 1967, Micromethods in neuropharmacology: An approach to the study of anesthetics, *Anesthesiology* **28:**54–64.

SAMPSON, S. R., and JAFFE, R. A., 1975, Excitatory effects of 5-hydroxytryptamine, veratridine and phenyl diguanide on sensory ganglion cells of the cat, *Life Sci.* **15:** 2157–2165.

SASAKI, K., and OTANI, J., 1962, Accommodation in motoneurons as modified by circumstantial conditions, *Jap. J. Physiol.* **12:**383–396.

SATO, M., AUSTIN, G. M., and YAI, H., 1967, Increase in permeability of the postsynaptic membrane to potassium produced by "Nembutal," *Nature (London)* **215:**1506–1508.

SATO, M., AUSTIN, G., YAI, H., and MARUHASHI, J., 1968, The ionic permeability changes during acetylcholine-induced responses of aplysia ganglion cells, *J. Gen. Physiol.* **51:**321–345.

SAUBERMANN, A. J., GALLAGHER, M. L., and HEDLEY-WHYTE, J., 1974, Uptake, distribution, and anesthetic effect of pentobarbital-2-^{14}C after intravenous injection into mice, *Anesthesiology* **40:**41–51.

SCHMIDT, R. F., 1963, Pharmacological studies on the primary afferent depolarization of the toad spinal cord, *Pflugers Arch.* **277:**325–346.

SCHMIDT, R. F., 1964, The pharmacology of presynaptic inhibition, *Progr. Brain Res.* **12:**119–134.

SCHMIDT, R. F., 1971, Presynaptic inhibition in the vertebrate central nervous system, *Ergebn Physiol.* **63:**20–101.

SCHOEPFLE, G. M., 1957, Pentothal block of single nerve fibers and subsequent revival by means of anodal polarization, *Fed. Proc.* **16:**114.

SCHOENENBERGER, G. A., CUENI, L. B., MONNIER, M., and HATT, A. M., 1972, Humoral transmission of sleep. VII. Isolation and physical chemical characterization of the "Sleep Inducing Factor Delta," *Pflugers Arch. Ges. Physiol.* **338:**1–17.

SCHOLFIELD, C. N., and HARVEY, J. A., 1975, Local anesthetics and barbiturates: Effects on evoked potentials in isolated mammalian cortex, *J. Pharmacol. Exp. Ther.* **195:**522–531.

SCHOLFIELD, C. N., 1977, Prolongation of post-synaptic inhibition by barbiturates, *Br. J. Pharmacol.* **59:**507P.

SCHON, F., and KELLY, J. S., 1975, Selective uptake of ^{3}H-β-alanine by glia-association with the glial uptake system for GABA, *Brain Res.* **86:**243–257.

SEEMAN, P., 1972, The membrane action of anesthetics and tranquilizers, *Pharmacol. Rev.* **24:**583–655.

SEYAMA, I., and NARAHASHI, T., 1975, Mechanism of blockade of neuromuscular transmission by pentobarbital, *J. Pharmacol. Exp. Ther.* **192:**95–105.

SHAPOVALOV, A. I., 1963, Intracellular microelectrode investigation of effects of anesthetics on transmission of excitation in the spinal cord, *Fed. Proc., Trans. Suppl.* **23:**113–116.

SMAJE, J. C., 1976, General anaesthetics and the acetylcholine-sensitivity of cortical neurones, *Br. J. Pharmacol.* **58:**359–366.

SNYDER, S. H., and BENNET, J. P., 1976, Neurotransmitter receptors in the brain: Biochemical identification, *Ann. Rev. Physiol.* **38:**153–176.

SOMJEN, G. G., 1963, Effects of ether and thiopental on spinal presynaptic terminals, *J. Pharmacol. Exp. Ther.* **140:**396–402.

SOMJEN, G. G., and GILL, M., 1963, The mechanism of the blockade of synaptic transmission in the mammalian spinal cord by diethyl ether and by thiopental, *J. Pharmacol. Exp. Ther.* **140:**19–30.

STAIMAN, A., and SEEMAN, P., 1974, The impulse blocking concentrations of anesthetics, alcohols, anticonvulsants, barbiturates, and narcotics on phrenic and sciatic nerves, *Canad. J. Physiol. Pharmacol.* **52:**535–550.

STERIADE, M., WYZINSKI, P., and HALLE, J., 1974, Input-output organization of the motor cortex and its alterations during sleep and waking, in: *Basic Sleep Mechanisms* (O. Petre-Quadens and J. Schlag, eds.), Academic Press, New York.

SURIA, A., and COSTA, E., 1975, Action of diazepam, dibutyryl cGMP, and GABA on presynaptic nerve terminals in bull frog sympathetic ganglia, *Brain Res.* **87:**102–106.

TAN, A. T., 1975, Effects of amino acid transmitters on synaptosomal Cl fluxes, *Neurosci. Abst.* **1:**377.

TEBECIS, A. K., and DIMARIA, A., 1972, A re-evaluation of the mode of action of 5-hydroxytryptamine on lateral geniculate neurones: Comparison with catecholamines and LSD, *Exp. Brain Res.* **14:**480–490.

THESLEFF, S., 1956, The effect of anaesthetic agents on skeletal muscle membrane, *Acta Physiol. Scand.* **37:**335–349.

THOMSON, T. D., and TURKANIS, S. A., 1973, Barbiturate-induced transmitter release at a frog neuromuscular junction. *Br. J. Pharmacol.* **48:**48–58.

THORNTON, J. A., WHELPTON, D., and BROWN, B. H., 1963, The effect of general anaesthetic agents on nerve conduction velocities. *Br. J. Anaesth.* **40:**583–587.

VALDMAN, A. V., and ARUSHANYAN, E. B., 1967, The influence of analgetic drugs on segmental and suprasegmental inhibition, *Prog. Brain Res.* **20:**223–242.

VAN GILDER, J. C., and O'LEARY, J. L., 1971, Effect of Nembutal anesthesia upon Purkinje cell activation in the cat, *Electroenceph. Clin. Neurophysiol.* **30:**173–188.

VESELYUNENE, M. A., GUTMAN, A. M., and LESENE, V. A., 1971, Effect of Nembutal upon the inhibitory wave of antidromically evoked potential in the motor cortex of the cat, *Farmakol. Toksikol.* **5:**520–522.

WAHLSTROM, G., 1966, Differences in anaesthetic properties between the optical antipodes of hexobarbitol in the rat, *Life Sci.* **5:**1781–1790.

WAHLSTROM, G., 1968, Differences in anaesthetic properties between the optical isomers of 5-(2-bromoallyl)-5-isopropyl-1-methylbarbituric acid (Enibomal NFN) in the rat, *Acta Pharmacol. Toxicol.* **26:**81–91.

WALL, P., 1958, Excitability changes in afferent fibre terminations and their relation to slow potentials, *J. Physiol. (Lond.)* **142:**1–21.

WAY, W. L., and TREVOR, A. J., 1971, Sedative-hypnotics, *Anesthesiology* **34:**170–182.

WEAKLY, J. N., 1969, Effect of barbiturates on 'quantal' synaptic transmission in spinal motoneurones, *J. Physiol. (Lond.)* **204:**63–77.

WEAKLY, J. N., ESPLIN, D. W., and ZABLOCKA, B., 1968, Criteria for assessing effects of drugs on postsynaptic inhibition, *Arch. Int. Pharmacodyn. Ther.* **171:**385–393.

WEINBERGER, J., NICLAS, J., and BERL, S., 1975, Differential effects of anticonvulsants on the active uptake of putative neurotransmitters by rat brain synaptosomes, *Neurosci. Abst.* **1:**402.

WESTMORELAND, B. F., WARD, D., and JOHNS, T. R., 1971, The effect of methohexital at the neuromuscular junction, *Brain Res.* **26:**465–468.

York, D. H., 1975, Amine receptors in CNS. II. Dopamine, in: *Handbook of Psychopharmacology,* Vol. 6 (L. L. Iversen, S. D. Iversen, and S. H. Snyder, eds.), Plenum, New York.
Zukin, S. R., Young, A. B., and Snyder, S. H., 1974, Gamma-aminobutyric acid binding to receptor sites in the rat central nervous system, *Proc. Nat. Acad. Sci.* **71**:4802–4807.

5

ALCOHOL AND HUMAN BEHAVIOR

Nancy K. Mello and Jack H. Mendelson

1. ALCOHOL: THE DRUG

There has been a rapid expansion of behavioral research on alcohol and alcoholism within the past 10 years. The relics of a complex mythology have begun to yield to empirical observations, and a clearer impression of some behavioral effects of alcohol has begun to emerge. However, the transition from mythology to an accurate descriptive phenomenology is still incomplete, and the neural mechanisms underlying the effects of alcohol are unknown. We now recognize that alcohol can change human behavior in many subtle and elusive ways that are modulated by experience and expectancy as well as by the drug itself. The nature of the behavioral change is often unpredictable because of the many factors that interact to determine the effect of drinking.

Several aspects of alcohol use and abuse and the effects of alcohol on human behavior are explored in this review. Since our current understanding of the behavioral consequences of alcohol intoxication is so limited, the view presented here may represent only an approximation of reality. We proceed from the substantive to the more speculative, a sequence that reflects, in part, the differences in methodological development of the biological and behavioral sciences. The pharmacological characteristics of alcohol and how it is absorbed and processed in man are well understood and provide the basis for our subsequent treatise. Physiological tolerance for and dependence upon alcohol are described and compared with other addicting drugs. Contemporary patterns of alcohol use, including polydrug use, are then discussed.

Nancy K. Mello and *Jack H. Mendelson* • Alcohol and Drug Abuse Research Center, Harvard Medical School—McLean Hospital, Belmont, Massachusetts.

The second section focuses upon alcohol abuse and alcohol addiction. Current hypotheses concerning the development of alcohol problems are summarized. Several factors that are believed to maintain and perpetuate alcohol abuse are described, and the behavioral and medical consequences of chronic alcoholism are reviewed. Since alcohol addiction is similar in many ways to other forms of drug addiction, some of the commonalities and differences between these related phenomena are described.

In the third and final section, we selectively review recent studies of the effects of alcohol on several related behavioral variables. The spectrum of behavioral effects of alcohol is not completely covered by the categories of sociability and mood, aggression and sexual function, and memory and sleep. However, these categorical areas have been the primary topics of concern for a number of investigators. This review of behavioral studies is not exhaustive; rather, certain studies have been selected to illustrate some of the dominant trends and issues in the field. This review is often critical, and it is evident that interpretation of some behavioral data is seriously compromised by basic problems in experimental design and methodology. Some limitations of the studies are described, and possible sources of discrepant findings are suggested.

Whatever conclusions may be drawn from this review, one theme is dominant: we need to learn much more about every aspect of the behavioral effects of alcohol. Eventual progress will require some combination of new ways of thinking about behavior, some different and more incisive questions, and improved methodologies in the behavioral sciences. The development of new approaches to the study of alcohol and behavior will require consistent long-term research support and a stable commitment to this area of inquiry by investigators and funding agencies alike.

1.1. Alcohol: Its Absorption, Metabolism, and Degradation

Ethanol is a relatively simple organic molecule that is produced by the fermentation processes of microorganisms. The basic ingredients necessary to produce alcohol (sugar, water, yeast, oxygen, warmth, and an appropriate acid–base balance) have probably existed since paleolithic times. The circumstances surrounding man's early discovery of alcohol are unknown but have inspired considerable speculation. Prehistoric alcohol was probably fermented from honey, fruits, and grains. The process of distillation, the production of high ethanol concentration beverages through condensation of alcohol vapor, was developed during the first century A.D. (Forbes, 1948; Roueche, 1960).

Ethanol is rapidly absorbed, primarily from the small intestine, and distributed throughout the fluid compartments of the body. Once alcohol attains equilibrium, its concentration in body tissues is directly proportional to their water content. Regional concentrations of alcohol are dependent in part on regional differences in water concentration.

The liver is the primary site of alcohol detoxification and metabolic degradation; only about 2 to 10% of beverage alcohol is excreted by the kidneys and lungs (Isselbacher and Greenberger, 1964). There are no pharmacological agents currently available that can significantly increase the rate of alcohol metabolism or attenuate the acute intoxicating effects of alcohol (cf. Mendelson *et al.*, 1974; McNamee *et al.*, 1975; Noble *et al.*, 1973, 1975). Pharmacological tolerance for alcohol may be associated with a transient increase in the rate of alcohol metabolism in both alcohol addicts and normal drinkers (cf. discussion in Section 1.2).

The rate of alcohol absorption into the blood is influenced by several factors in the beverage and in the consumer. Both alcohol concentration and congener content affect absorption. The rate of absorption increases with increasing *ethanol concentrations,* up to a maximum of about 40%. Consequently, distilled spirits are absorbed much more rapidly than wine or beer (Haggard *et al.*, 1941; Lolli and Meschieri, 1964; Newman and Abramson, 1942*a*,*b*).

The rate of alcohol absorption decreases with increasing concentrations of *congeners.* Congeners are impurities in beverage alcohol and include vitamins, organic and amino acids, minerals, salts, sugars, and low concentrations of fusel oils (higher alcohols) that can be relatively toxic (Murphree, 1971; Leake and Silverman, 1971). Distilled spirits have a higher congener content than wine or beer, and the congener content has been shown to increase as a function of aging (Liebmann and Scherl, 1949).

Another factor that slows the rate of alcohol absorption is the presence of *food* in the stomach. Any variable that may retard the emptying time of the stomach will also delay the rate of alcohol absorption.

Rapid drinking will produce a higher concentration of alcohol in blood than slowly sipping an equivalent amount of alcohol (Moskowitz and Burns, 1975). Consumption of an equal amount of alcohol in the form of wine, beer, or whiskey will produce equivalent blood alcohol levels *and* equivalent behavioral effects (Kalant *et al.*, 1975).

Since alcohol is uniformly distributed throughout the body fluids following absorption, *body weight* also influences blood alcohol concentration. For example, a 180-lb man will have a lower blood alcohol level than a 130-lb man after consuming the same amount of alcohol under the same conditions.

These several factors that may interact to accelerate or retard the rate of alcohol absorption make it impossible to accurately predict blood alcohol concentrations following alcohol ingestion. However, it has been estimated that the usual legal limit of intoxication (100 mg alcohol per 100 ml blood) occurs after drinking 6 oz of distilled spirits on an empty stomach. The behavioral level of intoxication is a function of the concentration of alcohol in the blood. A blood alcohol level of 30 to 50 mg/100 ml may be associated with a pleasant feeling of tranquility and mild sedation. A blood alcohol level of about 100 mg/100 ml may result in motor discoordination. Blood alcohol levels above 100 mg/100 ml produce obvious intoxication in normal (nontolerant) drinkers. Confusion, disorientation, and stupor can follow the ingestion of large quantities of alcohol and blood alcohol concentrations above 500 mg/100 ml may be fatal.

The alcohol molecule possesses an ideal oil–water partition coefficient for effectively passing through the epithelial lining of capillaries into the extracellular tissue space of the brain. Following absorption from the gastrointestinal tract, alcohol in neural tissue achieves equilibrium with blood ethanol concentrations. The absolute level of ethanol in neural tissue may be somewhat higher or lower than in blood depending upon relative concentration of lipid, protein, and water in the specific sites involved, as well as the degree of vascularization of regions of the brain. Although ethanol is lipid soluble, its solubility is not high enough to result in trapping of the ethanol molecule in lipid compartments. Thus, movement of ethanol into and out of neural tissue is virtually unimpeded (Oldendorf, 1974).

The mechanisms by which alcohol affects the brain in order to produce the behavioral expression of intoxication is unknown. Recent evidence suggests that alcohol acts primarily on the reticular-activating system that regulates the activity of the cerebral cortex and subcortical structures (Kalant, 1970; Seixas and Eggleston, 1973). It was once thought that the signs of intoxication reflected a hierarchical disruption of central nervous system function, progressing from structures that control complex cognitive and motor behaviors and critical faculties to structures that control essential life functions such as breathing.

It has been difficult to establish the precise mechanism of action on neurochemical mechanisms that regulate ethanol-induced changes in behavior. A variety of *in vitro* and *in vivo* studies have shown that extraordinarily large concentrations of ethanol are necessary to inhibit neurochemical processes involved in metabolism, electrolyte transport, and neurotransmitter activity (Kalant, 1970).

There has been some recent evidence that physiological doses of ethanol have specific effects on some transmitter mechanisms. A decrease in norepinephrine turnover in the hypothalamus, brain stem, and telencephalon was found following administration of acute doses of ethanol to rat (Pohorecky, 1974). However, following chronic administration of ethanol for a period of 2 weeks, an acceleration of norepinephrine turnover was found as contrasted to baseline, acute, and chronic ethanol-ingestion conditions. A study of the time course of norepinephrine turnover during ethanol withdrawal revealed that maximal changes occurred 8 hr following cessation of alcohol availability. Moreover, the largest changes in norepinephrine turnover were found in the brain stem in contrast to other regions of the central nervous system. These findings with rat are of particular interest since the neurochemical changes observed parallel the time course that corresponds to physiological processes associated with withdrawal symptoms in humans. Clinical observations indicate that tremor and psychomotor agitation are most likely to occur within 8 to 24 hr following cessation of drinking (Victor and Adams, 1953; Isbell *et al.*, 1955; Mendelson, 1964). Therefore, it is possible that maximal norepinephrine turnover found in rat brain stem 8 hr after alcohol withdrawal may contribute to the CNS hyperexcitability following CNS depression during chronic drinking.

Effects of alcohol on levels of divalent cations in brain may be important in producing changes in behavior (Ross *et al.*, 1974). Following injection of 1.5 mg/kg of ethanol intraperitoneally, a significant decrease in calcium levels was found in hypothalamus, hippocampus, corpus striatum, and cerebral cortex. Ross and his associates also found that administration of morphine produced a significant decrease in calcium content in the same regions of the central nervous system. These data suggest that some common mechanisms may be involved in both ethanol- and morphine-induced alterations in neurochemical processes in the central nervous system.

Redos and his colleagues (1976) found that acute doses of alcohol induced a 95% depletion of cerebellar guanosine 3,5-cyclic monophosphate (cyclic GMP) in rat. Significant depletion of cyclic GMP occurred 1 hr following administration of the acute dose of alcohol. The degree of cyclic GMP depletion was related to the dose of ethanol administered and was correlated with blood alcohol levels. Although the role of cyclic GMP in neurochemical function remains to be determined, the authors suggest that it may be important in mediation of acetylcholine effects and also function as an antagonist of cyclic AMP activity. Moreover, since a significant depletion of cyclic GMP occurred in rat cerebellum at blood ethanol levels that are associated with mild to moderate intoxication in man, it is possible that signs of intoxication such as ataxia and dysarthria may be associated with alcohol-induced changes in cyclic GMP levels (Redos *et al.*, 1976).

In addition to its effects on the central nervous system, alcohol may also produce *peripheral physiological changes* such as dilation of the peripheral blood vessels, resulting in a sensation of warmth and skin flushing, muscular relaxation, and stimulation of gastric secretion and peristalsis. Recent evidence suggests that some of the physiological changes produced by alcohol may be accentuated by idiosyncratic and perhaps genetic factors. For example, flushing and peripheral vasodilatation following alcohol ingestion has been shown to occur with greater frequency and intensity in Orientals than in Occidentals. Studies of infant responses to alcohol indicate that this phenomenon is not due to cultural, cognitive, or experiential factors (Wolfe, 1972). These findings were confirmed in a comparison between 24 Oriental and 24 Occidental adult subjects following a small acute dose of alcohol. Skin flushing, decreased blood pressure, and complaints of subjective discomfort occurred in Oriental subjects at blood alcohol levels that produce little effect in most Occidental subjects (Ewing *et al.*, 1974).

A differential reactivity to alcohol as a function of genetic influences should not be confused with the hypothesis that differences in the rate of alcohol metabolism may account for the high incidence of alcohol problems among certain ethnic subgroups such as Eskimos and Indians. This hypothesis has not been confirmed and relevant data are inconsistent and conflicting.

In 1971, Fenna and his associates reported that Canadian Eskimos and Indians metabolize ethanol at significantly lower rates than Caucasians. More recent studies indicate that both Tarahumara Indians (Zeiner *et al.*, 1976) and Ojibwas (Reed *et al.*, 1976) metabolize alcohol more rapidly than Caucasian controls. In more detailed studies, Bennion and Li (1976) measured rates of ethanol metabolism in 30 American Indians and Caucasians using sensitive gas-chromatographic techniques for assessing ethanol concentrations in blood. The subjects were in good health and apparently had no evidence of chronic nutritional deficiencies. Blood alcohol data were expressed in terms of amount of ethanol metabolized *per unit of body weight* during fixed intervals of time. Bennion and Li found that the mean rate of alcohol metabolism was almost identical in the Caucasians and American Indians (Bennion and Li, 1976). In addition, these investigators examined alcohol dehydrogenase activity and isoenzyme patterns in hepatic biopsy specimens obtained from 7 Indians and 6 Caucasians and found no differences between groups in these indices. It was concluded that tolerance to ethanol cannot be explained on the basis of differences in rates of ethanol metabolism. However, Bennion and Li (1976) did find a positive correlation between rate of ethanol metabolism and past history of alcohol intake. Individuals with past histories of heavy alcohol intake had higher rates of ethanol catabolism than subjects who reported past histories of little or no alcohol intake. This finding is consistent with data that significant increments in rates of ethanol metabolism may be induced in alcohol addicts during heavy drinking (Mendelson *et al.*, 1965).

1.2. Alcohol Tolerance

Tolerance to alcohol can develop as a function of prolonged exposure, just as tolerance develops to many psychoactive drugs of abuse. Tolerance is inferred when progressively higher doses of alcohol are required through time to produce comparable subjective and behavioral effects. Three types of tolerance have been identified that are common to alcohol addiction and to other forms of drug addiction: behavioral tolerance, pharmacological tolerance, and cross-tolerance to other potentially addictive drugs (Seevers and Deneau, 1963).

Pharmacological tolerance for alcohol is inferred from an alcohol-induced increase in the rate of alcohol metabolism, both in alcoholics and in controls, as a function of the amount and duration of alcohol ingestion (Iber *et al.*, 1969; Mendelson *et al.*, 1965). This alcohol-induced acceleration of alcohol metabolism appears to be transient and does not persist long after cessation of drinking. However, the consistent consumption of as much as a quart of bourbon per day may result in unexpectedly low levels of alcohol in the blood (Mello and Mendelson, 1970*a*, 1972). A transient alcohol-induced increase in metabolic rate is consistent with the finding that the rate of ethanol metabolism in *abstinent* alcoholics and normal drinkers is not significantly different (Carpenter, 1940; Harger and Hulpieu, 1956; Jacobsen, 1952; Mendelson, 1968; Mendelson *et al.*, 1965; Newman, 1941).

Behavioral tolerance has been observed in alcohol addicts *and* in moderate drinkers, under certain conditions (Goodwin *et al.*, 1971). One illustration of behavioral tolerance for alcohol is the fact that an alcohol addict can consume between $^4/_5$ and 1 qt of bourbon per day without signs of gross intoxication (Mello, 1972, 1973; Mello and Mendelson, 1970*a*, 1972). A number of investigators have observed that alcohol may not induce significant impairments in the performance of behavioral tasks by tolerant individuals even when blood alcohol levels are twice the legal limit of intoxication, i.e., above 200 mg/100 ml (Carpenter, 1962; Doctor *et al.*, 1966; Mello, 1972, 1973; Talland *et al.*, 1964*a,b*; Talland, 1966). The dramatic behavioral tolerance for alcohol shown by the alcohol addict cannot be accounted for by a more rapid or effective capacity to metabolize alcohol. Alcoholics can perform very well on difficult tasks at the time that their blood alcohol levels are above 200 mg/100 ml (Mello, 1972, 1973). These findings converge to suggest that the adaptive processes subserving tolerance occur in the central nervous system as well as at a metabolic level.

Although alcohol tolerance is a striking phenomenon, the opiate or barbiturate addict develops a far greater degree of drug tolerance on a relative dosage basis. For example, barbiturate addicts may ingest 20 to 30 times the usual hypnotic dose over a 24-hr period. Heroin addicts may show similar increases in heroin self-administration, and many voluntarily go through heroin withdrawal in order to reduce tolerance and thereby lower their daily maintenance dose requirements (Goldstein *et al.*, 1968). In the alcohol addict, the lethal level of alcohol dosage remains close to that for normal drinkers and blood alcohol concentrations above 500 to 600 mg/100 ml can result in severe respiratory depression. Despite behavioral tolerance, the alcohol addict rarely develops blood alcohol levels above 450 mg/100 ml.

Alcohol tolerance is often accompanied by *cross-tolerance*, which is defined as a reduced responsivity to other drugs. It has been shown that sober alcoholics metabolize a number of drugs more rapidly than normal controls (Kater *et al.*, 1968). There are several reports that alcohol addicts require far larger doses of anesthesia to induce a surgical level of anesthesia than nonaddict patients (Bloomquist, 1959; Lee *et al.*, 1964). The alcohol addict may also show cross-tolerance to other potentially addictive drugs such as barbiturates, hypnotics, and sedatives (Seevers and Deneau, 1963). However, no cross-dependence has been shown between alcohol and opiate narcotics (Goldstein *et al.*, 1968). The alcohol addict also shows tolerance for many toxic alcohols and is able to ingest these in amounts that would be fatal for a nonalcoholic (Mendelson *et al.*, 1957). Cross-tolerance for other drugs only occurs in the *sober* alcohol addict. In an intoxicated individual, many drugs contribute to the effects of alcohol and the alcohol addict may metabolize other drugs more slowly than normal controls (Rubin *et al.*, 1970).

1.3. Alcohol Dependence

Alcohol is an addicting drug and prolonged abuse can result in physical dependence upon alcohol. Upon cessation of heavy drinking, a characteristic pattern of signs and symptoms occurs that constitute the alcohol withdrawal syndrome and defines the condition of alcohol dependence. The biological mechanisms underlying the expression of the alcohol withdrawal syndrome and of drug abstinence syndromes generally are unknown. The development of physical dependence is thought to be multiply determined by a complex interaction of neural, endocrine, and metabolic variables (Mendelson, 1971). Most attempts to account for the characteristic psychomotor and autonomic hyperactivity associated with drug withdrawal syndromes have postulated a heightened central nervous system excitability. This heightened CNS excitability has been attributed to a rebound effect following drug-induced depression of neural activity (Jaffe, 1970, 1975; Mendelson, 1971). There is considerable neurophysiological evidence that is consistent with the notion that the central nervous system becomes more excitable during drug withdrawal (Jaffe, 1970, 1975; Mendelson, 1971).

The clinical expression of the alcohol withdrawal syndrome may include tremor, profuse sweating, gastrointestinal disorders, nystagmus, hyperreflexia, sleep disturbances, hallucinations, and, occasionally, seizures. The usual alcohol withdrawal syndrome occurs between 12 and 72 hr following cessation of drinking, although the time course and severity are quite variable (Victor, 1966; Victor and Adams, 1953). Remission of the major symptoms is usually complete within 3 to 5 days. The common alcohol withdrawal syndrome is generally similar to a mild barbiturate, opiate, and nonbarbiturate–sedative withdrawal syndrome (Essig, 1968).

The critical determinants of the onset of the alcohol withdrawal syndromes are unclear since either a relative decrease in blood alcohol levels or the abrupt cessation of drinking may precipitate a withdrawal syndrome. The severity and duration of alcohol withdrawal syndromes also do not appear to be directly related either to the volume of alcohol ingested or to the duration of a drinking episode. It appears that the pattern of drinking may be more important than the duration of drinking in determining the expression of the alcohol abstinence syndrome (Mello and Mendelson, 1970*a*, 1977).

Alcohol withdrawal is not an all-or-none phenomenon. During the course of chronic drinking, alcohol addicts may experience wide fluctuations in blood alcohol levels as a function of periodicity of alcohol intake and alterations in the rate of absorption and metabolism of alcohol. The tremulousness associated with alcohol withdrawal may occur during alcohol consumption after a *relative* fall in blood alcohol level (Isbell *et al.*, 1955; Victor and Adams, 1953; Mello and Mendelson, 1970*a*, 1972). It is not possible to arbitrarily define a critical blood level at which the alcohol withdrawal syndrome is either initiated or suppressed. For example, alcohol addicts with blood alcohol levels as high as 300 mg/100 ml may experience severe abstinence symptoms when blood alcohol levels fall to 100 mg or to only 50 mg/100 ml.

It is important to distinguish the common alcohol withdrawal syndrome from *delirium tremens*. Even though delirium tremens is a distinct and specific disorder, which occurs quite infrequently, the term is often erroneously used as a generic description of alcohol withdrawal states. Delirium tremens usually occurs later than the common alcohol withdrawal syndrome, i.e., 72 to 96 hr after cessation of drinking. It may be preceded by tremulousness and is often preceded by seizure disorders (Victor and Adams, 1953; Victor, 1966). Delirium tremens is characterized by profound confusion, disorientation, delusional states, and hallucinatory episodes in addition to motor and autonomic dysfunction (Victor and Adams, 1953). Confusional states and delirium are rarely seen in the common alcohol withdrawal syndrome. Patients with delirium tremens frequently do have profuse sweating, tachycardia, hyperreflexia, mild to severe tremulousness, hypertension, and fever.

There are a number of recent comprehensive reviews of the clinical expression of the alcohol withdrawal syndrome (Victor, 1973; Gross *et al.*, 1974; Mello and Mendelson, 1977). More detailed information concerning the clinical expression and treatment of the alcohol withdrawal syndrome as well as a discussion of the current theories concerning the nature of alcohol dependence can be found in these reports.

1.4. Drinking Behavior: Alcohol Use and Abuse

There is little question that the recreational use of alcohol is common in this country. It is of some historical interest that the estimated consumption of alcohol in 1830 was twice that estimated for 1970 (Rorabaugh, 1976). A recent survey of American drinking practices estimates that two-thirds of all American adults use alcohol occasionally, although there are considerable regional variations both in beverage preference and in the amount of alcohol usually consumed (Cahalan *et al.*, 1969). This survey included 2746 representative individuals, of whom 32% reported total abstinence. Some possible determinants of abstinence have been examined by Goodwin and co-workers (1969*c*).

Contemporary use of alcohol continues a long tradition in Western society. Records of early civilizations show that alcohol was used in religious ceremonies, in medical treatments, and in many aspects of daily life.

Ambivalent attitudes about alcohol use have apparently existed almost as long as alcohol itself. Festival drunkenness was usually condoned, but there were always warnings against excessive secular use of alcohol. One of the oldest temperance tracts, entitled "The Wisdom of Ani" was written in Egypt about 3000 years ago (Roueche, 1960). The Old and New Testaments, and the ancient writings of Greece, Rome, India, Japan, and China all contain warnings against excessive drinking. In some cultures, alcohol was considered to be the gift of the gods. It was believed that the gods could use wine to cause madness or to create enhanced pleasure and awareness (Younger, 1966). As religious beliefs changed, alcohol itself came to be imbued with autonomous powers, and some animistic thinking about alcohol still persists.

The goals of temperance movements and the penalties imposed for drinking have varied in different cultures at different times. The American Temperance Movement of the 1830s urged abstinence only from distilled spirits (Gusfield, 1962). This objective was later expanded to an effort to ban all alcoholic beverages; a goal officially accomplished in 1920 by the 18th Amendment. National Prohibition was repealed in 1933 as it became obvious that legal sanctions were ineffective in controlling alcohol abuse or in changing the fact that many people like to drink.

There has been a recurrent pattern of moral and legal concerns throughout the centuries that reflects societal attitudes about alcohol use and abuse. One frequently debated issue has been whether the bartender or the drinker should be held responsible for adverse consequences of drinking. A law promulgated by King Khammurabi between 2285 and 2243 B.C. reads in translation: "If riotous persons assemble in the house of a wine merchant, and those riotous persons she sees as not and drives to the palace, that wine merchant shall be put to death" (Emerson, 1908, p. 12). Apparently females held the role of tavern keeper and wine merchant in Khammurabi's kingdom. More recently, the State Supreme Court of California decided that if a bartender knowingly serves an intoxicated person and that person later causes injury to others, the bar owner may be held responsible (1971). In 1976, this ruling was modified to release the tavern keeper from liability for injuries received by a patron after drinking during obvious intoxication. However, third parties who may be injured by the drinker may sue the tavern keeper for damages sustained. Several states have these so-called dram shop laws making it a misdemeanor to furnish alcoholic beverages to common drunkards or obviously intoxicated persons. Interpretation and enforcement of dram shop laws varies considerably between states.

Spontaneous changes in drinking patterns do occur. In the 1969 survey of American drinking patterns, 12% of the respondents were categorized as "heavy" drinkers (Cahalan *et al.*, 1969). The definition of "heavy" drinkers included persons who drank almost daily, or once a week, and often consumed five or more drinks per occasion (Cahalan *et al.*, 1969). A follow-up survey, conducted 3 years after the initial survey, indicated that there was considerable change in the composition of the "heavy," "moderate," and "infrequent" drinking groups. Fifteen percent of the sample had either moved out of or into the "heavy" drinking group (Cahalan and Room, 1974). These observations of rapid changes in drinking patterns suggest that "heavy" drinking does not invariably progress to alcohol abuse or alcoholism.

The several problems associated with compilation of a meaningful volume–frequency index of alcohol consumption (Cahalan *et al.*, 1969; Knupfer, 1966) have never been effectively overcome. Even though the total quantity of alcohol consumed over a particular time interval may be equivalent, the extent to which drinking is spaced or concentrated within a brief period reflects distinctly different drinking patterns. In contrast to the "heavy" drinker, an alcohol addict may drink between 24 to 32 oz of distilled spirits per day in increments of 2 or 3 oz per occasion (Mello, 1972; Nathan *et al.*, 1970). The length of a drinking spree may vary from a few days to a few weeks, depending upon the resources and the health of the drinker.

In this society, alcohol problems have long been associated with social stigma, which has precluded obtaining accurate indices of the incidence or prevalence of the problem. Official estimates of the number of alcoholics in this country have tended to vary between 5 million and 15 million. It appears unlikely that the accuracy of estimates of alcoholism incidence and prevalence is likely to improve in the near future. The many factors that contribute to denial of alcohol problems persist (Keller, 1962) and are perhaps overcompensated for by politically or economically motivated tendencies to inflate the estimate. However, whether 7 or 17% of the adult population has drinking problems, there can be no denial of the social cost to the afflicted individuals and their families. In its most severe form, chronic alcoholism is associated with disruption of the normal family relationships, job loss, progressive diminution of earning capacity, compromised physical and psychological health, and decreased life expectancy. A violent death or a suicide may terminate this progressive isolation and alienation from self and society (Goodwin, 1973; Robbins *et al.*, 1959; Tinklenberg, 1973; Waller, 1972).

A fuller discussion of the definitions of and criteria for alcoholism, its developmental course, and clinical expression, will be described in Section 2 of this review.

1.5. Polydrug Use Involving Alcohol

The tradition of categorizing drug abusers in terms of the type of drug abused is now being challenged by an increasing awareness of multiple drug use. It is not clear whether the accumulating impressions of prevalent polydrug abuse represent a genuine change in drug use patterns or primarily reflect a more objective and intensive examination of this problem (Ball *et al.*, 1975; Benvenuto *et al.*, 1975; Gould and Kleber, 1974; Green *et al.*, 1975). Alcoholism was once thought to be a problem that was distinct from opiate abuse, barbiturate abuse, or the abuse of stimulants or tranquilizers. Now it appears that heroin addicts, stabilized on methadone, engage in a diverse pattern of polydrug abuse, and alcohol and cocaine are among the preferred substances (Bourne, 1975; Kaufman, 1975; Langrod, 1970; Maddux and Elliott, 1975; Raynes *et al.*, 1975; Schut *et al.*, 1973; Woody *et al.*, 1975). The combined abuse of alcohol and barbiturates (Devenyi and Wilson, 1971; Freed, 1973) and alcohol abuse and marihuana use (Fisher and Brickman, 1973; Tec, 1973) has also been reported. Consequently, it appears that alcohol is often one component of nonopiate polydrug abuse. It has been estimated that between 22% (Benvenuto *et al.*, 1975) and 30% (Bourne, 1975) of polydrug abusers also abuse alcohol.

It has been very difficult to determine the prevalence of nonopiate polydrug abuse and the nature of multiple drug use patterns. The term "nonopiate polydrug abuse" is commonly used to refer *both* to the abuse of medically prescribed, psychoactive drugs such as tranquilizers and barbiturates, as well as to the abuse of recreational and illicit drugs, such as alcohol, marihuana, hallucinogens, inhalants, and cocaine (Bourne, 1975). These complex overlapping use and abuse patterns defy any simple categorization.

Recognition that alcohol may no longer be the exclusive agent of abuse for some substantial proportion of the drug-abusing population points to a need for more information about interactions between drugs of abuse. At present, we do not know whether the combined availability of alcohol and other drugs of abuse such as methadone, barbiturates, and marihuana changes the use patterns of any or all of these agents. It is possible that the combined availability of several drugs would facilitate overall drug use. Alternatively, it is conceivable that use of one drug might be modulated or attenuated by the simultaneous use of a second or third drug. At present, there is virtually no information about common use patterns or the subjective and objective effects of multiple drug use. However, an alcohol-induced increase in tobacco smoking has been well documented (Griffiths *et al.*, 1976; Dreher and Fraser, 1967; Maletzky and Klotter, 1974).

There is a vast literature in which the acute effects of alcohol have been compared with the effects of other drugs on various measures of performance and subjective reactions. Moskowitz *et al.* (1972) have recently reviewed studies that compare the effects of alcohol with the effects of marihuana on skills related to driving. Although both drugs impair response measures that are important for skilled performance, these are often different response measures.

A number of compounds have been shown to interact with and to facilitate the effects of alcohol (Forney and Hughes, 1968, 1970; Kissin, 1974). Studies of the combined effects of alcohol and marihuana on various measures of perception and psychomotor performance appear to indicate that some, but not all, functions are more impaired by alcohol plus marihuana than by either drug alone (Manno *et al.*, 1971, 1974). Low social doses of marihuana plus alcohol do not always produce significant impairment in experienced users (Macavoy and Marks, 1975). The more frequent finding is that combined effects of alcohol and marihuana produce greater impairments on a variety of tasks than either drug alone (Burford *et al.*, 1975; Goode, 1973). The combined effects of alcohol and marihuana appear to produce greater impairments in actual automobile driving performance than either alcohol or marihuana alone (Smiley *et al.*, 1975).

Most drugs of abuse have been shown to have some adverse medical consequences following heavy chronic use. The medical consequences associated with chronic alcohol abuse are discussed in Section 2.5 of this review. Currently, there is no information available on the chronic effects of the combined use of alcohol and one or more other drugs. Bourne (1975) has suggested that "the chronic endemic use of nonopiate" drugs may, in the long run, "represent a greater threat to society" than the more visible and publicized problem of heroin addiction (Bourne, 1975, p. 206). The adverse consequences of polydrug abuse involving alcohol and the comparative toxicity of chronic alcoholism and chronic nonopiate polydrug abuse remain to be determined.

2. ALCOHOL ABUSE AND ALCOHOL ADDICTION

2.1. Definitions

Alcohol abuse and alcoholism denote stages on a continuum of severity from problem drinking to chronic alcohol addiction. Since a continuing lack of consensus concerning an adequate definition of either alcoholism or alcohol abuse affects both the conceptualization and medical management of these problems, some discussion of the nature of the disagreements is necessary. Most definitions include repetitive excessive drinking that results in injury to an individual's health, adequate social function, or both. However, there are considerable variations in the criteria for each component of this definition. Only recently has there been some progress in developing more precise definitions that include objective criteria for differential diagnosis of alcoholism and facilitate the early identification of problem drinking (National Council on Alcoholism, 1972).

Most definitions of alcohol abuse and alcoholism emphasize either sociocultural or pharmacological considerations. The World Health Organization used sociocultural criteria to define abnormal drinking as that form of drinking that transgresses the normal social and dietary habits of the specific community involved (World Health Organization, 1955). Since there is enormous variation in acceptable drinking habits within and between countries, such sociocultural definitions do not have general applicability. For example, heavy drinking in a society that condones heavy drinking would not constitute alcohol abuse, whereas consumption of any alcohol in an abstinent society would be defined as alcohol abuse. No commonalities between groups of "abnormal" drinkers in different societies could be assumed and comparisons would be difficult.

The use of diagnostic criteria for alcoholism that are based on pharmacological criteria of addiction, tolerance, and physical dependence is one way to resolve the numerous problems associated with sociocultural definitions. Tolerance and physical dependence are used to objectively define the abuse of, and addiction to, other drugs that affect the central nervous system (see also discussion in Section 1). A pharmacological definition of alcoholism has the advantage of referring to observable events (i.e., the alcohol withdrawal syndrome) and permits selection of comparable patients for research and treatment evaluation. However, a pharmacological definition is limited in that it applies only to the alcohol addict and does not include the early problem drinker. The extent to which physical dependence upon alcohol occurs among middle and upper socioeconomic classes is unknown. The "skid row" alcoholic accounts for an estimated 3 to 5% of persons with alcohol problems (*Alcohol and Health,* 1971).

Reliance upon predominantly sociocultural or pharmacological definitions of alcohol addiction appears to influence the subsequent response to that problem by society. As long as alcoholism was considered a form of moral transgression and social deviancy, public drunkenness was dealt with in the criminal justice system. Although legal sanctions and moral pressures have never provided an adequate remedy for alcohol problems, a moralistic view of the alcoholic has limited interest in biomedical research on alcoholism. The introduction of pharmacological criteria for alcoholism has led to a gradual acceptance of the idea that alcoholism is an illness and a medical problem. Associated with this change in attitude has been an increase in biomedical research on alcoholism and attention to the medical aspects of the problem. Traditionally, physicians have often been reluctant to treat alcoholics for a variety of reasons, and it has also been difficult for alcoholics to gain admission to general hospitals. Today, however, many medical insurance plans will provide reimbursement for inpatient hospitalization and outpatient treatment of alcoholism.

Although few would deny the numerous medical consequences of alcoholism, there is still considerable controversy about whether or not alcoholism should be considered a disease. This recurrent controversy appears to revolve around a misunderstanding of the basic assumptions of a disease model of alcoholism. Critics complain that a disease model implies a linear physical causality without sufficient attention to the social and psychological factors. Actually, a disease model assumes that expression of the disorder depends upon an interaction between the individual (the host), the agent of the disease (alcohol), and the environment in which the disease process develops. Most disease processes cannot be explained on the basis of any specific factor within these three categories. Even infectious disease is more often closely related to host–resistance factors and environmental variables than to the presence or even the virulence of any given infectious agent (Mendelson, 1970, 1971; Mendelson and Stein, 1966). The factors that place certain individuals at high risk for development of alcoholism cannot yet be specified. However, there is little question that this disorder is determined by an interaction between many factors in the environment, the individual, and the drug itself.

2.2. Antecedents of Alcoholism

No single psychological, social, or biological variable has yet been shown to predict the development of problem drinking or to uniquely differentiate alcoholics from nonalcoholics. Repetitive heavy alcohol consumption can lead to the development of alcoholism in anyone, irrespective of age; individual personality characteristics; or educational, cultural, religious, ethnic, or socioeconomic background. The only reliable similarity among alcoholic individuals is repetitive drinking to intoxication, tolerance for, and physical dependence upon, alcohol. Among the prevalent hypotheses as to why some individuals develop alcohol problems and some do not, the roles of genetic, demographic, socioeconomic, and personality variables have been most thoroughly examined. Some evidence relating to each of these alleged predisposing factors will be described.

2.2.1. *Personality Variables*

There is no evidence that alcoholism is associated with any consistent or unique constellation of personality variables. Yet the search for the "alcoholic personality" continues unabated. The persistent appeal of a personality-based formulation resides in its all-encompassing simplicity and fundamental untestability. Personality-related characteristics such as depression, dependency, immaturity, hostility, and isolation have been associated with the development of alcoholism in the psychiatric literature. There are countless theories that attempt to conceptualize alcoholism in terms of psychodynamic variables, psychosocial development, etc. A comprehensive review of various psychological theories of alcoholism was prepared in 1959 by Zwerling and Rosenbaum. Since that time, aside from some relabeling of the same basic ideas, there has been little in the way of novel or substantive revisions of the various psychological theories. For the most part, these theories have been difficult to examine experimentally.

2.2.2. *Genetic Influences*

Although many individuals develop alcohol problems independently of a family history of alcoholism, the importance of genetic influences in the genesis of this disorder has been suggested by several recent studies

(Goodwin *et al.*, 1973*b*, 1974*b*; Schuckit *et al.*, 1972). Alcoholism appears to occur at a higher rate among relatives of alcoholics than in the general population, however, identification of the relative contribution of familial learning factors and genetic variables has always been a difficult methodological problem. Recently, Goodwin and co-workers have been able to examine these issues in individuals who were separated from their biological parents soon after birth and raised by nonrelatives, without subsequent contact with the biological parents. These studies were conducted in Denmark, where there is a centralized national registry of adoptions, psychiatric hospitalization, and criminal records. No such registry of information is maintained in the United States.

Fifty-five men whose biological parents had a hospital diagnosis of alcoholism were compared to a group of 67 control adoptees. These groups were matched with respect to reports of drinking problems and several other psychiatric and psychosocial factors. The rate of alcoholism in the group with an alcoholic biological parent was almost four times that of the control group. The experimental group also had a divorce rate three times higher than the control group. However, the two groups were equivalent with respect to diagnosed depression, anxiety, neurosis, sociopathy, and drug addiction and the incidence of these factors was low (Goodwin *et al.*, 1973*b*).

The drinking patterns of the parents of the adoptees were also studied in an effort to determine if learning factors may have influenced these findings. Possible or definite alcoholism was found in 13% of the foster parents of the experimental group and in 22% of the foster parents of the control group. However, there was no significant correlation between the drinking patterns of the adoptees and the presence or absence of alcoholism in their foster parents (Goodwin *et al.*, 1973*b*).

The influence of alcoholic or nonalcoholic foster parents on the incidence of alcoholism in children separated from one biological parent has been examined in two studies (Schuckit *et al.*, 1972; Goodwin *et al.*, 1974*b*). Children with one alcoholic biological parent, raised by a nonalcoholic parent, were compared with children with nonalcoholic biological parents who were raised by an alcoholic adopted parent. In 54 cases, the mother was the biological parent shared by the proband and by the half-sibling. It was found that alcoholism in half-siblings was associated with alcoholism in biological parents and not with being raised by an alcoholic parent. The development of alcoholism in both full and half-siblings was predicted with greater reliability by alcoholism in the biological parent than by any of the environmental factors examined (Schuckit *et al.*, 1972).

These findings were confirmed and extended in a similar study that compared the adopted sons of biological alcoholic parents with their brothers who were raised by the alcoholic biological parent (Goodwin *et al.*, 1974*b*). Both groups had comparable high rates of alcoholism of 25 and 17%, but the length of time spent with the alcoholic parent did not appear to be associated with development of alcoholism. The severity of the parent's alcoholism, as indicated by the number of hospitalizations, was positively related to the development of alcoholism in the offspring. These data suggest that exposure to an alcoholic biological or foster parent does not necessarily increase the risk of the development of alcoholism in the offspring (Schuckit *et al.*, 1972; Goodwin *et al.*, 1974*b*).

Comprehensive reviews of the issue of alcoholism and genetic factors have been published by Goodwin (1971*b*, 1976).

2.2.3. *Demographic and Socioeconomic Variables*

Although the studies of Goodwin and Schuckit have shown that childhood exposure to an alcoholic parent figure is less important for the development of alcoholism than having an alcoholic biological parent, a broader examination of socioeconomic and demographic variables indicates that alcoholism is not equally distributed across all strata of society. The largest proportion of problem drinkers appears to be persons of lower economic status who live in urban areas (Cahalan *et al.*, 1969; Mulford, 1964). The highest rates of alcohol-related problems were found in urban males, under 25, both single and divorced, who usually reported disrupted childhood and a transition from rural to urban living. The proportion of heavy drinkers among white and black males was comparable (22 vs. 19%) whereas black women showed a considerably higher rate of heavy drinking (11%) than white women (4%). Estimates of alcohol abuse prevalence rates based on arrested or hospitalized alcoholic populations show a higher rate of severe drinking problems among ghetto-reared black males (Robins and Guze, 1971). Bourne (1973) has reviewed some historical and cultural factors that may contribute to this pattern of alcoholism among urban blacks. American Indian and Eskimo populations have also been shown to be at high risk for the development of alcoholism (*Alcohol and Health,* 1971).

Data from longitudinal studies suggest that the same childhood patterns predict drinking problems for ghetto-reared blacks and whites. Adult drinking problems in both groups appear to be associated with early school problems, delinquency, drug use, and broken homes. These data have been interpreted to suggest that attention to *early* school problems might avert the subsequent progression of school failure and dropout, early drug exploration, and adolescent delinquency (Robins and Guze, 1971). Despite the disproportionate representation of alcohol problems among the economically disadvantaged, it is important to recognize that none of these factors permit reliable prediction of the development of problem drinking. Alcohol problems can develop in anyone who drinks alcohol to excess.

2.2.4. *Alcoholism in Women*

The actual rate of alcohol problems among women is unknown. Most available information about alcoholism has been obtained from the study of male alcoholics. Recently, the question of possible differences between alcoholic men and women has received somewhat more attention and critical reviews of the existing literature on the female alcoholic have been provided by Schuckit (1972), Schuckit and Morrissey (1976), Lindbeck (1972), and Beckman (1975).

Schuckit and Morrissey (1976) conclude that it is not possible to make generalizations about the female alcoholic. The literature does not appear to support the hypothesis that factors presumably unique to women, such as hormonal fluctuations, and concerns with femininity and sex roles are causally related to the development of alcoholism. The course of development and pattern of expression of alcohol problems appear to be influenced more by social class and socioeconomic status than by sex differences. It appears that there may be as many differences between female alcoholics as a function of social class and socioeconomic status as between female and male alcoholics. The age of onset of drinking problems is often similar in male and female alcoholics. However, alcoholism in women often occurs secondary to depressive illness and is accompanied by more suicidal behavior than is shown in males.

Schuckit and Morrissey (1976) attribute the inconsistencies in the existing literature to a failure to compare women and male alcoholics in the context of differences between men and women in the general population. They emphasize the importance of controlling for underlying psychiatric disorder, socioeconomic status, occupational status, and marital status in any effort to compare female and male alcoholics.

2.3. Development of Alcohol Dependence*

Little is known about the critical factors that lead to the development of alcohol dependence, defined by the alcohol withdrawal syndrome. However, it is now agreed that alcohol withdrawal signs and symptoms occur solely as a function of cessation of drinking in those individuals who have consumed enough alcohol over a long enough period of time. Both the quantity of alcohol and the minimum time course necessary for development of alcohol dependence in man are unknown. It is usually assumed that physical dependence upon alcohol develops after some years of heavy drinking, but it is not possible to examine this assumption by direct experimental observation. Self-report data, with all of its inherent unreliability, appears to be the only way to try to reconstruct the time course of the development of alcohol dependence. In a study of 129 alcoholics, it was found that the volume of alcohol consumed was not a consistent predictor of either the time course of development of alcohol dependence *or* the acute expression of most with-

* Clinical signs and symptoms associated with the alcohol withdrawal syndrome are described in Section 1.3 of this review.

drawal signs and symptoms (Mello and Mendelson, 1976). Data shown in Fig. 1 indicate that a minimum of 2 years of heavy drinking usually preceded the development of withdrawal signs and symptoms. For the vast majority (72% of the sample studied) at least 5 years or more of heavy drinking were required for the development of alcohol dependence.

The time course of development of alcohol dependence appeared to be independent of the alcohol concentration of the preferred beverage, e.g., whiskey vs. wine or beer. However, these data did offer tentative support for the notion that abuse of low alcohol content beverages, such as wine and beer, may result in some delay in the development of physical dependence, as compared with the abuse of whiskey. The frequency of early onset of withdrawal signs and symptoms was lower in the wine and beer drinkers studied. However, there is no question that alcohol addiction does result if sufficient alcohol is consumed in any beverage form, regardless of alcohol concentration. In the sample studied, "sufficient" alcohol appeared to be as little as 1 pint of whiskey, 1 qt of beer, or 4/5 of wine per day. Most whiskey drinkers reported drinking between 4/5 and 1 qt of whiskey per day (Mello and Mendelson, 1976).

It is interesting to compare these human data with studies of animal models of alcohol dependence (cf. Mello, 1973*a*, 1976, 1977 for review). Alcohol withdrawal signs and symptoms have been produced in rodents in as little as 3 to 5 days (Goldstein, 1972; Majchrowicz, 1975). Alcohol depend-

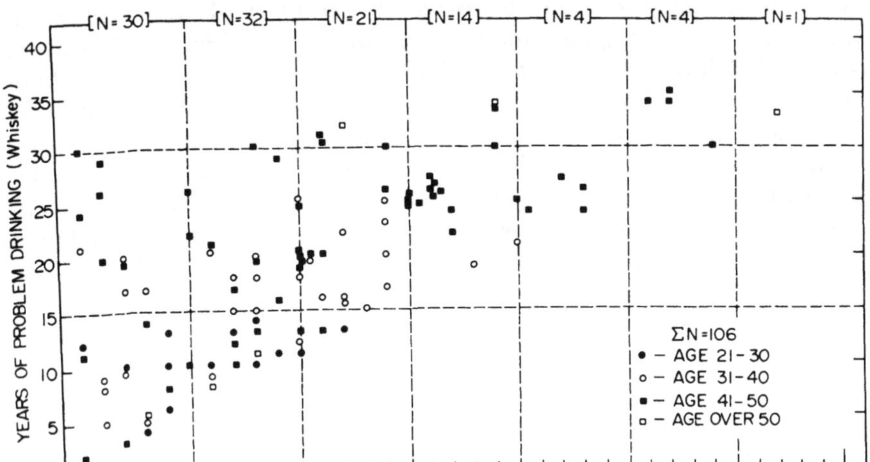

FIG. 1. Time course of the development of alcohol dependence. Self-report data from 106 alcohol addicts describing the latency between the initiation of problem drinking (whiskey) and the development of withdrawal signs and symptoms. The circles and squares indicate the age of the subject at the time of the interview (lower right corner). The total number of subjects appearing in each 5-year column is indicated at the top of the figure. From Mello and Mendelson, 1976.

ence has been produced in primates within 10 days to 2 weeks (Ellis and Pick, 1971; Pieper *et al.*, 1972). Each of these animal models required maintenance of relatively high blood alcohol levels throughout the period of observation.

It is of some historical interest that the causal role of alcohol in the production of alcohol abstinence phenomena was questioned until about 25 years ago. Although alcohol withdrawal phenomena have been described in the medical literature since 1787 (Lettsom, 1787; Sutton, 1813; Pearson, 1813), it was generally believed that an interaction between malnutrition, intercurrent illness, and the toxic effects of alcohol abuse accounted for the alcohol abstinence syndrome. It was not until 1953 that the clinical study of Victor and Adams (1953) demonstrated that cessation of drinking *per se* resulted in the alcohol withdrawal syndrome. These findings were subsequently confirmed in experimental studies in man in 1955 (Isbell *et al.*, 1955) and in 1964 (Mendelson, 1964). Today, there is little question that cessation of drinking by an alcohol addict may result in the characteristic pattern of withdrawal signs and symptoms known as the alcohol abstinence syndrome.

The factors that contribute to the onset and severity of withdrawal signs and symptoms are not fully understood. Observations of alcohol withdrawal signs and symptoms following a period of experimental drinking in an inpatient research ward suggest that both the duration of alcoholism and the pattern of drinking may be more important in determining the expression of withdrawal signs and symptoms than the volume of alcohol consumed (Mello and Mendelson, 1970*a*, 1976, 1977). For example, it was rather surprising to find that following cessation of drinking, 20% or more of the sample studied exhibited tremor, nystagmus, and GI symptoms, even when very low average blood alcohol levels (below 50 mg/100 ml) were maintained throughout a period of experimental drinking (Mello and Mendelson, 1976). Clarification of the determinants of the alcohol withdrawal syndrome in its several variants awaits further research. Blood alcohol levels, duration of drinking, pattern of drinking, intercurrent illness, conditioning and learning factors, and expectancies about withdrawal, are probably only part of the total matrix which affects the expression of alcohol abstinence (Mello and Mendelson, 1976, 1977).

2.4. Possible Factors That Maintain Alcohol Addiction

There is little objective information about the factors that maintain alcohol abuse or any other form of drug abuse. In the absence of data, speculations have ranged from the plausible to the absurd. In the era when alcoholism was seen as a moral issue reflecting character weakness, the view that alcohol abuse is a hedonistic pursuit was seldom challenged. This notion, like much of the conventional wisdom about alcoholism, was based in part on the assumption that alcohol abuse continually produced pleasurable effects for the alcoholic comparable to the effects of mild intoxication for the moderate social drinker. The cumulation of evidence that chronic inebriation is not a suspended state of carefree euphoria and relaxation has changed the perception of alcoholism by biomedical scientists (see discussion in Sections 3.2 and 3.3). Apparently many nonscientists continue to suspect that alcohol abuse produces sustained gratification and they believe that calling alcoholism a disease has merely dignified irresponsible and uncontrolled pleasure seeking.

A second hypothesis is that alcoholics continue to drink to avoid withdrawal signs and symptoms that may occur following an abrupt reduction of blood alcohol concentration. This is a plausible hypothesis that has been advanced to account for other forms of drug abuse. However, this hypothesis is not supported by the available evidence. If the avoidance of withdrawal signs is the factor that motivates an alcoholic to continue drinking, it would be expected that he would drink consistently and maintain stable blood alcohol levels during a drinking spree. However, both human alcohol addicts (Mello and Mendelson, 1972; Nathan *et al.*, 1971*a,b*) and primates (Woods *et al.*, 1971; Winger and Woods, 1973) show a marked cyclicity in alcohol self-administration. Despite the attendant discomfort of partial withdrawal signs, the alcoholic does not invariably respond to this condition by increased drinking (Mello and Mendelson, 1972). There is considerable variability in individual drinking patterns and aside from a tendency to drink early in the morning after a period of sleep and abstinence, the distribution of drinking within a day, or within a week, seems to be determined by the conditions necessary to obtain alcohol (cf. Mello, 1972).

The relationship between physical dependence upon alcohol and reinitiation of alcohol self-administration after a period of abstinence is poorly understood. It has been difficult to examine the assumption that physical dependence is one aspect of an addict's motivation for drug use. Logically, it is difficult to account for the reinitiation of an addictive drinking sequence, after a prolonged period of sobriety, in terms of physical dependence on alcohol. Presumably, whatever factors first prompted excessive drinking before the development of physical dependence continue to affect the resumption of abusive drinking.

Another hypothesis often advanced to account for the perpetuation of drinking is the notion of "craving," which implies that once an alcoholic starts to drink, "he is compelled to continue until he reaches a state of severe intoxication" (Mardones, 1963). This explanation is inherently circular since the concept of "craving" is defined by the behavior that it is invoked to explain. There has been no empirical support for the notion of alcohol "craving" on the basis of direct experimental observations of alcoholics given alcohol and clinical material (cf. Mello, 1975, for review). Although this construct appears to be of limited utility, it has long formed the basis for the usual therapeutic goal of total abstinence in the treatment of the alcoholic patient and has been the source of considerable confusion in the literature on alcoholism.

The term "psychological dependence" represents another hypothesis about why an alcoholic continues to abuse alcohol. This term is imprecisely defined and usually is used to refer to the motivational factors that underlie drug-seeking behavior *and* to the psychological effects of drug use. A confusion between the antecedent motivation and the effects of drug use reflects our current limited understanding of the factors that initiate and maintain a drinking episode.

At present, there are no satisfactory explanations for the repetition of excessive drinking and alcohol withdrawal episodes, despite the totally predictable adverse medical, social, economic, and often legal consequences. Immediate rather than the long-range consequences of alcohol abuse appear to control drinking behavior, however, even these immediate consequences do not appear to be "positive" in the sense that moderate drinking may be positive for the normal social drinker. The possible contribution of physical dependence upon alcohol to the reinitiation of drinking after a period of sobriety has not been determined. It is very unlikely that the condition of physical dependence in the sober alcoholic influences subsequent drinking behavior in the same way that the presence or absence of food deprivation affects food-seeking behavior. The resumption of addictive drinking after a period of abstinence probably reflects many interacting social, environmental, and psychogenic factors. Clinical observations of affluent or employed alcoholics suggest these individuals often plan a 2- to 3-week drinking spree in the same way others might plan a vacation. Interpersonal or emotional stress does not invariably precipitate a drinking spree (Mello, 1972), and the antecedents of each drinking episode probably vary, even for an individual alcoholic.

Equally puzzling are the conditions under which an initial exposure to alcohol becomes translated into alcohol abuse and alcoholism. Many alcoholics report a vivid recollection of their first drink (Kuehnle, *et al.*, 1974); however, this recollection is not necessarily positive. More frequently, the first drink was associated with extreme intoxication, nausea, vomiting, and some despondency—a series of consequences that do not appear to invite repetition. Aversive consequences of an initial drug exposure are not unique to alcohol, but also occur after opiate and barbiturate use (Jaffe, 1975). Moreover, *chronic* alcohol and opiate abuse both appear to be associated with the development of progressive dysphoria, anxiety, irritability, and aggressivity (Haertzen and Hooks, 1969; McNamee *et al.*, 1968; Mello, 1972; Mirin *et al.*, 1975, 1976; Nathan *et al.*, 1971*b*). The continuation of drug use that produces adverse consequences *during* intoxication seems antithetical to the idea that drug use is maintained by positive or "rewarding" consequences.

These data on the adverse initial and chronic consequences of alcohol and drug use have important implications for study of the behavioral basis of drug abuse. It is possible that drugs are used to induce some change in subjective state, and the direction of change—up or down—may be far less important than the change itself. If the stimulus properties of drugs are more important than the specific qualities of these stimuli, then it may be useful to think of drug self-administration within a more general framework of stimulus self-administration (Mello, 1977). A stimulus self-administration hypothesis could account for multiple drug use patterns involving drugs with demonstrably different pharmacological effects, e.g., methadone + alcohol, marihuana + alcohol, amphetamines + barbiturates, etc. Anecdotal accounts of polydrug use suggest that the goal is to achieve a rapid change in state and the direction of change may be of secondary importance. Wikler and Rasor (1953) were perhaps the first to suggest the importance of state change in maintaining opiate abuse. Opiate addicts reported that they used drugs to "get off the normal" (Wikler and Rasor, 1953).

The hypothesis that alcohol and drug self-administration could be thought of as stimulus self-administration is consistent with contemporary concepts about the nature of reinforcement in the basic literature on the experimental analysis of behavior (Morse and Kelleher, 1970, 1977). The traditional tendency to think about reinforcers in terms of the alleged properties of events, rather than in terms of the functional relations between events and behavior, has been persuasively challenged by Morse and Kelleher (1977). In their formulation, the defining characteristics of reinforcers and punishers are how they change behavior, rather than in terms of the inherent properties of the reinforcing or punishing stimulus event. The same stimulus may have either reinforcing or punishing effects, i.e., increase or decrease behavior, depending upon the conditions under which it is presented. Within this framework, the alleged stimulus properties of an event, such as alcohol-induced nausea, anxiety, and dysphoria, do not distract from the behavioral observation that these events are part of the total stimulus complex that apparently maintains alcohol abuse. This aspect of human drug use has provocative parallels with basic behavioral data obtained on primates. It has been found that the same electric shock event that can maintain escape and avoidance behavior may, under certain conditions, be self-administered by the same monkey. Response-produced shock was first reported by Kelleher *et al.* in 1963, and has now been observed in many laboratories, across several species, and has been shown to be a reliable and persistent phenomenon (cf. Morse and Kelleher, 1970; McKearney, 1972; Mello, 1977, for review). These findings on response-produced shock have recently been extended to response-produced narcotic antagonist administration in opiate-dependent monkeys (Woods *et al.*, 1975).

These data on response-produced shock and response-produced antagonist administration in opiate-dependent monkeys challenge prevailing assumptions about what constitutes a "positive" and an "aversive" event and argue strongly that it is not the inherent properties of an event *per se*, but the way in which the event is scheduled that determines the subsequent effect on behavior. The alcoholic and the drug addict apparently schedule drug use and its consequences in such a way that the behavior is maintained. One way to try to analyze that schedule is to examine and compare spontaneous patterns of alcohol and drug self-administration. Whether this approach will yield a way to determine factors that could be manipulated to change the basic schedule, and hence the drug abuse pattern, remains to be determined.

It is important to recognize that many nonpharmacological factors also contribute to the perpetuation of alcohol abuse (Orcutt, 1975; Orcutt and Biggs, 1975). Behavioral analysis of patterns of substance use and their consequences is also one approach to the study of nonpharmacological factors. The role of social influences and peer pressure in adolescent patterns of alcohol and drug misuse have been described by Jessor and Jessor (1975). The complex interactions of nonpharmacological factors in drug dependence have been eloquently described by Freedman (1972).

2.5. Medical Consequences of Alcoholism

Detailed discussions of the medical consequences of alcoholism appear in reviews by Mendelson (1975), Seixas *et al.* (1975), and Kissin and Begleiter (1974). A brief overview of some of the major medical problems associated with chronic alcoholism will be described in this section.

There is little question that prolonged abuse of alcohol has toxic effects on several organ systems and secondary adverse effects on metabolic processes. *Liver damage* is one of the earliest and most profound consequences of excessive alcohol use (Lieber *et al.*, 1971; Isselbacher and Carter, 1971). Liver disease is a potentially fatal condition, which may also be associated with derangements of central nervous system function (Victor, 1974). Alcohol has been shown to produce transient development of fatty liver in normal drinkers in as short a period as 2 days (Rubin and Lieber, 1968*a*). Alcohol-induced fatty liver may progress to alcoholic hepatitis or potentially fatal cirrhosis of the liver in the chronic alcoholic. Although alcohol abuse almost invariably produces fatty liver, not all alcoholics develop cirrhosis. The variables that predispose some alcoholics to the development of cirrhosis are unknown. An experimental model of alcoholic cirrhosis in the baboon exposed to alcohol over a 4-year period has recently been developed by Lieber, Rubin and co-workers (Rubin and Lieber, 1974; Lieber *et al.*, 1975; Lieber and DeCarli, 1974). The availability of this animal model should permit clarification of the determinants of alcoholic cirrhosis.

Alcohol abusers frequently develop recurrent *gastritis* and *pancreatitis* (Isselbacher and Carter, 1971; Pirola and Lieber, 1974). Gastritis may progress to gastric or duodenal ulcers that in turn may lead to potentially fatal gastrointestinal bleeding. Pancreatitis is also a potentially lethal condition. The mechanism of pancreatitis production is unknown (Webster, 1975; Dreiling, 1975). However, individuals with Type IV hyperlipidemia are at greater risk for development of pancreatitis (Frederickson *et al.*, 1967). It has been observed that alcoholics with genetically determined primary hypertriglyceridemia develop striking lipid abnormalities during experimentally induced intoxication (Mendelson and Mello, 1973). Alcohol-induced elevations in triglyceride levels have also been found in normal drinkers who have a familial Type IV disorder, but no history of alcohol abuse (Ginsberg *et al.*, 1974).

Excessive alcohol use may also interfere with the absorption of essential nutrients and vitamins into the blood from the small intestine. Alcohol addicts often have a compromised nutritional status associated with poor diet and a nutritional malabsorption syndrome.

Nutritional deficiencies and malabsorption syndromes are also associated with a variety of *neurological* disorders often seen in chronic alcoholics. It is not clear whether disorders of central nervous system function associated with chronic alcohol abuse result primarily from the direct toxic action of alcohol or from a combination of alcohol abuse and poor nutrition. Prolonged alcohol intake, even in the presence of an adequate diet, may result in impairment of eye muscle control due to nerve dysfunction. This condition is usually readily reversible following cessation of excessive alcohol use. However, it may also indicate a potentially serious condition that can progress to permanent incapacity, Wernicke's disease, and Korsakoff's psychosis. These disorders are characterized by a profound impairment of memory and deranged thinking processes. Alcoholic neuropathies may involve vagus and sympathetic nerve degeneration associated with hoarseness, weakness of voice, dysphasia, and autonomic nervous system dysfunction; a clinical picture that may also herald the development of Wernicke's disease (Novak and Victor, 1974). Many other forms of "organic brain disorders" associated with alcohol abuse and nutritional deficiencies are often seen in chronic alcohol addicts, particularly in older individuals. Comprehensive reviews of the clinical symptoms and pathological changes associated with these diseases of the nervous system have been prepared by Victor (1975) and Dreyfus (1974).

The question of whether or not alcohol exerts a direct toxic effect on neural tissue, independent of any nutritional disorder, remains to be answered. Tewari and Noble (1971) reported an alcohol-induced inhibition of protein synthesis in the brains of mice chronically exposed to alcohol, and have more recently extended their findings to rats (Noble and Tewari, 1975). A decrease in the *in vitro* incorporation of radioactive leucine into brain ribosomes was observed in animals that consumed a 10% alcohol solution for 10 days or more. An even greater derangement in brain protein synthesis was seen in animals physically dependent upon alcohol, after alcohol withdrawal (Noble and Tewari, 1975). These findings have been confirmed and extended by *in vivo* studies of mice exposed to a 10% alcohol solution for 4 to 8 weeks (Fleming *et al.*, 1975). Acute alcohol administration consistently results in a decreased capacity for cerebral synthesis of protein in both *in vivo* and *in vitro* studies with experimental animals (cf. Noble and Tewari, 1977 for review). However, it remains to be determined if alcohol intake produces alterations in protein synthesis in the human central nervous system, and if changes in protein synthesis are associated with changes in CNS function and behavior.

Peripheral neuropathies are also associated with chronic alcohol abuse. These involve compromised function of motor and sensory nerves in the arms and legs and are characterized by pain, impaired movement and coordination, and, eventually, muscle wasting. This condition is often reversible in the presence of an adequate diet and cessation of alcohol abuse (Mayer, 1966; Myerson, 1971).

Prevailing impressions about the relation between alcohol and *cardiac function* have evolved from a belief that alcohol is beneficial and acts as a coronary artery vasodilator to a concern that alcohol is toxic and compromises cardiac efficiency. There is cumulating evidence that alcohol may contribute directly to a form of cardiac myopathy, independent of thiamine deficiency or related nutritional imbalance. Alcoholic cardiomyopathy is characterized by enlargement of the heart, congestive heart failure, and pulmonary vascular congestion (Gunnar *et al.*, 1975; Talbott, 1975). The process by which alcohol may compromise cardiac function is unknown. Alcohol is a mild cardiac depressant and has been shown to decrease left ventricular contractibility and eventually to reduce the mechanical efficiency of the left ventricle (Regan *et al.*, 1975). There is suggestive evidence that clinically normal, alcoholic patients show abnormalities of cardiac function that are similar to, but quantitatively less than, a group with demonstrable cardiomyopathy (Spodick *et al.*, 1972).

The significance of these data on the possible cardiac toxicity of alcohol for the overall incidence of heart disease remains to be evaluated. Just as in the case of cirrhosis, the majority of alcohol users apparently do not develop cardiac myopathy and the factors that place some persons at high risk are unknown (Burch and Giles, 1974). Prospective studies have shown that habitually abstinent individuals have a greater chance of developing coronary artery disease than moderate drinkers (Klatsky *et al.*, 1974). It was also found that *former* drinkers were more prone to develop myocardial infarction than drinkers *or* nondrinkers (The Framingham Heart Study, 1966).

The possible contribution of alcohol abuse to the development of certain types of *cancer* has become a subject of considerable concern. Alcohol has been associated with cancer of the liver, the esophagus, the head and neck, and several other areas. Cancer victims, primarily patients with Hodgkins disease and othe lymphomas, may be intolerant of alcohol and develop local painful reactions soon after drinking. A comprehensive review of the current state of knowledge about alcohol and cancer has been provided by Kissin and Kaley (1974). They emphasize that the apparently significant relation between alcohol and cancer does not necessarily indicate a causal relationship, and the evidence that alcohol is an etiological factor in cancer is less compelling than the evidence implicating smoking (Kissin and Kaley, 1974).

Considerably more research will be required before a definite association can be disconfirmed or validated.

Many alcohol addicts and alcohol abusers may also have disorders of affect or overt psychosis. There is little evidence that a causal relationship exists between alcoholism and a number of *psychiatric conditions* but rather the relationship appears to be associational. Even the "alcoholic paranoid state" has yet to be shown to be a unique psychosis that is caused by or even aggravated by alcohol abuse. Although some individuals with neurotic and psychotic affective disorders may abuse alcohol, many other individuals with symptoms of these disorders do not drink heavily and may even be abstinent from alcohol. The traditional notion that depression is the "underlying basis" for alcohol abuse has not been clinically validated and has not generated uniquely effective therapies for alcoholism. It has also been difficult to relate the appearance of so-called "pathological intoxication" to a specific pharmacological effect of alcohol on the central nervous system (Mello and Mendelson, 1975).

Recently, there has been a renewed concern about the effect of alcohol on *fetal development,* which has paralleled an awareness of the deleterious effects of heroin addiction and methadone maintenance on offspring of opiate-dependent mothers (Wilson *et al.*, 1973; Zelson *et al.*, 1971; Stone *et al.*, 1971). The idea that maternal drinking may have an adverse effect on infant development has a long history. Prescriptions against drinking during pregnancy have been attributed to Aristotle, as well as to the Old Testament, and became a focus of concern in England between 1720 and 1865. The fluctuating status of these beliefs and the virtual disappearance of attention to this issue during Prohibition have been reviewed by Warner and Rosett (1975).

In 1973, Jones and co-workers reported a similar pattern of cranial, facial, limb, and cardiovascular defects associated with deficient prenatal growth onset and delayed development in eight children born to chronic alcoholic mothers. Jones and colleagues (1974) later determined that there was a 17% perinatal mortality among the offspring of 23 alcoholic women and of the survivors, 44 had borderline to moderate mental deficiency and 32 had abnormal physical features. Recent prospective studies indicate a higher incidence of morphological and functional abnormalities, as well as gross retardation in infants of heavy drinkers as compared to children of abstainers and moderate drinkers (Warner and Rosett, 1975; Rosett *et al.*, 1976). Heavy drinkers were defined according to Cahalan's criteria, i.e., at least 5 or 6 drinks on one occasion and a minimum average of 1.5 drinks per day. In the population studied, average consumption was 4 oz of alcohol per day and a quarter of the heavy drinkers consumed 8 to 16 oz per day. Of the 282 infants evaluated by a pediatrician, only 30% of the infants of heavy drinkers were normal as contrasted with 67% of the children of mothers who drank rarely. Children of heavy drinkers also had a statistically significantly greater frequency of congenital abnormalities, growth abnormalities, and functional abnormalities than the children of rare drinkers (Rosett *et al.*, 1976). Heavy drinkers received counseling throughout pregnancy and in those women who significantly reduced their alcohol consumption, 6 of 8 infants were diagnosed as normal. The authors interpret these observations to suggest that abstinence or marked reduction of alcohol use during the second half of pregnancy can lower risk to the offspring (Rosett *et al.*, 1976). To date, the effects of moderate social drinking during pregnancy on the physical and developmental capacities of the infant are unknown. It is of interest to note that an animal model of the fetal alcohol syndrome has recently been reported in the beagle dog (Ellis *et al.*, 1977*a,b*).

3. BEHAVIORAL EFFECTS OF ALCOHOL

The effects of alcohol on a variety of subjective variables and objective measures will be described in the remainder of this review. The available evidence suggests that most behavioral effects of alcohol are not an invariant, precisely predictable, function of alcohol dosage or blood alcohol levels. In addition to the variables discussed in Section 1.1, many nonpharmacological factors such as expectancy, experience with alcohol, and motivation to perform accurately, may act singly or in combination to modulate the observed effects of alcohol on behavior. The nonpharmacological factors that are alleged to influence subjective aspects of intoxication have been extremely difficult to identify and examine in isolation, but psychological variables obviously contribute to patterns of drug use and abuse. Provocative discussions of nonpharmacological factors in drug use and drug dependence have been provided by Freedman (1972), Hollister *et al.* (1975), and Orcutt (1975). In heavy drinkers and alcohol addicts, the development of behavioral tolerance for alcohol may further influence the objective and subjective effects of alcohol intoxication. Considerably more alcohol is required to produce impairments on objective measures of performance in tolerant alcohol abusers.

The effects of acute doses of alcohol on *psychomotor performance* have concerned many investigators over many years. The relevant literature prior to 1962 has been reviewed by Carpenter. The effects of alcohol on driving skills have recently been reviewed by Moskowitz (1971) and co-workers (1974). In general, the available evidence indicates that many objective measures of psychomotor performance deteriorate linearly with increasing blood alcohol levels (Sidell and Pless, 1971; Evans *et al.*, 1974; Franks *et al.*, 1976). An inverse linear relationship between alcohol dosage and performance decrements has been observed in normal drinkers over an alcohol dose range of 0.54, 0.75, and 1.0 g/kg, which yielded peak blood alcohol levels of 69, 92, and 113 mg/100 ml, respectively (Franks *et al.*, 1976). An acute alcohol dose of 25, 40, 55, and 70 ml/70 kg, which yielded peak blood alcohol levels of 17, 42, 61, and 89 mg/100 ml, respectively, also resulted in a linear decrement in performance on a pursuit meter and a wobble board (Evans *et al.*, 1974). Performance decrements on a number of psychomotor tasks were observed in a blood alcohol range relevant to the social drinking experience of normal drinkers.

The common impression that beer and wine are less intoxicating than distilled spirits appears to be incorrect. Kalant and co-workers (1975) examined the effects of a standard dose of alcohol (1.3 g/kg), administered in the form of rye whiskey, beer, and sparkling wine, on sensorimotor tasks and physiological variables in normal drinkers. No significant differences among the effects of these three alcoholic beverages on sensory, motor, or physiological measures were observed at any blood alcohol level. Peak blood alcohol levels ranged between 90 and 120 mg/100 ml. The relevant variable influencing performance appeared to be blood alcohol concentration as a function of dose of alcohol ingested, and not the type of beverage consumed (Kalant *et al.*, 1975).

Studies of the effects of alcohol on subjective states and interpersonal variables have yielded more equivocal results. Problems in devising sensitive and adequate methods continue to limit the generality of results obtained. Empirical findings that are contrary to folk wisdom and common knowledge about the behavioral effects of alcohol have had an almost imperceptible influence on attitudes about alcohol. Entrenched belief systems continue to limit the types of questions that are asked and the acceptance of new ideas. The contest between old beliefs and new information is most sharply drawn in the area of treatment of alcohol problems (Kalb and Propper, 1976; Mello, 1975).

Beyond problems of adequate measurement and fixed attitudes, wide differences in alcohol dosage and drinking experience of the subjects studied have contributed to the apparent inconsistency and confusion in the behavioral literature. In previous reviews, we have tried to simplify this situation by suggesting that the effects of alcohol intoxication on sociability and subjective feelings of well being are different for the normal drinker and for the alcohol addict (Mello, 1968, 1972; Mello and Mendelson, 1975). This formulation has the unfortunate, and probably erroneous, implication that there is no overlap between normal drinkers and alcoholics on the dimension of alcohol-induced changes in affective states. Probably a more accurate formulation is that the transition from sobriety *to* intoxication-related elation *to* intoxication-related depression is alcohol-dose-related in *both* groups. Increased depression has been observed in normal drinkers at high doses of alcohol (6 to 8 oz) (Williams, 1966). Alcohol addicts commonly ingest between 26 and 32 oz of distilled spirits a day (or the equivalent), and the depression and anxiety usually observed is also probably dose related. In other words, the alcohol addict may require considerably higher doses of alcohol than the normal drinker to produce comparable subjective effects across a range of changes in subjective experience and interpersonal reactivity. Insofar as the subjective effects appear to be predominantly elation in normal drinkers and depression in alcoholics, this in turn may reflect the relative doses of alcohol commonly consumed.

3.1. The Effects of Alcohol on Sociability

Alcohol has always been regarded as a social facilitator. Alcohol enhancement of conviviality and social function is a dominant theme in contemporary advertising, and has ample precedent throughout art history. The cocktail party effect on social interaction is so familiar that objective study of this obvious phenomenon would seem unlikely to yield new information. However, over the past 10 years, a number of investigators have examined the interrelations between alcohol intoxication and social interactions. In clinical research studies, in which alcoholic subjects were employed as their own control during periods of sobriety and alcohol intoxication, it was possible to make repeated observations of the same individual and/or group of individuals through time. Some of the early studies in this area have been reviewed in detail previously (Mello, 1972), and since that time a number of increasingly sophisticated research designs have evolved that attempt to clarify both the effect of alcohol on sociability *and* that of sociability on alcohol consumption.

The complex structure of the alcoholic "bottle gang" as a sociological phenomenon was described in 1968 by Rubington. Subsequently, several investigators have replicated and confirmed the basic observation that alcohol can serve as a focus for formation of a cohesive, although transient, social group. Mutual support and sharing of resources to obtain alcohol appear to characterize the skid-row alcoholic social organization (Wolin and Steinglass, 1974).

The early clinical research attempted to determine if patterns of spontaneous social interaction were correlated with drinking behavior (Mendelson *et al.*, 1968; Weiner *et al.*, 1971; Steinglass and Weiner, 1971). Alcoholic volunteers lived on a clinical research ward for several weeks and were observed during a baseline period, an episode of chronic drinking, and a postdrinking control period. All the clinical research studies to be described use a design in which each subject served as his own control. Some parallels with the street "bottle gang" were observed on the clinical research ward insofar as one member of the group assumed the role of alcohol provider and other subjects consumed most of the alcohol provided (Mendelson *et al.*, 1968). Interpersonal discord and stress were more often correlated with cessation of drinking than with an exacerbation of drinking. Observations of related alcoholics, e.g., father and son pairs, before, during, and after a period of chronic intoxication also showed reduction of drinking following an external stress or painful interpersonal interaction (Weiner *et al.*, 1971).

Clinical observations of a series of family pairs, father and son, brothers, and unrelated alcoholics suggested that intoxication did *not* necessarily increase sociability, but rather the condition of drunkenness or relative sobriety was the basis for one member of the pair assuming a more dominant role in the dyadic interaction patterns (Weiner *et al.*, 1971; Steinglass and Weiner, 1971; Steinglass and Wolin, 1974).

Nathan and co-workers were first to extend these observations of spontaneous social interaction during alcohol intoxication in an attempt to determine if experimentally controlled social isolation would affect the amount of alcohol consumed (Nathan *et al.*, 1970, 1971*a,b*; Nathan and O'Brien, 1971). Twenty alcoholic subjects were studied in small groups on a clinical research ward during three successive periods: a prealcohol baseline, a period of alcohol availability, and alcohol withdrawal. Subjects worked at a simple operant task to obtain points for alcohol or socialization (20 ml of bourbon or 15 min out of isolation). During drinking periods of 6, 12, and 18 days, a 3-day period of free socialization was alternated with a 3-day period of isolation, and this sequence continued throughout all phases of the study. Only two subjects spent points earned to break the period of isolation. The majority of subjects drank about the *same* amount during periods of socialization and periods of isolation; only five subjects drank slightly less during isolation.

Subsequently, Nathan and co-workers introduced a bar and a bartender and an unpredictable sequence of socialization and isolation to ensure that knowledge of the sequence of the experimental conditions did not determine the results. The subjects studied tended to socialize considerably more at the bar than had previous groups, but they drank somewhat less. These subjects did spend more points to socialize during and after the drinking period than the previous group, however, this occurred primarily during the first isolation period of the drinking phase. As points became exhausted, most subjects chose to spend accumulated points for alcohol rather than for socialization (Nathan *et al.*, 1971*a*).

These data suggest that given a choice between buying alcohol and social interaction, most alcoholics prefer to spend their resources for alcohol. Significant enhancement or reduction of drinking did not occur as a function of changes in socialization conditions. These findings appear to be at variance with studies in which drinking cost a period of nonsocialization (Bigelow *et al.*, 1974; Griffiths *et al.*, 1974*a*). However, differences in the conditions of social isolation and the group available for social interaction seriously limit comparisons between these studies. One major procedural difference between studies of Bigelow, Griffiths, and colleagues and all other clinical research studies reviewed is that their alcoholic subjects were studied sequentially rather than together, and their interaction opportunities were usually with seven other psychiatric patients (diagnosis not specified) who were not intoxicated at the time.

Bigelow, Griffiths, and co-workers reported that if a time-out from social activities was made contingent upon alcohol ingestion, the drinking of chronic alcoholics was suppressed. When 10 or 15 min of "isolation" immediately followed each drink, drinking was suppressed to about half of baseline levels (Bigelow *et al.*, 1974). Under conditions where the subjects' privileges were also restricted (i.e., no television and no reading), contingent time-out from social interaction (40 min) was even more effective in suppressing alcohol intake in comparison to baseline. However, it is important to note that during time-outs from social interactions, subjects were still exposed to social stimulation since they could listen to, observe, and be close to other individuals. These variables make it rather difficult to interpret the resulting data, since the presence and absence of social interaction was not clearly tested in this design. The authors conclude that "drinking in alcoholics is not only related to social interactions but is actually reinforced and maintained by social interactions" (Griffiths *et al.*, 1974*a*). Alternatively, it would appear that social interaction opportunities were most important when alcoholics had nothing else to do, i.e., when privileges were restricted. Subsequently, four alcoholic subjects were given an opportunity to choose between talking and interacting with others for 20 min or receipt of a small amount of money (10 to 35 cents) (Griffiths *et al.*, 1975). Twelve daily choice trials were given at 20-min intervals under conditions where four drinks were consumed during the first 2 hr of each session with four more drinks during the second 2 hr of each session. The rationale for assuming an equivalence between the monetary and social reinforcers was not described. However, all four subjects chose socialization over money for a significantly greater number of sessions when alcohol was available than when a nonalcoholic beverage was available. In summary, when socialization does not involve a choice between alcohol and social interaction, socialization may be more attractive than money and socialization may be more attractive than drinking if drinking involves isolation with nothing to do.

Griffiths and co-workers (1974*b*) observed that spontaneous rates of social interaction of five alcoholic subjects were substantially higher on days when ethanol was available than when ethanol was not available. Essentially the same acceleration of social interaction was observed whether alcohol was presented in an irregular sequence or over several successive days. Increased interaction during drinking was also found in a large sample of alcoholic individuals interacting with each other. Thornton and co-workers (1976) examined the social interaction behavior of a series of 98 male alcoholics over 6 weeks during which a 1-week control period was followed by a 4-week interval wherein subjects made hourly decisions (between 9 a.m. and 9 p.m.) to drink or not to drink 1 or 2 oz of distilled spirits. This period of alcohol availability was followed by a 1-week postdrinking period. Of the 98 patients studied, 43 voluntarily abstained from alcohol during the entire 4-week drinking period. The remaining 55 patients drank from 2 oz to the maximum allowed (26 oz) per day. Social interaction behavior was observed and recorded 33 times daily at approximately half-hour intervals over the entire 6 weeks of the program. In the final data analysis, abstainers were compared to 25 heavy drinkers who consumed more than 10 oz per day on the average (Thornton *et al.*, 1976).

It was found that the abstainers maintained a constant level of socializing throughout the various phases of the study. Heavy drinkers showed a significant increase in socializing during the first drinking week that decreased only slightly during the final 3 weeks of alcohol availability. When alcohol was no longer available, socializing again sharply declined in this group ($p < .01$). Within both the abstaining and the heavy drinking group, those subjects who were most "extroverted" socialized more than subjects who were most "introverted" as assessed by Form A of the Eysenck Personality Inventory. However, there was no indication that the socialization behavior of introverted alcoholics was more affected by the drinking than that of the extroverted. The investigators concluded that increases in social interaction associated with alcohol consumption were comparable for introverted and extroverted alcoholics. "Extroverted alcoholics socialized at significantly higher rates than introverted alcoholics," in both drinking and abstinent groups across all phases of the study (Thornton *et al.*, 1976).

The implicit assumption in most of the foregoing studies is that alcohol consumption is maintained to some extent by intoxication-related changes in affective state. Pliner and Cappell have compared conditions of social and solitary drinking with respect to the affective consequences of intoxication (1974). In describing their rationale for this study, Pliner and Cappell object to a procedure that involves completing an adjective checklist after drinking and assuming that the results reflect the effects of alcohol on mood without regard to the particular circumstances in which the self-ratings were made. A group of 60 male and 60 female volunteers were compared with respect to alcohol versus placebo in a social group versus a solitary drinking condition. Of subjects who drank in groups, those given alcohol became significantly more friendly, less unhappy, less bored, and more euphoric than placebo subjects as determined by self-reports on a Clyde Mood Scale. No comparable changes were reported by subjects who drank either alcohol or placebo in isolation, with a single exception that solitary alcohol subjects reported a significant increase in aggressive feelings. Breathalyzer readings were about 50 mg/100 ml for both groups. It was concluded that social or solitary conditions affect the qualitative perceptions of intoxication and determine whether the reported emphasis is on affective changes or on physical symptoms (Pliner and Cappell, 1974).

3.2. The Effects of Alcohol on Mood

Study of the effects of alcohol on mood has been complicated by a number of interacting factors. One problem is the difficulty of devising adequate measures of affect that in fact reflect the mood states presumably tested. Since mood changes can only be assessed by subjective reports, the assumption that a subject's verbal behavior has some relationship to actual feeling states cannot be satisfactorily established with reference to any objective criteria. Variables related to the cooperativeness, expectancy, and compliance of the subject may influence answers on a mood assessment inventory as much as or more than the presence or absence of alcohol. No satisfactory resolution of this problem appears imminent and most investigators have been forced to rely on a combination of several apparently sensitive instruments and global clinical impressions.

Russell and Mehrabian (1975) have recently reviewed a diverse literature interpreted to suggest that alcohol use is at least partially motivated by its ability to change emotion. They emphasize that another problem in the measurement of alcohol effects has been the ambiguity and inconsistency with which emotional states have been defined. Russell and Mehrabian (1975) conclude that the emotional impact of the given dose of alcohol may depend upon the environmental setting, the drinker's prior mood, and underlying personality. To the extent that most research has neglected examination of all of these variables in relation to alcohol, findings in this area are at best inconclusive (Russell and Mehrabian, 1975).

The pervasive assumption that the effects of alcohol on mood are well known and beneficial has also impeded the study of alcohol effects. The traditional view that alcoholics are inveterate hedonists, disregarding all for the pursuit of alcohol-related pleasures, illustrates a prevalent attitude toward, and expectancy about, the behavioral effects of alcohol. However, this belief has not been supported by the empirical findings. Part of the confusion about the behavioral effects of alcohol may also derive from the assumption that a drinking experience for an alcoholic is the same as that for a normal drinker. In fact, small doses of alcohol may have very little effect for the behaviorally tolerant alcoholic and some euphorogenic effects for the social drinker. However, within each individual's range of alcohol tolerance, increasing doses of alcohol may be associated with an increase in dysphoria. The intensity of intoxication-related negative affect probably varies as a function of experience with alcohol, the pattern, volume and duration of drinking, and the social context of drinking. However, it is important to recognize that given sufficient amounts of alcohol, both social drinkers (Warren and Raynes, 1972; Williams, 1966) and alcohol addicts (Mayfield, 1968; Mendelson, 1964; McNamee *et al.*, 1968; Tamerin and Mendelson, 1969; Tamerin *et al.*, 1970; Mello and Mendelson, 1972; Nathan and O'Brien, 1971; Nathan *et al.*, 1970, 1971*a,b*, 1972; Wolin and Mello, 1973, Nagarajan *et al.*, 1973) have reported or exhibited signs of increasing depression, anxiety, and affective discomfort (cf. Mello, 1972, for review). Usually, the severity of dysphoria and anxiety tends to increase in alcoholics as heavy drinking continues (Alterman *et al.*, 1975). Comparable dysphoric changes as a function of prolonged heroin intoxication have also been reported in heroin addicts (Mirin *et al.*, 1976). However, despite the overall increase in depression, irritability, and anxiety, heroin addicts reported a transient sense of well being associated with each successive heroin dose. It is possible that a comparable transient perception of well-being accompanies the initiation of each successive episode of intoxication for the alcoholic during a drinking spree (cf. Davis, 1971). Euphoria has been reported in normal couples studied in a semistructured social drinking situation (Smith *et al.*, 1975). Peak blood alcohol levels ranged between 67 and 100 mg/100 ml. But, there was no consistent relationship between blood alcohol levels and emotional responsivity. Anxiety and depression were not diminished following drinking in these subjects.

The efficacy of alcohol as a "tension reducer" has also been questioned. Steffen *et al.* (1974) examined the relationship between blood alcohol levels, reported subjective distress, and electromyographic activity recorded from the frontalis muscle. Four alcoholic subjects were studied over a 12-day drinking period during which they had free access to bourbon. Blood alcohol levels were positively correlated with reports of subjective distress, but there was no relation between subjective distress and the electromyographic response. Blood alcohol levels were significantly negatively correlated with muscle tension. Since muscle tension was not correlated with subjective reports of disturbance and each subject was affected in different ways by increasing blood alcohol levels, these data further illustrate the problems with employing an overinclusive definition of tension.

In 1972, Cappell and Herman critically reviewed data relevant to the hypothesis that alcohol consumption can be accounted for by its "tension reduction" effects. Acute alcohol administration did not result in a demonstrable diminution of tension in the animal and human studies examined. Cappell and Herman (1972) conclude that even if alcohol did reduce tension, this would not necessarily mean that alcohol is consumed for its tension-reducing effects. Tension reduction could be one of several reinforcing consequences of alcohol consumption.

Higgins and Marlatt (1973) examined the other side of the alcohol-tension equation and attempted to manipulate levels of anxiety and determine the effect of anxiety on consumption of alcohol by alcoholics and social drinkers. In order to disguise the purpose of the study, subjects were asked to rate the taste of brandy, port, and beer according to a series of adjectives that appeared sequentially in the window of a subject-operated memory drum. Subjects were told they would be asked to evaluate how drinks taste before and after the electrical stimulation. Anxiety was manipulated by establishing different expectancies about the nature of the electrical stimulation. One group of subjects was told that they would occasionally receive mild shocks to excite their sense of touch. A second group was told that they would receive painful electric shocks and were shown a formidable electronic console. Although subjects exposed to the elaborate shock apparatus expressed anxious concern about the prospect of being shocked, there were no significant differences in the amount of alcohol consumed under the low- and high-anxiety conditions within either the alcoholic group or the social drinking group. However, the alcoholic group did drink more than twice as much as the normal drinking group in the 55-min test period. Estimated blood alcohol levels were about 60 mg/100 ml for the alcoholics and 20 mg/100 ml for the social drinkers. Higgins and Marlatt (1973) conclude that even if alcohol is able to alleviate tension and reduce arousal, "this does not necessarily imply that states of arousal and anxiety have a causative relation to the initiation of drinking" (p. 432).

Miller and co-workers (1974) have also examined the effect of stress (personal criticism and confrontation with social, martial, or vocational inadequacies) on 10 min of operant performance for a small dose of alcohol in eight alcoholic and eight control subjects. The effectiveness of the stress experience was inferred from the significant increase in pulse rate observed in both groups. Alcoholics worked for alcohol at a higher rate than nonalcoholics under both stress and nonstress conditions. All alcoholics increased rate of response for alcohol after stress conditions, whereas six of the social drinkers decreased responding. Although the difference between the two groups was significant, stress did not result in a statistically significant increase in operant rate of the alcoholic subjects over nonstress conditions. The actual amount of alcohol earned, the blood alcohol levels, and the effect of drinking on subsequent performance were not described.

It appears that experimentally induced "stress" does not necessarily result in increased alcohol consumption in alcoholics or in social drinkers (Higgins and Marlatt, 1973; Miller *et al.*, 1974). These experimental data are concordant with clinical observations that interpersonal or situational stress may be accompanied by cessation rather than acceleration of drinking in a clinical research setting (cf. Mello, 1972, for review). If stress is an important modulator of alcohol consumption, it has been difficult to demonstrate in experimental situations. Since the efficacy of alcohol in reducing tension has also been repeatedly challenged (Cappell and Herman, 1972; Steffen *et al.*, 1974), it appears unlikely that "tension reduction" is a viable explanatory construct to account for alcohol abuse. Much remains to be learned about the nature of the reinforcing consequences of alcohol abuse.

3.3. The Effects of Alcohol on Aggression

Since prolonged ingestion of alcohol appears to increase feelings of dysphoria, despondency, and social isolation, it is perhaps not surprising that alcohol intoxication is associated with the facilitation and perhaps the induction of violent and aggresssive behavior (Tinklenberg, 1973). Studies of criminal homicides indicate that more than half of the offenders had ingested large quantities of alcohol before commission of the crime (Wolfgang, 1958). Similar findings have been obtained in studies of assaultive behaviors, armed robbery with aggravated assault, and a variety of other crimes of violence (Shupe, 1954; Tinklenberg, 1973).

In a review of the association between alcoholism and suicide, and homicide and drinking, Goodwin (1973) indicated that both killer and victim commonly were drinking, often to the point of intoxication, immediately before the event, but few murderers are alcoholics. Suicide is substantially more frequent among alcoholics than in the general population. Although about one-quarter of all suicide victims (both alcoholics and nonalcoholics) drink immediately before death, little is known about the role of intoxication in suicides.

The high concordance between automobile accidents and alcohol abuse is well known (Waller, 1972). Traffic fatalities associated with alcohol abuse are probably a complex combination of alcohol-induced impairment of driving skills, enhanced risk-taking, and an overt expression of anger and violence.

The earlier literature on the effects of alcohol on aggressive behavior in man and animals has been summarized by Carpenter and Armenti (1972). These reviewers were unable to discern a clear pattern of alcohol effects on aggression, in part because of variations in definitions of criteria for aggressive behavior.

In the past 12 years of clinical research studies of alcohol addicts given access to alcohol for several days or weeks, it has been consistently observed that alcohol intoxication is associated with a dramatic increase in interpersonal aggression spanning a continuum from verbal insults and sarcasm to threats of physical assault, actual physical assault, severe temper tantrums, and on occasion, self-destructive behavior (Mendelson and Mello, 1974; Tamerin and Mendelson, 1969). These clinical impressions have also been confirmed by others (Nathan *et al.*, 1970, 1972; Steinglass and Wolin, 1974).

There have been a series of studies on the effects of alcohol on aggressive behavior in nonalcoholic social drinkers that appear to support the impression that alcohol facilitates the expression of aggression. Boyatzis (1974, 1975) has analyzed videotapes of aggressive behavior exhibited by social drinkers during 4-hr experimental cocktail parties. A self-reported history of aggressive behavior was correlated with the expression of interpersonal aggression after heavy drinking. Even under optimal social drinking conditions, physical and verbal assaultive behavior during intoxication has been reported (Smith *et al.*, 1975).

Taylor and Gammon (1975) have recently reported that the expression of physical aggression in response to deliberate provocation was directly related to the quantity of alcohol ingested. Four groups of 10 subjects each were randomly assigned to one of four alcohol conditions: a high or low dose of bourbon or vodka (0.5 or 1.5 oz/40 lb body weight). Subjects were told they were competing with a subject in an adjoining room at a task involving reaction time. At the beginning of each of 21 trials, the subject could select any of 10 intensities of shock to be delivered to his opponent. Subjects were told that shock would be delivered at the end of each trial to whichever member of the pair was slowest in reacting. In fact, the frequency of wins, losses, and amounts of shock received were controlled by the experimenter. Provocation was defined in terms of level of shock received. The intensity of shock each subject selected to deliver to his opponent increased as a function of provocation. It was found that a small dose of alcohol tended to inhibit, and a large dose provoked the expression of aggressive behavior. However, the actual blood alcohol levels achieved were not reported (Taylor and Gammon, 1975). These data confirmed and extended previous observations of these investigators in a comparable experimental paradigm (Shuntich and Taylor, 1972).

Taylor and co-workers have also compared the effects of alcohol and of marihuana on the expression of aggression using similar procedures (Taylor *et al.*, 1976). Aggression was again measured by the intensity of the shock the subject set for his opponent to receive. Subjects were not told the amount or type of drug administered. A high oral dose of marihuana (0.3 mg/kg) decreased the tendency to initiate aggressive behavior, whereas a high dose of alcohol (1.5 oz/40 lb) increased the tendency to initiate aggressive behavior using these measures.

Marlatt and co-workers have argued that the studies of Taylor and Boyatzis are not conclusive evidence of the role of alcohol in the facilitation of aggression since the role of expectancy of alcohol consumption was not controlled (Lang *et al.*, 1975). These investigators suggest that alcohol may be an acceptable excuse for aggressive acting out, and if so, awareness of alcohol ingestion could be as important as the drug effect in determining the expression of aggression. Marlatt and co-workers have assembled a convincing case for the importance of the role of expectancy in determining aggressive behavior in an ingenious and well-controlled study in social drinkers (Lang *et al.*, 1975).

In order to examine the role of expectancy in the effects of alcohol on behavior, 48 subjects were told they would receive alcohol and 48 subjects in another group were told they would receive tonic. In fact, half of each group was given alcohol and the other half was not. Half of the subjects within each subgroup were then insulted prior to exposure to a task that involved the administration of electric shocks to another person in the context of a "teaching" exercise. Blood alcohol levels varied between 96 and 98 mg/100 ml in all subjects that received alcohol. However, expressed aggression, defined as intensity and duration of shocks administered to another, was greater in subjects who expected to consume alcohol than in those who expected to consume only tonic. These data, summarized in Fig. 2, show that those who expected their drinks to contain alcohol, regardless of the actual alcohol content, administered longer and more intense shocks to the other person than those who expected to consume only nonalcoholic drinks (Lang *et al.*, 1975). Subsequently, most subjects estimated that they had consumed

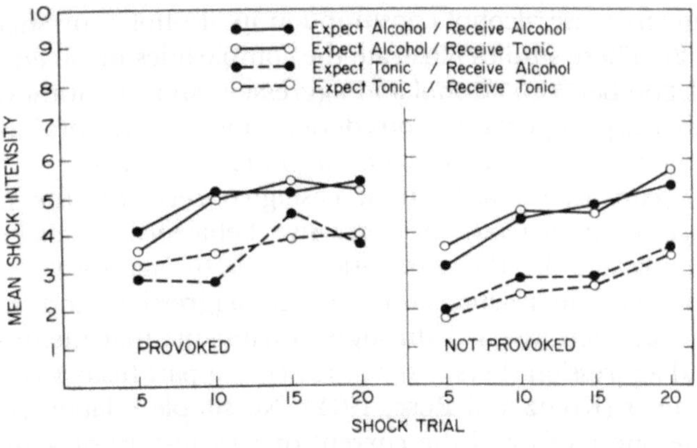

FIG. 2. The effects of alcohol and expectancy on aggressive behavior. Mean shock intensity delivered by provoked and nonprovoked subjects (based on intensities for each subject averaged over blocks of five shock trials). Subjects who expected alcohol delivered more intense shocks to another person, irrespective of beverage actually received, than subjects who did not expect alcohol. The effect of expectancy was statistically significant ($p < .001$). From Lang *et al.*, 1975.

some alcohol, however those who expected alcohol estimated a higher intake than those who did not (4.58 oz vs. 1.25 oz). Although subjects could not *taste* the difference between vodka and placebo at a rate better than chance, those who had actually received alcohol estimated a higher alcohol intake than those who received tonic (3.60 oz vs. 2.23 oz). A blood alcohol level of 90 mg/100 ml should be easily discriminable from placebo for a social drinker. Consequently, the significant effect of expectancy on this measure of aggression is an intriguing datum.

In a subsequent study, employing a similar procedure with shock duration and intensity as the measure of aggression, it was found that subjects who were insulted and given no opportunity to retaliate drank more than subjects who were insulted and did have an opportunity to retaliate (Marlatt *et al.*, 1975). Alcohol was administered in a taste-rating task designed to make subjects believe that the purpose of the study was to examine variables that affected ability to discriminate taste differences in wines. Blood alcohol levels averaged about 20 mg/100 ml. Although provoked subjects did not drink significantly more wine than control subjects, provoked subjects who were permitted to aggress against another drank significantly less than provoked subjects denied the opportunity to retaliate. The authors argue that these data may be most parsimoniously interpreted in terms of individual feelings of loss of personal control over a situation that in turn may be associated with increased alcohol consumption. Insults prior to drinking (Marlatt *et al.*, 1975) and anticipating evaluations following a period of drinking (Higgins and Marlatt, 1975) both were associated with increases in alcohol consumption. These data are at variance with reports that stress does not consistently increase alcohol consumption in alcoholics or social drinkers (cf. Section 3.2). These studies illustrate the complexities involved in trying to clarify the relation between alcohol and aggression and the numerous control procedures that are important. Considerably more behavioral research on these issues will be required before a clear pattern emerges.

In recent years, there has been increasing concern with the study of the possible *biological concomitants* of aggressive behavior. Testosterone levels have been implicated in the expression of both aggressive and sexual behavior. The possible relationship between aggression and testosterone levels in man has been assessed through instruments that measure feelings of hostility and aggression (Persky *et al.*, 1971) or a past history of aggression and violent crimes (Kreuz and Rose, 1972). No simple relationship between plasma testosterone levels and the current or past history of aggression has been indicated by these studies. Data obtained on primates presents a more consistent indication that androgen levels can modulate and influence aggressive behavior. Rose and his associates have shown that plasma testosterone is correlated with rank in a dominance hierarchy and with aggression frequency in male rhesus monkeys (Rose *et al.*, 1971). Changes in social environment, i.e., access to receptive females, have also been shown to change plasma testosterone levels (Rose *et al.*, 1972). Subsequent exposure to and defeat by a group of males was associated with a precipitous fall in plasma testosterone levels to 80% below baseline. Plasma testosterone levels increased above baseline when receptive females were again provided (Rose *et al.*, 1972).

Several investigators have attempted to analyze the interrelationship among both chronic and acute alcohol intake, aggressive behavior, and androgen function. Mendelson and Mello (1974) studied nine alcohol addicts before, during, and after an 11- or 12-day spontaneous drinking period. Blood samples for analysis of testosterone were collected at 8 a.m. each morning. Testosterone shows a small diurnal variation and levels tend to be highest in the morning upon awakening (Rose *et al.*, 1972). It was found that plasma testosterone levels were suppressed during chronic alcohol intoxication in eight of the nine subjects. The one subject who did not show significant changes in plasma testosterone levels drank very little alcohol. Following cessation of drinking, six of the nine subjects showed an increase in testosterone levels over that observed during the alcohol-available period. However, there was no invariant relationship between testosterone levels and the overt expression of aggression. Six instances of aggression that involved physical assault and/or temper tantrums were observed during the drinking period. Only two aggressive episodes were associated with suppressed testosterone levels.

Dotson *et al.* (1975) have examined the effects of cocktail party drinking on testosterone. Testosterone levels remained within the normal range in normal drinkers given acute doses of alcohol during a cocktail party situation over a period of 3 hr. However, there was a slight depression in postparty testosterone values as compared to preparty values. Aggression during the party was not reported. However, blood alcohol levels and smoking were correlated with scores on a Buss–Durkee Hostility inventory given to each subject before drinking.

A serious methodological problem with most studies that have attempted to correlate testosterone with aggressive behavior is that investigators have relied upon a single daily sample or infrequent samples separated by relatively long periods of time. Depending upon the point at which the sample for testosterone was collected, testosterone levels could be greatly elevated or greatly depressed with respect to control samples. The reason for this is that testosterone has a marked circhoral variation as well as a diurnal variation that accounts for approximately 20% of the overall variance. In addition, testosterone has a very short half-life of an estimated 7 min (Southern *et al.*, 1965). Consequently, unless repeated testosterone samples are taken and temporally correlated with the observed behaviors, it is virtually impossible to conclude anything about testosterone levels and aggressive behavior.

Techniques are currently available to permit collection of plasma samples for the analysis of integrated testosterone and other hormone levels at 20-min intervals through the use of a nonthrombogenic pump attached to a venous catheter that can be left in place for up to 24 hr (DeLacerda *et al.*, 1973). This technological advance potentially permits more precise temporal correlation of hormonal fluctuations and behavior.

Figure 3 illustrates the effects of an acute dose of alcohol (2.4 mg/kg) on testosterone and luteinizing hormone levels, assessed by this technique, in a single subject. Blood samples were collected at consecutive 20-min intervals over 6 hr prior to and following oral alcohol administration. Serial determinations of testosterone and luteinizing hormone in 16 healthy adult males supported previous findings of the suppressive effects of alcohol on testosterone in alcoholics (cf. Mendelson and Mello, 1974; Mendelson *et al.*, 1976). Testosterone fell significantly during the ascending limb of the blood alcohol curve as contrasted to prealcohol levels. Luteinizing hormone levels did not change significantly during the ascending blood alcohol curve but were significantly elevated at the peak of the blood alcohol curve, i.e., about 109 mg/100 ml. Control studies indicated that neither elapsed time nor activity levels could account for the changes observed (Mendelson *et al.*, 1976).

The mechanism of alcohol-induced suppression of testosterone is unknown. Since luteinizing hormone levels did not fall prior to testosterone suppression, it is unlikely that this phenomenon can be accounted for by an ethanol-induced central suppression of gonadotrophin secretion. Rather, the rapid fall in testosterone following alcohol intake suggests that alcohol acts peripherally to inhibit testosterone production in the gonads as suggested by Van Thiel *et al.* (1974). The change in testosterone levels could also be accounted for by alterations in the rate of testosterone transformation in the liver (Rubin *et al.*, 1976), but this would require a very rapid induction of

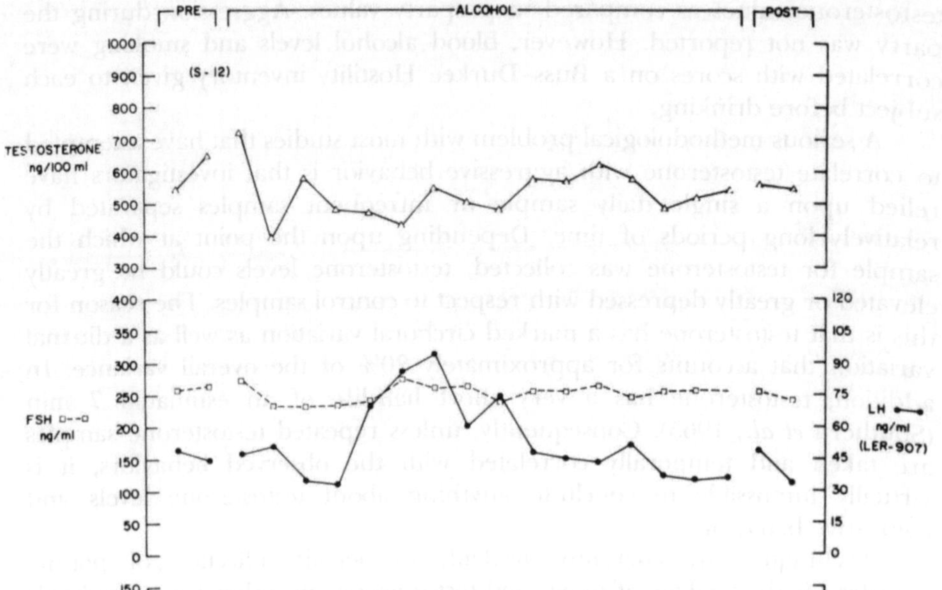

FIG. 3. The effect of alcohol on circhoral variations in plasma testosterone, luteinizing hormone, and follicle-stimulating hormone levels in a normal adult male. An acute dose of alcohol of 2.4 mg/kg was given over 15 min and serial determinations of hormonal levels prior to and following alcohol administration were carried out at consecutive 20-min intervals. From J. H. Mendelson (unpublished).

regulating enzyme systems (Mendelson *et al.*, 1976). The possible behavioral correlates of these hormonal changes remain to be determined. The effects of alcohol and other drugs on testosterone and on other pituitary–gonadal hormones have recently been reviewed by Mendelson *et al.* (1977).

3.4. The Effects of Alcohol on Sexual Function

The effect of alcohol on sexual function has been the subject of many anecdotes that usually concur with Shakespeare's classic observation that alcohol intoxication evokes desire but compromises sexual performance. These anecdotal impressions are supported by data that indicate that moderate to high doses of ethanol (2.4 to 3.2 mg/kg) may abolish the ejaculatory reflex in dogs (Gantt, 1952; Hart, 1968). Clinical observations further suggest that chronic alcohol abuse may impair sexual function through a disruption of gonadal function. In 1926, Silvestrini reported the occurrence of testicular atrophy and gynecomastia in male alcoholics who also had evidence of liver disease. This observation was subsequently confirmed by many others, and recent studies show that gynecomastia and testicular atrophy reflect a derangement in androgen metabolism (Galvao-Teles *et al.*, 1973). Testosterone is the most active and potent androgen in human males, and relative levels of testosterone significantly affect libidinal function and influence the intensity of sexual desire. The literature on alcoholism has consistently described the male alcoholic as experiencing diminished heterosexual desire and activity (Levine, 1955) and often sexual impotence (Lemere and Smith, 1973). However, exceptions to this general impression of sexual problems in alcoholics have also been reported (Burton and Kaplan, 1968).

Clarification of the effects of alcohol and other psychoactive drugs on human sexuality clearly requires detailed studies of measurable aspects of sexual behavior prior to, during, and following drug administration. Impediments to this important type of research have recently developed and are currently enforced through a congressional edict.* In a curious combination of politics and prudery, Representative Michel of Illinois persuaded his colleagues in Congress to enact special legislation to stop federal funding for studies of the effects of drugs on sexual behavior conducted by H. B. Rubin and colleagues at the University of Southern Illinois School of Medicine. Representative Michel contended that this work was "offensive to the sensibilities of most Americans." † Mr. Michel's well-publicized expressions of outrage coincided with the period immediately before an election, and his constituents returned him to office.

In addition to establishing an unfortunate precedent in which congressional representatives presume to determine the course of scientific inquiry, without consideration of scientific merit or qualified peer review, this legislation also ensures that our understanding of the effects of psychoactive drugs on human sexuality will remain anecdotal for some time to come. Fortunately, several studies on the effects of alcohol on sexual behavior were completed prior to the congressional embargo (Briddell and Wilson, 1976; Farkas and Rosen, 1976; Rubin and Henson, 1976; Wilson and Lawson, 1976*a*). Anyone unaware of the congressional furor would be unlikely to find much to offend, outrage, or excite the prurient interest in these reports.

In each study, penile tumescence was measured in the presence and absence of erotic stimuli. Farkas and Rosen (1976) studied 16 male college students during four successive sessions in which subjects were given no alcohol or brought to a blood alcohol level of 25, 50, or 75 mg/100 ml. Subsequently, subjects were attached to a heart rate and penile gauge measurement apparatus. After stable recordings were obtained, 5 min of

* H.R. 13172, section 404, Second Supplemental Appropriations Bill, 1976.

† Congressional Record, April 13, 1976, H 3299.

music was followed by a 15-min erotic film. The same film was used during each of the four sessions that were separated by 2 to 7 days. The degree of penile tumescence observed appeared to habituate to this constant stimulus, although tonic heart rate did not. At the lowest blood alcohol level (25 mg/100 ml), there was an increase in maximum penile diameter above control sessions. However, the rate of penile tumescence tended to decrease as blood alcohol levels increased, and blood alcohol levels of 50 and 75 mg/100 ml also depressed the diameter of increase in tumescence below baseline. Subjective estimates of erection paralleled the physiological data and were highest at a blood alcohol level of 25 mg/100 ml and lowest at 75 mg/100 ml. Despite the repetition of the same erotic stimulus over the four sessions, tonic heart rate continued to rise as a linear function of alcohol dose (Farkas and Rosen, 1976).

Rubin and Henson (1976) also studied 16 young adult males and examined the effects of low (0.5 or 0.6 ml/kg), moderate (1.0 or 1.2 ml/kg), or high (1.5 or 1.8 ml/kg) doses of alcohol on the following variables: sexual arousal and response to erotic motion pictures, ability to voluntarily inhibit arousal to the same film, and ability to become voluntarily aroused in the absence of overt erotic stimuli. Nonsexual matching-to-sample tasks were interpolated between erotic stimulus presentations and also provided a measure of nonsexual performance. Meticulous attention to experimental details ensured that drinks were consumed, that urination could be accomplished without removal of the penile transducer, that subjects could communicate with the experimenters without compromising their privacy, and that subjects were in fact attending to the film presentation. Six erotic motion pictures, each of about 10 min duration, focused upon a variety of heterosexual acts. A control session was followed by three drug evaluation sessions, each of which were separated by 7-day intervals. Each subject saw four different films twice, initially with instructions to relax and subsequently with instructions to inhibit any sensations of sexual arousal. After presentation of four films under the inhibition instructions, subjects were then asked to fantasize in the absence of any film and attempt to become sexually aroused over a 10-min period.

It was found that even low doses of alcohol significantly reduced mean erections. The first drink produced a decrease from 51 to 45% of maximum, whereas the third drink produced a decrease from 48 to 23% of maximum. The mean latency to full erection was not significantly affected until the last drink when it increased significantly from about 1.5 to 3 min. Illustrative data are shown in Fig. 4. These data indicate that although small and moderate amounts of alcohol had little or no effect on elicited arousal, large amounts usually had a considerable depressive effect. However, blood alcohol concentrations as high as 106 to 156 mg/100 ml did not completely eliminate the ability to become aroused. Moreover, these data suggest that the primary effect of lower amounts of alcohol was on the maintenance of tumescence rather than on the speed of development of arousal or the

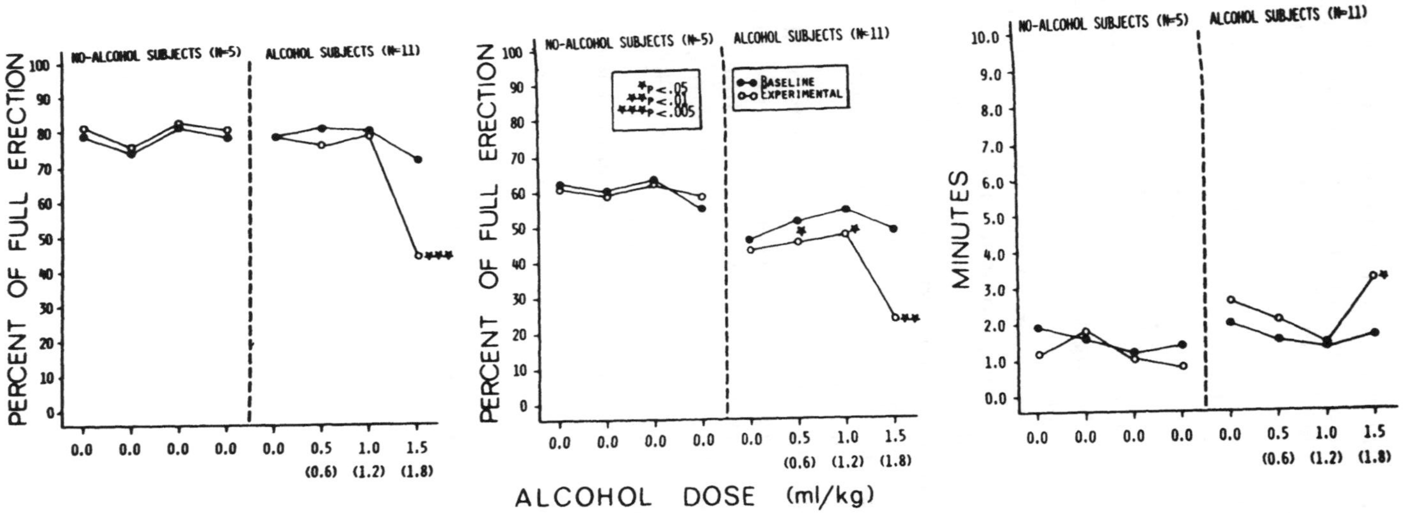

FIG. 4. The effect of alcohol on sexual arousal in men. Mean peak erections (left panel), mean average erection (center panel), and mean latencies to 20% of full erection (right panel) developed by subjects to each of four erotic films when under relax instructions during both the baseline condition (i.e., the mean of sessions 1 and 3, "closed" circles) and the experimental condition (i.e., session 2, "open" circles) are presented as a function of the cumulative alcohol dosage ingested during the experimental conditions. The four dosages depicted for both the no-alcohol subjects (left side of each panel) and the alcohol subjects (right side of each panel) correspond, from left to right, with the presentation of films 1, 2, 3, and 4. The "stars" indicate probabilities for significant one-tailed t-tests resulting from the dependent measures analysis. From Rubin and Henson, 1976.

degree of erection attained. The three levels of alcohol intoxication did not significantly impair subjects' ability to voluntarily inhibit sexual arousal even though there was some nonsignificant deterioration in control after a moderate amount of alcohol.

Of the 11 subjects, 6 reported that they believed that alcohol enhanced their sexual responding prior to the experiment and they maintained this belief at the end. This report illustrates the difficulty in reconciling objective and subjective information about sexual behavior. Rubin and Henson (1976) conclude that "an individual whose threshold for penile erection and/or ejaculation has been raised by the ingestion of alcohol may consider this depressant effect to be an enhancement of sexual abilities because it increases the time available for sexual stimulation of his partner that could well increase the probability of her being brought to orgasm. To him, the depressant effect of alcohol leads to enhancement of his abilities." We have obtained comparable reports of altered sexual function from male heroin addicts in Hong Kong, where many youth initiate and maintain heroin abuse in part because it improves their sexual performance by delaying time to ejaculation (Mendelson and Mello, 1975).

Briddell and Wilson (1976) have examined the effects of alcohol and expectancy concerning the sexual effects of alcohol on penile tumescence. Forty-eight undergraduate students were shown segments from erotic films and penile tumescence (amplitude, rate, and duration of response) were measured with a mercury strain gauge apparatus. After a single adaptation session, subjects were given one of four alcohol doses (.08, 0.4, 0.8 or 1.2 gm/kg) and assigned to an expectancy condition. Blood alcohol levels prior to measurement of penile tumescence averaged 0, 35, 67 or 95 mg/100 ml.

The expectancy instruction that alcohol would increase *or* decrease sexual arousal did not affect responsivity. Most subjects had preconceived ideas about the effects of alcohol which were not influenced by the expectancy manipulation (Briddell and Wilson, 1976). Increasing doses of alcohol did result in a significant decrease in penile tumescence in all subjects, consistent with data obtained by Farkas and Rosen (1976) and Rubin and Henson (1976).

The effects of alcohol on sexual arousal in women have long been the subject of anecdote and speculation. The availability of a vaginal photoplethysmograph to monitor pressure pulse and vaginal blood volume, permits objective measurement of one physiological correlate of sexual arousal in women. Wilson and Lawson (1976*a*) examined the effects of alcohol on vaginal pulse pressure during an erotic film and a neutral control film in 16 undergraduate and graduate students. One of four doses of alcohol was administered (.05, .25, .50, .75) and average initial blood alcohol levels were .63, 25, 48, and 79 mg/100 ml. The possible effects of expectancy were manipulated by telling subjects that alcohol would increase or decrease their levels of sexual arousal.

As in the study of effects of expectancy and alcohol on male sexual arousal (Briddell and Wilson, 1976), female subjects did not agree with the instructional set and the expectancy manipulation was not effective in modifying arousal levels. Data showed a negative linear relationship between increasing blood alcohol levels and sexual arousal, measured by vaginal pulse pressure. This effect was obtained despite the fact that most subjects predicted that alcohol would increase sexual arousal levels. These data indicate that increasing alcohol intoxication in both men and women results in progressively reduced sexual arousal in response to erotic films (Wilson and Lawson, 1976*a*; Briddell and Wilson, 1976).

Since most subjects studied believed that alcohol increases sexual arousal (Briddell and Wilson, 1976; Wilson and Lawson, 1976*a*), the effects of expectancy of drinking on sexual arousal were studied in 40 undergraduate males (Wilson and Lawson, 1976*b*). Subjects were shown two erotic films, depicting a heterosexual and a male homosexual interaction and penile tumescence was measured with a strain gauge. Half the subjects were told they would receive vodka and tonic prior to the movies and a second group was told they would only receive tonic. In fact, half of each of the two groups received only tonic and the remaining half received vodka and tonic. The average blood alcohol level in subjects who received alcohol was 40 mg/100 ml. Subjects who believed that they had consumed alcohol, irrespective of whether their drinks in fact contained alcohol, showed greater levels of sexual arousal measured by penile tumescence, than subjects who believed they drank only tonic (Wilson and Lawson, 1976*b*). These data confirm and extend the previous observations that subjects who expected to consume alcohol became significantly more aggressive than subjects who believed that they would consume a nonalcoholic beverage, irrespective of the actual alcohol content of their drinks (Lang *et al.*, 1975).

The *hormonal concomitants* of sexual arousal and the effects of alcohol on hormonal changes have not been studied. In the preceding section on the effects of alcohol on aggression, the relationship between testosterone levels and aggressive behavior was discussed. Because the repertoire of behaviors associated with procreative function and aggression are so closely linked in a number of animal species, it has been postulated that the biological mechanisms that regulate sexual function must also be associated with the processes of aggression. In animals, there is substantial evidence that testosterone levels not only co-vary with but perhaps determine and regulate aggressive and sexual behaviors (Rose *et al.*, 1972; Floody and Pfaff, 1974). Evidence from human studies is less definitive regarding the regulatory actions of sex hormones on sexual and aggressive behavior, in part because of the previously discussed methodological problems involved in temporally correlating hormonal changes with behavior. However, there has been one report of a hormonal correlate of sexual arousal in human males. Laferla *et al.* (1976) collected blood samples from normal males during exposure to erotic stimuli and correlated pituitary–gonadal hormones with sexual arousal. It was found that increments in circulating luteinizing hormone levels and follicle-stimulating hormone levels occurred in normal males during periods of sexual arousal. The elevation in luteinizing hormone levels was directly related to the duration of sexual arousal. This important study represents the first occasion on which serial hormone levels were determined over short intervals of time and correlated with standardized presentation of erotic stimuli. These data suggest that there may be a significant relationship between libidinal drive and plasma luteinizing hormone levels in human males. Hopefully, political considerations will not prevent continued explorations in this important area. Technology has now progressed to the point where elucidation of the interrelationship between behavioral and biological events is increasingly promising.

3.5. The Effects of Alcohol on Memory

Studies of the effects of alcohol on memory function account for only a small part of the vast literature on the mechanisms of memory (cf. John, 1967). Examination of the effects of alcohol on memory has yielded inconsistent and often inconclusive results. Before discussing alcohol and memory function, we will consider some general problems in the studies to be reviewed that contribute to the equivocal status of this area.

One persistent problem has been an inconsistency in *definitions* of "memory." The inconsistent use of definitions makes it difficult to compare data from different laboratories. For example, "short-term" memory has been variously defined as 5 sec, 5 min, and 30 min. Since the temporal definition of memory span is essential to an assessment of memory function, the prevailing disregard for consistency is surprising. For the most part, research on this problem has been conducted by investigators who are expert in the area of alcoholism rather than expert in the assessment of memory function and conversant with the conceptual and methodological issues in that field.

Beyond the issue of consistent definitions of "memory," numerous *methodological differences* further contribute to the discrepant findings and often preclude valid comparisons between studies. Obvious methodological differences that could influence data interpretation are variables such as: task composition and difficulty, alcohol dose, blood alcohol level achieved, conditions of alcohol administration (fasting, other drug use, etc.), the interval between successive tests, the presence or absence of cues, and practice effects. Less obvious variables that may also influence the results obtained are the subjects' motivation, attention to the test material, and behavioral tolerance for and experience with alcohol. Because these variables have been ignored and neglected in the design and interpretation of many of the studies to be reviewed, we will discuss the possible impact of these omissions on data obtained.

3.5.1. Motivation

Apparently, most investigators assume that their subjects will try to perform as well as possible on whatever tasks are presented. Often subjects are paid for their participation in the study. However, this payment is rarely made contingent upon performance accuracy. There is no reason to assume that paid volunteers will consistently perform at the upper limit of their capacity unless they are specifically paid to do so, i.e., unless the accuracy of their performance results in a task-specific reinforcement. Student volunteers and alcohol addicts both might perform better if they were immediately reinforced for accurate performance. We believe that differences in the conditions of reinforcement for accurate performance are probably the most important factors accounting for differences in performance on memory tasks during sobriety and during intoxication. Of course, it is essential to establish that the reinforcement offered is an *adequate reinforcement.* Pennies and candy may not be effective reinforcements for college students. Alcohol appears to be the only reinforcement that will consistently maintain performance in alcoholic subjects during intoxication (cf. Mello, 1973; Tamerin *et al.*, 1971).

3.5.2. Attention

Although it seems obvious that the subjects' attention to the stimuli to be recalled is essential for the evaluation of any drug intervention on subsequent recall, most investigators have not attempted to control this variable. Some have attempted to manipulate attention in an ingenious way by presenting materials to be recalled that are intrinsically interesting to the subject, e.g., erotic movies (Goodwin *et al.*, 1970). However, distractability, fatigue, boredom, and lack of motivation to perform well all can influence attention. In behavioral techniques, an *observing response* is often required of a human or animal subject to ensure that the subject attends to the discriminative stimulus upon which the subsequent performance is based. An observing response requirement could be adapted for nonautomated procedures without great effort (cf. Honig, 1966).

3.5.3. Behavioral Tolerance

Most investigators have been insensitive to the possible effects of behavioral tolerance upon the subjects' reaction to alcohol. The duration of alcohol-induced tolerance is unknown, but it has been shown to occur in social drinkers as well as alcoholics (cf. Sec. 1.2). Consequently, the assumption that it is valid to compare an alcoholic who has been sober for 1 day with an alcoholic who has been sober for 3 weeks, or an alcoholic who is intoxicated, is unreasonable and naive.

Finally, within the broad category of "alcoholic," determination of the normal, sober, intellectual status of the subject prior to examining the effects of acute or chronic doses of alcohol has been frequently neglected. Since some alcoholics may develop severe and persistent impairments of cognitive function, as a function of prolonged nutritional deficiency (cf. Victor, 1975; Dreyfus, 1974), establishing baseline performance capacity before examining the effect of alcohol is essential.

3.5.4. Clinical Observations of Memory Function Associated with Alcohol

Excessive alcohol use has been associated with several types of impaired memory function. These memory impairments fall along a continuum of severity (if not a continuum of process) from a transient disruption of memory function to a chronic and incapacitating amnestic disorder. *Wernicke's Korsakoff syndrome* is the most severe and persistent amnestic disorder associated with a combination of chronic alcohol abuse and chronic nutritional deficiency. This memory disorder is characterized by an amnesia for recent events, an apparent inability to acquire any new information, and a relatively clear recall of events during childhood and adolescence (Victor *et al.*, 1959). The memory defect in Korsakoff's psychosis has been described in a series of ingenious and careful studies by Talland (1965) and Cermak and Butters (1973). Damage to midline thalamic nuclei (medial–dorsal nucleus) and the mammaliary bodies has been observed in postmortem examinations of these patients (Victor *et al.*, 1971).

A second type of memory disorder that may accompany heavy intoxication is a transient global memory loss called the alcoholic *blackout* (Goodwin *et al.*, 1969*a,b*). During alcohol intoxication, the subject professes total amnesia for a series of events that culminate in "finding himself" in an unexpected or unfamiliar situation. Information concerning blackouts has been based upon retrospective reports obtained during periods of relative sobriety. Clearly, if the blackout involves unacceptable or threatening situations, it is impossible to adequately differentiate between intentional denial and genuine dissociation in a clinical interview. Frequently, however, these dissociative reactions are not accompaniments of unacceptable behavior, and the blackout is usually a frightening experience for the individual.

The alcoholic blackout is not restricted to the alcohol addict. Normal drinkers have also reported blackouts during intoxication. Goodwin *et al.* (1969*b*) have attempted to identify the circumstances that favor the development of blackouts through interviews with 100 alcoholics. Neglect of meals, gulping drinks, and a history of head trauma were among the factors that sometimes preceded the occurrence of a blackout. The degree of intoxication alone does not reliably predict the occurrence of a blackout.

Blackouts may last for an hour or several days. Since most blackouts end in sleep, estimates of the length of time involved are necessarily imprecise, however, most subjects can report when a blackout began (Goodwin *et al.*,

1969*a*; Goodwin, 1971*a*; Ryback, 1970). The importance of distinghishing between an "enbloc" memory loss (defined as amnesia with a definite onset point, involving memory loss for significant events and ending with a sense of lost time), and a "fragmentary" memory loss (wherein awareness of forgetting occurs in response to a reminder) emerged from the studies of Goodwin and colleagues. Several of their subjects volunteered that drinking seemed to improve their recall for events experienced during a previous drinking episode. Some deliberately drank to facilitate recall. This clinical phenomenon has now been subjected to experimental study and is considered to be one aspect of *state-dependent learning*.

The fragmentary absence of recall of some events during a subsequent period of sobirety is a third form of memory dysfunction associated with alcohol intoxication. In some instances, events during intoxication (such as hiding money or alcohol) are only recalled during a subsequent period of intoxication and therefore can be described as state-dependent effects. The observation that behavior learned during a drug state may not occur during a nondrug state, then reoccur during reinstitution of a drug state has been demonstrated in experimental animals and in man (cf. Overton, 1972, for review). Simply stated, responses established under specific conditions are most easily elicited once these conditions are reestablished.

Clinically, the dissociative effect of alcohol is most often expressed by a failure to recall the aversive consequences of drinking (e.g., depression, anxiety, illness) during a subsequent period of sobriety. Alcohol addicts form positive expectancies about a forthcoming drinking experience, and following a period of chronic intoxication they tend to recall their experience in terms of the predrinking expectancy, rather than the actual events (McGuire *et al.*, 1966; McNamee *et al.*, 1968; Tamerin *et al.*, 1970). The implications of this dissociative phenomenon for the treatment of the alcoholic were first noted in 1962 by Diethelm and Barr. Alcoholic patients interviewed under conditions of acute intoxication talked more freely and described emotions, especially guilt and hostility, that they had not discussed during sobriety. Usually these patients forgot the content of the interviews once they became sober again.

Alcohol-induced state-dependent effects have not been demonstrated for all forms of memory tasks (Overton, 1972) but have been shown to occur in normal medical students (Goodwin *et al.*, 1969*d*) and normal army volunteers (Petersen, 1977) as well as in alcoholic individuals. Petersen (1977) has attempted to determine the influence of cues on alcohol-state-dependent learning. Four groups of army volunteers, assigned to alcohol, placebo, alcohol–placebo, or placebo–alcohol conditions over 2 successive days were given tasks that required either cued or unaided recall. On a cued recall task, subjects were asked to visualize noun triplets in a particular *context*, e.g., "dress–ring–candle" in the context of a wedding. Then they were asked to rate the image on semantic differential scales, good–bad and strong–weak. On the second day, they were given the context word (e.g., wedding) for 20 noun triplets and were asked to recall the other 3 words used to form the image. This task was compared with free recall of 16 nouns and the cued and uncued recall of a categorized list of 48 words. Alcohol dosage was 1.0 ml/kg and mean blood alcohol levels were about 88 mg/100 ml within 0.5 hr after drinking.

There was no evidence of state-dependent learning for the context-cued recall task or for the cued portion of the category recall tasks. State-dependent learning of the unaided recall tasks did occur. Petersen (1977) suggests that altering the drug state also alters the cognitive cues used for the retrieval process and suggests that recall can be enhanced either by presenting material in the same drug state as existed at the time of learning or by providing cues if it is known how the material was organized at the time of learning. Although most previous studies have included tasks with variations in the meaningfulness of the stimuli, the specific role of cues was not investigated (Goodwin *et al.*, 1969*d*). Petersen's (1977) data suggest that the fragmentary dissociative memory loss that may occur during intoxication represents difficulties in retrieval rather than in acquisition or retention of information.

A number of investigators have studied alcohol-state-dependent learning of specific tasks by alcoholics, and these studies have recently been reviewed by Goodwin (1974). In one illustrative study, 32 alcoholic subjects were tested over a 2-day period, during which they were given alcohol both days, placebo both days, or alcohol and placebo, or placebo and alcohol. Subjects were given 8 to 10 oz of 80-proof vodka over a 1-hr period, an amount equivalent to 1.2 gm/kg. Memory problems included a word-association task, a word-recall task, and a word-recognition task. All subjects were able to perform well during alcohol intoxication. It was found that learning acquired during alcohol intoxication was recalled somewhat better during reintoxication than during sobriety (Goodwin *et al.*, 1974*a*). Goodwin and co-workers noted that their alcoholic volunteers were tolerant to alcohol and showed little or no behavioral intoxication at this alcohol dose. They suggest that intoxication may be a less distinctive and novel state for the alcoholics than for the nonalcoholics and novelty may favor drug-induced dissociation (Goodwin, 1974; Goodwin *et al.*, 1974*a*). Since these alcoholic subjects did not show state-dependent effects at the same alcohol dosage as normal subjects (cf. Goodwin *et al.*, 1969*d*), the authors conclude that alcoholics are not more susceptible to alcohol-induced dissociation than nonalcoholics.

Exactly the opposite conclusion was reached by Weingartner and Faillace (1971) after comparing the performance of five alcoholics and closely matched controls on word association and free-recall word tasks. Nonalcoholic subjects did not show state-dependent effects on tasks involving recall of free associations, but both groups showed state-dependent effects on free recall of learned words (Weingartner and Faillace, 1971). The design and the dose of alcohol (1.239 g/kg) were similar to that of Goodwin and co-workers (1974*a*) but a longer interval intervened between initial learning and retesting (48 hr). Also, Weingartner and Faillace (1971) administered alcohol 2 hr after lunch. Blood alcohol levels were not reported. However, Weingartner and Faillace (1971) emphasize the difficulties involved in comparing the effects of alcohol in alcoholic and nonalcoholic subjects, since a behaviorally effective dose for alcoholics produced nausea and vomiting in controls.

Since behavioral tolerance for alcohol is a powerful determinant of effective dosage, it is probably unrealistic to conclude that alcoholics or normal controls are differentially susceptible to state-dependent effects. The presence or absence of cues to recall may prove to be the most reliable predictor of alcohol-induced state dependence in any subject.

3.5.5. Alcohol and Short-Term Memory

Relatively low doses of alcohol have been shown to disrupt visual short-term memory at delays of 5.5 sec to 1 min in *normal* drinkers (Carpenter and Ross, 1965). Jones (1973) reports that 1.32 ml/kg alcohol impaired immediate, short-term, and long-term free recall of word lists in normal subjects in comparison to prealcohol baseline performance and placebo controls. Moreover, immediate memory was more impaired on the ascending than on the descending limb of the blood alcohol curve at the same blood alcohol level (90 mg/100 ml). Short-term memory was impaired by alcohol throughout the period of testing. Unfortunately, the temporal definition of immediate and short-term memory and the rationale for these designations were not described. Apparently, immediate memory was the recall of a 12-word list, presented over 24 sec, within 1 min after its conclusion. Presentations of six lists with recall periods and other intervals occupied about 10 min. Short-term memory was the recall of words from any of the six lists presented within 5 min, i.e., a span of 30 sec to a possible 15 min. No information was provided about the distribution of words recalled from the first and last lists; only the serial position within each list was analyzed. Despite the vague definitions of the constructs studied, a significant impairment of "memory" by alcohol was clearly demonstrated.

Tarter and co-workers (1971) have also shown that an alcohol dose of 1.1 ml/kg (which yielded blood alcohol levels of about 80 mg/100 ml) can disrupt performance on a variety of perceptual, motor, and short-term memory tasks in nonalcoholic subjects. However, practice or familiarity with the task prevented an alcohol-induced disruption on the second test. Subjects first tested under placebo conditions were not significantly impaired by alcohol during the second test, 48 hr later. Subjects in an alcohol–placebo sequence improved performance on the second test session. These investigators also state that there was no systematic increase in impairment with increasing task complexity as a function of the initial dose of alcohol. These data suggest that *practice* can have a very important role in overcoming the adverse properties of alcohol (Tarter *et al.*, 1971).

Studies of the effects of alcohol on short-term memory in *alcoholics* have yielded inconsistent findings. Most of the procedural and methodological problems discussed at the beginning of this section have contributed to these inconsistencies.

Several investigators have argued that if alcohol disrupts short-term memory in alcoholics with a clinical history of "blackouts," this could account for the phenomenon of blackouts during intoxication. If information was lost from short-term memory storage, it would not subsequently be available from long-term memory storage, so that intoxication could result in a period of global memory loss. Despite the early findings of Goodwin and co-workers (1970) and Tamerin and colleagues (1971), this hypothesis has not been supported by subsequent studies (Goodwin *et al.*, 1973; Mello, 1973; Parker *et al.*, 1974).

Goodwin and co-workers (1970) compared five alcoholic subjects who gave a history of frequent blackouts with five alcoholic controls on tests of immediate (2 min), short-term (30 min) and remote (24 hr) memory after administering 16 to 18 oz of 86-proof bourbon over 4 hr. Subjects had fasted for 5 hr and consumed 6 oz in the 1st hr and 4 oz per hour for the next 3 hr, a dose of about 2.4 g/kg. An impairment of "short-term" memory was seen *only* in the five subjects with a history of frequent blackouts. This impairment began between the 2nd and 3rd hr of drinking when average blood alcohol levels were about 280 mg/100 ml. These five subjects were also unable to recall and recognize stimuli 24 hr later. Immediate memory was unimpaired for recall of toys and recall of 1-min scenes from erotic movies. Unfortunately, no assessments of memory function were made in either group before *or* after intoxication. Control observations to establish that memory function in the two groups did not differ during sobriety is critical for interpretation of these data, since so little is known about why some alcoholics develop blackouts and some do not. No information is available to rule out the possibility that alcohol-induced blackouts reflect an underlying neuropathological process, such as impaired temporal lobe function, that is accentuated by intoxication.

Each of Goodwin's subjects was continuously monitored by EEG recordings from the parietal and temporal lobe during the memory study (Freemon *et al.*, 1971). There was no evidence of spike activity or paroxysmal discharges in any subject during intoxication. In most subjects, maximum slowing of the EEG occurred concomitantly with maximum blood alcohol levels. There appeared to be no correlation between the time course of memory loss and the time course of EEG slowing. There were no differences in EEG recordings of those individuals who had short-term memory loss and those who did not. The investigators point out that although EEG slowing could be detected with only two leads, it is possible that subjects with memory loss might have shown epileptiform activity in areas that were not studied. Subsequent control studies on two additional subjects did not reveal epileptiform activity during intoxication (Freemon *et al.*, 1971).

Tamerin and co-workers (1971) also reported that alcohol significantly impairs short-term visual memory at 5 sec and 5 min in alcoholics with a history of blackouts at blood alcohol levels above 200 mg/100 ml. Short-term memory was assessed with a picture recall and visual spatial recognition task. Two problems limited generalizations from the Tamerin study. These investigators did not examine the effect of alcohol on memory function in alcoholics *without* a clinical history of blackouts. Therefore, the extent to which blackout history and alcohol might interact uniquely to affect memory function was not determined. A second problem was that subjects were reinforced for performance with cigarettes in a situation where alcohol was freely available. It has been consistently observed that alcohol addicts show minimal interest in working for cigarettes, money, and reinforcers other than alcohol during alcohol intoxication (Mello, 1972).

Subsequent reports by Mello (1973*b*), Goodwin *et al.* (1973*a*), and Parker *et al.* (1974) challenge the notion that alcohol has a specific effect on short-term memory that could account for the alcoholic blackout. Mello (1973*b*) compared the performance of alcoholics with and without a history of blackouts during sobriety and acute and chronic alcohol intoxication and found no impairment of short-memory in either group under any condition (Mello, 1973*b*, 1976*b*). Of the 20 subjects studied, 13 reported a history of erratic blackouts of several hours to several days duration during heavy intoxication. Short-term memory function was examined with a delayed matching-to-sample procedure. The subject's task was to choose which one of four visual comparison stimuli was identical to a sample stimulus. The delay between the sample sitmulus offset and the onset of the comparison stimuli defined the span of "short-term" memory. Since there were no spatial cues, correct matching after a delay interval necessarily required recall of the sample stimulus. The length of the delay interval increased with each correct match trial and decreased with each incorrect trial in 4-sec increments. The possible delay intervals ranged between 0 and 6 min. Attention to the sample stimulus was ensured by requiring the subject to initiate each trial by making an observing response. Motivation to perform well was aided by requiring completion of four correct trials before four error trials to earn a single token. Each token was exchangeable for one cigarette or 15 min of television time during the prealcohol baseline and for 1 oz of alcohol during the alcohol availability period. Data for four representative subjects are shown in Fig. 5.

Alcoholics with a blackout history did not differ from control subjects in the accuracy of performance on delayed matching-to-sample tasks at comparable blood alcohol levels. Seven of the blackout subjects and four control subjects actually improved matching-to-sample performance during intoxication as compared with the predrinking baseline. Four of the five blackout subjects, whose peak blood alcohol levels exceeded 200 mg/100 ml, improved their performance over baseline. The absence of an alcohol-induced impairment of matching-to-sample performance in blackout subjects in comparison to alcoholic controls, at blood alcohol levels above 200 mg/100 ml, was

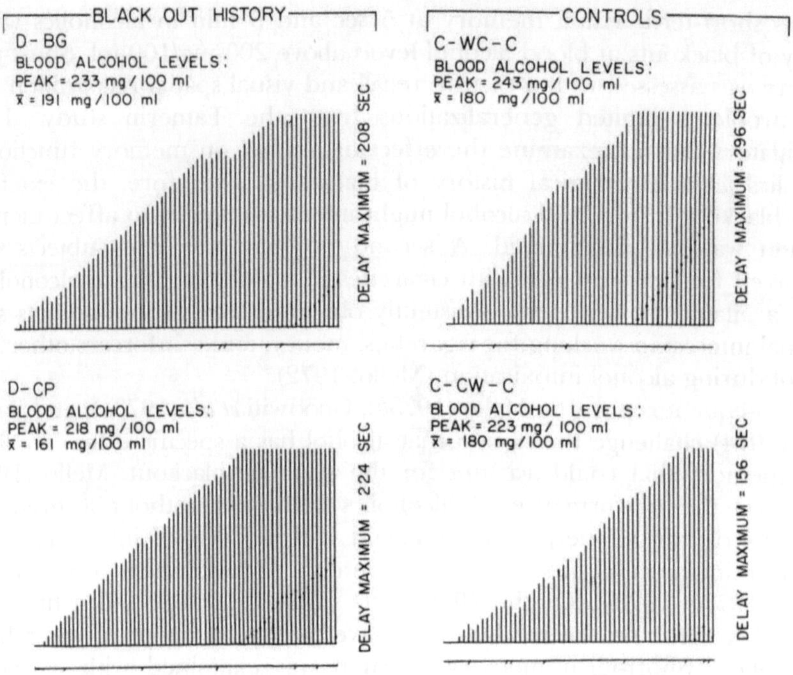

FIG. 5. The effect of alcohol on short-term memory. An analog readout of the delay interval on successive matching-to-sample trials is shown for four representative subjects with peak blood alcohol levels above 200 mg/100 ml. The two subjects shown on the left reported a history of blackouts, and the two subjects shown on the right were alcoholic controls. The mean and peak blood alcohol levels for each subject are shown at the upper left of each block. The vertical bars in the top trace of each row represent the delay between the sample stimulus offset and the comparison stimulus onset of each successive trial. Once the recorder pen in the upper trace reached the limit of its excursion, it reset and continued up the same line until the delay interval terminated. This is indicated by the small dots superimposed on the vertical lines. The maximum delay reached by each subject during the 2.5 hr session is shown at the right of each histogram. The maximum delays are a function of the amount of time that each subject spent at the machine. Errors are indicated by downward deflections of the baseline pen. Each error is followed by a 4-sec decrease in the sample-to-match delay interval, shown as a shorter line on the upper trace. Each correct response is followed by a 4-sec increase in the match-to-sample delay interval, shown as a longer line on the upper trace. From Mello, 1973*b*, reprinted with permission.

consistently observed during a 10- to 12-day period of chronic intoxication (Mello, 1976*b*). These findings are consistent with the earlier studies of Talland on the effects of chronic intoxication in alcoholics (Talland, 1966; Talland *et al.*, 1964).

A comparable study of the effects of alcohol (1 to 3.5 g/kg) on matching-to-sample performance in nonaddicted rhesus monkeys also failed to show an alcohol-induced impairment of short-term memory (Mello, 1971). The consistent accurate performance on a matching-to-sample task by heavily intoxicated alcoholics illustrates the behavioral tolerance for alcohol that characterizes this addictive disorder. The fact that subjects in this study were reinforced with alcohol for accurate performance is probably the most important factor that accounts for differences in performance on short-term memory tasks during intoxication in this study and studies reporting an alcohol-induced impairment (Tamerin *et al.*, 1971; Lisman, 1974; Nathan *et al.*, 1972).

Goodwin and colleagues (1973*a*) examined the performance of 32 alcoholics on word-list recall after 8 to 10 oz of vodka consumed within a 1-hr period (1.2 g/kg). All subjects reported a history of blackouts. Recall and recognition were examined after 30 min and again after 24 hr. The alcohol and placebo groups did not differ in their ability to recall and recognize the test words. Blood alcohol levels were not reported.

Parker and co-workers (1974) compared the performance of alcoholics with matched nonalcoholic controls under conditions of sobriety and two doses of alcohol (0.5 and 1.1 g/kg). The 12 alcoholic subjects had been withdrawn from alcohol for 3 weeks prior to the study. Testing sessions were separated by 1 week and alcohol was administered between 8 and 9 a.m. after an overnight fast. Forward digit span, reverse digit span, and free recall of a 30-word list were studied. No significant differences between alcoholics and controls were observed during sobriety. Alcohol administration significantly impaired registration, recall, and organization of information in both groups. Performance on digit span and free recall deteriorated with increasing doses of alcohol. The investigators conclude that "memory deficits are a pervasive concomitant of alcohol intoxication, but the acute effects of alcohol do not differentiate alcoholics from nonalcoholics" (Parker *et al.*, 1974, p. 826). They suggest that the findings are not consistent with the notion that memory loss during intoxication is a specific predictor of the alcoholic blackout. Subjects were not specifically reinforced for accurate performance but appeared to the investigators to be "trying hard to perform." It is possible that the 3-week period of abstinence resulted in a decrease of behavioral tolerance for alcohol that accounted for the profound effect of alcohol on the tasks studied.

3.5.6. *Alcohol Effects on Information Processing*

Most investigators have been primarily concerned with determining whether or not intoxication produces discernible deficits in memory function. Recently there have been several ingenious studies of alcohol effects on information processing. This approach allows a closer examination of some identifiable components of information transfer that comprise the global construct of memory.

Moskowitz and Murray (1976*a*) have reported that alcohol significantly impairs the *rate* at which information is transferred from the initial sensory information storage system into short-term memory. Studies used a backward masking technique in which a brief presentation of a visual target stimulus (15 msec) is followed, after some interstimulus interval, by a masking stimulus that interferes with the image of the first stimulus and thereby blocks the transfer of this information into short-term memory. By varying the interval between the target and the masking stimulus and determining the relative amount of information reported, the *rate* of this stage of information processing can be measured. These conditions were compared with a no-mask condition, in which subjects had ample time to transfer target stimulus data into short-term memory. This control permitted the investigators to determine if there was a source of impairment other than a decrement in central processing time.

Twelve subjects were given a placebo, 0.4 g/kg vodka, or 0.8 g/kg vodka after a 4-hr fast. Actual blood alcohol levels were not reported. Subjects reported fewer stimuli correctly after alcohol than after no alcohol at all masking interstimulus intervals. These data were interpreted to indicate that alcohol reduced the amount of information that was read out of an immediate visual information storage system. Alcohol had no effect under conditions where there was no backward masking, which suggests that alcohol primarily affects the rate of transfer from the immediate visual storage system, iconic memory.

Iconic memory refers to a rapidly fading visual image that persists after termination of a brief visual stimulus. In a second experiment, Moskowitz and Murray (1976*b*) examined the influence of alcohol on the decay rate of information in the iconic memory storage system itself. Assessment of the rate of decay of information from iconic memory involved the tachistoscopic presentation of a matrix of 12 letters. Subjects were instructed to report only the top row of three rows of four letters at the sound of a tone. Subjects were trained for eight 1-hr training sessions of approximately 150 trials. The 3 experimental test days (placebo and low- and high-dose alcohol, 0.4 and 0.8 g/kg) were at 1-week intervals. Stimulus–tone intervals of 1, 50, 150, 400, and 750 msec were presented in an ascending order for 6 subjects and a descending order for 6 subjects. The amount of information retained in iconic memory rapidly decreased as a function of time (stimulus–tone interval) under all conditions. Alcohol did *not* affect the rate at which information was dissipated from iconic memory. Alcohol did decrease the average number of letters correctly reported; however, this decrease was constant at each stimulus–tone interval and is not a measure of memory decay rate (Moskowitz and Murray, 1976*b*). The nature of this alcohol-induced deficit is unclear since no alcohol impairment of information acquisition or storage capacity was found previously. No deficit in recall occurred after alcohol under the unmasked condition, i.e., when there was no effort to interfere with transfer of information from iconic memory to short-term memory (Moskowitz and Murray, 1976*a*).

Previous studies from Moskowitz' laboratory have shown that performance requiring a division of attention between two or more information inputs is sensitive to impairment at blood alcohol concentrations as low as 15 mg/100 ml (Moskowitz and Sharma, 1974; Moskowitz *et al.*, 1974; Moskowitz, 1971). Since divided attention probably involves a serial, rather than a parallel, processing of information sampled alternately from the various sources, an alcohol-induced reduction in information processing rate would produce a decreased capacity to handle information for more than one channel. The mechanism of an alcohol-induced reduction in the rate of information processing is unknown (Moskowitz and Murray, 1976*a*).

Tharp and co-workers (1974) used auditory and visual stimulus recognition tasks in an effort to determine which stage of information processing was primarily affected by alcohol. In all tasks studied, it appeared that alcohol disrupted organization and selection of the correct response, an impairment the investigators compared to a "slip of the tongue." Increases in reaction time, errors, or both, depending upon the specific task conditions, were the basis for this conclusion. Since a blood alcohol level of about 100 mg/100 ml did not change interaction and additivity patterns among the task-related treatment variables, the investigators concluded that perception (stimulus preprocessing and encoding) was not qualitatively affected by alcohol (Tharp *et al.*, 1974).

3.5.7. *Persistence of Memory and Cognitive Deficits in Alcoholics*

Whether or not alcohol abuse can eventually produce persistent deficits in cognitive and memory function is a question that has never been completely resolved. Investigators concerned with these issues have been forced to rely upon comparisons between chronic alcoholics and "matched" controls. Information about the alcoholics' premorbid level of functioning is almost never available and it is difficult to determine the contribution of age, intercurrent illness, or simple lack of interest to the performance pattern observed. Some investigators have attempted to follow the recovery of function after an episode of intoxication by administering repeated tests. The extent to which recovery may in fact reflect the effect of practice on similar tests is seldom considered. Another problem of design and interpretation relates to adequate evaluation of the subject population. This is especially important since chronic alcoholism combined with malnutrition may lead to permanent and irreversible disorders of cognitive and memory function (Victor, 1975; Dreyfus, 1974).

Given these several limitations, the available clinical evidence suggests that memory impairments associated with alcohol intoxication are transient and usually recover within 3 to 4 weeks after cessation of drinking. Allen *et al.* (1971) report that recovery of memory function, assessed by free recall of word lists, occurred within 13 days after withdrawal from alcohol. The criterion used for recovery was the performance of a control group. Weingartner *et al.* (1971) also observed that after a 3-week period of hospitalization, alcoholic subjects were able to retain verbal information as well as controls. Cermak and Ryback (1976) report that within 1 month of hospitalization, older alcoholics were able to perform on a short-term memory distractor test at a level comparable to younger alcoholics, whereas immediately following hospital admission, the same individuals performed as poorly as alcoholic Korsakoff's patients. The average age of the older alcoholic patients was 58 and the average age of the younger group was 28.

Jones (1971) and Jones and Parsons (1972) compared alcoholics with controls on various measures of cognitive function to determine if real deficits exist. Thirty alcoholics were compared with controls on a nonverbal measure of intelligence (the Advanced Ravens Progressive Matrices) and a verbal intelligence measure (the Shipley–Hartford). Those alcoholics who reported a severe alcohol problem of about 3-years duration did better than those individuals who reported an alcohol problem of 15-years duration, even though both groups were matched for age. Both groups of alcoholics performed more poorly than controls on the spatial but not on the verbal intelligence tests (Jones, 1971). These findings were replicated and extended in a comparison of 26 alcoholics with controls on the same verbal and nonverbal measures of intelligence and a Halstead category test that involves visual–spatial abstraction. Deficits in abstracting ability appeared to be restricted to visual–spatial tasks. Alcoholics did not differ from controls in tasks that involved verbal abstracting capacities (Jones and Parsons, 1972).

3.6. The Effects of Alcohol on Sleep

The study of sleep in man is a broad and complex field of inquiry, of which examination of the effects of alcohol and other psychoactive drugs accounts for only a very small part. Comprehensive reviews of some of the major questions and ideas in the field have been provided by Feinberg and Evarts (1969) and Snyder (1971). There have been several recent reviews of the effects of alcohol on sleep, primarily in alcoholic individuals (Gross *et al.*, 1971, Gross and Hastey, 1976; Williams and Salamy, 1972). This selective review will consider only a few of the main questions and findings in this area.

The notion that alcohol improves sleep has remained an almost unquestioned aspect of the common knowledge about alcohol. The fact that alcohol is usually classified as a central nervous system depressant is concordant with this view. Alcohol addicts frequently complain of recurrent insomnia, even during sobriety, and often attribute their excessive drinking to an effort to combat this insomnia. However, as interest in the electroencephalographic analysis of the effects of drugs on sleep patterns increased, the usual assumptions about the effects of alcohol have been consistently challenged.

Alcohol intoxication and alcohol withdrawal appear to adversely affect the quality of sleep according to EEG criteria derived from studies of "normal" individuals. It is generally agreed that "poor sleep" is characterized by any deviation from normal REM sleep activity and by a relative decrease in slow-wave sleep. However, alcohol does appear to reduce the latency of sleep onset.

3.6.1. Alcohol Intoxication

Some effects of alcohol on sleep occur consistently in social drinkers and alcohol addicts. Most prominent of these effects is that acute or chronic doses of alcohol reduce *rapid eye movement (REM) sleep* below the "normal" percentage of 20 to 25% of total sleep. Gresham *et al.* (1963) first reported this effect in seven normal adults following an acute alcohol dose of 1 g/kg. An alcohol-related reduction in REM time was subsequently reported by Yules and co-workers (1966*a*, 1967). An alcohol dose of 1 g/kg produced a decrease in REM time whether alcohol was given 45 min or 4 hr before subjects went to bed. However, since the 4-hr delay resulted in an effectively lower dose of alcohol upon retiring, the magnitude of the effect was less (Yules *et al.*, 1967). Comparable effects of acute doses of alcohol have been reported in normal subjects by Knowles *et al.* (1968) and by Rundell and co-workers (1972). REM reduction after an acute dose of alcohol has also been observed in cats (Yules *et al.*, 1966*b*).

The pattern of alcohol-induced REM changes was quite consistent across studies. A REM reduction during the first half of the night was usually followed by a compensatory increase during the second half of the night. In some instances, total REM activity was unchanged (cf. Rundell *et al.*, 1972). However this pattern may be specific to isolated acute doses of alcohol. Rundell and co-workers (1972) have compared the effects of single and repeated doses of alcohol (0.9 g/kg after a 4-hr fast) on the sleep patterns of 17 normal volunteers. Blood alcohol levels at bedtime averaged between 75 and 77 mg/100 ml. There appeared to be some adaptation to the effects of alcohol over 3 consecutive nights, since a significant REM suppression during the first half of the night only occurred on the first alcohol night and not on the subsequent alcohol nights.

Most studies of alcoholic subjects during chronic intoxication also reveal an alcohol-related depression of REM sleep (Greenberg and Pearlman, 1967; Gross and Goodenough, 1968; Johnson, 1971; Johnson *et al.*, 1970; Gross *et al.*, 1973; Zarcone *et al.*, 1975). During a long period of chronic intoxication, there may be considerable variation in the degree of total REM suppression. The observed variations are not systematic and do not appear to be consistently related to changes in blood alcohol level (Wolin and Mello, 1973; Johnson, 1971; Johnson *et al.*, 1970).

An alcohol-related decrease in REM activity is often associated with *sleep fragmentation,* defined by frequent awakenings, frequent EEG stage changes, and brief sleep periods. Behavioral evidence of sleep fragmentation in 50 alcoholic subjects was reported by Mello and Mendelson (1970*b*) and EEG correlates of sleep fragmentation have been observed by Johnson (1971) and

Gross *et al.* (1971). An increase in ocular activity during non-REM sleep after moderate alcohol ingestion has also been reported (McIntosh *et al.*, 1975). Most investigators have noted that sleep fragmentation increases even more during alcohol withdrawal (Gross *et al.*, 1973; Johnson, 1971).

Studies of the effects of alcohol on *slow-wave sleep* have yielded conflicting data. In normal subjects, alcohol does not appear to change slow-wave sleep significantly. After acute or repeated alcohol doses, slow-wave sleep tended to decrease slightly during the second half of the night (Rundell *et al.*, 1972). In alcoholics, alcohol has been reported to suppress (Johnson *et al.*, 1970) and to facilitate slow-wave sleep (Gross and Goodenough, 1968; Gross *et al.*, 1973). Some recent evidence suggests that differences in baseline slow-wave sleep activity may account for these descrepant findings.

Gross and Hastey (1975*a*) reported that alcoholic subjects with 20 to 40% slow-wave sleep during a drug-free baseline showed an *increase* of slow-wave sleep over 4 days of heavy drinking, whereas those subjects with less than 20% slow-wave sleep during baseline showed a further *reduction* of slow-wave sleep during alcohol intoxication. However, Gross and Hastey (1975*a*) note that when drinking continued beyond 4 days, slow-wave sleep activity tended to decrease even in those subjects with a high baseline slow-wave sleep who showed an initial increase in slow-wave sleep level during intoxication.

Wagman and Allen (1975) reported an increase in slow-wave sleep following ingestion of 18 and 26 oz of alcohol over 5 consecutive days of drinking. The effects of 32 oz of alcohol were examined for at least 1 day. Alcoholic subjects were recruited from emergency ward admissions, stabilized on alcohol or librium for 3 days, then withdrawn for 7 days before alcohol was administered. In contrast to Gross and Hastey's subjects (1975*a*), these subjects had relatively low slow-wave sleep activity during baseline (3%). The basis for these discrepancies between laboratories and in successive studies by the same investigators is not immediately apparent from an examination of the published papers (cf. Wagman and Allen, 1975; Gross and Hastey, 1975*a*). In an earlier report, Gross and co-workers (1973) suggested that discrepancies between their findings and those of other investigators relate primarily to the length of recovery periods allowed after subjects were admitted to the hospital. Gross' subjects had 3 to 6 weeks of good nutrition and supervised abstinence without other medication before baseline measures began.

The confounding influences of differences in baseline observations undoubtedly also account for much of the confusion in the literature on the effects of alcohol withdrawal on sleep activity. Some investigators have used a single-day baseline (Johnson *et al.*, 1970) and other investigators have studied acute admissions to an emergency ward, which precludes the possibility of obtaining any baseline measures (Gross *et al.*, 1966; Greenberg and Pearlman, 1967; Gross and Goodenough, 1968). Data so acquired indicated a severe disruption of a hypothetical normal sleep pattern and dramatic increases in REM activity. However, it is difficult to determine whether intercurrent illness, lack of adaptation to the experimental procedures, or an alcohol abstinence syndrome was primarily responsible for the observed sleep disruptions.

3.6.2. *Alcohol Withdrawal*

It is important to recognize that both alcohol intoxication and withdrawal of alcohol in physically dependent individuals can result in sleep disturbances. Clinical observations have consistently suggested that *insomnia* is a characteristic of the alcohol abstinence syndrome (Victor and Adams, 1953; Victor, 1966, 1973). Contrary to this prevailing clinical impression, abrupt cessation of drinking did not invariably produce an initial insomnia in 50 alcoholics following 7 to 62 days of spontaneous drinking (Mello and Mendelson, 1970*b*). These behavioral studies of sleep patterns in alcoholics further indicated that hallucinosis occurred as a concomitant of the alcohol abstinence syndrome and independent of an antecedent or concurrent state of insomnia (Mello and Mendelson, 1970*b*). The dissociation between insomnia and hallucinosis during alcohol withdrawal was surprising since insomnia, and attendant REM deprivation, were thought to be essential for the development of hallucinations. It was hypothesized that REM deprivation was followed by a compensatory rebound of REM activity which, if it exceeded 50% of total sleep time, might overflow into the waking state as hallucinatory behavior (Fisher and Dement, 1963).

The extent to which a temporal continuity between reports of dreams and hallucinations may reflect a neurophysiological continuity has long been a subject of speculation. In childhood hallucinosis, episodes that begin with a nightmare often extend into a frightening hallucinatory experience (Mack, 1970). Similarly, in alcoholics, intensely disturbing nightmares during withdrawal are sometimes closely followed by hallucinations (Gross *et al.*, 1966; Greenberg and Pearlman, 1967). Feinberg and Evarts (1969) have reviewed studies relevant to the idea first advanced by Hughlings Jackson and William James that dreams are associated with neurophysiologic processes that are also related to some types of hallucinations occurring in the waking state. Evarts (1962) has synthesized several ideas about the origins of hallucinations into a single hypothesis, i.e., that some hallucinations correlate with a process similar to one that occurs during sleep, which involves an increased neural discharge of brain structures involved in waking perception. Feinberg and Evarts (1969) have proposed a model to account for REM-associated delirium and drug withdrawal. They suggest that after an initial drug-induced REM suppression, chronic drug use is accompanied by a return to REM baseline levels through some unspecified compensatory mechanism. The subsequent REM overshoot during drug withdrawal then may facilitate the eruption of hallucinosis.

A temporal association between alcohol withdrawal, hallucinations, and a high percentage of REM sleep has been observed by several investigators (Johnson *et al.*, 1970; Gross *et al.*, 1966). Gross and Goodenough (1968) also report that two patients in alcohol withdrawal who did not develop hallucinations also did not show an elevation of REM activity. However, the notion that drug-induced REM reduction is inevitably followed by REM rebound has now been challenged (Feinberg *et al.*, 1974; Gross and Hastey, 1975*b*). Only subjects with no discernible REM activity during 4 to 6 days of alcohol intoxication show a significant REM rebound during withdrawal (Gross and Hastey, 1975*b*). The assumption that there is an isomorphism between dreams and REM activity is no longer accepted since awakenings from non-REM sleep also yield reports of mental activity (Berger, 1969; Snyder, 1971).

A reexamination of the relationship between EEG sleep measures, dreams, and hallucinations in alcohol addicts during a sequence of sobriety, 11 or 12 days of spontaneous drinking, and alcohol withdrawal suggested that there is no invariant association between vivid dreams and hallucinatory episodes and REM activity (Wolin and Mello, 1973). Of the 14 subjects studied, 11 reported a history of hallucinations during alcohol withdrawal. Clinical interviews focusing upon dream reports and hallucinatory experiences were conducted with each subject each day at the same time and for the same length of time throughout the study. A series of perceptual tasks were also administered. Data obtained did not support the notion that there may be a continuum of sequential changes progressing from perceptual alterations to illusions to vivid dreams to hallucinations during chronic intoxication and withdrawal. An alcohol-induced suppression of REM activity, followed by REM hyperactivity during alcohol withdrawal, was not consistently observed. Out of 26 hallucinatory events observed, 20 were associated with an antecedent REM suppression or with insomnia, but there were no invariant relationships between hallucinosis and REM activity. Most important, hallucinations were observed *during intoxication* as well as during alcohol withdrawal.

The major effect of alcohol intoxication was to increase the relative frequency of dream reports among both the hallucinators and the vivid dreamers (Wolin and Mello, 1973). However, neither dream occurrence nor dream intensity appear to be systematically related to alcohol dosage. Although there were no consistent dose–response relationships between alcohol intake, dreams, and hallucination intensity, a qualitative change in reported dream content was observed. Of the 12 subjects who reported dreams during withdrawal, 9 described an intense kinesthetic dream experience. Withdrawal hallucinations also involved tactile and kinesthetic delusions (Wolin, 1973). The currently available evidence suggests that hallucinations cannot be explained solely on the basis of changes in REM activity. The mechanisms underlying hallucinatory behavior during alcohol intoxication and alcohol withdrawal are unknown.

3.6.3. Sleep of Abstinent Alcoholics

Several investigators have attempted to determine if alcohol-related sleep disturbances persist in alcoholics during periods of sustained sobriety. In a study of the long-term sleep patterns of sober alcoholics, Allen and co-workers (1971*b*) found that REM sleep remains fragmented and slow-wave sleep is suppressed with respect to normal values over many weeks. Adamson and Burdick (1973) also observed fragmentation and a persistent depression of slow-wave sleep in 10 subjects after 1 to 2 years of abstinence. Wagman and Allen (1975) studied 20 male alcoholics who were abstinent members of Alcoholics Anonymous over 3 consecutive nights and found that suppression of slow-wave sleep can be seen for at least 3.5 weeks after the initiation of abstinence. In the sample studied, recovery to normal values was complete after 200 weeks.

Gross and co-workers (1975) have suggested that a persistent reduction in slow-wave sleep following alcohol withdrawal could be an indication of residual functional tolerance for, and physical dependence upon, alcohol. This hypothesis was tested by examining subjects treated for alcohol withdrawal over a 3-week period and then administering alcohol for 5 or 7 days. Evaluation of EEG sleep patterns, behavioral levels of intoxication, and pulse rate suggested to the authors that those alcoholics with a lower baseline slow-wave sleep reacquired alcohol tolerance at a higher rate than the group with the higher baseline level of slow-wave sleep. The investigators acknowledge that these findings are preliminary since the sample size was small, and indicate that further studies are in progress to examine this hypothesis (Gross *et al.*, 1975).

Sleep changes as a function of age may also contribute to the appearance of persistent sleep problems in sober alcoholics. Johnson (1971) has noted that the sleep of alcoholics is more like the sleep of elderly people than nonalcoholic subjects of equivalent age. Alcoholics take longer to fall asleep, have more stage 1 sleep and more changes in sleep stage, reach the first REM period more quickly, and have dramatically less stage 4 sleep than nonalcoholic persons of their age (Johnson, 1971). Lester and co-workers (1973) were concerned with the possible confounding influence of age differences on sleep patterns of alcoholics. EEG sleep profiles of sober alcoholics were compared with age-matched controls and the effects of 2 days of *ad lib* drinking on the sleep of 17 chronic alcoholics was subsequently studied. During sobriety, the alcoholic patients had significantly more REM and stage 1 sleep and less stage 3 sleep than control subjects. The alcoholic subjects also showed significantly more sleep fragmentation, arousals, and changes in sleep stages than controls. However, this difference was only significant during the second half of the baseline sleep nights. The average duration of the interval between successive REM periods was shorter for alcoholics than for controls and accounts for the increased amount of REM activity in alcoholic subjects. The duration of REM episodes did not differ between the two groups.

During the 2-day drinking period subjects achieved average blood alcohol levels of 157 and 159 mg/100 ml. On the first alcohol night, time awake, stage 1, and REM were all decreased and slow wave sleep was increased. After single and repeated doses of alcohol, alcoholics and normal subjects in both age groups showed depressed REM activity, reduced intervals between REM cycles, enhanced slow-wave sleep, and reduced latency of sleep onset. It may be that the reduction in latency of sleep onset accounts for the prevalent subjective impression that alcohol improves sleep. The major difference between alcoholics and age-matched controls was in the under 40 age group: each control subject had some stage 4 sleep but six of the eight alcoholics had no stage 4 sleep. It is important to note that the alcoholics studied had been abstinent for at least 3 weeks, maintained good nutritional status, and were in good health (Lester *et al.*, 1973). Consequently, the sleep changes observed probably can be attributed to the effects of alcohol and not to withdrawal signs or intercurrent illness.

In summary, both acute and chronic doses of alcohol are associated with a disruption of sleep in both normal and alcoholic subjects according to EEG and behavioral criteria. The prevalent assumption that alcohol improves sleep has received virtually no support from experimental studies. The hypothesis that alcohol-suppressed REM during intoxication, followed by a REM rebound during withdrawal, could account for behavioral disruptions such as hallucinations has not been supported, either for alcohol or for other drugs.

Few clear patterns have emerged from the recent profusion of data on the effects of alcohol on sleep patterns in alcoholics. The literature on the effects of alcohol on sleep in alcoholics contains many discrepancies and inconsistencies. Among the many methodological differences that may contribute to the inconsistent findings are: differences in the clinical status of alcoholics at the time of study; differences in duration and adequacy of baseline measures; differences in absolute alcohol dosage per day; differences in spontaneous or programmed alcohol administration paradigms; differences in the hours per day that subjects are allowed access to alcohol; differences in age of the subjects; differences in duration of alcoholism. Even if data were collected under more uniform conditions, procedures for EEG analysis vary considerably from laboratory to laboratory. It is generally acknowledged that hand scoring of EEG records is qualitative rather than quantitative, and even an experienced scorer may "read" a record differently on successive occasions. The technology of automatic sleep staging by computer is evolving (cf. Johnson, 1971; Lubin *et al.*, 1969; Itil *et al.*, 1969), but it is not yet available to all sleep laboratories. Since computer scoring seldom yields information in the same format as hand scoring, and since considerable variation still exists in the interpretation of spectral analysis, coherence, values, etc., it is perhaps surprising that any consistent findings have emerged. The process by which alcohol produces disruptive effects on sleep behavior is not known.

4. CONCLUSIONS

The effects of alcohol on human behavior are diverse and complex, and rarely in accord with traditional beliefs. Alcohol use has long been associated with a real or imagined enhancement of many aspects of human behavior. The common perception of alcohol's positive and beneficial effects has led to the assumption that the abuse of alcohol also involves a magnification and perpetuation of the satisfaction of social drinking. In fact, alcohol abuse often results in a distortion of many of the simplest alcohol-related pleasures. The once positive effects of alcohol are often transformed into their antithesis. The casual drinker who evolves into an alcohol abuser crosses an intangible line into a realm of continuing expectancy rather than fulfillment.

The illusion of sustained gratification appears to be shared by abusers of many psychoactive drugs. As Freedman (1972, p. 25) has expressed it:

> In enhancing our purposes with chemicals, we seem, nevertheless, to be intrinsically limited in the extent to which we can endure chemical pleasures. I have often wondered whether the fact that drugs rarely sustain their initial allure and promise was a mischievous and malevolent trick of nature. Whatever the problems of design, there do appear to be intrinsic biological and biosocial limits upon the extent to which the chemically induced moment of pleasure can be sustained and woven into a fabric of viable social life. We can readily give up our lease on reality, but apparently it is difficult to gain ownership of paradise!

It is, in part, the inconstancy and unpredictability of the behavioral effects of alcohol that defies our best efforts to describe and understand it. As our current concepts evolve toward greater precision and depth, and we begin to define and examine behavioral events in terms of their consequences rather than in terms of arbitrary labels and entrenched beliefs, the puzzle of alcohol abuse may unfold into a more comprehensible pattern.

ACKNOWLEDGMENTS

Preparation of this review was supported in part by Grant DA 4RG010 from the Special Action Office of Drug Abuse Prevention, Executive Office of the President, Washington, D.C., and the National Institute on Drug Abuse, ADAMHA, and by Grant DA 01676-01 from the National Institute on Drug Abuse, ADAMHA. We thank Francine Fein, Doris Lindgren, and Virginia Davis for excellent assistance in all phases of manuscript preparation.

5. REFERENCES

Adamson, J., and Burdick, J. A., 1973, Sleep of dry alcoholics, *Arch. Gen. Psychiat.* **28:**146–149.

Alcohol and Health, First Special Report to Congress, Publ. No. DHEW 72-9099, 1971, U.S. Govt. Printing Office, Washington, D.C.

Allen R. P., Faillace, L. A., and Reynolds, D. M., 1971*a*, Recovery of memory functioning in alcoholics following prolonged intoxication, *J. Nerv. Ment. Dis.* **153:**417–423.

Allen, R. P., Wagman, A., Fallice, L. A., and McIntosh, M., 1971*b*, Electroencephalographic (EEG) sleep recovery following prolonged alcohol intoxication in alcoholics, *J. Nerv. Ment. Dis.* **153:**424–433.

Alterman, A. I., Gottheil, E., and Crawford, H. D., 1975, Mood changes in an alcoholism treatment program based on drinking decisions, *Am. J. Psychiat.* **132:**1032–1037.

Ball, J. C., Graff, H., and Chien, K., 1975, Changing world patterns of drug abuse, 1945–1974, *Int. J. Clin. Pharmacol.* **12:**109–113.

Beckman, L. J., 1975, Women alcoholics: A review of social and psychological studies, *J. Stud. Alc.* **36:**797–824.

Bennion, L. J., and Li, T-K., 1976, Alcohol metabolism in American indians and whites: Lack of racial differences in metabolic rate and liver alcohol dehydrogenase, *N. Engl. J. Med.* **294:**9–13.

Benvenuto, J. A., Lau, J., and Cohen, R., 1975, Patterns of nonopiate/polydrug abuse: Findings of a national collaborative research project, in: *Problems of Drug Dependence*, Proceedings of the 37th Annual Scientific Meeting, Committee on Problems of Drug Dependence, National Academy of Sciences-National Research Council, Washington, D.C., pp. 234–254.

Berger, R. J., 1969, The sleep and dream cycle, in: *Sleep, Physiology and Pathology* (A. Kales, ed.), pp. 17–32, J. B. Lippincott, Philadelphia.

Bigelow, G., Liebson, I., and Griffiths, R., 1974, Alcoholic drinking: Suppression by a brief time-out procedure, *Behav. Res. Ther.* **12:**107–115.

Bloomquist, E. R., 1959, Addiction, addicting drugs, and the anesthesiologist. *JAMA* **171:**518–523.

Bourne, P. G., 1973, Alcoholism in the urban negro population, in: *Alcoholism: Progress in Research and Treatment* (P. G. Bourne and R. Fox, eds.), pp. 211–226, Academic Press, New York.

Bourne, P. G., 1975, Polydrug abuse—Status report on the federal effort, in: *Developments in the Field of Drug Abuse: National Drug Abuse Conference* (E. Senay, V. Shorty, and H. Alksen, eds.), pp. 197–207, Schenkman, Cambridge, Mass.

Boyatzis, R. E., 1974, The effect of alcohol consumption on the aggressive behavior of men, *Q. J. Stud. Alcohol* **35:**959–972.

Boyatzis, R. E., 1975, The predisposition toward alcohol-related interpersonal aggression in men, *J. Stud. Alcohol* **36:**1196–1207.

Briddell, D. W., and Wilson, G. T., 1976, Effects of alcohol and expectancy set on male sexual arousal, *J. Abnorm. Psychol.* **85**(2):225–234.

Burch, G. E., and Giles, T. D., 1974, Alcoholic cardiomyopathy, in: *The Biology of Alcoholism*, Vol. 3, *Clinical Pathology* (B. Kissin and H. Begleiter, eds.), pp. 435–460, Plenum, N.Y.

Burford, R., French, I. W., and LeBlanc, A. E., 1975, The combined effects of alcohol and common psychoactive drugs: I. Studies on human pursuit tracking capability, in: *Alcohol, Drugs and Traffic Safety* (S. Israelstam and F. Lambert, eds.), pp. 423–431, Addiction Research Foundation of Ontario, Toronto, Canada.

Burton, G., and Kaplan, K. M., 1968, Sexual behavior and adjustment of married alcoholics, *Q. J. Stud. Alcohol* **29:**603–609.

Cahalan, D., and Room, R., 1974, *Problem Drinking Among American Men*, Monograph No. 7, Rutgers Center of Alcohol Studies, New Brunswick, New Jersey.

Cahalan, D., Cisin, I. H., and Crossley, H. M., 1969, *American Drinking Practices: A National Study of Drinking Behavior and Attitudes,* Monograph No. 6, Rutgers Center of Alcohol Studies, New Brunswick, New Jersey.

Cappell, H., and Herman, P. C., 1972, Alcohol and tension reduction: A review. *Q. J. Stud. Alcohol* **33:**33–64.

Carpenter, J. A., 1962, Effects of alcohol on some psychological processes, *Q. J. Stud. Alcohol* **23:**274–314.

Carpenter, J. A., and Armenti, N. P., 1972, Some behavioral effects of alcohol on man, in: *The Biology of Alcoholism,* Vol. 2, *Physiology and Behavior* (B. Kissin and H. Begleiter, eds.), pp. 510–543, Plenum, New York.

Carpenter, J. A., and Ross, B. M., 1965, Effect of alcohol on short-term memory, *Q. J. Stud. Alcohol* **26:**561–579.

Carpenter, T. M., 1940, The metabolism of alcohol: A review, *Q. J. Stud. Alcohol* **1:**201–226.

Cermak, L. S., and Butters, N., 1973, Information processing deficits of alcoholic Korsakoff patients, *Q. J. Stud. Alcohol* **34:**1110–1132.

Cermak, L. S., and Ryback, R. S., 1976, Recovery of verbal short-term memory in alcoholics, *J. Stud. Alcohol* **37:**46–52.

Davis, D., 1971, Mood changes in alcoholic subjects with programmed and free-choice experimental drinking, in: *Recent Advances in Studies of Alcoholism* (N. K. Mello and J. H. Mendelson, eds.), pp. 596–618, U.S. Govt. Printing Office Publ. No. (HSM) 71-9045, Washington, D.C.

DeLacerda, L., Kowarski, A., Johanson, A. J., Athanasiou, R., and Migeon, C. J., 1973, Integrated concentration and circadian variation of plasma testosterone in normal men, *J. Clin. Endocrinol. Metab.* **37:**366–371.

Devenyi, P., and Wilson, M., 1971, Abuse of barbiturates in an alcoholic population, *Canad. Med. Assoc. J.* **104:**219–221.

Diethelm, O., and Barr, R. M., 1962, Psychotherapeutic interviews and alcohol intoxication, *Q. J. Stud. Alcohol* **23:**243–251.

Doctor, R. G., Naitoh, P., and Smith, J. C., 1966, Electroencephalographic changes and vigilance behavior during experimentally induced intoxication with alcoholic subjects, *Psychosom. Med.* **28:**605–615.

Dotson, L. E., Robertson, L. S., and Tuchfeld, B., 1975, Plasma alcohol, smoking, hormone concentrations and self-reported aggression; a study in a social-drinking situation, *J. Stud. Alcohol* **36:**578–586.

Dreher, K. F., and Fraser, J. G., 1967, Smoking habits of alcoholic out-patients. I., *Int. J. Addict.* **2:**259–270.

Dreiling, D. A., 1975, Alcoholism, alcoholic pancreatitis, and pancreatic secretion, *Ann. N. Y. Acad. Sci.* **252:**187–199.

Dreyfus, P. M., 1974, Diseases of the nervous system in chronic alcoholics, in: *The Biology of Alcoholism,* Vol. 3, *Clinical Pathology* (B. Kissin and H. Begleiter, eds.), pp. 265–290, Plenum, New York.

Ellis, F. W., and Pick, J. R., 1971, Ethanol intoxication and dependence in rhesus monkeys, in: *Recent Advances in Studies of Alcoholism* (N. K. Mello and J. H. Mendelson, eds.), pp. 401–412, U.S. Govt. Printing Office Publ. No. (HSM) 71-9045, Washington, D.C.

Ellis, F. W., Pick, J. R., and Sawyer, M., 1977*a*, Effects of ethanol administration during pregnancy on fetal development in beagle dogs, *Fed. Proc.* **36**(3):285, Abstract.

Ellis, F. W., Pick, J. R., and Saywer, M., 1977*b*, Ethanol dose–response relationships in a beagle model of fetal alcohol syndrome, Paper presented at NIAAA Workshop on the Fetal Alcohol Syndrome, San Diego, February 12–14, 1977.

Emerson, E. R., 1908, *Beverages Past and Present,* Vol. 1, Putnam, New York/London.

Essig, C. F., 1968, Alcohol and related addicting drugs, in: *Alcoholism, The Total Treatment Approach* (R. J. Catanzaro, ed.), pp. 58–69, Charles C Thomas, Springfield, Ill.

Evans, M. A., Martz, R., Rodda, B. E., Kiplinger, G. F., and Forney, R. B., 1974,

Quantitative relationship between blood alcohol concentration and psychomotor performance, *Clin. Pharmacol. Ther.* **15**:253–260.

Evarts, E. V., 1962, A neurophysiologic theory of hallucinations, in: *Hallucinations* (L. J. West, ed.), pp. 1–13, Grune & Stratton, New York.

Ewing, J. A., Rouse, B. A., and Pellizzari, E. D., 1974, Alcohol sensitivity and ethnic background, *Am. J. Psychiat.* **131**:206–210.

Farkas, G. M., and Rosen, R. C., 1976, Effect of alcohol on elicited male sexual response, *J. Stud. Alcohol* **37**:265–272.

Feinberg, I., and Evarts, E. V., 1969, Some implications of sleep research for psychiatry, in: *Neurobiological Aspects of Psychopathology* (J. Zubin and C. Shagass, eds.), pp. 334–393, Grune & Stratton, New York.

Feinberg, I., Hibi, S., Cavness, C., and March, J., 1974, Absence of REM rebound after barbiturate withdrawal, *Science* **185**:534–535.

Fenna, D., Mix, L., Schaefer, O., and Gilbert, J. A. L., 1971, Ethanol metabolism in various racial groups, *Canad. Med. Assoc. J.*, **105**:472–475.

Fisher, C., and Dement, W. C., 1963, Studies on the psychopathology of sleep and dreams, *Am. J. Psychiat.* **119**:1160–1168.

Fisher, G., and Brickman, H. R., 1973, Multiple drug use of marihuana users, *Dis. Nerv. Sys.* **34**:40–43.

Fleming, E. W., Tewari, S., and Noble, E. P., 1975, Effects of chronic ethanol ingestion on brain amino acyl-*t*-RNA synthetases and *t*-RNA, *J. Neurochem.* **24**:553–560.

Floody, O. R., and Pfaff, D. W., 1974, Steroid hormones and aggressive behavior: Approaches to the study of hormone-sensitive brain mechanisms for behavior, in: *Aggression*, Vol. 52 (S. H. Frazier, ed.), pp. 149–185, Res. Publ. ARNMD, Williams & Wilkins, Baltimore.

Forbes, S. H. D., 1948, *Short History of the Art of Distillation*, Leiden.

Forney, R. B., and Hughes, F. W., 1968, *Combined Effects of Alcohol and Other Drugs*, Charles C Thomas, Springfield, Ill.

Forney, R. B., and Hughes, F. W., 1970, Interaction between alcohol and psychopharmacologic drugs, in: *International Encyclopedia of Pharmacology and Therapy*, Vol. 2, Section 20, Alcohol and Derivatives, pp. 445–464, Pergamon Press, New York.

Franks, H. M., Hensley, V. R., Hensley, W. J., Starmer, G. A., and Teo, R. K. C., 1976, The relationship between alcohol dosage and performance decrement in humans, *J. Stud. Alcohol* **37**:284–297.

Fredrickson, D. S., Levy, R. I., and Lees, R. S., 1967, Fat transport in lipoproteins—An integrated approach to mechanisms and disorders, *N. Engl. J. Med.* **276**:32–44, 94–103, 148–156, 215–226, 273–281.

Freed, E. X., 1973, Drug abuse by alcoholics: A review, *Int. J. Addict.* **8**:451–473.

Freedman, D. X., 1972, Non-pharmacological factors in drug dependence, in: *Drug Abuse: Nonmedical Use of Dependence Producing Drugs* (S. Btesh, ed.), pp. 25–34, Plenum, New York.

Freemon, F. R., Goodwin, D. W., Halikas, J. A., and Othmer, E., 1971, An electroencephalographic study of memory loss during alcohol intoxication, *Dis. Nerv. Sys.* **32**:848–852.

Galvao-Teles, A., Anderson, D. C., Burke, C. W., Marshall, J. C., Corker, C. S., Brown, R. L., and Clark, M. L., 1973, Biologically active androgens and oestradiol in men with chronic liver disease, *Lancet* **7796**:173–177.

Gantt, W. A., 1952, Effect of alcohol on the sexual reflexes of normal and neurotic male dogs, *Psychosom. Med.* **14**:174–181.

Ginsberg, H., Olefsky, J., Farquhar, J. W., and Reaven, G. M., 1974, Moderate ethanol ingestion and plasma triglyceride levels, *Ann. Int. Med.* **80**:143–149.

Goldstein, A., Aronow, L., and Kalman, S. M., 1968, *Principles of Drug Action*, Harper & Row, New York.

GOLDSTEIN, D. B., 1972, Relationship of alcohol dose to intensity of withdrawal signs in mice, *J. Pharmacol. Exp. Ther.* **180:**203–215.

GOODE, E., 1973, The major drugs of use among adolescents and young adults, in: *Drugs and Youth* (E. Harms, ed.), pp. 33–72, Pergamon Press, New York.

GOODWIN, D. W., 1971*a*, Blackouts and alcohol induced memory dysfunction, in: *Recent Advances in Studies of Alcoholism* (N. K. Mello and J. H. Mendelson, eds.), pp. 508–536, U.S. Govt. Printing Office Publ. No. (HSM) 71-9045, Washington, D.C.

GOODWIN, D. W., 1971*b*, Is alcoholism hereditary? A review and critique, *Arch. Gen. Psychiat.* **25:**545–549.

GOODWIN, D. W., 1973, Alcohol in suicide and homicide, *Q. J. Stud. Alcohol* **34:**144–156.

GOODWIN, D. W., 1974, Alcoholic blackout and state dependent learning, *Fed. Proc.* **33:**1833–1835.

GOODWIN, D. W., 1976, *Is Alcoholism Hereditary?*, Oxford Univ. Press, New York.

GOODWIN, D. W., CRANE, J. B., and GUZE, S. B., 1969*a*, Phenomenological aspects of the alcoholic blackout, *Brit. J. Psychiat.* **115:**1033–1038.

GOODWIN, D. W., CRANE, J. B., and GUZE, S. B., 1969*b*, Alcoholic blackouts: A review and clinical study of 100 alcoholics, *Am. J. Psychiat.* **126:**191–198.

GOODWIN, D. W., JOHNSON, J., MAHER, C., RAPPAPORT, A., and GUZE, S. B., 1969*c*, Why people do not drink: A study of teetotalers, *Comp. Psychiat.* **10:**209–214.

GOODWIN, D. W., POWELL, B., BREMER, D., HOINE, H., and STERN, J., 1969*d*, Alcohol and recall: State-dependent effects in man, *Science* **163:**1358–1360.

GOODWIN, D. W., OTHMER, E., HALIKAS, J. A., and FREEMON, F., 1970, Loss of short term memory as a predictor of the alcoholic "blackout," *Nature (London)* **227:**201.

GOODWIN, D. W., POWELL, B., and STERN, J., 1971, Behavioral tolerance to alcohol in moderate drinkers, *Am. J. Psychiat.* **127:**1651–1653.

GOODWIN, D. W., HILL, S. Y., POWELL, B., and VIAMONTES, J., 1973*a*, Effect of alcohol on short term memory in alcoholics, *Br. J. Psychiat.* **122:**93–94.

GOODWIN, D. W., SCHULSINGER, F., HERMANSEN, L., GUZE, S. B., and WINOKUR, G., 1973*b*, Alcohol problems in adoptees raised apart from alcoholic biological parents, *Arch. Gen. Psychiat.* **28:**238–243.

GOODWIN, D. W., POWELL, B., HILL, S. Y., LIEBERMAN, W., and VIAMONTES, J., 1974*a*, Effect of alcohol on "dissociated" learning in alcoholics, *J. Nerv. Ment. Dis.* **158:**198–201.

GOODWIN, D. W., SCHULSINGER, F., MOLLER, N., HERMANSEN, L., WINOKUR, G., and GUZE, S. B., 1974*b*, Drinking problems in adopted and nonadopted sons of alcoholics, *Arch. Gen. Psychiat.* **31:**164–169.

GOULD, L. C., and KLEBER, H. D., 1974, Changing patterns of multiple drug use among applicants to a multimodality drug treatment program, *Arch. Gen. Psychiat.* **31:**408–413.

GREEN, M. H., NIGHTINGALE, S. L., and DUPONT, R. L., 1975, Evolving patterns of drug abuse, *Ann. Int. Med.* **83:**402–411.

GREENBERG, R., and PEARLMAN, C., 1967, Delirium tremens and dreaming, *Am. J. Psychiat.* **124:**133–142.

GRESHAM, S. C., WEBB, W. B., and WILLIAMS, R. L., 1963, Alcohol and caffeine: Effect on inferred visual dreaming, *Science* **140:**1226–1227.

GRIFFITHS, R., BIGELOW, G., and LIEBSON, I., 1974*a*, Suppression of ethanol self-administration in alcoholics by contingent time-out from social interactions, *Behav. Res. Ther.* **12:**327–334.

GRIFFITHS, R., BIGELOW, G., and LIEBSON, I., 1974*b*, Assessment of effects of ethanol self-administration on social interactions in alcoholics, *Psychopharmacologia (Berlin)* **38:**105–110.

GRIFFITHS, R., BIGELOW, G., and LIEBSON, I., 1975, Effect of ethanol self-administration on choice behavior: Money vs. socializing, *Pharmacol. Biochem. Behav.* **3:**443–446.

GRIFFITHS, R., BIGELOW, G., and LIEBSON, I., 1976, Facilitation of human tobacco self-administration by ethanol: A behavioral analysis, *J. Exp. Anal. Behav.* **25:**279–292.

GROSS, M. M., and GOODENOUGH, D. R., 1968, Sleep disturbances in the acute alcoholic psychoses, in: *Clinical Research in Alcoholism* (J. O. Cole, ed.), pp. 132–147, American Psychiatric Association, Washington, D.C.

GROSS, M. M., and HASTEY, J. M., 1975*a*, The relation between baseline slow wave sleep and the slow wave sleep response to alcohol in alcoholics, in: *Alcohol Intoxication and Withdrawal: Experimental Studies,* II, Vol. 59, *Advances in Experimental Medicine & Biology* (M. M. Gross, ed.), pp. 467–475, Plenum, New York.

GROSS, M. M., and HASTEY, J. M., 1975*b*, A note on REM rebound during experimental alcohol withdrawal in alcoholics, in: *Alcohol Intoxication and Withdrawal: Experimental Studies,* II, Vol. 59, *Advances in Experimental Medicine &Biology* (M. M. Gross, ed.), pp. 509–513, Plenum, New York.

GROSS, M. M., and HASTEY, J. M., 1976, Sleep disturbances in alcoholism, in: *Alcoholism: Interdisciplinary Approaches to an Enduring Problem* (R. E. Tarter and A. A. Sugarman, eds.), pp. 257–307, Addison-Wesley, Reading, Mass.

GROSS, M. M., GOODENOUGH, D. R., TOBIN, M., HALPERT, E., LEPORE, D., PERLSTEIN, A., SIROTA, M., DIBIANCO, J., FULLER, R., and KISHNER, I., 1966, Sleep disturbance and hallucinations in the acute alcoholic psychoses, *J. Nerv. Ment. Dis.* **142:**493–514.

GROSS, M. M., GOODENOUGH, D. R., HASTEY, J. M., ROSENBLATT, S. M., and LEWIS, E., 1971, Sleep disturbances in alcohol intoxication and withdrawal, in: *Recent Advances in Studies of Alcoholism* (N. K. Mello and J. H. Mendelson, eds.), pp. 317–397, U.S. Govt. Printing Office Publ. No. (HSM) 71-9045, Washington, D.C.

GROSS, M. M., GOODENOUGH, D. R., HASTEY, J. M., and LEWIS, E., 1973, Experimental study of sleep in chronic alcoholics before, during and after four days of heavy drinking, with a non-drinking comparison, in: *Alcoholism and the Central Nervous System* (F. A. Seixas and S. Eggleston, eds.), *Ann. N. Y. Acad. Sci.* **215:**254–265.

GROSS, M. M., LEWIS, E., and HASTEY, J. M., 1974, Acute alcohol withdrawal syndrome, in: *The Biology of Alcoholism,* Vol. 3, *Clinical Pathology* (B. Kissin and H. Beglieter, eds.), pp. 191–263, Plenum, New York.

GROSS, M. M., HASTEY, J. M., LEWIS, E., and YOUNG, N., 1975, Slow wave sleep and carry-over of functional tolerance and physical dependence in alcoholics, in: *Alcohol Intoxication and Withdrawal: Experimental Studies,* II, Vol. 59, *Advances in Experimental Medicine & Biology* (M. M. Gross, ed.), pp. 477–493, Plenum, New York.

GUNNAR, R. M., DEMAKIS, J., RAHIMTOOLA, S. H., SINNO, M. Z., and TOBIN, J. R., JR., 1975, Clinical signs and natural history of alcoholic heart disease, *Ann. N. Y. Acad. Sci.* **252:**264–272.

GUSFIELD, J. R., 1962, Status conflicts and the changing ideologies of the American temperance movement, in: *Society, Culture and Drinking Patterns* (D. J. Pittman and C. R. Snyder, eds.), pp. 101–120, Wiley, New York.

HAERTZEN, C. A., and HOOKS, N. T., 1969, Changes in personality and subjective experience associated with the chronic administration and withdrawal of opiates, *J. Nerv. Ment. Dis.* **148:**606–614.

HAGGARD, H. W., GREENBERG, L., and LOLLI, G., 1941, The absorption of alcohol with special reference to its influence on the concentration of alcohol appearing in the blood, *Q. J. Stud. Alcohol* **1:**684.

HARGER, R. N., and HULPIEU, H. R., 1956, The pharmacology of alcohol, in: *Alcoholism* (G. N. Thompson, ed.), pp. 103–232, Charles C Thomas, Springfield, Ill.

HART, B. L., 1968, Effects of alcohol on sexual reflexes and mating behavior in the male dog, *Q. J. Stud. Alcohol* **29:**833–844.

HIGGINS, R. L., and MARLATT, G. A., 1973, Effects of anxiety arousal on the consumption of alcohol by alcoholics and social drinkers, *J. Consult. Clin. Psychol.* **41:**426–433.

HIGGINS, R. L., and MARLATT, G. A., 1975, Fear of interpersonal evaluation as a determinant of alcohol consumption in male social drinkers, *J. Abnorm. Psychol.* **84:**644–651.

HOLLISTER, L. E., OVERALL, J. E., and GERBER, M. L., 1975, Marihuana and setting, *Arch. Gen. Psychiat.* **32:**798–801.

HONIG, W. K., ed., 1966, *Operant Behavior: Areas of Research and Application,* Appleton-Century-Crofts, New York.

IBER, F., KATER, R. M., and CARULI, M., 1969, Differences in the rate of ethanol metabolism in recently drinking alcohol and non-alcoholic subjects, *Am. J. Clin. Nutr.* **22:**1608–1617.

ISBELL, H., FRASER, H., WIKLER, A., BELLEVILLE, R., and EISENMAN, A., 1955, An experimental study of the etiology of rum fits and delirium tremens, *Q. J. Stud. Alcohol* **16:**1–33.

ISSELBACHER, K. J., and CARTER, E. A., 1971, Effects of alcohol on liver and intestinal function, in: *Recent Advances in Studies of Alcoholism* (N. K. Mello and J. H. Mendelson, eds.), pp. 42–58, U.S. Govt. Printing Office Publ. No. (HSM) 71-9045, Washington, D.C.

ISSELBACHER, K. J., and GREENBERGER, N. J., 1964, Metabolic effects of alcohol on the liver, *N. Engl. J. Med.* **270:**351–356, 402–410.

ITIL, T. M., SHAPIRO, D. M., FINK, M., and KASSENBAUM, D., 1969, Digital computer classifications of EEG sleep stages, *Electroenceph. Clin. Neurophysiol.* **27:**76–83.

JACOBSEN, E., 1952, The metabolism of ethyl alcohol, *Pharmacol. Rev.* **4:**107–135.

JAFFE, J. H., 1970, Drug addiction and drug abuse, in: *The Pharmacological Basis of Therapeutics* (L. S. Goodman and A. Gilman, eds.), pp. 276–313, Macmillan, New York.

JAFFE, J. H., 1975, Drug addiction and drug abuse, in: *The Pharmacological Basis of Therapeutics* (L. S. Goodman and A. Gilman, eds.), 5th Ed., pp. 284–324, Macmillan, New York.

JESSOR, R., and JESSOR, S. L., 1975, Adolescent development and the onset of drinking: A longitudinal study, *J. Stud. Alcohol* **36:**27–51.

JOHN, E. R., 1967, *Mechanisms of Memory,* Academic Press, New York.

JOHNSON, L. C., 1971, Sleep patterns of alcoholics, in: *Recent Advances in Studies of Alcoholism* (N. K. Mello and J. H. Mendelson, eds.), pp. 288–316, U.S. Govt. Printing Office Publ. No. (HSM) 71-9045, Washington, D.C.

JOHNSON, L. C., BURDICK, J. A., and SMITH, J., 1970, Sleep during alcohol intake and withdrawal in the chronic alcoholic, *Arch. Gen. Psychiat.* **22:**406–418.

JONES, B. M., 1971, Verbal and spatial intelligence in short and long term alcoholics, *J. Nerv. Ment. Dis.* **153:**292–297.

JONES, B. M., 1973, Memory impairment on the ascending and descending limbs of the blood alcohol curve, *J. Abnorm. Psychol.* **82:**24–32.

JONES, B. M., and PARSONS, O. A., 1972, Specific vs. generalized deficits of abstracting ability in chronic alcoholics, *Arch. Gen. Psychiat.* **26:**380–384.

JONES, K. L., SMITH, D. W., ULLELAND, C. N., and STREISSGUTH, A. P., 1973, Pattern of malformation in offspring of chronic alcoholic mothers, *Lancet* **1:**1267–1271.

JONES, K. L., SMITH, D. W., STREISSGUTH, A. P., and MYRIANTHOPOULOUS, N. C., 1974, Outcome in offspring of chronic alcoholic women, *Lancet* **1:**1076–1078.

KALANT, H., 1970, Effects of ethanol on the nervous system, in: *Alcohols and Derivatives,* Vol. 1, Section 20, *International Encyclopedia of Pharmacology and Therapeutics* (J. Tremolieres, ed.), pp. 189–236, Pergamon Press, New York.

KALANT, H., LEBLANC, A. E., WILSON, A., and HOMATIDIS, S., 1975, Sensorimotor and physiological effects of various alcoholic beverages, *Canad. Med. J.* **112:**953–958.

KALB, M., and PROPPER, M. S., 1976, The future of alcohology: Craft or science? *Am. J. Psychiat.* **133:**641–645.

KATER, R. M. H., ZEIVE, D., TOBON, F., ROGGIN, G. M., and IBER, F. L., 1968, Heavy drinking accelerates drugs' breakdown in liver, *JAMA* **206:**1709.

KAUFMAN, H., 1975, Multidrug abuse: Definition and determinants, in: *Problems of Drug Dependence,* Proceedings of the 37th Annual Scientific Meeting, Committee on Problems of Drug Dependence, National Academy of Sciences-National Research Council, Washington, D.C., pp. 218–233.

KELLEHER, R. T., RIDDLE, W. C., and COOK, L., 1963, Persistent behavior maintained by unavoidable shocks, *J. Exp. Anal. Behav.* **6:**507–517.

KELLER, M., 1962, The definition of alcoholism and the estimation of its prevalence, in:

Society, Culture and Drinking Patterns (D. J. Pittman and C. R. Snyder, eds.), pp. 310–329, Wiley, New York.

KISSIN, B., 1974, Interactions of ethyl alcohol and other drugs, in: *The Biology of Alcoholism*, Vol. 3, *Clinical Pathology* (B. Kissin and H. Begleiter, eds.), pp. 109–161, Plenum, New York.

KISSIN, B., and BEGLEITER, H., eds., 1974, *The Biology of Alcoholism*, Vol. 3, *Clinical Pathology*, Plenum, New York.

KISSIN, B., and KALEY, M. M., 1974, Alcohol and cancer, in: *The Biology of Alcoholism*, Vol. 3, *Clinical Pathology* (B. Kissin and H. Begleiter, eds.), pp. 481–511, Plenum, New York.

KLATSKY, A. L., FRIEDMAN, G. D., and SIEGELAUG, A. B., 1974, Alcohol consumption before myocardial infarction, *Ann. Int. Med.* **81**:294–301.

KNOWLES, J. B., LAVERTY, S. G., and KUECHLER, H. A., 1968, Effects of alcohol on REM sleep, *Q. J. Stud. Alcohol* **29**:342–349.

KNUPFER, G., 1966, Some methodological problems in the epidemiology of alcoholic beverage usage: Definition of amount of intake, *Am. J. Public Health* **2**:237–242.

KREUZ, L. E., and ROSE, R. M., 1972, Assessment of agressive behavior and plasma testosterone in a young criminal population, *Psychosom. Med.* **34**:321–332.

KUEHNLE, J. C., ANDERSON, W. H., and CHANDLER, E., 1974, Report on first drinking experience in addictive and nonaddictive drinkers, *Arch. Gen. Psychiat.* **31**:521–523.

LAFERLA, J. J., ANDERSON, D. L., and SCHALACH, D. S., 1976, Psychoendocrine response to visual erotic stimulation in human males, *Psychosom. Med.* **38**:62 (Abst.).

LANG, A. R., GOECKNER, D. J., ADESSO, V. J., and MARLATT, G. A., 1975, Effects of alcohol on aggression in male social drinkers, *J. Abnorm. Psychol.* **84**:508–518.

LANGROD, J., 1970, Secondary drug use among heroin users, *Int. J. Addict.* **5**:611–635.

LEAKE, C. D., and SILVERMAN, M., 1971, The chemistry of alcoholic beverages, in: *The Biology of Alcoholism*, Vol. 1, *Biochemistry* (B. Kissin and H. Begleiter, eds.), pp. 575–612, Plenum, New York.

LEE, T. K., CHO, M. H., and DOBKIN, A. B., 1964, Effects of alcoholism, morphinism and barbiturate resistance on induction and maintenance of general anesthesia. *Canad. Anaesth. Soc. J.* **11**:354–381.

LEMERE, F., and SMITH, J. W., 1973, Alcohol-induced sexual impotence, *Am. J. Psychiat.* **130**:212–213.

LESTER, B. K., RUNDELL, O. H., COWDEN, L. C., and WILLIAMS, H. L., 1973, Chronic alcoholism, alcohol and sleep, in: *Alcohol Intoxication and Withdrawal: Experimental Studies*, Vol. 35, *Advances in Experimental Medicine and Biology* (M. M. Gross, ed.), pp. 261–279, Plenum, New York.

LETTSOM, J. C., 1787, Some remarks on the effects of lignum quassil amare, *Memoirs Med. Soc. London* **1**:151–165.

LEVINE, J., 1955, The sexual adjustment of alcoholics—A clinical study of a selected sample, *Q. J. Stud. Alcohol* **16**:675–680.

LIEBER, C. S., RUBIN, E., and DECARLI, L. M., 1971, Chronic and acute effects of ethanol on hepatic metabolism of ethanol, lipids and drugs: Correlation with ultrastructural changes, in: *Recent Advances in Studies of Alcoholism* (N. K. Mello and J. H. Hendelson, eds.), pp. 3–41, U.S. Govt. Printing Office Publ. No. (HSM) 71-9045, Washington, D.C.

LIEBER, C. S., and DECARLI, L. M., 1974, An experimental model of alcohol feeding and liver injury in the baboon, *J. Med. Prim.* **3**:153–163.

LIEBER, C. S., DECARLI, L. M., and RUBIN, E., 1975, Sequential production of fatty liver, hepatitis, and cirrhosis in sub-human primates fed ethanol with adequate diets, *Proc. Nat. Acad. Sci.* **72**(2):437–441.

LIEBMANN, A. J., and SCHERL, B., 1949, Changes in whiskey while maturing, *Ind. Eng. Chem.* **41**:534.

LINDBECK, V. L., 1972, The woman alcoholic: A review of the literature, *Int. J. Addict.* **7**:567–580.

Lisman, S. A., 1974, Alcoholic "blackout": State-dependent learning? *Arch. Gen. Psychiat.* **30:**46–53.

Lolli, G., and Meschieri, L., 1964, Mental and physical efficiency after wine and ethanol solutions ingested on an empty and on a full stomach, *Q. J. Stud. Alcohol* **25:**535–540.

Lubin, A., Johnson, L. C., and Austin, M. T., 1969, Discrimination among states of consciousness using EEG Spectra, *Psychophysiology* **6:**122–132.

Macavoy, M. G., and Marks, E. F., 1975, Divided attention performance of cannabis users and non-users following cannabis and alcohol, *Psychopharmacologia (Berlin)* **44:**147–152.

Mack, J. E., 1970, *Nightmares and Human Conflict,* Little, Brown, Boston.

Maddux, J. F., and Elliott, B., 1975, Problem drinkers among patients on methadone, *Am. J. Drug Alc. Abuse* **2:**245–254.

Majchrowicz, E., 1975, Induction of physical dependence upon ethanol and the associated behavioral changes in rats, *Psychopharmacologia (Berlin)* **43:**245–254.

Maletzky, B. M., and Klotter, J., 1974, Smoking and alcoholism, *Am. J. Alc.* **131:**445–447.

Manno, J. E., Kiplinger, G. F., Scholz, N., Forney, R. B., and Haine, S. E., 1971, The influence of alcohol and marihuana on motor and mental performance, *Clin. Pharmacol. Ther.* **12:**202–211.

Manno, J. E., Manno, B. R., Kiplinger, G. F., and Forney, R. B., 1974, Motor and mental performance with marihuana: Relationship to administered dose of delta-9-tetrahydrocannabinol and its interaction with alcohol, in: *Marihuana, Effects on Human Behavior* (L. L. Miller, ed.), pp. 45–72, Academic Press, New York.

Mardones, J., 1963, The alcohols, in: *Physiological Pharmacology* (W. S. Root and F. G. Hoffmann, eds.), pp. 99–183, Academic Press, New York.

Marlatt, G. A., Kosturn, C. F., and Lang, A. R., 1975, Provocation to anger and opportunity for retaliation as determinants of alcohol consumption in social drinkers, *J. Abnorm. Psychol.* **84:**652–659.

Mayer, R. F., 1966, Peripheral nerve conduction in alcoholics, in: *Alcoholism: A Symposium on Recent Advances in Biological and Behavioral Research* (J. H. Mendelson, ed.), *Psychosom. Med.* **28:**475–483.

Mayfield, D. G., 1968, Psychopharmacology of alcohol. II. Affective tolerance in alcohol intoxication. *J. Nerv. Ment. Dis.* **146:**322–327.

McGuire, M. T., Mendelson, J. H., and Stein, S., 1966, Comparative psychosocial studies of alcoholic and non-alcoholic subjects undergoing experimentally induced ethanol intoxication, *Psychosom. Med.* **28:**13–25.

McIntosh, M., Funderburk, F., Wagman, A., and Allen, R., 1975, Ocular activity in the quiet sleep of chronic alcoholics, *Biol. Psychiat.* **10:**329–332.

McKearney, J. W., 1972, Schedule-dependent effects: Effects of drugs, and maintenance of responding with response-produced electric shocks, in: *Schedule-Effects: Drugs, Drinking, and Aggression* (R. M. Gilbert and J. D. Keehn, eds.), pp. 3–25, Univ. of Toronto Press, Toronto.

McNamee, H. B., Mello, N. K., and Mendelson, J. H., 1968, Experimental analysis of drinking patterns of alcoholics: Concurrent psychiatric observations, *Am. J. Psychiat.* **124:**1063–1069.

McNamee, H. B., Mendelson, J. H., and Korn, J., 1975, Fenmetozole in acute alcohol intoxication in man, *Clin. Pharmacol. Ther.* **17:**735–737.

Mello, N. K., 1968, Some aspects of the behavioral pharmacology of alcohol, in: *Psychopharmacology: A Review of Progress, 1957–1967* (D. H. Efron, ed.), pp. 787–809, U.S. Govt. Printing Office PHS Publ. No. 1863, Washington, D.C.

Mello, N. K., 1971, Alcohol effects on delayed matching to sample performance by rhesus monkey, *Physiol. Behav.* **7:**77–101.

Mello, N. K., 1972, Behavioral studies of alcoholism, in: *The Biology of Alcoholism,* Vol. 2, *Physiology and Behavior* (B. Kissin and H. Begleiter, eds.), pp. 219–291, Plenum, New York.

MELLO, N. K., 1973*a*, A review of methods to induce alcohol addiction in animals, *Pharmacol. Biochem. Behav.* **1**:89–101.

MELLO, N. K., 1973*b*, Short-term memory function in alcohol addicts during intoxication, in: *Alcohol Intoxication and Withdrawal: Experimental Studies,* Proceedings 30th International Congress on Alcoholism and Drug Dependence (M. M. Gross, ed.), pp. 333–344, Plenum, New York.

MELLO, N. K., 1975, A semantic aspect of alcoholism, in: *Biological and Behavioral Approaches to Drug Dependence* (H. D. Cappell and A. E. LeBlanc, eds.), pp. 73–87, Addiction Research Foundation of Ontario, Toronto.

MELLO, N. K., 1976*a*, Animal models for the study of alcohol addiction, *Psychoneuroendocrinology,* **1**:347–357.

MELLO, N. K., 1976*b*, Effects of chronic alcohol intoxication on "short-term memory" function in alcohol addicts, in preparation.

MELLO, N. K., 1977, Stimulus self-administration: Some implications for the prediction of drug abuse liability, in: *Predicting Dependence Liability of Stimulant and Depressant Drugs* (P. Thompson and K. R. Unna, eds.), pp. 243–260, University Park Press, Baltimore.

MELLO, N. K., and MENDELSON, J. H., 1970*a*, Experimentally induced intoxication in alcoholics: A comparison between programmed and spontaneous drinking. *J. Pharmacol. Exp. Ther.* **173**:101–116.

MELLO, N. K., and MENDELSON, J. H., 1970*b*, Behavioral studies of sleep patterns in alcoholics during intoxication and withdrawal. *J. Pharmacol. Exp. Ther.* **175**:94–112.

MELLO, N. K., and MENDELSON, J. H., 1972, Drinking patterns during work-contingent and noncontingent alcohol acquisition, *Psychosom. Med.* **34**:139–164.

MELLO, N. K., and MENDELSON, J. H., 1975, Alcoholism: A biobehavioral disorder, in: *American Handbook of Psychiatry* (M. Reiser, ed.), pp. 371–403, Basic Books, New York.

MELLO, N. K., and MENDELSON, J. H., 1976, The development of alcohol dependence: A clinical study, *McLean Hosp. J.* **1**:65–88.

MELLO, N. K., and MENDELSON, J. H., 1977, Clinical aspects of alcohol dependence, in: *Handbook of Experimental Pharmacology: Drug Addiction* (W. R. Martin, ed.), Springer-Verlag, Berlin/Heidelberg/New York (in press).

MENDELSON, J. H., ed., 1964, Experimentally induced chronic intoxication and withdrawal in alcoholics, *Q. J. Stud. Alcohol, Suppl. 2.*

MENDELSON, J. H., 1968, Ethanol-1-C^{14} metabolism in alcoholics and non-alcoholics, *Science* **159**:319–320.

MENDELSON, J. H., 1970, Biological concomitants of alcoholism, *N. Engl. J. Med.* **283**:24–32, 71–81.

MENDELSON, J. H., 1971, Biochemical mechanisms of alcohol addiction, in: *The Biology of Alcoholism,* Vol. 1, *Biochemistry* (B. Kissin and H. Begleiter, eds.), pp. 513–544, Plenum, New York.

MENDELSON, J. H., 1975, Alcohol abuse and alcohol-related illness, in: *The Cecil-Loeb Textbook of Medicine* (P. B. Beeson and W. McDermott, eds.), pp. 597–602, W. B. Saunders, Philadelphia.

MENDELSON, J. H., and MELLO, N. K., 1973, Alcohol-induced hyperlipedemia and beta lipoproteins, *Science* **180**:1372–1374.

MENDELSON, J. H., and MELLO, N. K., 1974, Alcohol, aggression and androgens, in: *Aggression,* Proc. ARNMD (S. H. Frazier, ed.), pp. 225–247, Williams & Wilkins, Baltimore.

MENDELSON, J. H., and MELLO, N. K., 1975, Plasma testosterone levels during chronic heroin use and protracted abstinence: A study of Hong Kong addicts, *Clin. Pharmacol. Ther.* **17**:529–533.

MENDELSON, J. H., and STEIN, S., 1966, The definition of alcoholism, in: *Alcoholism* (J. H. Mendelson, ed.), pp. 3–16, Little, Brown, Boston.

MENDELSON, J. H., WEXLER, D., LEIDERMAN, P., and SOLOMON, P., 1957, A study of addiction to nonethyl alcohols and other poisonous compounds, *Q. J. Stud. Alcohol* **18**:561–580.

MENDELSON, J. H., STEIN, S., and MELLO, N. K., 1965, Effects of experimentally induced intoxication on metabolism of ethanol-1-C^{14} in alcoholic subjects, *Metabolism* **14:**1255–1266.

MENDELSON, J. H., MELLO, N. K., and SOLOMON, P., 1968, Small group drinking behavior: An experimental study of chronic alcoholics, in: *The Addictive States* Res. Publ. Assoc. Nerv. Ment. Dis. (A. Wikler, ed.), pp. 399–430, Williams & Wilkins, Baltimore.

MENDELSON, J. H., ROSSI, A. M., BERNSTEIN, J. G., and KUEHNLE, J. C., 1974, Propranolol and behavior of alcohol addicts after acute alcohol ingestion, *Clin. Pharmacol. Ther.* **15:**571–578.

MENDELSON, J. H., ELLINGBOE, J., and KUEHNLE, J. C., 1976, Effects of alcohol and marihuana on plasma luteinizing hormone and testosterone, Proceedings 38th Annual Meeting, Committee on Problems of Drug Dependence, pp. 525–537, National Academy of Sciences-National Research Council, Washington, D.C.

MENDELSON, J. H., MELLO, N. K., and ELLINGBOE, J., 1977, Effects of alcohol on pituitary-gonadal hormones, sexual function, and aggression in human males, in: *Psychopharmacology, A Generation of Progress,* Raven Press, New York (in press).

MILLER, P. M., HERSEN, M., EISLER, R. M., and HILSMAN, G., 1974, Effects of social stress on operant drinking of alcoholics and social drinkers, *Behav. Res. Ther., Oxford,* **12:**67–72.

MIRIN, S. M., MEYER, R. E., and MCNAMEE, H. B., 1975, Psychopathology and mood during heroin use: Acute vs. chronic effects, in: *Problems of Drug Dependence,* Proceedings of the 37th Annual Scientific Meeting, Committee on Problems of Drug Dependence, National Academy of Sciences-National Research Council, Washington, D.C., pp. 300–319.

MIRIN, S. M., MCNAMEE, H. B., and MEYER, R. E., 1976, Psychopathology, craving and mood during heroin acquisition: An experimental study, *Int. J. Addict.* **11:**525–543.

MORSE, W. H., and KELLEHER, R. T., 1970, Schedules as fundamental determinants of behavior, in: *The Theory of Reinforcement Schedules* (W. N. Schoenfeld, ed.), pp. 139–185, Appleton-Century-Crofts, New York.

MORSE, W. H., and KELLEHER, R. T., 1977, Determinants of reinforcement and punishment, in: *Operant Behavior,* Vol. 2 (W. K. Honig and J. E. R. Staddon, eds.), pp. 174–200, Prentice-Hall, Englewood Cliffs, New Jersey.

MOSKOWITZ, H., 1971, The effects of alcohol on performance in a driving simulator of alcoholics and social drinkers, Institute of Transportation and Traffic Engineering, University of California at Los Angeles Technical Report UCLA—ENG—7205 (1971).

MOSKOWITZ, H.,and BURNS, M., 1975, Effects of rate of drinking on human performance, *J. Stud. Alcohol* **37:**598–605.

MOSKOWITZ, H.,and MURRAY, J. T., 1976*a*, Backward masking of visual information, *J. Stud. Alcohol* **37:**40–45.

MOSKOWITZ, H., and MURRAY, J. T., 1976*b*, Decrease of iconic memory after alcohol, *J. Stud. Alcohol* **37:**278–283.

MOSKOWITZ, H., and SHARMA, S., 1974, Effects of alcohol on peripheral vision as a function of attention, *Human Factors* **16:**174–180.

MOSKOWITZ, H., SHARMA, S., and SCHAPIRO, M., 1972, A comparison of the effects of marihuana and alcohol on visual function, in: *Current Research in Marihuana* (M. F. Lewis, ed.), pp. 129–150, Academic Press, New York.

MOSKOWITZ, H., DAILY, J., and HENDERSON, R., 1974, Acute tolerance to behavioral impairment by alcohol in moderate and heavy drinkers, Systems Development Corp., Santa Monica, California Technical Report HS-009-2-332 (1974).

MULFORD, H. A., 1964, Drinking and deviant drinking, *Q. J. Stud. Alcohol* **25:**634–650.

MURPHREE, H. B., 1971, The importance of congeners in the effects of alcoholic beverages, in: *Biological Basis of Alcoholism* (Y. Israel and J. Mardones, eds.), pp. 209–234, Wiley-Interscience, New York.

MYERSON, R. M., 1971, Effects of alcohol on cardiac and muscular function, in: *Biological Basis of Alcoholism* (Y. Israel and J. Mardones, eds.), pp. 183–208, Wiley-Interscience, New York.

NAGARAJAN, M., GROSS, M. M., KISSIN, B., and BEST, S., 1973, Affective changes during 6 days of experimental alcoholization and subsequent withdrawal, in: *Alcohol Intoxication and Withdrawal: Experimental Studies, Advances in Experimental Medicine and Biology*, Vol. 35 (M. M. Gross, ed.), pp. 351–363, Plenum, New York.

NATHAN, P. E., and O'BRIEN, J. S., 1971, An experimental analysis of the behavior of alcoholics and nonalcoholics during prolonged experimental drinking: A necessary precursor of behavior therapy? *Behav. Ther.* **2:**455–476.

NATHAN, P. E., TITLER, N. A., LOWENSTEIN, L. M., SOLOMON, P., and ROSSI, A. M., 1970, Behavioral analysis of chronic alcoholism: Interaction of alcohol and human contact, *Arch. Gen. Psychiat.* **22:**419–430.

NATHAN, P. E., O'BRIEN, J. S., and LOWENSTEIN, L. M., 1971*a*, Operant studies of chronic alcoholism: Interaction of alcohol and alcoholics, in: *Biological Aspects of Alcohol* (M. K. Roach, W. M. McIsaac, and P. J. Creaven, eds.), pp. 341–370, Univ. of Texas, Austin.

NATHAN, P. E., O'BRIEN, J. S., and NORTON, D., 1971*b*, Comparative studies of the interpersonal and affective behavior of alcoholics and non-alcoholics during prolonged experimental drinking, in: *Recent Advances in Studies of Alcoholism* (N. K. Mello and J. H. Mendelson, eds.), pp. 619–646, U.S. Govt. Printing Office Publ. No. (HSM) 71-9045, Washington, D.C.

NATHAN, P. E., GOLDMAN, M. S., LISMAN, S. A., and TAYLOR, H. A., 1972, Alcohol and alcoholics: A behavioral approach, *Trans. N. Y. Acad. Sci.* **34:**602–627.

NATIONAL COUNCIL ON ALCOHOLISM, 1972, Criteria for the diagnosis of alcoholism, *Am. J. Psychiat.* **129:**127–135.

NEWMAN, H. W., 1941, Acquired tolerance to ethyl alcohol, *Q. J. Stud. Alcohol* **2:**453–463.

NEWMAN, H. W., and ABRAMSON, M., 1942*a*, Absorption of various alcoholic beverages, *Science* **96:**43.

NEWMAN, H. W., and ABRAMSON, M., 1942*b*, Some factors influencing the intoxicating effect of alcoholic beverages, *Q. J. Stud. Alcohol* **3:**351.

NOBLE, E. P., and TEWARI, S., 1975, Ethanol and brain ribosomes, *Fed. Proc.* **34:**1942–1947.

NOBLE, E. P., and TEWARI, S., 1977, Metabolic aspects of alcoholism in the brain, in: *Metabolic Aspects of Alcoholism* (C. S. Lieber, ed.), pp. 149–185, University Park Press, Baltimore.

NOBLE, E. P., PARKER, E., ALKANA, R., COHEN, H., and BIRCH, H., 1973, Propranolol-ethanol interaction in man, *Fed. Proc.* **32:**724.

NOBLE, E. P., ALKANA, R. L., and PARKER, E. S., 1975, Ethanol-induced CNS depression and its reversal: A review, in: *Biomedical Research in Alcohol Abuse Problems,* Conference Proceedings. Non-Medical Use of Drugs Directorate, National Health and Welfare, Canada pp. 308–367, Halifax, Nova Scotia.

NOVAK, D. J., and VICTOR, M. C., 1974, The vagus and sympathetic nerves in alcoholic polyneuropathy, *Arch. Neurol.* **30:**273–284.

OLDENDORF, W. H., 1974, Drug penetration of the blood-brain barrier, in: *Narcotics and the Hypothalamus* (E. Zimmermann and R. George, eds.), pp. 213–222, Raven Press, New York.

ORCUTT, J. D., 1975, Social determinants of alcohol and marijuana effects: A systematic theory, *Int. J. Addict.* **10:**1021–1033.

ORCUTT, J. D., and BIGGS, D. A., 1975, Recreational effects of marihuana and alcohol: Some descriptive dimensions, *Int. J. Addict.* **10:**229–239.

OVERTON, D. A., 1972, State-dependent learning produced by alcohol and its relevance to alcoholism, in: *The Biology of Alcoholism: Physiology and Behavior* (B. Kissin and H. Begleiter, eds.), Vol. 2, pp. 193–217, Plenum, New York.

PARKER, E. S., ALKANA, R. L., BIRNBAUM, I. M., HARTLEY, J. T., and NOBLE, E. P., 1974, Alcohol and disruption of cognitive processes, *Arch. Gen. Psychiat.* **31:**824–828.

PEARSON, S. B., 1813, Observations on brain fever; delirium tremens, *Edinburgh Med. Surg. J.* **9:**326–332.

Persky, H., Smith, K. D., and Basu, G. K., 1971, Relation of psychologic measures of aggression and hostility to testosterone production in man, *Psychosom. Med.* **33:**265–277.

Petersen, R. C., 1977, Retrieval failures in alcohol state dependent learning, *Psychopharmacologia (Berlin),* in press.

Pieper, W. A., Skeen, M. J., McClure, H. M., and Bourne, P. G., 1972, The chimpanzee as an animal model for investigating alcoholism, *Science* **176:**71–73.

Pirola, R. C., and Lieber, C. S., 1974, Acute and chronic pancreatitis, in: *The Biology of Alcoholism,* Vol. 3, *Clinical Pathology* (B. Kissin and H. Begleiter, eds.), pp. 359–402, Plenum, New York.

Pliner, P., and Cappell, H., 1974, Modification of affective consequences of alcohol: A comparison of social and solitary drinking, *J. Abnorm. Psychol.* **83:**418–425.

Pohorecky, L. A., 1974, Effects of ethanol on central and peripheral noradrenergic neurons, *J. Pharmacol. Exp. Ther.* **189:**380–391.

Raynes, A., Patch, V. D., and Judson, B., 1975, Polydrug abuse in Boston, in: *Developments in the Field of Drug Abuse: National Drug Abuse Conference* (E. Senay, V. Shorty, and H. Alksen, eds.), pp. 250–253, Schenkman, Cambridge, Mass.

Redos, J. D., Catravas, G. N., and Hunt, W. A., 1976, Ethanol-induced depletion of cerebellar guanosine 3,5-cyclic monophosphate, *Science* **193:**58–59.

Reed, T. K., Kalant, H., Gibbins, R. J., Kapur, B. M., and Rankin, J. G., 1976, Alcohol and acetaldehyde metabolism in Caucasians, Chinese and Amerinds, *Canad. Med. Assoc. J.* **115:**851–855.

Regan, T. J., Ettinger, P. O., Oldewurtel, H. A., and Haider, B., 1975, Heart cell responses to ethanol, *Ann. N. Y. Acad. Sci.* **252:**250–263.

Robbins, E., Murphy, G., Wilkerson, R., Gasner, S., and Kayes, J., 1959, Some clinical considerations in the prevention of suicide based on a study of 134 successful suicides, *Am. J. Public Health* **49:**888.

Robins, L. N., and Guze, S. B., 1971, Drinking practices and problems in urban ghetto populations, in: *Recent Advances in Studies of Alcoholism* (N. K. Mello and J. H. Mendelson, eds.), pp. 825–842, U.S. Govt. Printing Office Publ. No. (HSM) 71-9045, Washington, D.C.

Rorabaugh, W. J., 1976, Estimated U. S. alcoholic beverage consumption, 1790–1860, *J. Stud. Alcohol* **37:**357–364.

Rose, R. M., Haladay, J. W., and Bernstein, I. S., 1971, Plasma testosterone, dominance rank and aggressive behaviour in male rhesus monkeys, *Nature (London)* **231:**366–368.

Rose, R. M., Gordon, P. P., and Bernstein, I. S., 1972, Plasma testosterone levels in the male rhesus: Influences of sexual and social stimuli, *Science* **178:**643–645.

Rosett, H. L., Ouellette, E. M., and Weiner, L., 1976, A pilot prospective study of the fetal alcohol syndrome at the Boston City Hospital. Part I: Maternal drinking, *Ann. N. Y. Acad. Sci.* **273:**118–122.

Ross, D. H., Medina, M. A., and Cardenas, H. L., 1974, Morphine and ethanol: Selective depletion of regional brain calcium, *Science* **186:**63–65.

Roueche, B., 1960, *The Neutral Spirit: A Portrait of Alcohol,* Little, Brown, Boston.

Rubin, H. B., and Henson, D. E., 1976, Effects of alcohol on male sexual responding, *Psychopharmacologia* **47:**123–134, 1976.

Rubin, E., and Lieber, C. S., 1968*a*, Alcohol-induced hepatic injury in non-alcoholic volunteers, *N. Engl. J. Med.* **278:**869–876.

Rubin, E., and Lieber, C. S., 1968*b*, Hepatic microsomal enzymes in man and rat: Induction and inhibition by ethanol, *Science* **162:**690–691.

Rubin, E., and Lieber, C. S., 1974, Fatty liver, alcoholic hepatitis and cirrhosis produced by alcohol in primates, *N. Engl. J. Med.* **290:**128–135.

Rubin, E., , Gang, H., Misra, P., and Lieber, C. S., 1970, Inhibition of drug metabolism by acute ethanol intoxication: A hepatic microsomal mechanism, *Am. J. Med.* **49:**800–806.

Rubin, E., Altman, K., Gordon, G. G., and Southren, A. L., 1976, Prolonged ethanol consumption increases testosterone metabolism in the liver, *Science* **191:**563–564.

Rubington, E., 1968, The bottle gang, *Q. J. Stud. Alcohol* **29:**943–955.

Rundell, O. H., Lester, B. K., Griffiths, W. J., and Williams, H. L., 1972, Alcohol and sleep in young adults, *Psychopharmacologia* **26:**201–218.

Russell, J. A., and Mehrabian, A., 1975, The mediating role of emotions in alcohol use, *J. Stud. Alcohol* **36:**1508–1536.

Ryback, R. S., 1970, Alcohol amnesia: Observations on seven drinking inpatient alcoholics, *Q. J. Stud. Alcohol* **31:**616–632.

Schuckit, M., 1972, The alcoholic woman: A literature review, *Psychiat. Med.* **3:**37–43.

Schuckit, M. A., and Morrissey, E. R., 1976, Alcoholism in women: Some clinical and social perspectives, in: *Alcoholism in Women and Children* (M. Greenblatt and M. A. Schuckit, eds.), pp. 5–35, Grune & Stratton, New York.

Schuckit, M. A., Goodwin, D. A., and Winokur, G., 1972, A study of alcoholism in half siblings, *Am. J. Psychiat.* **128:**1132–1136.

Schuntich, R. J., and Taylor, S. P., 1972, The effects of alcohol on human physical aggression, *J. Exp. Res. Personal.* **6:**34–38.

Schut, J., File, K., and Wohlmuth, T., 1973, Alcohol use by narcotic addicts in methadone maintenance and treatment. *Q. J. Stud. Alcohol* **34:**1356–1359.

Seevers, M. H., and Deneau, G. A., 1963, Physiological aspects of tolerance and physical dependence, in: *Physiological Pharmacology* (W. S. Root and F. G. Hofmann, eds.), pp. 565–640, Academic Press, New York.

Seixas, F. A., and Eggleston, S., eds., 1973, *Alcoholism and the Central Nervous System, Ann. N. Y. Acad. Sci.* **215**.

Seixas, F. A., Williams, K., and Eggleston, S., eds., 1975, *Medical Consequences of Alcoholism, Ann. N. Y. Acad. Sci.* **252**.

Shuntich, R. J., and Taylor, S. P., 1972, The effects of alcohol on human physical aggression, *J. Exp. Res. Personal.* **6:**34–38.

Shupe, L. M., 1954, Alcohol and crime. A study of the urine alcohol concentration found in 882 persons arrested during or immediately after commission of a felony, *J. Criminal Law Criminol.* **44:**661.

Sidell, F. R., and Pless, J. E., 1971, Ethyl alcohol: Blood levels and performance decrements after oral administration to men, *Psychopharmacologia* **19:**246–261.

Silvestrini, R., 1926, Gynecomastia in men with cirrhosis of the liver, *La Reforma Med.* **142:**701–704.

Smiley, A., LeBlanc, A. E., French, I. W., and Burford, R., 1975, The combined effects of alcohol and common psychoactive drugs: II. Field studies with an instrumented automobile, in: *Alcohol, Drugs, and Traffic Safety* (S. Israelstam and F. Lambert, eds.), pp. 433–438, Addiction Research Foundation of Ontario, Toronto.

Smith, R. C., Parker, E. S., and Noble, E. P., 1975, Alcohol and affect in dyadic social interaction, *Psychosom. Med.* **37:**25–40.

Snyder, F., 1965, Progress in the new biology of dreaming, *Am. J. Psychiat.* **122:**377.

Southren, A. L., Tochimoto, S., Carmody, N. C., and Isurugi, K., 1965, Plasma production rates of testosterone in normal adult men and women and in patients with the syndrome of feminizing testes, *J. Clin. Endocrinol. Metab.* **25:**1441–1450.

Spodick, D. H., Pigott, V. M., and Chirife, R., 1972, Preclinical cardiac malfunction in chronic alcoholism, *N. Engl. J. Med.* **287:**677–680.

Steffen, J. J., Nathan, P. E., and Taylor, H. A., 1974, Tension-reducing effects of alcohol: Further evidence and some methodological considerations, *J. Abnorm. Psychol.* **83:**542–547.

Steinglass, P., and Weiner, S., 1971, Familial interactions and determinants of drinking behavior, in: *Recent Advances in Studies of Alcoholism* (N. K. Mello and J. H. Mendelson, eds.), pp. 687–705, U.S. Govt. Printing Office Publ. No. (HSM) 71-9045, Washington, D.C.

Steinglass, P., and Wolin, S., 1974, Explorations of a systems approach to alcoholism: Clinical observations of a simulated drinking gang, *Arch. Gen. Psychiat.* **31:**527–532.

Stone, M. L., Salerno, L. J., Green, M., and Zelson, C., 1971, Narcotic addiction in pregnancy, *Am. J. Obstet. Gynecol.* **109:**716–723.

Sutton, T., 1813, *Tracts on Delirium Tremens, on Periodonitis and Other Inflammatory Afflictions*, Thomas Underwood, London.

Talbott, G. D., 1975, Primary alcoholic heart disease, *Ann. N. Y. Acad. Sci.* **252:**235–236.

Talland, G. A., 1965, *Deranged Memory*, Academic Press, New York.

Talland, G. A., 1966, Effects of alcohol on performance in continuous attention tasks, *Psychosom. Med.* **28:**596–604.

Talland, G. A., Mendelson, J. H., and Ryack, P., 1964*a*, Experimentally induced chronic intoxication and withdrawal in alcoholics, Part 4, Tests of motor skills, *Q. J. Stud. Alcohol, Suppl.* 2, 53–73.

Talland, G. A., Mendelson, J. H., and Ryack, P., 1964*b*, Experimentally induced chronic intoxication and withdrawal in alcoholics, Part 5, Tests of attention, *Q. J. Stud. Alcohol, Suppl.* 2, 74–86.

Tamerin, J. S., and Mendelson, J. H., 1969, The psychodynamics of chronic inebriation: Observations of alcoholics during the process of drinking in an experimental group setting. *Am. J. Psychiat.* **125:**886–889.

Tamerin, J. S., Weiner, S., and Mendelson, J. H., 1970, Alcoholics' expectancies and recall of experiences during intoxication, *Am. J. Psychiat.* **126:**1697–1704.

Tamerin, J. S., Weiner, S., Poppen, R., Steinglass, P., and Mendelson, J. H., 1971, Alcohol and memory: Amnesia and short-term function during experimentally induced intoxication, *Am. J. Psychiat.* **127:**1659–1664.

Tarter, R. E., Jones, B. M., Simpson, C. D., and Vega, A., 1971, Effects of task complexity and practice on performance during acute alcohol intoxication, *Percept. Mot. Skills* **33:**307–318.

Taylor, S. P., and Gammon, C. B., 1975, Effects of type and dose of alcohol on human physical aggression, *J. Personal. Soc. Psychol.* **32:**169–175.

Taylor, S. P., Vardaris, R. M., Rawtich, A. B., Gammon, C. B., Cranston, J. W., and Lubetkin, A. I., 1976, The effects of alcohol and delta-9-tetrahydrocannabinol on human physical aggression, *Aggress. Behav.* **2:**153–161.

Tec, N., 1973, A clarification of the relationship between alcohol and marihuana, *Br. J. Addict.* **68:**191–195.

Tewari, S., and Noble, E. P., 1971, Chronic effects of ethanol on brain protein synthesis, in: *Recent Advances in Studies of Alcoholism* (N. K. Mello and J. H. Mendelson, eds.), pp. 107–122, U.S. Govt. Printing Office Publ. No. (HSM) 71-9045, Washington, D.C.

Tharp, V. K., Rundell, O. H., Lester, B. K., and Williams, H. L., 1974, Alcohol and information processing. *Psychopharmacologia (Berlin)* **40:**33–52.

The Framingham Heart Study; Habits and Coronary Heart Disease, 1966, U.S. Govt. Printing Office PHS Publ. No. 1515, U.S. National Heart Institute, Washington, D.C.

Thornton, C. C., Alterman, A. I., Skoloda, T. E., and Gottheil, E., 1976, Drinking and socializing in "introverted" and "extroverted" alcoholics, *Ann. N. Y. Acad. Sci.* **273:**481–487.

Tinklenberg, J. R., 1973, Alcohol and violence, in: *Alcoholism: Progress in Research and Treatment* (P. Bourne and R. Fox, eds.), pp. 195–210, Academic Press, New York.

Van Thiel, D. H., Lester, R., and Sherins, R. J., 1974, Hypogonadism in alcoholic liver disease: Evidence for a double defect, *Gastroenterology* **67:**1188–1199.

Victor, M., 1966, Treatment of alcoholic intoxication and the withdrawal syndrome: A critical analysis of the use of drugs and other forms of therapy, *Psychosom. Med.* **28:**636–650.

Victor, M., 1973, The role of hypomagnesemia and respiratory alkalosis in the genesis of alcohol-withdrawal symptoms, *Ann. N. Y. Acad. Sci.* **215:**235–248.

Victor, M., 1974, Neurologic changes in liver disease, in: *Brain Dysfunction in Metabolic Disorders, Res. Publ. Assoc. Nerv. Ment. Dis.* (F. Plum, ed.), pp. 1–12, Raven Press, New York.

VICTOR, M., 1975, Nutrition and diseases of the nervous system (including psychiatric disorders), *Prog. Food Nutr. Sci.* **1:**145–172.

VICTOR, M., and ADAMS, R. D., 1953, The effect of alcohol on the nervous system, *Res. Publ. Assoc. Nerv. Ment. Dis.* **32:**526–573.

VICTOR, M., TALLAND, G. A., and ADAMS, R. D., 1959, Psychological studies of Korsakoff's psychosis: I. General intellectual functions, *J. Nerv. Ment. Dis.* **128:**528–537.

VICTOR, M., ADAMS, R. D., and COLLINS, G. H., 1971, *The Wernicke–Korsakoff Syndrome. A Clinical and Pathological Study of 245 Patients, 82 with Post-mortem Examinations,* F. A. Davis, Philadelphia.

WAGMAN, A. M. I., and ALLEN, R. P., 1975, Effects of alcohol ingestion and abstinence on slow wave sleep of alcoholics, in: *Alcohol Intoxication and Withdrawal: Experimental Studies II. Advances in Experimental Medicine and Biology* (M. M. Gross, ed.), Vol. 59, pp. 453–466, Plenum, New York.

WALLER, J. A., 1972, Factors associated with alcohol and responsibility for fatal highway crashes, *Q. J. Stud. Alcohol* **33:**160–170.

WARNER, R. H., and ROSETT, H. L., 1975, The effects of drinking on offspring, an historical survey of the American and British literature, *J. Stud. Alcohol* **36:**1395–1420.

WARREN, G. H., and RAYNES, A. E., 1972, Mood changes during three conditions of alcohol intake, *Q. J. Stud. Alcohol* **33:**979–989.

WEBSTER, P. D., III, 1975, Secretory and metabolic effects of alcohol on the pancreas, *Ann. N. Y. Acad. Sci.* **252:**183–186.

WEINER, S., TAMERIN, J. S., STEINGLASS, P., and MENDELSON, J. H., 1971*b*, Familial patterns in chronic alcoholism: A study of a father and son during experimental intoxication, *Am. J. Psychiat.* **127:**1646–1651.

WEINGARTNER, H., and FAILLACE, L. A., 1971, Alcohol state dependent learning in man, *J. Nerv. Ment. Dis.* **153:**395–406.

WEINGARTNER, H., FAILLACE, L. A., and MARKLEY, H. G., 1971, Verbal information retention in alcoholics, *Q. J. Stud. Alcohol* **32:**293–303.

WIKLER, A., and RASOR, R. W., 1953, Psychiatric aspects of drug addiction, *Am. J. Med.* **14:**566–570.

WILLIAMS, A. F., 1966, Social drinking, anxiety and depression, *J. Personal. Soc. Psychol.* **3:**689–693.

WILLIAMS, H. L., and SALAMY, A., 1974, Alcohol and sleep, in: *The Biology of Alcoholism,* Vol. 2, *Physiology and Behavior* (B. Kissin and H. Begleiter, eds.), pp. 436–484, Plenum, New York.

WILSON, G. T., and LAWSON, D. M., 1976*a*, Effects of alcohol on sexual arousal in women, *J. Abnorm. Psychol.* **85**(5):489–497.

WILSON, G. T., and LAWSON, D. M., 1976*b*, Expectancies, alcohol, and sexual arousal in male social drinkers, *J. Abnorm. Psychol.* **85:**587–594.

WILSON, G. S., DESMOND, M. M., and VERINAUD, W. M., 1973, Early development of infants of heroin addicted mothers, *Am. J. Dis. Child.* **126:**457–462.

WINGER, G. D., and WOODS, J. H., 1973, The reinforcing property of ethanol in the rhesus monkey: I. Initiation, maintenance, and termination of intravenous ethanol-reinforced responding, in: *Alcoholism and the Central Nervous System* (F. A. Seixas and S. Eggleston, eds.), *Ann. N. Y. Acad. Sci.* **215:**162–175.

WOLFE, P. H., 1972, Ethnic differences in alcohol sensitivity, *Science* **175:**449–450.

WOLFGANG, M. E., 1958, *Patterns in Criminal Homicide,* Univ. of Pennsylvania Press, Philadelphia.

WOLIN, S. J., 1973, Hallucinations during experimental intoxication, in: *Alcohol Intoxication and Withdrawal: Experimental Studies:* Vol. 35, *Advances in Experimental Medicine and Biology* (M. M. Gross, ed.), pp. 305–319, Plenum, New York.

WOLIN, S. J., and MELLO, N. K., 1973, The effects of alcohol on dreams and hallucinations in alcohol addicts, in: *Alcoholism and the Central Nervous System* (F. A. Seixas and S. Eggleston, eds.), *Ann. N. Y. Acad. Sci.* **215:**266–302.

WOLIN, S. J., and STEINGLASS, P., 1974, Interactional behavior in an alcoholic community, *Med. Ann. D. C.* **43:**183–187.

WOODS, J. H., IKOMI, F. I., and WINGER, G. D., 1971, The reinforcing properties of ethanol, in: *Biological Aspects of Alcoholism* (M. K. Roach, W. N. McIsaac, and P. J. Creaven, eds.), pp. 371–388, Univ. of Texas Press, Austin.

WOODS, J. H., DOWNS, D. A., and VILLARREAL, J. E., 1973, Changes in operant behavior during deprivation- and antagonist-induced withdrawal states, in: *Bayer Symposium IV, Psychic Dependence,* pp. 114–121.

WOODS, J. H., DOWNS, D. A., and CARNEY, J., 1975, Behavioral functions of narcotic antagonists: Response-drug contingencies, *Fed. Proc.* **34:**1777–1784.

WOODY, G. E., O'BRIEN, C. P., and GREENSTEIN, R., 1975, Misuse and abuse of diazepam: An increasingly common medical problem, *Int. J. Addict.* **10:**843–848.

WORLD HEALTH ORGANIZATION, 1955, Expert Committee on Alcohol, First Report, Geneva: WHO Technical Report Series, No. 84.

YOUNGER, W., 1966, *Gods, Men and Wine,* The Wine and Foods Society, World Publ. Co., Cleveland.

YULES, R. B., FREEDMAN, D. X., and CHANDLER, K. A., 1966*a*, The effect of ethyl alcohol on man's electroencephalograph sleep cycle, *EEG Clin. Neurophysiol.* **20:**109–111.

YULES, R. B., OGDEN, J. A., GAULT, F. P., and FREEDMAN, D. X., 1966*b*, The effect of ethyl alcohol on electroencephalographic sleep cycles in cats, *Psychonomon. Sci.* **5:**97–98.

YULES, R. B., LIPPMAN, M. E., and FREEDMAN, D. X., 1967, Alcohol administration prior to sleep, the effect on EEG sleep states, *Arch. Gen. Psychiat.* **16:**94–97.

ZARCONE, V., BARCHAS, J., HODDES, E., MONTPLAISIR, J., SACK, R., and WILSON, R., 1975, Experimental ethanol ingestion: Sleep variables and metabolites of dopamine and serotonin in the cerebrospinal fluid, in: *Alcohol Intoxication and Withdrawal: Experimental Studies,* II, Vol. 59, *Advances in Experimental Medicine and Biology* (M. M. Gross, ed.), pp. 431–451, Plenum, New York.

ZEINER, A. A., PAREDES, A., and COWDEN, L., 1976, Physiologic responses to ethanol among the Tarahumara Indians, *Ann. N. Y. Acad. Sci.* **273:**151–159.

ZELSON, C., RUBIO, E., and WASSERMAN, E., 1971, Neonatal narcotic addiction: 10 year observation, *Pediatrics* **48:**178–189.

ZWERLING, I., and ROSENBAUM, M., 1959, Alcohol addiction and personality, in: *American Handbook of Psychiatry* Vol. I (S. Arieti, ed.), pp. 623–644, Basic Books, New York.

6

CANNABIS: STRUCTURE–ACTIVITY RELATIONSHIPS

R. Duane Sofia

1. INTRODUCTION

Cannabis sativa or marihuana most likely is one of man's oldest and most widely used drugs (Mikuriya, 1969). The earliest record of its use and description was in China in 2737 B.C. Its use as an intoxicant spread to India and North Africa and from there to Europe, probably as a result of the expedition of Napoleon during his Egyptian campaign around 1800. In the Western Hemisphere marihuana has been known for centuries in South and Central America, but it was not used in the United States to any significant degree until the early 1900s.

Throughout its journeyman history the main interest in marihuana has been in its euphoria-inducing or intoxicating properties. To achieve this state marihuana has been eaten, prepared as a "tea" and drunk (Segelman *et al.*, 1974), sniffed, and more prevalently smoked as long as medical history has been recorded, and it is currently used by millions of people throughout the world (Grinspoon, 1971). In addition, cannabis was a very valuable medicine to physicians throughout the world (Mikuriya, 1969) and was available in the United States in 28 various "over-the-counter" and ethical pharmaceuticals (Sasman, 1938) used for a variety of maladies including pain relief, epilepsy, asthma, cough, insomnia, and melancholia.

At present marihuana is an illegal substance in the United States according to the Federal Marihuana Tax Act of 1937, which prohibits its

R. Duane Sofia • Biological Research, Wallace Laboratories, Cranbury, New Jersey 08512.

cultivation, possession, distribution, and use. Passage of this legislation and the subsequent removal of marihuana from the U.S. Pharmacopeia list of therapeutic substances in 1942 (Zunin, 1969) sharply reduced research into the chemistry and pharmacology as well as clinical utility of this plant.

2. NATURALLY OCCURRING CANNABINOIDS

2.1. Chemistry

As Mechoulam (1973) points out, however, although the amount of research conducted in cannabinoid chemistry during these years was limited to a few investigators, many important achievements were realized culminating in the isolation, structural elucidation, and partial synthesis of a pure crystalline cannabinoid substance from the plant material (Gaoni and Mechoulam, 1964) from which tetrahydrocannabinol or THC was obtained. The structural formulas and two numbering systems used to describe the tetrahydrocannabinols are shown below. The formal numbering system

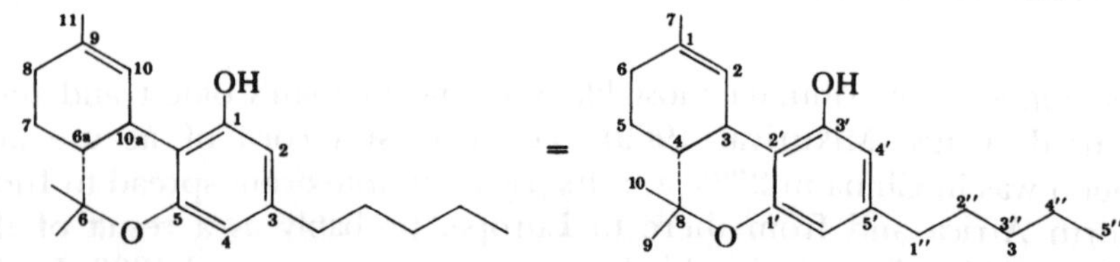

adopted by the American Chemical Society is the standard arrangement for pyran-type compounds and will be used throughout this chapter. However, for cannabinoids that are not pyrans this numbering system technically should not be used. The system preferred by Mechoulam (1970) assumes the cannabinoids are substituted monoterpenoids, which has the advantage that one particular carbon atom in a given molecule retains the same number in any chemical or metabolic transformation.

Since 1964 several naturally occurring cannabinoids have been isolated from marihuana (Gaoni and Mechoulam, 1971; Vree *et al.*, 1972; de Zeeuw *et al.*, 1972; Fetterman and Turner, 1972; de Zeeuw *et al.*, 1973), the structures for which are shown in Fig. 1.

The major pharmacologically active constituent of marihuana, which has been shown to mimic completely the activity of crude marihuana both in animals and in man, is Δ^9-THC (Mechoulam, 1973; Paton, 1975). Yields from both extraction of THC from plant material as well as its total synthesis were low, costly, and time consuming. However, synthetic processes for several of these naturally occurring cannabinoids have been scaled up, which has resulted in yields of large quantities (Petrzilka and Sikemeier, 1967), thereby spawning research interests once again.

Table 1

Metabolites of Naturally Occurring Cannabinoids

Cannabinoid	Metabolite	Species	Reference
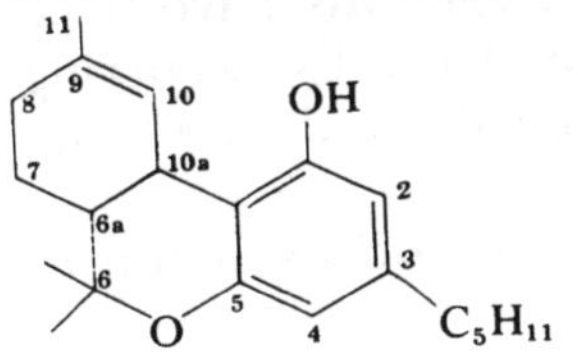	11-OH	Rabbit	Nilsson *et al.* (1970)
		Rat	Wall (1971)
			Burstein and Kupfer (1971)
		Mouse	Christensen *et al.* (1971)
		Monkey	Ho *et al.* (1972*b*)
		Man	Lemberger *et al.* (1970)
	8-OH(α or β)	Rabbit	Wall (1971)
Δ^9-THC	8α,11-$(OH)_2$	Rat	Wall (1971)
	8β,11-$(OH)_2$		Wall (1971)
		Mouse	Ho *et al.* (1972*b*)
		Monkey	Christensen *et al.* (1971)
	11-COOH,1″-OH	Rabbit	Burstein *et al.* (1972)
	11-COOH,2″-OH		
	1,11-Diacetyl	Rat	Mikes *et al.* (1971)
	8-Keto	Monkey	Gurny *et al.* (1972)
	9,10-Epoxide		
	11,3″-$(COOH)_2$	Rat	Nordqvist *et al.* (1974)
	3″-OH	Dog	Nordqvist and Widman (1975)
	4″-OH		
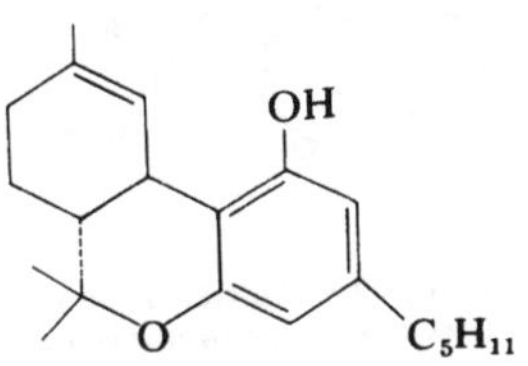	11-OH	Rabbit	Burstein *et al.* (1970)
		Rat	Foltz *et al.* (1970)
		Mouse	Christensen *et al.* (1971)
		Monkey	Ho *et al.* (1972*b*)
	7α,11-$(OH)_2$	Rat	Wall (1971)
	7β,11-$(OH)_2$		
	1″-OH	Dog	Maynard *et al.* (1971)
	3″-OH		
Δ^8-THC	7-OH(α or β)	Monkey	Gurny *et al.* (1972)
	7-Keto		
	1-O-CH_3-11-OH	Rat	Estevez *et al.* (1973)
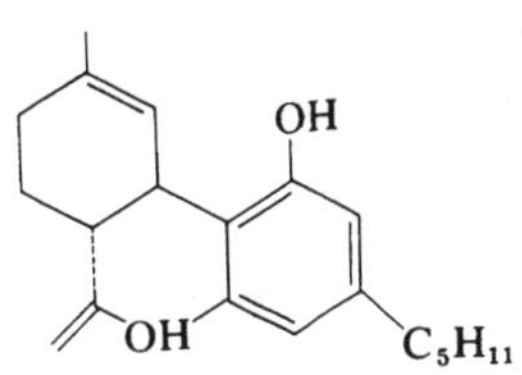	11-OH	Rat	Nilsson *et al.* (1973*b*)
		Man	Wall *et al.* (1975)
	3″-OH	Rat	Nilsson *et al.* (1973*b*)
CBD			
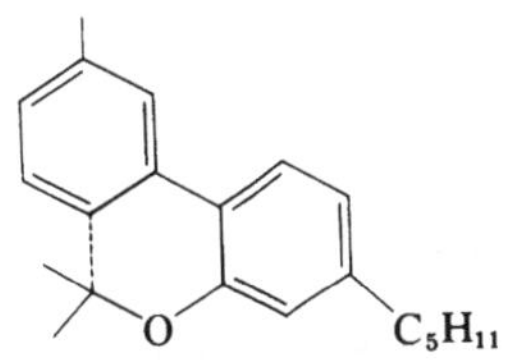	11-OH	Rat	Widman *et al.* (1971)
		Man	Wall *et al.* (1975)
	2′-OH		
	3′-OH	Rat	Widman *et al.* (1971)
	4′-OH	Rabbit	Burstein and Varanelli (1975)
	5′-OH	Mouse	
CBN			

2.2. Metabolism

Table 1 reveals that an extensive number of investigations have been conducted to determine the metabolic fate of various naturally occurring cannabinoids. The primary metabolites of each cannabinoid are their 11-OH derivatives.

King and Forney (1967) have studied the absorption and excretion of

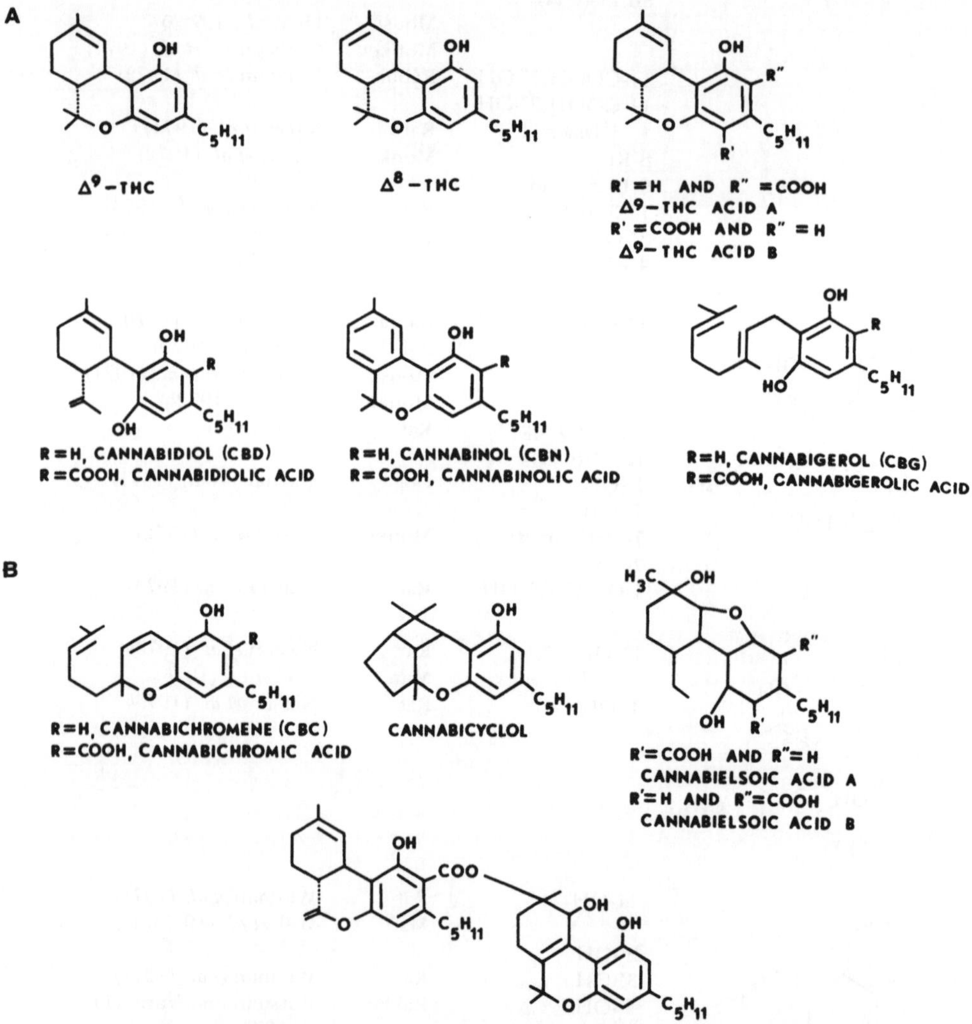

FIG. 1. Structure of naturally occurring cannabinoids isolated from marihuana. (A) Cannabinoids with a pentyl side chain. (B) Cannabitriol ester of cannabidiolic acid. (C) Cannabinoids with a propyl side chain. (D) Cannabinoids with a methyl side chain.

THC and CBN in rats after oral or intraperitoneal administration. Their results led them to conclude that each of these substances are largely absorbed from the gastrointestinal tract and that biliary excretion was important in their elimination. More recently, Widman *et al.* (1971 and 1974*b*) and Siemens and Kalant (1975) have confirmed that the bile is the major route of elimination in the rat for Δ⁹-THC since 60 to 70% of the dose was eliminated within 3 to 6 hr as unchanged drug or highly polar metabolites. Similar findings have been reported for both Δ⁸- and Δ⁹-THC in the monkey (Just *et al.*, 1975).

Klausner and Dingell (1971) have also demonstrated that Δ⁹-THC is eliminated by rats in a biplasic manner. During the first 2-hr period immediately after administration of [^{14}C]Δ⁹-THC, total body radioactivity declined very rapidly with a half-life of 0.5 hr. Over the next 50 hr total body ^{14}C declined much more slowly with a calculated $t_{1/2}$ of 21 hr. These data confirm similar findings in rat (Agurell *et al.*, 1969), mouse (Ryrfeldt and Ramsay, 1973), and man (Christiansen and Rafaelsen, 1969; Lemberger *et al.*, 1970). Metabolism of CBD and 11-OH-Δ⁹-THC also follow this same

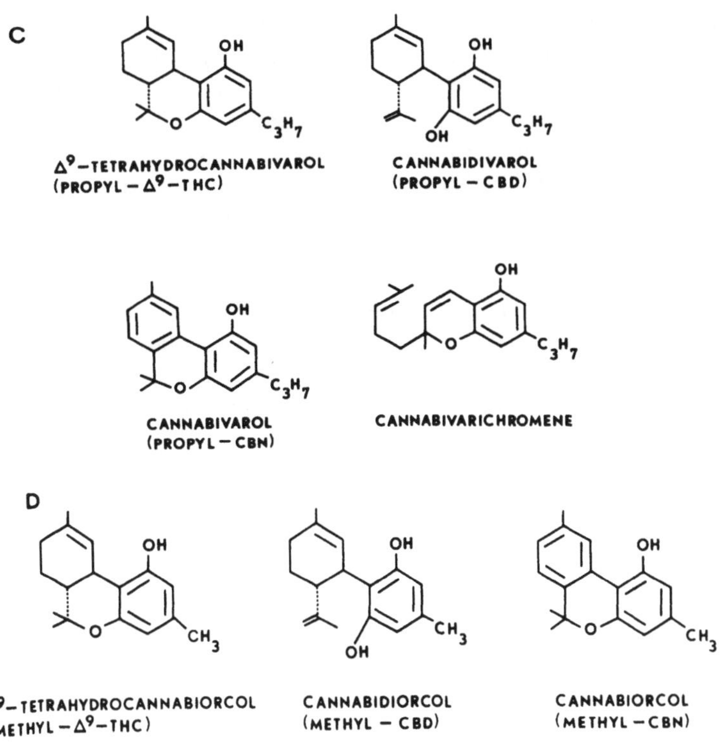

FIG. 1. *(continued)*

pattern (Lemberger *et al.*, 1972, 1973; Nilsson *et al.*, 1973*a,b*). Klausner and Dingell (1971) suggested that two pools of THC are formed after dosing, with the first being readily available for metabolism, while the more slowly metabolized THC might exist in a pool whose availability is decreased because of distribution into more slowly perfused tissues such as adipose and brain (Ho *et al.*, 1970, 1973*a*; Kreuz and Axelrod, 1973) or intracellular and plasma protein binding (Wahlqvist *et al.*, 1970; Klausner *et al.*, 1971 and 1975; Widman *et al.*, 1973, 1974*a*).

Comparative studies to determine blood levels of Δ^9-THC and its metabolites in tolerant and nontolerant rats (Ho *et al.*, 1973*b*; Siemens and Kalant, 1974) and pigeons (McMillan *et al.*, 1973) revealed no significant differences. Hence, tolerance development to specific effects of THC does not appear to be metabolic in origin.

Several investigators (Mechoulam, 1970; Foltz *et al.*, 1970; Christensen *et al.*, 1971; Truitt, 1971; Gill *et al.*, 1973; Lemberger *et al.*, 1972) have shown that the major metabolic product of Δ^9-THC, i.e., 11-OH-Δ^9-THC, is responsible for the pharmacological activity of the parent compound when administered systemically. Their conclusions are based on the rapid conversion of Δ^9-THC to its 11-OH derivative and direct administration of the metabolite itself. On the other hand, administration of the metabolic inhibitors SKF 525-A or chloramphenicol (Sofia and Barry, 1970, 1972; Adams and Sofia, 1973; Sofia, 1974) significantly enhanced the depressant and lethal effects of Δ^9-THC in mice and rats, which would suggest the unchanged drug to be more active. Subsequent to this it has been demonstrated both *in vitro* (Burstein and Kupfer, 1971; Dingell *et al.*, 1973) and *in vivo* (Gill and Jones, 1972; Estevez *et al.*, 1974; Siemens *et al.*, 1975) that SKF 525-A does indeed inhibit THC metabolism significantly. Hence, with all these data the only conclusion that can be drawn at this time is that THC is at least as effective as its primary metabolite.

Finally, several studies have been reported on the distribution of Δ^8- or Δ^9-THC in rabbit (Agurell *et al.*, 1970), mouse (Ryrfeldt and Ramsay, 1973), monkey (Just *et al.*, 1975), and rat (Ho *et al.*, 1970; Klausner and Dingell, 1971; Willinsky *et al.*, 1974). All are in good agreement, demonstrating that within 2 hr of administration of radiolabeled THC, elimination of metabolites via the kidney and feces is reflected by large amounts of radioactivity in these tissues as well as in the liver, spleen, gastrointestinal tract, adrenals, fat, and lungs. However, the brain and spinal cord exhibited the lowest level of radioactivity of all tissues. Despite these very low concentrations the drug does persist in the brain for several days, largely in the form of metabolites (Ho *et al.*, 1972*a*). This low level of activity is surprising since THC is a very lypophilic substance, a physiochemical property promoting passage through the blood-brain barrier. Furthermore, higher concentrations in the central nervous system might be expected since the drug has prominent effects on functions of central origin.

2.3. Pharmacology

The pharmacology of marihuana and its constituents, especially Δ^9-THC, has been the subject of many recent review articles and books (Paton and Crown, 1972; Mechoulam, 1973; Nahas, 1973; Truitt and Braude, 1974; Paton, 1975). Hence, this section will deal with only more recent studies in which various naturally occurring cannabinoids were studied.

2.3.1. *Effects on Behavior*

The effects of cannabis and its derivatives on the central nervous system are manifested by marked behavioral changes in animals. The general pattern appears to be a mixture of depressant and stimulatory effects. Barry and Kubena (1969), for instance, have shown that a 2.0 mg/kg dose of Δ^9-THC produced an initial increase in spontaneous locomotor activity followed by marked depression. Similarly, Garriott *et al.* (1967) reported that analogs of CBN and Δ^9-THC suppressed spontaneous locomotor activity during the first half hour after administration, while the latter increased activity prior to its depressant action. Similarly, Δ^8-, Δ^9-, and their 11-OH metabolite have also been shown to produce an initial period of hyperactivity followed by depression when administered to both mice and rats (Holtzman *et al.*, 1969; Christensen *et al.*, 1971; Truitt, 1971; Brown, 1972). Similarly, Moreton and Davis (1970) studied the effect of daily intraperitoneal administration of 25.0 mg/kg of Δ^9-THC on spontaneous locomotor activity in mice. On the first day, a biphasic response of stimulation during the 1st hour and depression during the 2nd hour after dosing was reported. By the 4th day tolerance to the stimulant action had developed, whereas the depressant component persisted for 11 days. Finally, the antiaggressive activity of Δ^9-THC was comprehensively studied by Dubinsky *et al.* (1973). These investigators confirmed earlier reports that intraperitoneal administration of Δ^9-THC markedly inhibits isolation-induced aggression in mice (ED_{50} = 4.0 mg/kg), electroshock-induced fighting in mice (ED_{50} = 22.0 mg/kg) and rats (ED_{50} = 14.9 mg/kg), and mouse-killing behavior of rats (ED_{50} = 4.9 mg/kg). Interestingly, the increased excitability and aggressivity in rats induced by bilateral septal lesions was potentiated 1 hr after doses of 10.0 to 40.0 mg/kg of Δ^9-THC, but significantly attenuated 3 hr after doses of 20.0 to 80.0 mg/kg, thus confirming the mixed stimulant and depressant action of the drug. Recently, ten Ham and de Jong (1975) reported that doses of CBD as high as 40.0 mg/kg had no effect on isolation-induced aggression in mice. Mice made aggressive by isolation (ten Ham and van Noordwijk, 1973; ten Ham and de Jong, 1974) and naturally aggressive Chinese hamsters (ten Ham and van Noordwijk, 1973) were significantly inhibited by Δ^9-THC in an intraperitoneal dose range of 25.0 to 50.0 mg/kg compared with 5.0 and 10.0 mg/kg of Δ^9-THC. Moreover, these investigators reported a lack of tolerance to this effect after 30 daily administrations.

When administered to Rhesus and squirrel monkeys (Scheckel *et al.*, 1968) both Δ^8- and Δ^9-THC caused marked alterations in their behavior. Using a conditioned avoidance procedure (lever pressing to delay electric shocks to their feet), the response rate was reduced 50% after intraperitoneal doses of 4.0 or 8.0 mg/kg of Δ^9- but not Δ^8-THC. However, as the dose of each cannabinoid was increased to 16.0, 32.0, or 64.0 mg/kg, a stimulant effect was observed, i.e., it increased the lever pressing rate to approximately twice the control rate. A biphasic gross behavioral pattern similar to that observed on operant behavior was observed in squirrel monkeys after Δ^9-THC administration. Harris *et al.* (1972) have shown that by the fifth intravenous dose of 2.0 mg/kg of Δ^9-THC a 60% attenuation of the initial effect on avoidance responding and general behavior in Rhesus monkeys had developed and persisted over a 30-day dosing period.

More recently, Ferraro and Billings (1972) and Ferraro *et al.* (1972) reported that Δ^9-THC or equivalent amounts administered as a marihuana extract distillate produce quite similar dose-related behavioral changes in the chimpanzee under operant reinforcement. Moreover, decrements in temporal, visual, and auditory discrimination performances (Elsmore, 1972) as well as timing (Conrad *et al.*, 1972) were observed in both the chimpanzee and Rhesus monkey following oral administration of doses ranging from 0.125 to 16.0 mg/kg.

Grunfeld and Edery (1969) reported that after intraperitoneal administration of 20.0 mg/kg of either Δ^8- or Δ^9-THC conditioned avoidance responding (CAR) in a shuttle box by rats was equally depressed, while the unconditioned response appeared unaltered. On the other hand, Karniol and Carlini (1973*a*) have shown that in the rope climbing test, another CAR procedure, the conditioned response was more significantly depressed by Δ^9-THC (ED_{50} = 10.0 mg/kg) than Δ^8-THC (ED_{50} = 22.0 mg/kg). Likewise, the presence of Δ^9-THC during acquisition and extinction of a variable interval schedule behavior by rats caused suppression in a dose-related fashion over a range of 0 to 8.0 mg/kg (Ferraro *et al.*, 1974). Recently, Karniol *et al.* (1974) have confirmed that Δ^9-THC (1.25 to 5.0 mg/kg) caused a dose-dependent depression of fixed-interval response rate in rats after reinforcement. In addition, CBN was approximately one-eighth as potent as Δ^9-THC (10.0 versus 1.25 mg/kg) in this respect, which for the first time suggests that the former substance has biological activity. Moreover, when the two cannabinoids were combined, CBN clearly potentiated the depressant effects of Δ^9-THC. Similarly, Davis and Borgen (1974) have shown for the first time that an intraperitoneal dose of 25.0 mg/kg of CBD produced decreases in response rate by rats on variable-interval and fixed-interval schedules of food-reinforced operant behavior that received 1.0 and 3.0 mg/kg of Δ^9-THC. However, higher doses of CBD (50.0 and 100.0 mg/kg) reduced the response rate of rats in a dose-related manner. This is in contrast to the potentiating effect of CBD (10.0 and 40.0 mg/kg) on impairment of Δ^9-THC-treated rats (10.0 mg/kg) on rope climbing performance. Finally, preliminary studies reported by Borgen and Shumway (1974) have shown that Δ^9-THC, CBN, and CBD all significantly altered timing behavior in the rat. Furthermore, Corcoran *et al.* (1974) reported that intraperitoneal doses of 30.0 mg/kg of CBD, CBC, and CBG to rats caused symptoms similar to those observed after 5.0 mg/kg of Δ^8- or Δ^9-THC, including hypoactivity, abnormal stance, and hyperreactivity to noise or movement.

Suppression of conditioned avoidance responding (Delini-Stula, 1973) and schedule-controlled temporally spaced responding (Frankenheim, 1974) in rats by Δ^8-THC definitely points out the similar depressant properties of this substance to Δ^9-THC. Moreover, these same authors have also confirmed the rapid tolerance development (after two doses) to Δ^8-THC that has been reported for Δ^9-THC (Black *et al.*, 1970; Barry and Kubena, 1971).

Kubena and Barry (1972) have demonstrated that Δ^9-THC possesses distinctive stimulus characteristics that enable animals to learn differential responses based solely on whether they are under the influence of the drug or vehicle. Table 1 shows the results in animals trained to respond after 4.0 mg/kg injection of Δ^9-THC or the vehicle condition. When other pharmacological agents, including tranquilizers, sedative–hypnotics, stimulants, and CBN or CBD were given in place of Δ^9-THC the animals made the nondrug response. This state-dependent learning in the rat under the influence of Δ^9-THC has been corroborated by Jarbe and Henriksson (1973, 1974). The lack of generalization to Δ^9-THC was extended to several other drugs, but appeared to be interchangeable with Δ^8-THC. Hence, these authors conclude that this unique effect of marihuana and its major psychoactive constituents, Δ^8- and Δ^9-THC, of inducing state-dependent learning, for the first time, offers a means to characterize other substances with marihuana-like activity.

Frankenheim *et al.* (1971) have shown that both Δ^9-THC (0.3 to 3.0 mg/kg) and Δ^8-THC (3.0 to 10.0 mg/kg) cause significant and dose-dependent reduction in rates of key pecking by pigeons under a multiple fixed-ratio, fixed-interval (FR–FI) schedule of food presentation. Moreover, using a schedule that required the spacings of pecks 20 to 24 sec apart these substances decreased the ratio and disrupted the timing response. Intramuscular doses of CBN up to 180.0 mg/kg had no effect on these birds. Using similar methodology, McMillan *et al.* (1972) demonstrated in pigeons that tolerance develops rapidly to the effects of both THCs and that cross-tolerance between the two substances also develops. The effects of Δ^9-THC and 11-OH-Δ^9-THC following intravenous administration of 0.03 to 0.3 mg/kg to pigeons produced remarkably similar depressant effects on the rate of key pecking by pigeons in terms of degree and duration of action (Kosersky *et al.*, 1974). Moreover, tolerance developed within 8 days of repeated injection of 0.3 mg/kg of either substance and reciprocal cross-tolerance was also demonstrated between Δ^9-THC and its 11-OH metabolite.

2.3.2. Effects on Food Consumption

The evidence appears to be incomplete and conflicting concerning the effects of Δ^9-THC on food consumption by laboratory animals. In rats (Boyd *et al.*, 1963), monkeys (Scheckel *et al.*, 1968), and pigeons (McMillan *et al.*, 1970) the effect of Δ^9-THC on a food-rewarded task could not be distinguished from its effect on the consummatory response. More recently, Glick and Milloy (1972) have shown that food intake by rats increased following a 1.0 mg/kg dose of Δ^9-THC but decreased after 2.0 mg/kg. However, a great deal of evidence supports an anorexigenic action for Δ^9-THC (Borgen *et al.*, 1971; Manning *et al.*, 1971; Elsmore and Fletcher, 1972; Phillips *et al.*, 1972; Jarbe and Henriksson, 1973; Sjoden *et al.*, 1973) when given to laboratory animals acutely or daily for periods of up to 30 days in doses ranging from 4.0 to 200.0 mg/kg. Sofia and Barry (1974) directly compared the anorexic effects of Δ^9-THC and *d*-amphetamine SO_4 (*d*-AMP) in rats that had access to food for a 6-hr period each day. Table 2 reveals that following a single intraperitoneal dose both Δ^9-THC and *d*-AMP produced marked anorexic action over the feeding period, each in a dose-related manner, with *d*-AMP being approximately twice as potent. Moreover, rats treated with either the 2.5 or 5.0 mg/kg doses of Δ^9-THC still displayed significant anorexia 24 hr after dosing. Unlike Δ^9-THC, *d*-amphetamine-treated rats reliably increased their food intake, indicating a compensatory response. More recently, Sofia and Knobloch (1976) have demonstrated a potent general anorexic effect for CBN and CBD, each of which was approximately one-tenth as potent as Δ^9-THC. However, it was observed that unlike *d*-AMP, a preference for "sweet calories" (various concentrations of sucrose solutions) occurred during the overall anorexia induced by each of these cannabinoids, thus simulating what has been reported for humans following marihuana smoking (Allentuck and

TABLE 2

The Effect of Acute Doses of Δ^9-THC and d-AMP on Food Intake 0–6 and 24–30 Hours Postinjection

Treatment and intraperitoneal dose (mg/kg)	Change in food intake (mean ± SE in grams for 26 rats): Acute drug effect (day 2–day 1)	Carry-over effect (day 3–day 1)
Propylene glycol	−1.47 ± 0.29[b]	−0.48 ± 0.54
Δ^9-THC: 2.5 mg/kg	−6.32 ± 0.81[b]	−3.92 ± 0.65[b]
5.0 mg/kg	−10.89 ± 0.81[b]	−8.25 ± 1.54[b]
Distilled water	−1.34 ± 0.33[b]	−0.08 ± 0.43
d-AMP: 1.25 mg/kg	−4.31 ± 0.55[b]	3.00 ± 0.71[b]
2.5 mg/kg	−6.77 ± 0.60[b]	−1.20 ± 0.51[c]

[a] From Sofia and Barry, 1974.
[b] $p < 0.001$ when compared with predrug food intake.
[c] $p < 0.05$ when compared with predrug food intake.

Bowman, 1942; Ames, 1958; Abel, 1971) or oral consumption of Δ^9-THC (Hollister, 1971). Finally, Rating *et al.* (1972) reported a 50% reduction in food intake induced by a single intraperitoneal dose of 10.0 mg/kg of Δ^8-THC that persisted and gradually returned to predrug control levels following seven daily doses.

2.3.3. *Neuropharmacological Effects*

Bicher and Mechoulam (1968) reported that Δ^8- and Δ^9-THC in rabbits after an intravenous dose of 8.0 mg/kg caused increased motor activity and restlessness, accompanied by EEG alterations such as increased excitability of cortical neurons and midbrain structures as manifested by a lowering of the arousal response threshold and accentuation of the cortical beta rhythm. Likewise, Lipparini *et al.* (1969) reported that Δ^8-, Δ^9-THC, and CBD each induced a flattening of the EEG tracing, disrupting hippocampal theta rhythm, and gave rise to trains of high-voltage spikes and waves in the rabbit and rat after intravenous doses of 0.5 to 10.0 mg/kg. In addition, CBD also caused EEG synchronization. Willinsky *et al.* (1973) have confirmed these data and have also shown similar theta disruption, occurrence of neocortical spikes and waves, and inhibition of arousal in the rabbit for 1.0 mg/kg of 11-OH-Δ^8-THC and, to a lesser extent, after 30.0 mg/kg of CBN. Similarly, Segal (1974) reported that intracerebral implants in the rabbit brain of Δ^8- and Δ^9-THC, CBD, and 11-OH-Δ^8-THC induced voltage and frequency changes in the motor cortex or caudate nucleus when implanted into the dorsal or ventral hippocampus. Approximately 20.0 to 45.0 μg of either Δ^8- or Δ^9-THC produced equipotent effects, depending on the site of implant, where only 14 μg of 11-OH-Δ^8-THC were required to produce similar EEG changes. On the other hand, four times as much CBD (150.0 to 300.0 μg) was required for a similar degree of activity.

Moreton and Davis (1970) have shown that rats that were chronically implanted with electrodes in the frontal cortex, dorsal hippocampus, and neck muscles exhibited a marked diminution in the level of paradoxical and slow-wave sleep after a single intraperitoneal 10.0 mg/kg injection of Δ^9-THC, with tolerance to this action developing after the second dose. Moreover, rats that had been deprived of paradoxical sleep for 3 days and given the same dose of Δ^9-THC demonstrated inhibition of paradoxical sleep rebound. Further studies by Masur and Khazan (1970) reveal that after acute or chronic dosing, Δ^8- and Δ^9-THC both induced large spike discharges in both the REM sleep and awake states.

In the conscious cat, Lipparini *et al.* (1969) reported only a moderate synchronization of the EEG after a dose of 6.0 mg/kg ip, which was easily disturbed by external stimuli. Dose-dependent (0.5 to 4.0 mg/kg) hypersynchronism in the cat following intraperitoneal administration of Δ^9-THC was observed by Hockman *et al.* (1971), which was followed by high-voltage activity and high-amplitude spindles from the hippocampus, amygdal, and hypothalamus. On the other hand, Δ^8-THC induced polyphasic spiking and changes in the paradoxical sleep pattern of the cat with a trend toward lesser but longer episodes of paradoxical sleep after initially suppressing it (Wallach and Gershon, 1973). However, the investigators did not observe hyper- or desynchrony of the EEG at the doses of Δ^8-THC studied (1.0 mg/kg iv and 10.0 mg/kg ip). Finally, Segal and Kenney (1972) reported in the cat that Δ^9-THC causes activation of the EEG, whereas Δ^8-THC produces EEG depression.

Sampaio *et al.* (1967) clearly demonstrated that 0.5 mg/kg of Δ^9-THC given intravenously to the anesthetized dog markedly abolishes the linguomandibular reflex (polysynaptic) following electrical stimulation of the central end of the lingual nerve. This datum suggests that the trigeminal system might be involved in the action of Δ^9-THC. Lapa *et al.* (1968) tested the effects of Δ^9-THC on polysynaptic reflexes by recording potentials from either the superior sensory nucleus of the trigeminal nerve or the nerve itself as it enters the pons of the cat, by electrical stimulation of the lower eyelid causing a moderate contraction of the orbiculous muscle. They reported that a decrease in the amplitude of both pre- and postsynaptic potentials occurred after intravenous doses of 1.0 mg/kg. The most pronounced effect following Δ^9-THC administration appeared to be an impairment of impulse conduction along the presynaptic fibers instead of a central synaptic blockade. However, the investigators pointed out that blockade of synaptic transmission in other central areas may account for other neural effects of Δ^9-THC. More recently, Byck and Ritchie (1973) demonstrated that Δ^9-THC as well as its 11-OH metabolite inhibited the size of the compound action potential of the isolated nonmyelinated fibers of the vagus nerve of the rabbit in a dose-related and chloride-dependent manner. In cats, intravenous administration of Δ^9-THC (0.3 to 10.0 mg/kg) selectively inhibited evoked potentials from preganglionic splanchnic but not cervical sympathetic nerves in response to hypothalamic stimulation (Sigg *et al.*, 1973). Finally, a recent report by Kayaalp (1974) revealed that Δ^9-THC appears to block nerve conduction by interfering with the depolarization of motor nerve fibers and the terminals, i.e., the neuromuscular junction.

2.3.4. *Effects on Body Temperature*

Marked reductions in body temperature have been observed after single intraperitoneal or subcutaneous doses of Δ^8- or Δ^9-THC in the range of 5.0 to 200.0 mg/kg given to mice or rats (Holtzman *et al.*, 1969; Lomax, 1971; Rating *et al.*, 1972). Lomax (1971) demonstrated a dose-related hypothermia in rats with acute tolerance development after the second 10.0 mg/kg (ip) dose of Δ^9-THC. However, when the dose was elevated to 20.0 mg/kg the tolerance was overcome even after 15 daily injections. Paradoxically, after the sixth 20.0 mg/kg dose of Δ^9-THC there was a persistent hyperthermia. Hence, the speculation was raised that Δ^9-THC might possess a dual effect on thermoregulatory mechanisms in the cat with hypothermia being the predominant response. When tolerance develops to this activity of Δ^9-THC, the hyperthermic effect is unmasked. A dual effect on body temperature is consistent with the observation made by Kubena (1970) of a hyperthermic effect in rats following acute doses of Δ^9-THC. This dose-dependent bidirectional action of Δ^9-THC on body temperature in the rat has been corroborated by Sofia (1972). Low doses in the range studied (0.125 to 8.0 and 1.25 to 80.0 mg/kg, ip and oral, respectively) produced a persistent hyperthermic effect, while higher doses caused profound body temperature reductions.

More recently, Haavik and Hardman (1973*a*,*b*) and Liu (1974) have demonstrated a dose-related hypothermia not only for Δ^9-THC, but also for Δ^8-THC and their 11-OH derivatives following intravenous administration to either mice or monkeys. In general, the magnitude of effect for the parent substances was somewhat greater and persisted for a longer period of time when compared with their metabolites.

2.3.5. *Anticonvulsant Activity*

The anticonvulsant effects of parenterally or orally administered Δ^9-THC have been established by several investigators using a variety of models of experimentally induced seizures in various species of laboratory animals following acute dosing. Karler *et al.* (1974*a*) and Sofia *et al.* (1976) demonstrated protection against electroshock-induced seizures, while Boggan *et al.* (1973) were able to show a reduction in audiogenic seizure susceptibility in mice. Similarly, Δ^9-THC has also been shown to be highly effective against these types of seizures in the rat (Consroe and Man, 1973; Consroe *et al.*, 1973; McCaughran *et al.*, 1974) as well as against seizure activity evoked by electrical stimulation of the rat amygdala (Corcoran *et al.*, 1973). Small parenteral doses of Δ^9-THC (5.0 to 160.0 μg/kg) protected the baboon against photomyoclonic seizures (Killam and Killam, 1972), while ten Ham *et al.* (1975) reported an anticonvulsant effect for Δ^9-THC in gerbils that exhibit spontaneous epileptiform seizures. On the other hand, near toxic doses of Δ^9-THC had minimal or no protective effect against pentylenetetrazol-, strychnine-, or nicotine-induced seizures in mice or rats (Sofia *et al.*, 1975*a*; Consroe and Man, 1973; McCaughran *et al.*, 1974; Chesher and Jackson, 1974). In fact, Sofia *et al.* (1976) have shown an enhancement of the lethal and convulsant activity of pentylenetetrazol after Δ^9-THC and diphenylhydantoin. This pattern of activity displayed by Δ^9-THC, i.e., protection against electroshock-induced seizures and inactivity against chemically induced seizures closely parallels that reported for diphenylhydantoin. Finally, Karler *et al.* (1974*b*) and ten Ham *et al.* (1975) have reported that like so many other effects of Δ^9-THC, tolerance develops quite rapidly to its anticonvulsant activity at least in mice and gerbils, i.e., after three to six daily doses, respectively.

Other naturally occurring cannabinoids have been reported to show significant anticonvulsant activity in laboratory animals (Table 3). These data reveal that in general, Δ^8- and Δ^9-THC were equally effective anticonvulsant agents in both mice and rats. However, the 11-OH metabolite of Δ^9-THC was markedly more potent than the parent compound. On the other hand, CBD and CBN were less effective inhibitors of electroshock-induced convulsions. Finally, Consroe and Man (1973) also have shown that Δ^8- and Δ^9-THC were similar in potency for inhibiting audiogenic seizures in the rat, with ED_{50} values of 4.7 and 3.3 mg/kg, respectively.

2.3.6. *Analgesic Activity*

The analgesic activity of Δ^9-THC has been firmly established using a number of tests such as tail-flick, hot-plate, paw-pressure, and writhing tests in a variety of laboratory animals including the mouse, rat, rabbit, cat, dog, and monkey (Bicher and Mechoulam, 1968; Scheckel *et al.*, 1968; Kaymakcalan and Deneau, 1971; Dewey *et al.*, 1972; Buxbaum, 1972; Sofia *et al.*, 1973, 1975; Chesher *et al.*, 1973; Kaymakcalan *et al.*, 1974). Table 4 lists comparative oral ED_{50} values for Δ^9-THC, CBD, CBN, morphine SO_4, and aspirin using some of the above-mentioned tests. In general, Sofia *et al.* (1975) suggest that Δ^9-THC and morphine are equipotent in all tests. CBN, similar to aspirin, only significantly reduced the writhing syndrome in mice induced

TABLE 3

Anticonvulsant Activity of Various Cannabinoids in Electroshock-Induced Seizures

Test drug	Species	ED_{50}, mg/kg (±95% confidence limits)	Reference
Δ^9-THC	Mouse	54.5(35.4–84.1)	Sofia *et al.* (1976)
	Mouse	80.0(64.0–100.0)	Karler *et al.* (1973)
	Rat	58.0(36.2–92.8)	McCaughran *et al.* (1974)
	Rat	4.3(3.9–4.8)	Karler *et al.* (1974*c*)
	Rat[a]	4.2(2.2–7.8)	Consroe and Man (1973)
11-OH-Δ^9-THC	Mouse	14.0(11.0–16.0)	Karler *et al.* (1974*c*)
	Rat	3.4(2.5–4.7)	Karler *et al.* (1974*c*)
Δ^9-THC	Mouse	83.0(61.0–113.0)	Karler *et al.* (1974*c*)
	Mouse		Chesher and Jackson (1974)
	Rat	72.0(48.0–108.0)	McCaughran *et al.* (1974)
	Rat[a]	2.6(1.6–4.3)	Consroe and Man (1973)
CBD	Mouse	105.0(79.0–204.0)	Karler *et al.* (1973)
	Mouse	115.0(90.0–147.0)	Karler *et al.* (1974*c*)
	Mouse		Chesher and Jackson (1974)
CBN	Mouse	230.0(215.0–246.0)	Karler *et al.* (1973)
	Mouse		Chesher and Jackson (1974)

[a] These rats were susceptible to audiogenic-induced seizures. The drugs in this study were given iv, while in all the others the drugs were administered ip.

TABLE 4

Comparative ED_{50} Values for the Analgesic Effectiveness of Δ⁹-THC, CBN, CBD, Morphine SO_4, and Aspirin in Mice and Rats in Three Models of Experimentally Induced Pain

Test compound	Oral ED_{50} (± 95% confidence limits), mg/kg			
	Acetic-acid-induced writhing (mice)	Hot plate test (mice)	Randall–Selitto paw-pressure test (rats): Injected paw	Randall–Selitto paw-pressure test (rats): Uninjected paw
Δ^9-THC	4.2(2.5–7.1)	7.7(4.9–12.2)	4.0(2.0–8.0)	32.0(17.9–57.3)
CBN	35.0(19.1–64.5)	>400.0[b]	148.0(59.7–367.4)	>320.0
CBD	>400.0[b]	>400.0[c]	>320.0	>320.0
Morphine SO_4	2.9(1.2–3.8)	4.0(2.1–10.1)	5.1(2.4–10.7)	7.5(3.8–15.0)
Aspirin	130.0(82.3–205.5)	>800.0	200.0(111.0–360.0)	>800.0

[a] From Sofia *et al.*, 1976.
[b] One mouse died within a 30-min interval following oral dosing.
[c] Two mice died within a 30-min interval following oral dosing.

by acetic acid and increased the pain threshold of the inflamed hind paw of the rat. These results suggest that THC possesses narcotic-like analgesic activity like morphine, while CBN, like aspirin, might be a nonnarcotic agent. On the other hand, CBD did not produce a significant analgesic effect in any of the tests even after a very high dose, thus confirming earlier reports (Karniol and Carlini, 1973*b*; Chesher *et al.*, 1973).

The analgesic activities of Δ^8- and Δ^9-THC in the mouse hot-plate (Dewey *et al.*, 1972; Chesher *et al.*, 1973; Wilson and May, 1975) and writhing tests (Dewey *et al.*, 1972) were strikingly equipotent, even when tested at various times (20 to 180 min) after intraperitoneal, subcutaneous, or oral dosing. Chesher *et al.* (1973) reported an equivalent potency for pethidine (ED_{50} values of 5.0 to 7.0 mg/kg), which was six times more active than CBN, whose ED_{50} in the hot plate test was 32.5 mg/kg. More recently, Wilson and May (1975) have demonstrated that the 11-OH metabolites of both Δ^8- and Δ^9-THC were approximately five times more potent than the parent compounds and equipotent with morphine HCl (Table 5). These data, therefore, suggest that the derivatives may be the analgesically effective forms of Δ^8- and Δ^9-THC in mice. Moreover, the narcotic-like analgesia induced by 4.0 mg/kg of 11-OH-Δ^8-THC was completely antagonized by a 1.0 mg/kg subcutaneous dose of the narcotic antagonist naloxone when given 10 min prior to the cannabinoid. Compounds with an 8α-OH substitute retained some analgesic activity, while 8β-compounds were completely ineffective.

Finally, Hine *et al.* (1975*a,b*) reported that Δ^9-THC (2.0 to 10.0 mg/kg) but not CBD (10.0 mg/kg) administered 1 hr prior to an intraperitoneal injection of naloxone HCl significantly lessened the abstinence syndrome in

Table 5
Analgesic Activity of Various Tetrahydrocannabinol Derivatives[a]

Test compound	Subcutaneous ED_{50}, mg/kg (±95% confidence limits) mouse hot plate test
(−)-Δ⁹-THC	9.6(7.4–12.5)
(−)-11-OH-Δ⁹-THC	1.9(1.4–2.7)
(−)-8α-OH-Δ⁹-THC	4/10 Active @20.0
(−)-8α,11-Dihydroxy Δ⁹-THC	2/10 Active @20.0
(−)-8β-OH-Δ⁹-THC	Inactive @20.0
(−)-8β,11-Dihydroxy Δ⁹-THC	Inactive @20.0
(−) Δ⁸-THC	8.8(6.2–12.5)
(−)-11-OH-Δ⁸-THC	1.9(1.4–2.7)
Morphine HCl	1.2(0.9–1.3)

[a] From Wilson and May, 1975.

morphine-dependent rats, while Δ⁹-THC itself did not induce abstinence. Unlike the conventional treatment for narcotic withdrawal, i.e., methadone substitution or use of neuroleptics, Δ⁹-THC may be useful in that it has not been shown to induce physical dependence nor produce toxic side reactions (extrapyramidal effects, etc.). Based on these preliminary data these investigators suggest that this potentially useful effect of Δ⁹-THC should be further explored and extended to other cannabinoid structures.

2.3.7. *Effects on Neurotransmitter Substances*

Several investigators have reported that Δ⁹-THC caused increases in whole brain serotonin (5-hydroxytryptamine, 5-HT) in mice (Holtzman *et al.*, 1969; Welch *et al.*, 1971) and rats (Sofia *et al.*, 1971*a*; Schildkraut and Efron, 1971). In the rat, 20.0 mg/kg ip of Δ⁹-THC increased whole brain levels of 5-HT by 66% 30 min after drug administration (Sofia *et al.*, 1971*a*). The hypothalamus plus midbrain and cerebellum were the only brain regions where significant elevations were noticed. In addition, Δ⁹-THC clearly inhibited the synthesis rate of 5-HT but had no effect on the enzyme most responsible for its degradation, i.e., MAO. Finally, these investigators also demonstrated that Δ⁹-THC markedly inhibited the rate of reserpine-induced depletion of brain 5-HT, suggesting an alteration of the vesicular membrane surrounding stored 5-HT. In a subsequent report, Sofia *et al.* (1971*b*) reported inhibition by Δ⁹-THC (10^{-7} M) of the uptake of [^{14}C]-5-HT by crude rat brain homogenates (synaptosomes). Subsequently, Banerjee *et al.* (1975) and Johnson and Dewey (1975), using hypothalamic and forebrain synaptosomes, respectively, have confirmed the blockade of 5-HT uptake by Δ⁹-THC. Each of these investigators have also shown that Δ⁸-THC and CBD were more active than Δ⁹-THC. In addition, the 11-OH metabolites of Δ⁸-

and Δ^9-THC and CBN were also active, but not to the same extent in each study. Johnson and Dewey (1975) suggest that hydroxylation at position 11 decreases activity, whereas Banerjee *et al.* (1975) report no alteration.

Holtzman *et al.* (1969) found that whole mouse brain levels of norepinephrine (NE) were decreased after intraperitoneal doses of 1.0 to 50.0 mg/kg of Δ^9-THC, but increased after much higher doses (100.0 to 500.0 mg/kg) when measured 45 min after drug administration. Maitre *et al.* (1970) and Welch *et al.* (1971) reported that Δ^9-THC had no significant effect on endogenous brain levels of NE or dopamine (DA) in rats and mice, respectively. However, the formation of [^{3}H]-NE and [^{3}H]-DA from intravenously administered [^{3}H]tyrosine was enhanced by Δ^9-THC. A similar activity was also attributed to Δ^9-THC by Maitre *et al.* (1971). Ho *et al.* (1973*c*) suggest that this latter effect may be a result, in part, of an increase in the activity of tyrosine hydroxylase. Finally, Banerjee *et al.* (1975) have shown that Δ^9-THC noncompetitively inhibits accumulation of [^{3}H]-NE and [^{3}H]-DA into hypothalamic and striatal synaptosomal preparations, respectively. Moreover, 11-OH-Δ^9-THC, Δ^8-THC, and its 11-OH derivative, and CBD were equal in activity to Δ^9-THC on NE uptake, whereas CBN and cannabigerol, although active, were less effective.

Brown (1973) reports that a 10.0 mg/kg ip dose of Δ^9-THC produced a small but significant 14% increase in whole rat brain acetylcholine (Ach) levels 1 hr after dosing with a return to normal within 5 hr. Using a much higher dose of Δ^9-THC (100.0 mg/kg ip) Karbowski *et al.* (1975) reported increases of 75% in the whole mouse brain levels of Ach. Furthermore, Friedman and Gershon (1974) have shown that acute or chronic dosing with 5.0 to 20.0 mg/kg of either Δ^8- or Δ^9-THC significantly and in a dose-related way inhibited Ach synthesis in the striatum, hypothalamus, and cortex regions of the rat brain.

The effects of cannabinoids on γ-aminobutyric acid (GABA) are conflicting. Leonard (1971) reports that a single 100.0 mg/kg ip dose of Δ^8-THC produced a small but significant 12% decrease in rat whole brain GABA content during severe catalepsy. More recently, Edery and Gottesfeld (1975) have shown that repeated, but not single, ip doses of 20.0 mg/kg of Δ^8-THC daily for 14 days to rats caused a marked elevation in GABA content and decreased glutamic acid decarboxylase activity in the cerebellum. In addition, [^{3}H]-GABA uptake by crude cerebellar synaptosomes was enhanced, whereas Banerjee *et al.* (1975) reported inhibition into cerebral cortical preparations for not only Δ^8-THC but also for Δ^9-THC, 11-OH-Δ^8-THC, 11-OH-Δ^9-THC, CBD, CBN, and cannabigerol.

Dolby and Kleinsmith (1974) reported that 0.1 to 1.0 mg/kg of Δ^9-THC caused a 50.0 to 160.0% increase in mouse whole brain levels of cyclic AMP, while higher doses, i.e., 2.0 to 10.0 mg/kg, produced a 30.0 to 60.0% depression. Similar responses were also observed in dissected brain areas including the cortex, cerebellum, and medulla. On the other hand, Askew and Ho (1974) report no effect for Δ^9-THC (10.0 mg/kg iv) on cyclic AMP levels in various rat brain areas. However, its isomer, Δ^8-THC, did produce a significant increase of cyclic AMP in the midbrain region with a concomitant decrease in the activities of adenyl cyclase and cyclic nucleotide phosphodiesterase, suggesting a decreased turnover rate of cyclic nucleotide.

2.3.8. *Interaction with Other Drugs*

To know how Δ^9-THC interacts with other drugs appears to be imperative since the occasional and chronic use of marihuana is widespread throughout the world (*Marihuana and Health,* 1974). Hence, a greater number of individuals who ingest a variety of drugs for medicinal or other reasons are exposing themselves to still another drug interaction when they take in marihuana.

Garriott *et al.* (1968) have clearly demonstrated an enhancing action for Δ^9-THC on hexobarbital sleeping time in mice. Using spontaneous motor activity and prolongation of barbiturate sleeping time to measure drug interactions, Kubena and Barry (1970) have shown that intraperitoneal doses of 4.0 and 16.0 mg/kg of Δ^9-THC potentiate the depressant effect of both pentobarbital and barbital. Since the latter is virtually unmetabolized, these authors concluded along with others (Sofia and Barry, 1970; Adams and Sofia, 1973) that this interaction with Δ^9-THC was a synergistic effect in the central nervous system, while that for pentobarbital may be associated with inhibition of liver microsomal enzyme systems responsible for drug metabolism (Gill *et al.*, 1970; Siemens *et al.*, 1974). Coper and Fernandes (1973) and Chesher *et al.* (1974) have shown that not only Δ^8- and Δ^9-THC but also CBD and CBN significantly enhanced hexobarbital-induced sleeping time in mice, with CBD being more potent and CBN less potent than Δ^9-THC. These results have also been reflected by *in vitro* studies on hexobarbital metabolism (Fernandes *et al.*, 1973). Siemens *et al.* (1974) demonstrated that when added *in vitro* to normal rat liver microsomes Δ^9-THC, CBD, and CBN competitively inhibited pentobarbital metabolism, with CBD being more potent than Δ^9-THC or CBN. Coldwell *et al.* (1974) have carried out a series of very elegant experiments to determine the effect of various naturally occurring cannabinoids on the *in vivo* metabolism of pentobarbital in the rat. From these experiments they concluded that (1) Δ^8- and Δ^9-THC decreased the elimination of pentobarbital, (2) CBD inhibited its metabolism, (3) cannabigerol decreased the rate of pentobarbital absorption, and (4) CBN had little effect on any parameter measured. On the other hand, when given chronically, daily, for 6 days Sofia and Barry (1973) have shown that Δ^9-THC decreased the duration of both hexobarbital- and zoxazolamine-induced sleeping time in rats, indicating possibly that Δ^9-THC was an enzyme inducer. However, Dewey *et al.* (1970) demonstrated that five daily injections of Δ^9-THC to rats did not stimulate microsomal enzyme activity. Because of the chronic use of marihuana and the implication of drug interaction, this question of enzyme induction warrants clarification.

Phillips *et al.* (1971*a*) and Forney (1971) have shown that intraperitoneal injections of Δ^9-THC in a dose range of 1.25 to 40.0 mg/kg markedly potentiated sleeping time in rats given 3.0 g/kg of ethanol. In a subsequent study doses of THC ranging from 5.0 to 40.0 mg/kg caused a dose-related increase in the number of rats that slept after 2.0 g/kg of ethanol, which by itself did not induce loss of righting reflex. Moreover, with the combination of 1.0 g/kg of ethanol and any of the doses of Δ^9-THC, no sleeping times were recorded. However, Phillips *et al.* (1971*a*) made the observation that as the concentration of Δ^9-THC increased, the magnitude of ataxia and depression manifested in the rats also increased. More recently, Sofia and Knobloch (1973) confirmed the potentiating effect of Δ^9-THC on ethanol and hexobarbital in mice and extended it to seven additional clinically useful sedative–hypnotic drugs (Table 6).

Gill *et al.* (1970) and Chesher *et al.* (1974) reported a prolongation of ether anesthesia in mice following administration of cannabis extract equivalent to 10 mg of Δ^9-THC/kg. Moreover, it has been demonstrated that oral administration of a single dose of Δ^9-THC produces significant and dose-related decreases in minimum alveolar concentration requirements of the volatile anesthetics halothane (Stoelting *et al.* 1973) and cyclopropane (Vitez *et al.*, 1973) in the dog and rat, respectively. In addition, Sofia and Knobloch (1974) have shown that the anesthetic effects of thiopental, ketamine, and CT-1341, a new steroidal anesthetic (Althesin), were dramatically augmented and enhanced by pretreatment with Δ^9-THC. Hence, the fact that these interactions exist in laboratory animals strongly suggests the possibility of dose adjustment when general anesthesia is required for a marihuana user.

Increased spontaneous locomotor activity resulting from *d*-amphetamine SO_4 in mice (Garriott *et al.* 1967) and rats (Forney, 1971) was significantly augmented by Δ^9-THC pretreatment. On the other hand, Kubena and Barry (1970) reported that the stimulant action of methamphetamine in rats was not potentiated by Δ^9-THC. However, in mice, Phillips *et al.* (1971*b*) clearly demonstrate that the stimulant effect of methamphetamine and caffeine was enhanced and prolonged by Δ^9-THC. Finally, Grunfeld and Edery (1969) have shown that the depressant action of Δ^8- and Δ^9-THC in monkeys (0.5 mg/kg iv) and rats (10.0 mg/kg ip) could be reversed by the administration of 0.5 and 10.0 mg/kg of *dl*-amphetamine, respectively. Hence, a species difference is apparent for the interaction of Δ^9-THC and CNS stimulants.

3. SYNTHETIC CANNABINOIDS

3.1. $\Delta^{6a,10a}$-THC and Derivatives

While studying the chemistry of natural THC Adams and Baker (1940) prepared purely synthetic analogs that are not found in the plant and differ

TABLE 6

The Effect of Pretreatment with Δ^9-THC (20.0 mg/kg) or Its Vehicle on Various Sedative–Hypnotic Drugs in Mice[a]

Sedative–hypnotic drug	HD_{50} (±95% Confidence Limits)[b] Vehicle and drug	Estimated duration[c] (min) of LRR for HD_{50}	Δ^9-THC and drug	Estimated duration (min) of LRR for HD_{50}	Potency[d] ratio
Hexobarbital	39.0(32.5–46.8)	11.0	31.5(25.4–39.1)	28.0	1.24
Methaqualone	58.0(42.3–79.4)	29.0	32.6(26.1–40.7)	39.0	1.49[e]
Ethchlorvynol	63.9(51.1–79.9)	9.0	30.6(20.8–45.1)	36.0	2.09[e]
Paraldehyde	>500.0, <750.0	15.0	312.0(226.0–431.0)	16.0	>1.60, <2.40[d]
Ethanol	4900.0(4080.0–5880.0)	12.0	3140.0(2660.0–3710.0)	23.0	1.56[e]
Ethinamate	160.0(93.6–274.0)	48.0	48.2(33.2–69.9)	40.0	3.32[e]
Chloral hydrate	198.0(161.0–244.0)	22.0	93.0(64.1–134.9)	25.0	2.14[e]
Meprobamate	271.0(213.0–344.0)	70.0	155.0(107.0–225.0)	71.0	1.75[e]
Glutethimide	125.0(94.0–166.2)	33.0	72.5(49.0–107.2)	60.0	1.73[e]

[a] From Sofia and Knobloch, 1973.
[b] HD_{50} = hypnotic $dose_{50}$. At least three different doses of drug ($N = 8$ per dose) were used to determine the HD_{50}.
[c] Duration estimate obtained from dose-response curve. LRR = loss of righting reflex.
[d] Obtained by (vehicle and drug)/(Δ^9-THC and drug).
[e] Statistically significant difference ($p < 0.05$) between vehicle and drug and Δ^9-THC and drug HD_{50}s.

from the naturally occurring substances only by the position of the double bond in the alicyclic ring. The basic structure of this substance, called $\Delta^{6a,10a}$-THC (*n*-amyl substituent at position 3), is shown. They discovered that this

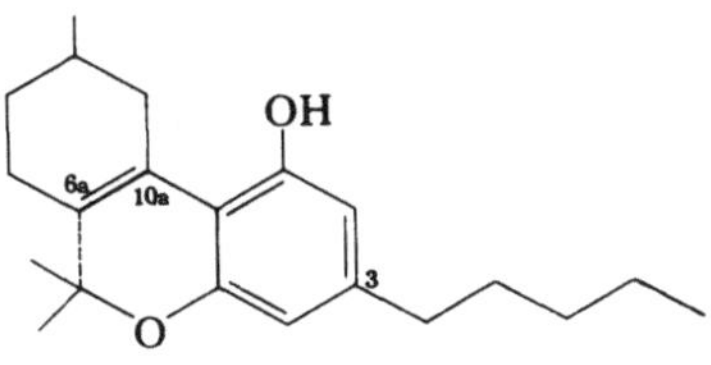

substance (named synhexyl in the United States and pyrahexyl in the United Kingdom) caused ataxia in dogs and corneal areflexia in rabbits similar to but substantially more potent than marihuana extracts. Subsequently, Loewe (1946) confirmed these findings and reported also that $\Delta^{6a,10a}$-THC induces catalepsy and some excitatory behavior in the rabbit. In a later investigation, Sampaio *et al.* (1967) demonstrated abolishment of the linguomandibular reflex in the dog without impairment of neuromuscular transmission following 1.0 mg/kg of pyrahexyl, suggesting a marked depressant action upon the trigeminal nuclei or related structures. Abel and Schiff (1969) have shown pyrahexyl to depress food intake by rats, increase time spent observing other animals outside the home cage, and not affect water consumption after six daily injections of 15.0 mg/kg, with the effects becoming more pronounced after each successive injection. After a single injection of 15.0 mg/kg of pyrahexyl to rats, a disruption of the suppressive effects of a conditioned stimulus with shock in a conditioned emotional response was observed (Abel, 1969). Measuring open field behavior in rats, Abel (1970) has shown that activity, measured as the number of squares crossed with both hind feet in the open field, was increased by 2.5 and 5.0 mg/kg but depressed by higher doses. Furthermore, rearing was also significantly decreased as the dose of drug was increased; however, grooming and defecation were not significantly affected. Hence, these data suggest that $\Delta^{6a,10a}$-THC very closely mimics the response of animals to injections of marihuana extracts or Δ^8- and Δ^9-THC.

In their synthetic series Adams and Baker (1940) were able to show that the pharmacological activity (dog ataxia test) varied greatly, depending on the substituent at position 3. Of the alkyl homologs prepared two compounds emerged as the most potent. The 1,2-dimethylheptylpyran (DMHP) derivative was observed to be superior in potency to the THC with a methyloctylpyran (MOP) side chain.

The pharmacology of these two substances, especially DMHP, has been studied rather extensively. Boyd *et al.* (1963) demonstrated depression of all measured aspects of behavior by DMHP (5.0 to 80.0 μg/kg) and MOP (20.0 to 320.0 μg/kg), except for one phase of a multiple FR–FI schedule in which rats exhibited a decreased ability to judge elapsed time accurately. Dagirmanjian and Boyd (1962) have reported that a 0.2 mg/kg dose of DMHP had no effect on the amplitude of the monosynaptic knee-jerk response, whereas 0.1

mg/kg markedly decreased the polysynaptic flexor reflex and the linguomandibular reflex progressively over a long period of time in the cat. A lower dose, 0.05 mg/kg, did not affect the flexor reflex but did depress the more sensitive linguomandibular reflex. MOP had a similar neuropharmacological profile, which was observed only after higher doses (0.5 mg/kg) and was of much shorter duration. Boyd and Merritt (1965 and 1966) have confirmed these activities of DMHP in the cat and have suggested that its depressant action on polysynaptic reflexes in the intact animal appears to be a result of (1) the summation of possible depressant actions along the neuroaxis from the reflex system itself to the level of the forebrain or (2) the depressant action at one or all facilitory regions including the reticular formation, primary sensory pathways, etc. Hence, these studies are supported by the experiments of Sampaio *et al.* (1967) on the dog linguomandibular reflex and its blockade by a cannabis extract and higher doses of Δ^9-THC (0.5 mg/kg). More recently, Haavik and Hardman (1973*a,b*) and Liu (1974) demonstrated a more potent and longer-lasting hypothermic effect for DMHP when compared with Δ^8- or Δ^9-THC, i.e., 2.0 to 5.0 mg/kg versus 32.0 to 50.0 mg/kg, when administered to mice or monkeys. Lemberger *et al.* (1973) have shown that in rabbits the plasma half-life for DMHP is much longer, and its pattern of excretion markedly differs from that reported for Δ^9-THC and may account for its greater potency and longer duration of action. Finally, Loev *et al.* (1973) have reported activities for DMHP that mimic Δ^9-THC such as analgesic, antiarthritic, antisecretory, and diuretic activities, some of which have also been observed by others (Winn *et al.*, 1976).

Because of the early structure–activity relationship (SAR) study of Adams (already summarized by Mechoulam, 1973) and the renewed interest in cannabinoids in general over the last several years, additional and more recent SAR investigations dealing with $\Delta^{6a,10a}$-THC analogs have been made. Table 7 reveals the results obtained by Loev *et al.* (1973). In the *n*-alkyl series with substitutions at position 3 of the aromatic ring, CNS depressant activity was more pronounced with longer chains, i.e., compounds 1, 2, and 3. When lower alkyl groups such as —CH_3 and —C_2H_3 were substituted on the side chain, potency was further enhanced as in the case of the 1-methylheptyl (5) and 1-ethylheptyl (7) derivatives. Moving the substituent to position 2 markedly inhibited activity (compound 8). On the other hand, increasing side-chain substitution to two alkyl groups further enhanced potency, as evidenced by the activity of the 1,2-dimethylheptyl (DMHP) (10) and 1,1-dimethylheptyl(12) derivatives. Interestingly, Loev *et al.* (1973) found the latter compound to be twice as potent as DMHP and 500 times as active as Δ^9-THC. Although the total number of carbon atoms in the side chain were identical, the branching pattern is important since the *n*-nonyl(3) and dibutylcarbonyl(13) analogs are substantially less active than DMHP. Compound 14, in which a double bond was introduced at position 1, did not affect potency. However, the side-chain substitution with an ether linkage

(15) was five times more active than compound 8, its corresponding methylene analog.

DMHP analogs in which various alkyl substitutions were made in the pyran ring resulted in drastically decreased CNS potency, although these substances still retained good activity. For instance, Table 7 reveals that replacement of the 9-CH_3 with —H (16) or —C_2H_5 (17), shifting the —CH_3 to C-8, or adding a —CH_3 to C-7 caused reductions in activity. These investigators point out that since the desmethyl compound (16) still retained substantial activity in these animals, i.e., decreased motor activity, it may be that formation of a 9-OH metabolite is not required. Acetylation (26), desmethylation (28), and more so, methylation (27) of the aromatic ring of DMHP markedly reduces activity. Similarly, the condensation products, 30 and 31, each had relatively weak activity. Finally, replacing the 6,6-dimethyl substitution with a carbonyl (35) or diethyl (33) markedly decreased CNS activity.

Consistent with potent activity of the 1,1-dimethylheptyl analog of $\Delta^{6a,10a}$-THC (12) reported by Loev *et al.* (1973), Stark and Archer (1975) and Page and West (1975) reported highly potent CNS activity for the cannabinoid *dl*-3-(1,1-dimethylheptyl)-6,6aβ,7,8,10aα-hexahydro-1-hydroxy-6,6-dimethyl-9*H*-dibenzo[b,d]pyran-9-one (nabilone), whose structure is shown

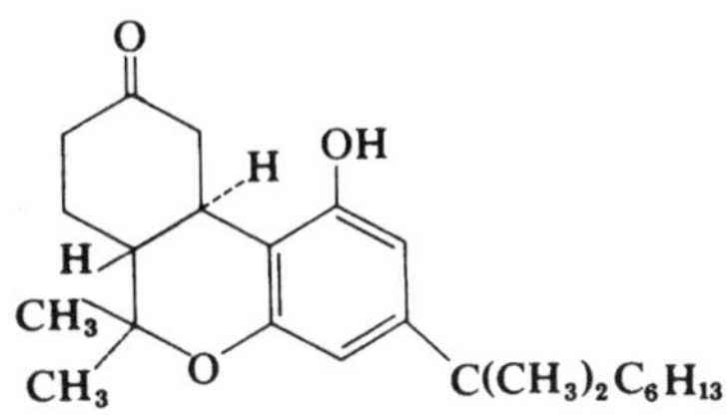

above. Nabilone was shown to inhibit rat muricide, septal-lesioned rat hyperactivity, and spontaneous locomotor activity in mice and to produce hypothermia in rats and ataxia in the dog. The least effective oral dose in rodents was 1.25 mg/kg, while in the dog observation test intravenous doses of <0.016 mg/kg were remarkably active.

In the first of a series of articles, Pars *et al.* (1976) reported on the synthesis and pharmacological activity of various nitrogen-containing cannabinoid analogs, i.e., benzopyranopyridines and benzopyranopyrroles. Table 8 reveals that DMHP had an MED_{50} of 0.075 mg/kg. The nitrogen analog of DMHP, compound 8, was substantially less active, having an MED_{50} of 1.0 mg/kg. Altering the side chain beginning with —CH_3 (7) as well as other substituents not shown in Table 8 even further reduced potency. When the ring position of the nitrogen of compound 8 was shifted (2) no significant change in potency was noticed. When different substitutions were made on the nitrogen of compound 8, remarkable changes in potency were observed (compounds 9–24). Substitution of a propargnyl group (22) markedly

TABLE 7
Pharmacological Activity of Various $\Delta^{6a,10a}$-THC Analogs[a]

Compound	Substituent	Relative CNS activity[b] Rat[c]	Dog[d]
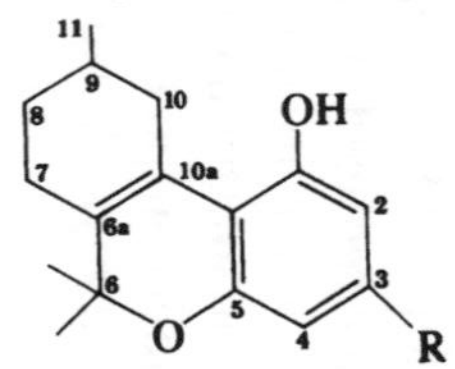	R		
1	$—C_5H_{11}$-*n*	0.5	0.1
2	$—C_6H_{13}$-*n*	1	1
3	$—C_9H_{19}$-*n*	4	0.1
4	$—CH(CH_3)C_5H_{11}$	20	9
5	$—CH(CH_3)C_6H_{13}$	100	18
6	$—CH(CH_3)C_7H_{15}$	50	1
7	$—CH(C_2H_5)C_6H_{13}$	100	—
8	$—CH_2CH(CH_3)C_5H_{11}$	2	—
9	$—CH(CH_3)CH(CH_3)C_4H_9$	100	22
10	$—CH(CH_3)CH(CH_3)C_5H_{11}$ (DMHP)	500	285, 42, 2[e]
11	$—CH(CH_3)CH(CH_3)C_6H_{13}$	100	10
12	$—C(CH_3)_2C_6H_{13}$	1000	12
13	$—CH(C_4H_9)_2$	<0.6	—
14	$—C(CH_3)=C(CH_3)C_5H_{11}$	500	—
15	$—OCH(CH_3)C_5H_{11}$	10	—
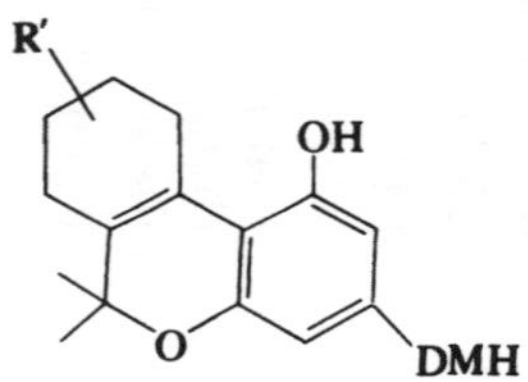	R′		

16		H		10	—
17		$9\text{-}C_2H_5$		20	—
18		$8\text{-}CH_3$		1	—
19		$7,9\text{-diCH}_3$		50	—

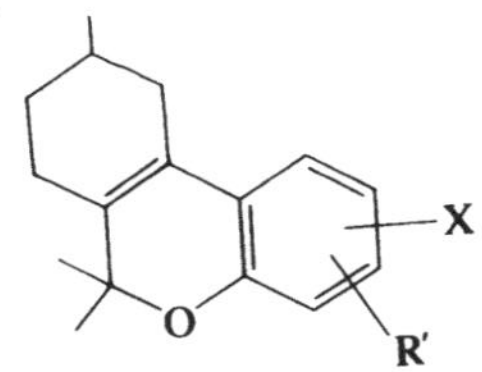

	R′	X		
26	3-DMH	$1\text{-OCH}_3\text{CO}$	>20	—
27	3-DMH	1-OCH_3	<0.4	—
28	3-DMH	H	1	—
29	2-DMH	3-OH	10	—
30	3-DMH	$1\text{-OH},2\text{-CH}_2\text{N(CH}_3)_2$	1	—
31	$3\text{-CH(C}_4\text{H}_9)_2$	$1\text{-OH},2\text{-CH}_2\text{N(CH}_3)_2\text{-HCl}$	<0.4	—

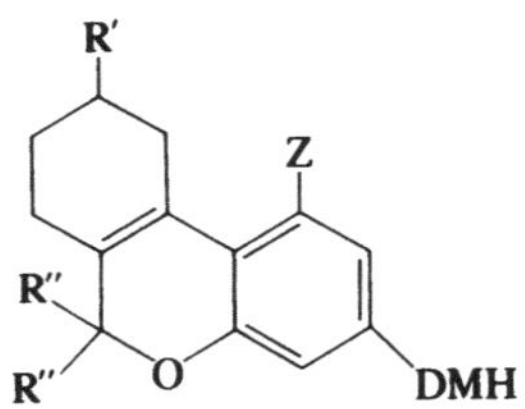

	R′	R″	Z		
32	—H	$—CH_3$	$—OCH_3CO$	>2	—
33	$—CH_3$	$—C_2H_5$	—OH	2	—
34	$—CH_3$	$—C_2H_5$	$—OCH_3CO$	0.5	—
35	$—CH_3$	=O	—OH	<0.1	—

[a] From Loev *et al.*, 1973.
[b] Relative to compound 2 used as the standard with respect to minimum oral dose producing overt side effects.
[c] Based on overt side effects observed after oral 50.0 mg/kg dose of compound 2.
[d] Reassessment of the dog ataxia data reported by Adams as summarized by Mechoulam (1973).
[e] Based on the evaluation of three different preparations of this substance.

TABLE 8

Pharmacological Activity of Various Nitrogen Analogs of the Cannabinoids[a]

Compound	Substituent			Mouse data[b]	
	R	R′	R″	MED_{50}[c]	LD_{50}
DMHP				0.075	63.0
N-5-Oxobenzopyrano[3,4-*c*]pyridines					
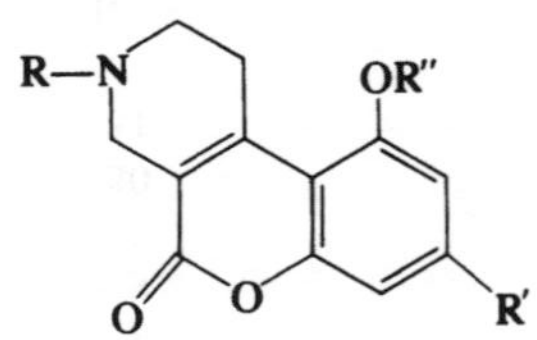					
1	—H	$—CH(CH_3)CH(CH_3)C_5H_{11}$	H	5.6	32.0
N-Benzopyrano[3,4-*c*]pyridines					
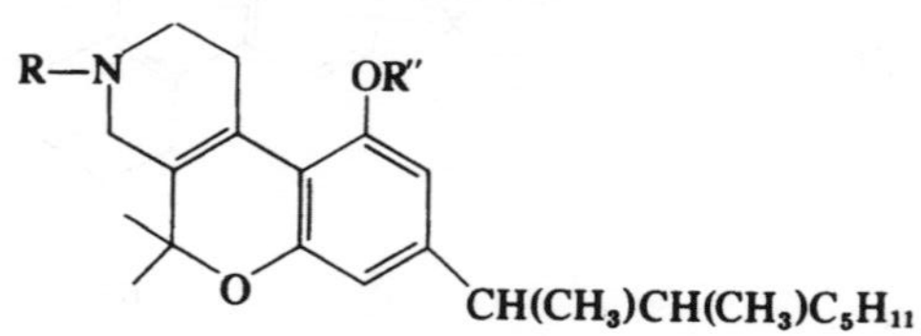					
2	$—CH_3$	—	H	1.8	>32.0
3	$—CH_2C{\equiv}CH$	—	H	18.0	>32.0

N-5-Oxobenzopyran-[3,4-*d*]pyridines

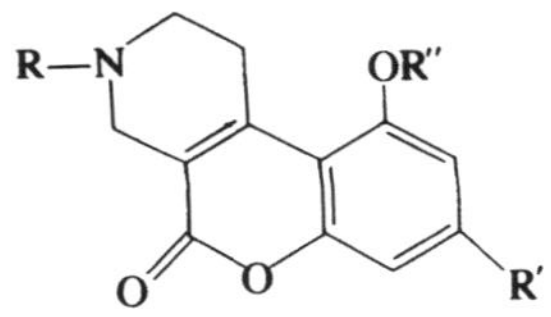

4	$—CH_3$	$—nC_5H_{11}$	H	5.6	56.0
5	$—CH_3$	$—CH(CH_3)C_{12}H_{25}$	H	3.2	>10.0
6	$—CH_2C{\equiv}CH$	$—CH(CH_3)CH(CH_3)C_5H_{11}$	H	1.8	>100.0

N-Methyl-benzopyrano[3,4-*d*]pyridines

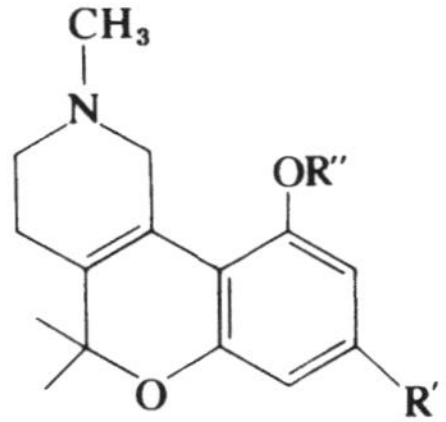

7	—	$—CH_3$	H	5.6	>32.0
8	—	$—CH(CH_3)CH(CH_3)C_5H_{11}$	H	1.2	>22.0

continued

TABLE 8—*continued*

Compound	Substituent: R	Substituent: R′	Substituent: R″	Mouse data[b]: MED_{50}[c]	Mouse data[b]: LD_{50}
N-Benzopyrano[3,4-*d*]pyridines					
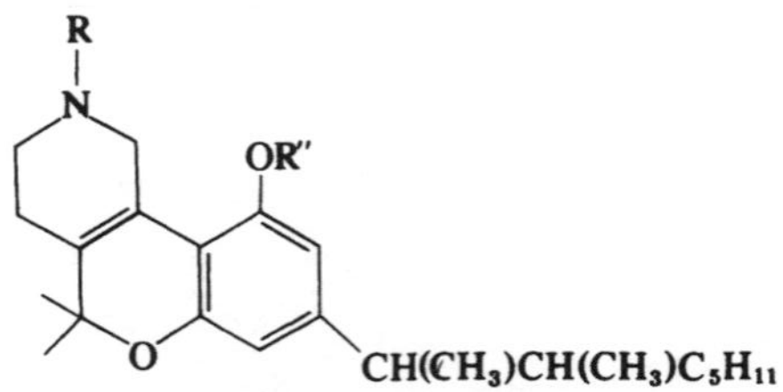					
9	—$CH_2C_6H_3$	—	—H	10.0	>32.0
10	—$COCH_3$	—	—H	5.6	>32.0
11	—C_2H_5	—	—H	5.6	>10.0
12	—nC_3H_7	—	—H	0.42	>3.2
13	—CO—◁	—	—H	10.0	>32.0
14	—CH_2—◁	—	—H	1.8	>10.0
15	—nC_5H_{11}	—	—H	1.8	>10.0
16	—CH_2—□	—	—H	0.56	25.0
17	—$CH_2CH_2C_6H_5$	—	—H	3.2	>10.0
18	—$CH_2CH{=}CH_2$	—	—H	0.75	>10.0
19	—$CH_2CH{=}CHCl$	—	—H	0.42	>32.0
20	—$CH_2CH{=}CHCl$(*cis*)	—	—H	0.42	>10.0
21	—$CH_2CH{=}CHCl$(trans)	—	—H	0.25	>10.0
22	$CH_2C{\equiv}CH$	—	—H	0.042	40.0
23	$CH_2C{\equiv}CH$	—	—$COCH_3$	0.18	>100.0
24	$CH_2C{\equiv}CCH_3$	—	—H	1.0	32.0

Quinuclidinyl analog					
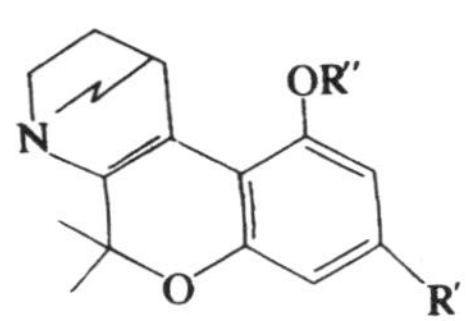					
25	—	$CH(CH_3)CH(CH_3)C_5H_{11}$	H	0.32	>32.0
Quaternary *N*-benzopyrano[3,4-*d*]pyridines					
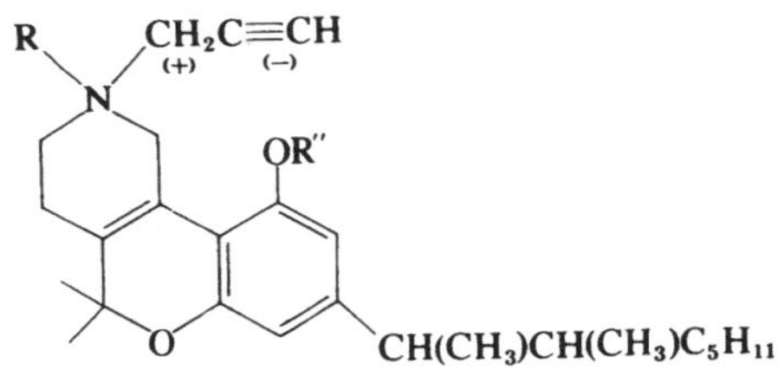					
26	$—CH_3$	—	H	5.6	56.0
27	$—CH_2C{\equiv}CH$	—	H	5.6	18.0
Pyrrolo analog					
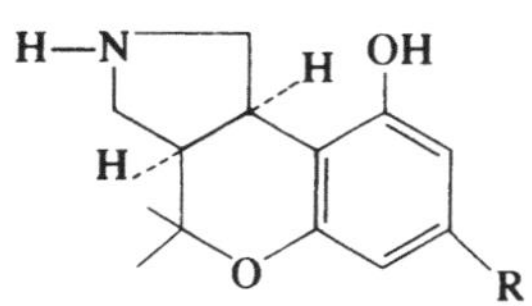					
28	$—CH(CH_3)CH(CH_3)C_5H_{11}$	—	—	10.0	56.0

[a] From Pars *et al.*, 1976.
[b] Doses expressed in mg/kg.
[c] MED_{50} is the minimum effective dose or that dose that elicits a given behavioral activity (mouse observational screen decreased locomotor activity and increased sensitivity to stimuli) in 50% of the animals after iv dosing.

elevated potency to the level of DMHP. Similarly, other three carbon substituents such as allyl and chlorallyl (18, 19–21) also greatly enhanced potency. Changing the side chain of 22 or acetylation of the phenolic —OH (23) reduced potency. Moreover, shifting of the ring position of the nitrogen (3), or quaternization of the nitrogen (26 and 27) of compound 22 was accompanied by a significant reduction in potency.

In a direct comparative study of compound 22 and DMHP Pars *et al.* (1976) found the general depressant effect of the former to be greater than that of the latter in the cat, dog, and rhesus monkey and less than that of the latter in the mouse. Both were equally effective depressants in potentiating hexobarbital sleeping time and in the inclined screen test in mice. Interestingly, at least part of the overt behavioral effects of these compounds may be mediated through the β-adrenergic system since effective blockade was achieved with dichloroisoproterenol, a powerful β-blocking agent.

When compared with morphine, compound 22 was more potent in phenylquinone writhing and less potent in the hot-plate and tail-flick tests for analgesia. Each were equally effective inhibitors of gastrointestinal mobility. In the morphine-dependent monkey, compound 22 precipitated abstinence and was found to possess narcotic–antagonist properties in the tail-flick test. Hence, compound 22 appears to be a partial agonist–antagonist similar to nalorphine and pentazocine.

Razdan *et al.* (1976*c*) have synthesized and tested water-soluble basic esters of the nitrogen analog of compound 22 mentioned above, of DMHP, and of the carboxylic DMHP analog in which the cyclohexane ring has been replaced by a cyclopentane ring. Table 9 reveals that formation of the basic esters of compound 1 markedly reduces their tranquilizing activity (rat motor activity and mouse fighting), with the effect being substantially greater for the hindered esters such as the α-methyl and α,α-dimethyl derivatives (compounds 3 and 4 compared with 2; 6 and 9 compared with 5 and 8, respectively). Substitution of a piperidino (2) or morpholino (8) group on the propargynl analog of DMHP still causes the compounds to retain analgesic effectiveness. Incorporation of an α-methyl group has little or no effect (6 and 9), whereas α,α-dimethyl substitution (4) markedly decreases analgesic activity. When the piperidine or morpholine moiety is replaced by a pyrrolidine or diethylamine substituent (not shown in Table 9) analgesic activity is eliminated. Likewise, replacing the DMH side chain on the aromatic ring with C_5H_{11} (7) or quaternization of the basic nitrogen (10) also eliminates overall activity. In general, the ester derivatives display selective analgesic and sedative–hypnotic activity compared with the parent phenolic derivative.

In the case of the basic esters of DMHP (Table 9) the analgesic activity of the γ-morpholinobutyrate (13) again is markedly greater than that of the parent phenol (11) and of codeine. All of these compounds were highly potent anticonvulsant agents, with the exception of the thiomorpholino analog (15). The homopiperidino derivative (14) displayed equal potency to diphenylhydantoin in a variety of anticonvulsant tests including supramaximal electroshock-, psychomotor electroshock-, and pentylenetetrazol-induced seizures.

On the other hand, basic esterification of the cyclopentane analog of DMHP (Table 9) markedly reduced or completely inhibited effects on rat motor activity. Analgesic activity was only slightly increased in the homopiperidino (18) and morpholino (20) derivatives, while the pyrrolidine (17) or replacement of the DMH side chain by —C_5H_{11} (19) caused reductions in potency. These substances have much less anticonvulsant activity than the DMHP derivatives, and more interesting, the homopiperidino analog is inactive (comparing 18 with 14). Based on these SAR investigations, Razdan *et al.* (1976*c*) concluded

> that (a) basic ester formation of the parent phenol retains biological activity, (b) formation of the ester can lead to greater selectivity of action, particularly the analgesic activity, and (c) SAR cannot be carried over from one series to another.

As an extension of these investigations Razdan *et al.* (1976*b*) have synthesized and tested various sulfur analogs of DMHP (thiopyranobenzopyrans and thienobenzopyrans). Table 10 shows that none of these sulfur analogs were particularly effective in the tests for tranquilization (rat motor activity and mouse fighting) with the exception of the α-methylpiperidinobutyryloxy ester of the thiopyrano[2,3-*c*][1]benzopyran (compound 7). However, the potent analgesic activity of the parent phenol of this series (5) was masked by its ester derivatives (6 and 7). This is in sharp contrast to the what was observed when the nitrogen and carbocyclic analogs were esterified with piperidino and morpholino moieties (Table 9). These data suggest that the size of the ring that contains sulfur is not important, but that the sulfur atom should be adjacent to the double bond in order to display pharmacological activity (1 and 5).

The effect of alkyl substitution in the alicyclic ring of sulfur (Razdan *et al.*, 1976*b*) and the carbocyclic (Razdan *et al.*, 1976*c*) analogs of DMHP has been studied by Razdan *et al.* (1976*a*). Methyl substitution at C-1 in the five-membered sulfur (2) and carbocyclic series (6) resulted in up to a 15-fold increase in analgesic activity, while the former caused a 10-fold elevation in sedative–hypnotic potency (2 compared with 1). However, the C-1 methyl analog in the five-membered carbocyclic series resulted in remarkably greater anticonvulsant activity without severely changing sedative–hypnotic potency. On the other hand, moving the methyl group from C-9 (DMHP) to C-10 did not markedly alter biological activity, thus confirming an earlier finding (Mechoulam, 1973). Hence, the authors suggest that these data point out that 9-methyl substitution in close proximity to the phenolic hydroxyl group selectively influences the activity of cannabinoids having a planar five-membered alicyclic ring.

In their original SAR study Adams and Baker (1940) uncovered the fact

TABLE 9

Pharmacological Activity of Various Basic Esters of DMHP and Its Propargyl and Cyclopentane Analogs[a]

Compound	R	Test[b]: Rat motor activity mg/kg (score)	Mouse fighting mg/kg (score)	Analgesia ED_{50}, mg/kg	Sedative–hypnotic mg/kg (TST)	Audiogenic seizure ED_{50}, mg/kg
Basic esters of propargyl analog of DMHP 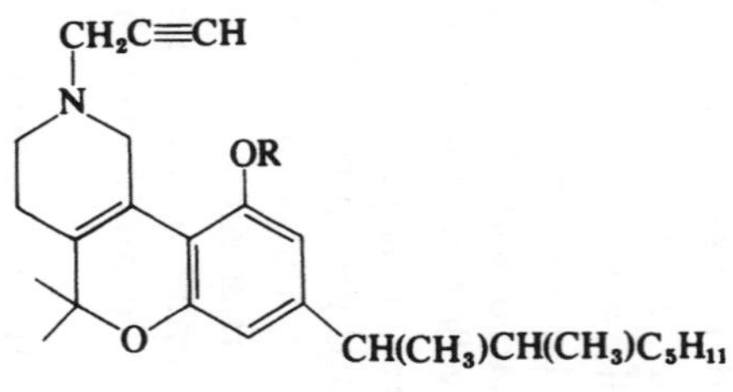						
1	—H	1 (+3)	1 (+2)	W (4.3) RTF (13.8) HP (7.7)	0.1 (+100)	—
2	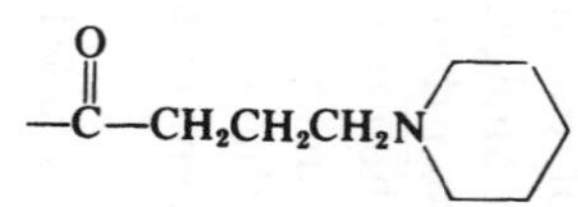	1 (+2)	5 (+2)	W (12.0) RTF (12.5) HP (4.2)	0.5 (+48)	—
3	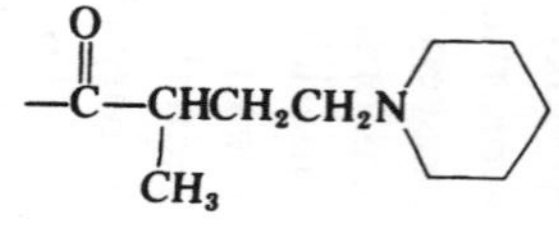	10 (+2)	Inactive @10	W (12.2) RTF (9.8)	0.5 (+45)	—

4	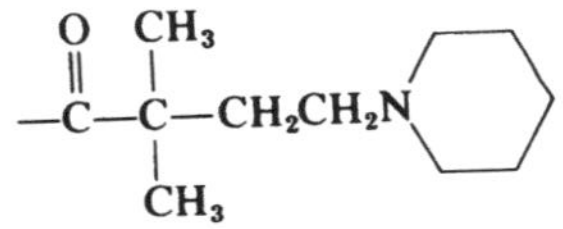	10 (+2)	Inactive @10	W (17.5) RTF (>20.0)	0.5 (+15)	—
5	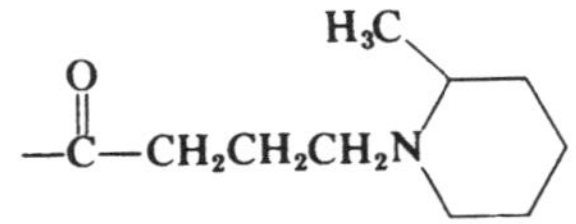	10 (+1)	10 (+1)	W (26.8)	0.5 (+92)	—
6	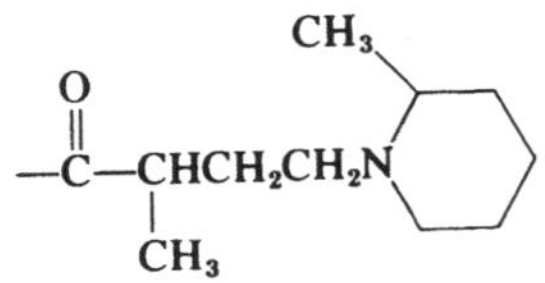	10 (+1)	Inactive @10	W (7.3) RTF (10.7)	0.5 (+38) 1.0 (+104)	— —
7	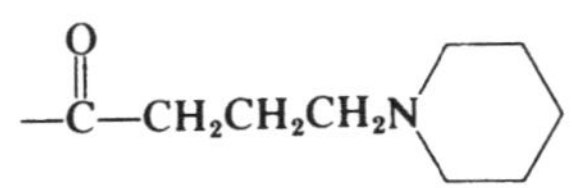 (DMH side chain replaced by C_5H_{11})	10 (+1)	5 (+1)	Inactive	—	—
8	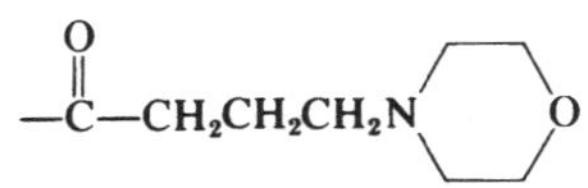	10 (+1)	5 (+2)	W (9.5) RTF (14.4)	1.0 (+30)	—
9	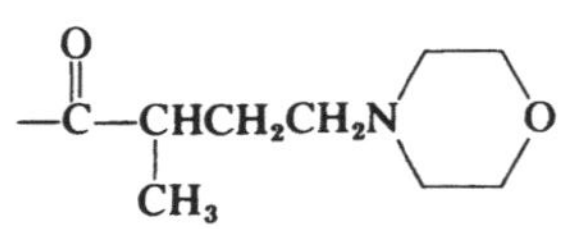	10 (+2)	10 (+1)	W (>10.0)	0.5 (+36)	—

continued

TABLE 9—*continued*

Compound	R	Test[b]: Rat motor activity mg/kg (score)	Mouse fighting mg/kg (score)	Analgesia ED_{50}, mg/kg	Sedative–hypnotic mg/kg (TST)	Audiogenic seizure ED_{50}, mg/kg
10	Bisquaternary salt of *8* $2CH_3I$	10 (+1)	10 (+2)	Inactive	—	—
Basic esters of DMHP 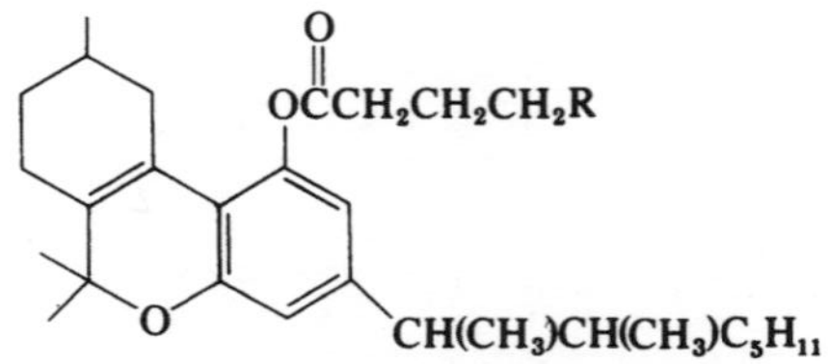						
11	—H	5 (+3)	10 (+3)	W (19.6) HP (12.4)	—	2.9
12	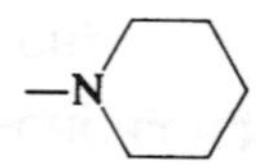 ·HCl	5 (+2)	10 (+2)	W (75.9)	—	2.8
13	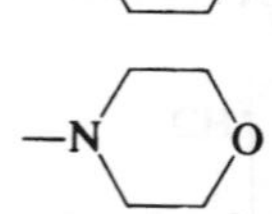 ·HBr	5 (+3)	10 (+2)	W (2.3) RTF (4.2) HP (0.5)	—	2.4
14	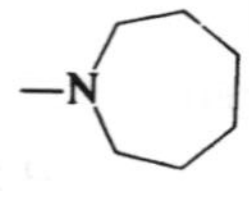	1 (+2)	5 (+2)	—	—	1.1
15	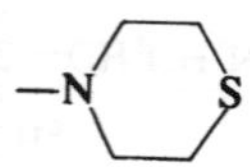	2 (+2)	—	—	—	*>100.0*

Basic esters of cyclopentane analog of DMPH 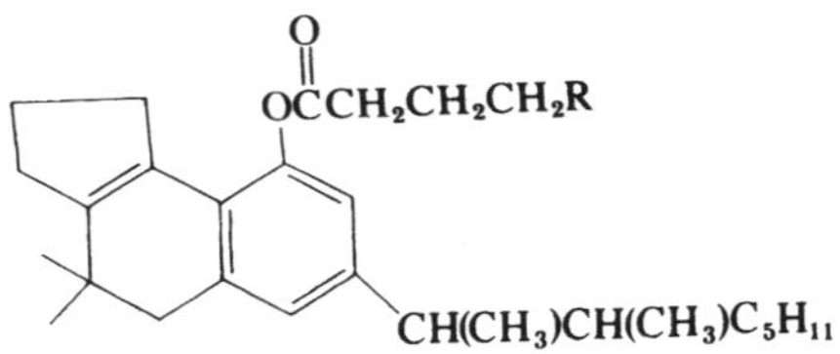						
16	—H	5 (+3)	5 (+2)	W (25.3) HP (45.1)	—	35.3
17	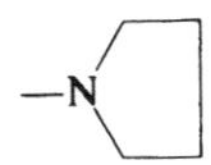 ·HCl	Inactive (a 5	Inactive (a 5	W (>20.0)	—	>100.0
	(DMH side chain replaced by C_5H_{11})					
18	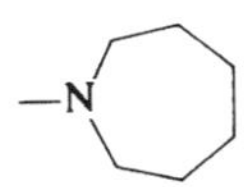 ·HCl	5 (+1)	10 (+1)	W (17.9) RTF (25.3)	—	>30.0
19	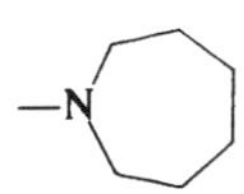 ·HCl	5 (+1)	5 (+1)	W (>20.0)	—	>100.0
	(DMH side chain replaced by C_5H_{11})					
20	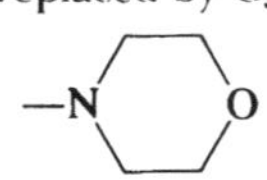	—	10 (+2)	W (13.4) HP (16.0)	—	60.0

[a] From Pars *et al.*, 1976.

[b] All drugs were administered orally. In the rat motor activity and mouse fighting tests +1, +2, and +3 correspond to inhibitions of 1–33%, 34–66%, and 67–100%, respectively. W, mouse writhing test; RTF, rat tail flick; and HP, mouse hot-plate tests for analgesia. TST = change in total sleep time.

TABLE 10
Pharmacological Activity of Various Sulfur Analogs (Basic Esters) of DMHP[a]

Compound	R	Test[b]: Rat motor activity mg/kg (score)	Test[b]: Mouse fighting mg/kg (score)	Test[b]: Analgesia ED_{50}, mg/kg
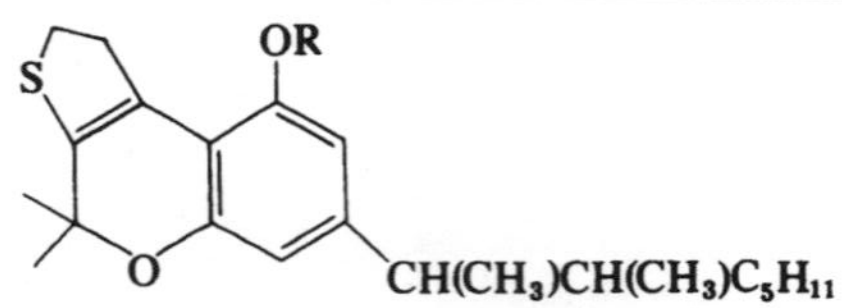				
1	—H	5 (+1)	10 (+2)	W (71.8) HP (12.1)
2	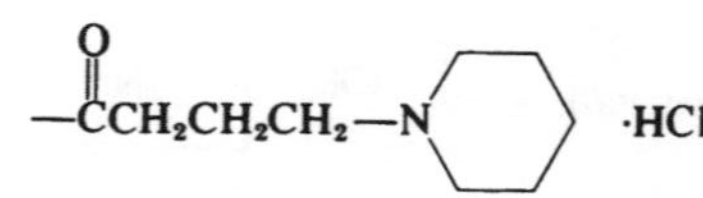	5 (+1)	10 (+2)	W (24.0)
3	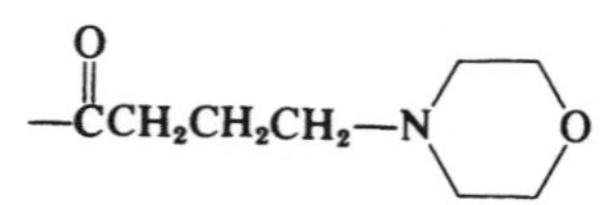	5 (+1)	10 (+2)	HP (>50.0)
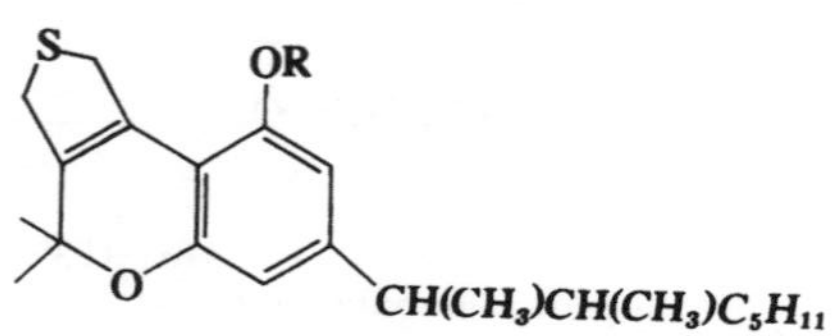				

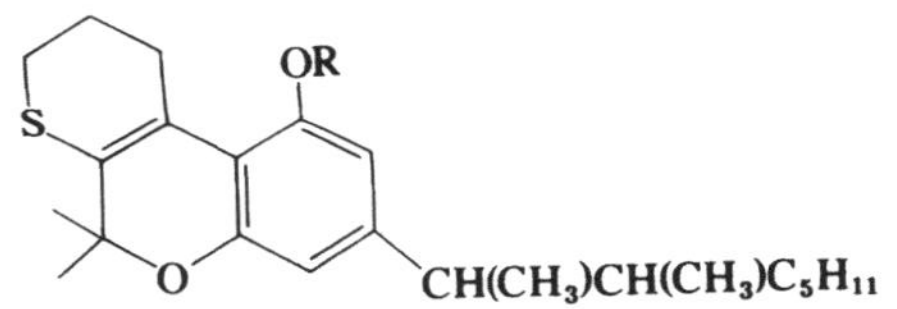

4	—H	5 (+1)	10 (+2)	W (51.7) HP (>120.0)
5	—H	5 (+1)	10 (+1)	W (8.6) HP (5.7) RTF (2.7)
6	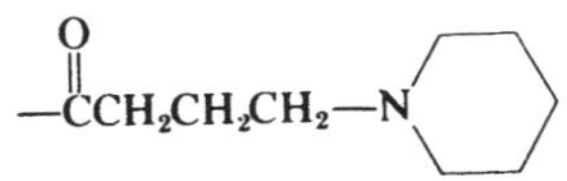 ·HCl	5 (+3)	5 (+1)	W (14.7)
7	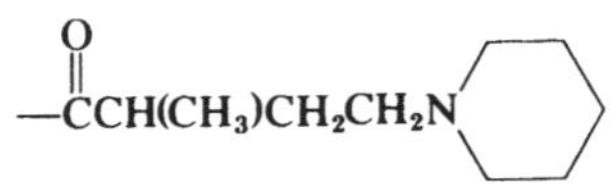 ·HCl	5 (+1)	10 (+3)	W (22.6)

continued

TABLE 10—*continued*

Compound	R	Test[b]		
		Rat motor activity mg/kg (score)	Mouse fighting mg/kg (score)	Analgesia ED_{50}, mg/kg
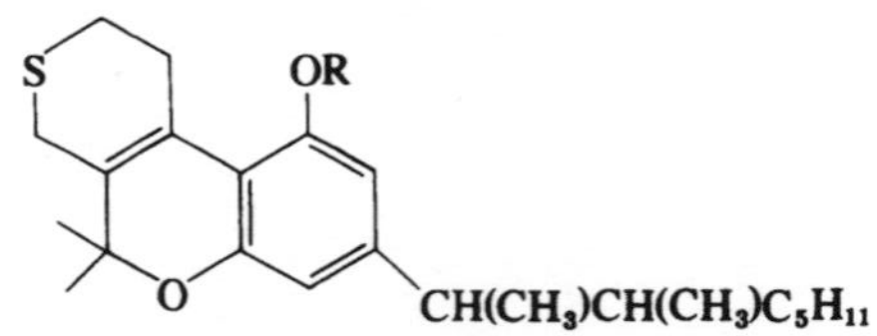 8	—H	10 (+1)	5 (+1)	W (>40.0) HP (>40.0)
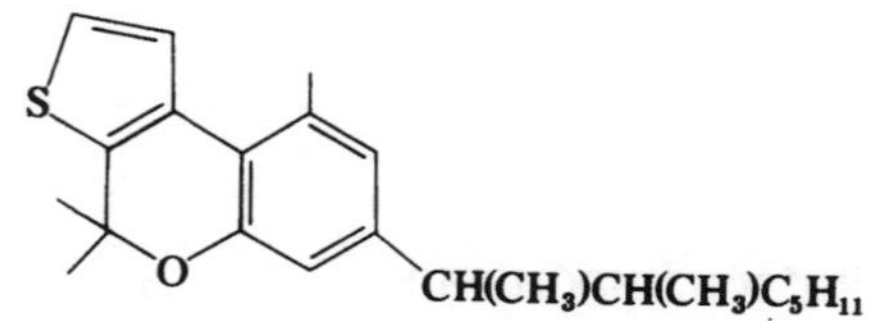 9	—H	5 (+1)	10 (+1)	W (>10.0)

[a] From Razdan *et al.*, 1976*b*.
[b] See Table 9 for explanation.

that alterations in the side chain of $\Delta^{6a,10a}$-THC, such as introduction of branched and linear aliphatic chains, profoundly influenced pharmacological activity, i.e., DMHP. As outlined above (Pars *et al.*, 1976; Razdan *et al.*, 1976*a–c*) incorporation of the 1,2-dimethylheptyl side chain into various carbocyclic and heterocyclic derivatives of $\Delta^{6a,10a}$-THC also affected biological activity. With this information at hand Winn *et al.* (1976) synthesized and tested $\Delta^{6a,10a}$-THCs and their nitrogen, sulfur, and carbocyclic analogs with an arylalkyl side chain substituent. The most potent analgesic compounds were (a) the 1-methyl-4(4-fluorophenyl)butyl derivatives of DMHP, its propargynl analogs including the basic esters and the methylated thienobenzopyran, (b) the 1,2-dimethyl-4(4-fluorophenyl)butyl derivates of DMHP and propargyl DMHP, and (c) the 1,2-dimethyl-4(4-pyridyl)butyl analog of DMHP. Maximum activity was achieved when the fluoro substitution was in the *para* position. Moreover, in tests for tranquilization, i.e., mouse fighting, rat motor activity, dog ataxia, and monkey antiaggression, the SAR nearly paralleled those for analgesia. Similar responses were observed for these compounds in reducing methamphetamine-induced hyperactivity in the rat as a measure of antipsychotic activity and sedative–hypnotic activity in the cat.

3.2. Δ^9- and Δ^8-THC Derivatives

Edery *et al.* (1972) and Loev *et al.* (1973) have reported that in rhesus monkeys and rats, respectively, changes in the side chain at C-3 in the aromatic ring caused increases in activity. These differences were not totally unexpected in light of the SAR investigations with $\Delta^{6a,10a}$-THC outlined above. The DMH derivatives of both Δ^8- and Δ^9-THC were 20 to 25 times more potent than the parent compounds in the rat (Loev *et al.*, 1973). Edery *et al.* (1972) reported that the onset occurs more rapidly while the duration of action is prolonged in rhesus monkeys for the DMH analogs of Δ^8- and Δ^9-THC. Moreover, acetylation of the phenolic hydroxyl group diminishes effectiveness, while the ether analogs display virtually no response. Activity in the monkey is markedly reduced or completely eliminated when a hydrogen on the aromatic ring of Δ^8- or Δ^9-THC is replaced with a carboxyl, carbomethoxyl, acetyl, acetoxyl, or alkyl substitution at C-4. On the other hand, alkyl substitution at C-2 on the same ring produces compounds that still retain activity.

Unlike $\Delta^{6a,10a}$-THC, only a few structural modifications of the terpenoid ring of Δ^8- and Δ^9-THC have been made. Isomeric mixtures of hexahydrocannabinol have been found to be active in the dog ataxia test while significantly altering behavior in the rhesus monkey (Mechoulam, 1973). In addition, the 10α- but not the 10β-hydroxy-Δ^8-THC was also active in these two species.

TABLE 11

Pharmacological Activity of Alkyl-Substituted Sulfur and Carbocyclic Analogs of DMHP[a]

Compound	Ring A	Test[b]: Mouse fighting mg/kg (score)	Test[b]: Analgesia ED_{50}, mg/kg	Test[b]: Sedative–hypnotic mg/kg (TST)	Test[b]: Audiogenic seizure mg/kg (score)
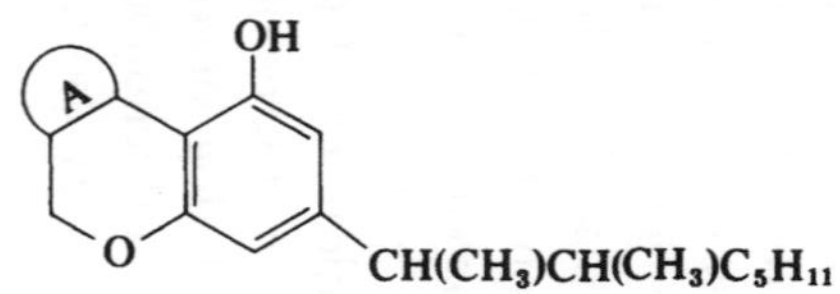					
1	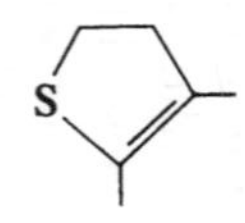	10 (+2)	W (71.8) HP (12.1)	2 (+31)	10 (+2)
2	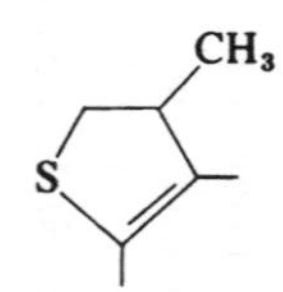	10 (+2)	W (4.7) HP (1.4)	0.25 (+50)	10 (+2)
3	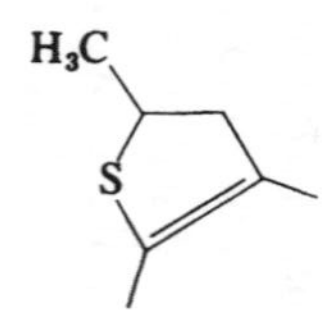	10 (+2)	W (34.0)	—	10 (+1)
4	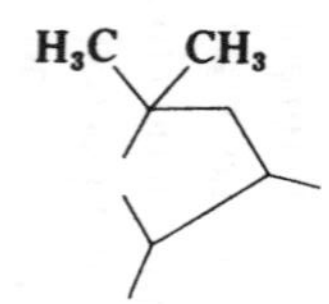	10 (+1)	W (>40.0)	—	10 (+1)

5	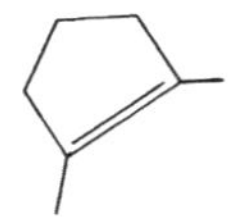	10 (+2)	W (25.3) HP (45.1)	1 (+65)	10 (+1)
6	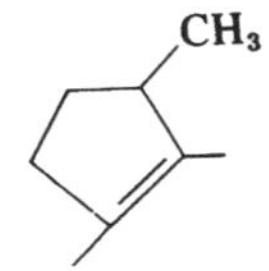	10 (+3)	W (13.3)	0.5 (+58)	10 (+3)
7	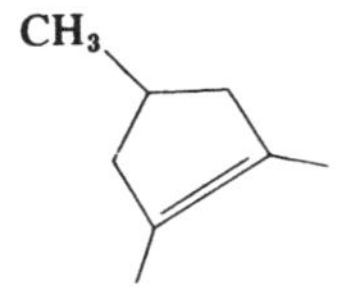	10 (+1)	W (22.6)	—	Inactive @10
8	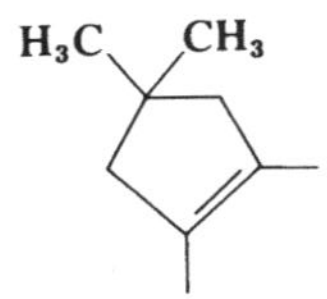	10 (+2)	W (>40.0) RTF (>40.0)	—	Inactive @10
9	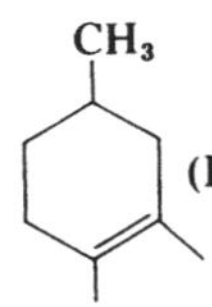 (DMHP)	10 (+3)	W (19.6) HP (12.4)	0.5 (+62)	10 (+3)
10	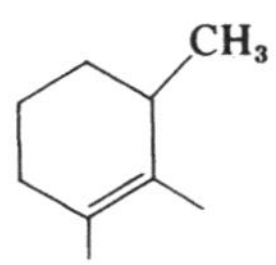	10 (+2)	W (10.5) HP (25.0)	0.5 (+54)	30 (+2)

[a] From Razdan *et al.*, 1976*a*.
[b] See Table 9 for explanation. For audiogenic seizures, +1, +2, and +3 correspond to scores for the mouse fighting.

Finally, Howes (1970) has reported on the activity of two water-soluble Δ^9-THC derivatives, one a basic ester and the other a basic ether. The ester

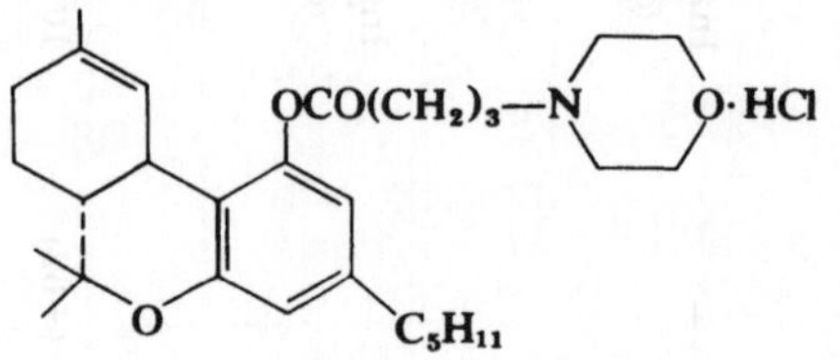

(as shown) produced similar but less pronounced effects than Δ^9-THC in the dog ataxia assay and in tests for analgesia. In addition, its onset of action was slower than Δ^9-THC, which was also observed by other investigators measuring the same parameters (Zitko *et al.*, 1972) or studying effects on operant behavior (Dykstra *et al.*, 1975). The basic ether was totally ineffective in all tests and may be related to the fact that this substance was not converted *in vitro* to Δ^9-THC as was the ester using a rat liver microsomal preparation.

4. SUMMARY AND CONCLUSIONS

The major psychoactive principle of marihuana is *l*-(*trans*)-Δ^9-tetrahydrocannabinol (Δ^9-THC), a highly viscous oil that is strongly lipophilic and totally insoluble in water. The diversity observed in the pharmacological activity of this substance described over the last several years has spawned a renewed interest in cannabinoid chemistry, which in turn has generated interest in other naturally occurring cannabinoids as well as in synthetic analogs. Structure–activity relationship (SAR) investigations have revealed some basic requirements for persistence of biological activity.

1. A benzopyran structure with a hydroxyl group at C-1 or C-3 and an alkyl group at C-3 or C-2 on the aromatic ring appears necessary. Activity was lost when the hydroxyl was placed at C-2 or C-4.
2. The aromatic hydroxyl must be free or esterified while an ether substitution inactivates the molecule.
3. Opening the pyran ring removes activity.
4. Increasing the length of the aliphatic chain on the aromatic ring considerably enhances activity. In addition, branching, i.e., a methyl or dimethyl at position 1 as well as 1,2-dimethylheptyl (DMHP), which appears optimal, also augments activity.
5. The terpenoid ring may be more drastically altered and retention of activity achieved. Other heterocyclic and carbocyclic rings containing nitrogen and sulfur may be exchanged for the terpenoid moiety. Substitution at C-1 or C-2 must be planar to the ring. Activity may also be observed if the C-11 methyl group is hydroxylated or

replaced with a hydrogen or ethyl group. In addition, hydroxylation at C-8 and alkyl substitution at C-7, C-8, or C-10 do not drastically impair biological activity.

Because of these extensive SAR investigations and the development of new cannabinoid molecular structures that possess more selective activity and/or less unwanted side effects, it does not seem unreasonable to assume that in the future a clinically effective therapeutic agent derived from these investigations will be available.

5. REFERENCES

ABEL, E. L., 1969, Effects of the marihuana homologue, pyrahexyl, on a conditioned emotional response, *Psychon. Sci.* **16:**44.

ABEL, E. L., 1970, Effects of the marihuana-homologue, pyrahexyl, on open field behaviour in the rat, *J. Pharm. Pharmacol.* **22:**785.

ABEL, E. L., 1971, Effects of marihuana on the solution of anagrams, memory and appetite, *Nature* **231:**260–261.

ABEL, E. L., and SCHIFF, B. B., 1969, Effects of the marihuana homologue, pyrahexyl, on food and water intake and curiosity in the rat, *Psychon. Sci.* **16:**38.

ADAMS, R., and BAKER, B. R., 1940, Structure of cannabidiol. VII. A method of synthesis of a tetrahydrocannabinol which possesses marihuana activity, *J. Am. Chem. Soc.* **62:**2405–2408.

ADAMS, H. R., and SOFIA, R. D., 1973, Interaction of chloramphenicol and Δ^1-tetrahydrocannabinol in barbital-anesthetized mice, *Experientia* **29:**181–182.

AGURELL, S., NILSSON, I. M., OHLSSON, A., and SANDBERG, F., 1969, Elimination of tritium-labelled cannabinols in the rat with special reference to the development of tests for the identification of cannabis users, *Biochem. Pharmacol.* **18:**1195–1201.

AGURELL, S., NILSSON, I. M., OHLSSON, A., and SANDBERG, F., 1970, On the metabolism of tritium-labelled Δ^1-tetrahydrocannabinol in the rabbit, *Biochem. Pharmacol.* **19:**1333–1339.

ALLENTUCK, S., and BOWMAN, K. M., 1942, The psychiatric aspects of marihuana intoxication, *Am. J. Psychiat.* **99:**248–251.

AMES, F., 1958, A clinical and metabolic study of acute intoxication with *Cannabis sativa* and its role in the model psychoses, *J. Ment. Sci.* **104:**972–999.

ASKEW, W. E., and HO, B. T., 1974, Effects of tetrahydrocannabinols on cyclic AMP levels in rat brain areas, *Experientia* **30:**879–880.

BANERJEE, S. P., SNYDER, S. H., and MECHOULAM, R., 1975, Cannabinoids: Influence on neurotransmitter uptake in rat brain synaptosomes, *J. Pharmacol. Exp. Ther.* **194:**74–81.

BARRY, H., III, and KUBENA, R. K., 1969, Acclimation to laboratory alters response of rats to Δ^1-tetrahydrocannabinol, in: *Proceedings of the 77th Annual Convention of the American Psychological Association*, Vol. 4, Part 2, pp. 865–866, American Psychological Association Press, Washington, D.C.

BARRY, H., III, and KUBENA, R. K., 1971, Repeated high doses of Δ^1-tetrahydrocannabinol enhance acquisition of shock avoidance in rats, in: *Proceedings of the 79th Annual Convention of the American Psychological Association*, Vol. 6, Part 2, pp. 747–748, American Psychological Association Press, Washington, D.C.

BICHER, H. I., and MECHOULAM, R., 1968, Pharmacological effects of two active constituents of marihuana, *Arch. Int. Pharmacodyn.* **172:**24–31.

BLACK, M. B., WOODS, J. H., and DOMINO, E. F., 1970, Some effects of (—)-Δ^9-*trans*-tetrahydrocannabinol and other cannabis derivatives on schedule-controlled behavior, *Pharmacologist* **12:**258.

BOGGAN, W. O., STEELE, R. A., and FREEDMAN, D. X., 1973, Δ^9-Tetrahydrocannabinol Effect on Audiogenic Seizure Susceptibility, *Psychopharmacologia* **29:**101–106.

BORGEN, L. A., and SHUMWAY, J., 1974, Comparative effects of Δ^9-tetrahydrocannabinol (Δ^9-THC), cannabidiol (CBD), and cannabinol (CBN) on timing behavior in rats, *Pharmacologist* **16:**260.

BORGEN, L. A., DAVIS, W. M., and PACE, H. B., 1971, Effects of synthetic Δ^9-tetrahydrocannabinol on pregnancy and offspring in the rat, *Tox. Appl. Pharmacol.* **40:**480–486.

BOYD, E. S., and MERITT, D. A., 1965, Effects of thiopental and a tetrahydrocannabinol derivative on arousal and recruiting in the cat, *J. Pharmacol. Exp. Ther.* **149:**138–145.

BOYD, E. S., and MERITT, D. A., 1966, Effects of barbiturates and a tetrahydrocannabinol derivative on recovery cycles of medial lemniscus, thalamus and reticular formation in the cat, *J. Pharmacol. Exp. Ther.* **151:**376–384.

BOYD, E. S., HUTCHINSON, E. D., GARDNER, L. C., and MERITT, D. A., 1963, Effects of tetrahydrocannabinols and other drugs on operant behavior in rats, *Arch. Int. Pharmacodyn.* **144:**533–554.

BROWN, H., 1972, Possible anticholinesterase-like effects of *trans*(—)Δ^8- and Δ^9-tetrahydrocannabinol as observed in the general motor activity of mice, *Psychopharmacologia* **27:**111–116.

BROWN, O. M., 1973, Effects of Δ^9-tetrahydrocannabinol (THC) on rat brain acetylcholine levels, *Pharmacologist* **15:**200.

BURSTEIN, S. H., and KUPFER, D., 1971, Hydroxylation of *trans*-Δ^1-tetrahydrocannabinol by a hepatic microsomal monooxygenase, *Chem. Biol. Interact.* **3:**316.

BURSTEIN, S., and VARANELLI, C., 1975, Transformations of cannabinol in the mouse, *Res. Comm. Chem. Pathol. Pharmacol.* **11:**343–354.

BURSTEIN, S. H., MENEZES, F., WILLIAMSON, E., and MECHOULAM, R., 1970, Metabolism of $\Delta^{1(6)}$-Tetrahydrocannabinol, an active marihuana constituent, *Nature* **225:**87–88.

BURSTEIN, S., ROSENFELD, J., and WITTSTRUCK, T., 1972, Isolation and characterization of two major urinary metabolites of Δ^1-tetrahydrocannabinol, *Science* **176:**422–423.

BUXBAUM, D. M., 1972, Analgesic activity of Δ^9-tetrahydrocannabinol in the rat and mouse, *Psychopharmacologia* **25:**275–280.

BYCK, R., and RITCHIE, J. M., 1973, Δ^9-Tetrahydrocannabinol: Effects on mammalian nonmyelinated nerve fibers, *Science* **180:**84–85.

CHESHER, G. B., DAHL, C. J., EVERINGHAM, M., JACKSON, D. M., MARCHANT-WILLIAMS, H., and STARMER, G. A., 1973, The effect of cannabinoids on intestinal motility and their antinociceptive effect in mice, *Br. J. Pharmacol.* **49:**588–594.

CHESHER, G. B., JACKSON, D. M., and STARMER, G. A., 1974, Interaction of cannabis and general anaesthetic agents in mice, *Br. J. Pharmacol.* **50:**593–599.

CHESHER, G. B., and JACKSON, D. M., 1974, Anticonvulsant effects of cannabinoids in mice: Drug interactions within cannabinoids and cannabinoid interactions with phenytoin, *Psychopharmacologia* **37:**255–264.

CHRISTENSEN, H. D., FREUDENTHAL, R. I., GIDLEY, J. T., ROSENFELD, R., BOEGLI, G., TESTINO, L., BRINE, D. R., PITT, C. G., and WALL, M. E., 1971, Activity of Δ^8- and Δ^9-Tetrahydrocannabinol and related compounds in the mouse, *Science* **172:**165–167.

CHRISTIANSEN, J., and RAFAELSEN, O. J., 1969, Cannabis metabolites in urine after oral administration, *Psychopharmacologia* **15:**60–63.

COLDWELL, B. B., BAILEY, K., PAUL, C. J., and ANDERSON, G., 1974, Interaction of cannabinoids with pentobarbital in rats, *Tox. Appl. Pharmacol.* **29:**59–69.

CONRAD, D. G., ELSMORE, T. F., and SODETZ, F. J., 1972, Δ^9-Tetrahydrocannabinol: Dose-related effects on timing behavior in chimpanzee, *Science* **175:**547–550.

Consroe, P. F., and Man, D. P., 1973, Effects of Δ^8- and Δ^9-Tetrahydrocannabinol on experimentally induced seizures, *Life Sci.* **13:**429–439.

Consroe, P. F., Man, D. P., Chin, L., and Picchioni, A. L., 1973, Reduction of audiogenic seizure by Δ^8- and Δ^9-Tetrahydrocannabinols, *J. Pharm. Pharmacol.* **25:**764–765.

Coper, H., and Fernandes, M., 1973, Interaction between cannabis and other drugs, in: *Bayer Symposium IV, Psychic Dependence* (L. Goldberg and F. Hoffmeister, eds.), pp. 135–141, Springer-Verlag, New York.

Corcoran, M. E., McCaughran, J. A., Jr., and Wada, J. A., 1973, Acute antiepileptic effects of Δ^9-tetrahydrocannabinol in rats with kindled seizures, *Exp. Neurol.* **40:**471–483.

Corcoran, M. E., Bolotow, I., Amit, Z., and McCaughran, J. A., Jr., 1974, Conditioned taste aversions produced by active and inactive cannabinoids, *Pharmacol. Biochem. Behav.* **2:**725–728.

Dagirmanjian, R., and Boyd, E. S., 1962, Some pharmacological effects of two tetrahydrocannabinols, *J. Pharmacol. Exp. Ther.* **135:**25–33.

Davis, W. M., and Borgen, L. A., 1974, Effects of cannabidiol and Δ^9-tetrahydrocannabinol on operant behavior, *Res. Comm. Chem. Pathol. Pharmacol.* **9:**453–462.

Delini-Stula, A., 1973, Suppression of conditioned avoidance behavior and the development of tolerance to Δ^8-Tetrahydrocannabinol and dimethylheptylpyran in rats, *Pharmakopsychiat. Neuro-Psychopharmacol.* **6:**189–197.

Dewey, W. L., Kennedy, J. S., and Howes, J. F., 1970, Some autonomic, gastrointestinal, and metabolic effects of two constituents of marihuana, *Fed. Proc.* **29:**650.

Dewey, W. L., Harris, L. S., and Kennedy, J. S., 1972, Some pharmacological and toxicological effects of 1-*trans*-Δ^8- and 1-*trans*-Δ^9-tetrahydrocannabinol in laboratory rodents, *Arch. Int. Pharmacodyn. Ther.* **196:**133–145.

de Zeeuw, R. A., Wijsbeek, J., Breimer, D. D., Vree, T. B., van Ginneken, C. A. M., and van Rossum, J. M., 1972, Cannabinoids with a propyl side chain in cannabis: Occurrence and chromatographic behavior, *Science* **175:**778–779.

de Zeeuw, R. A., Vree, T. B., Breimer, D. D., and van Ginneken, C. A. M., 1973, Cannabivarichromene, a new cannabinoid with a propyl side chain in cannabis, *Experientia* **29:**260–261.

Dingell, J. V., Miller, K. W., Heath, E. C., and Klausner, H. A., 1973, The intracellular localization of Δ^9-tetrahydrocannabinol in liver and its effects on drug metabolism *in vitro*, *Biochem. Pharmacol.* **22:**949–958.

Dolby, T. W., and Kleinsmith, L. J., 1974, Effects of Δ^9-tetrahydrocannabinol on the levels of cyclic adenosine 3′,5′-Monophosphate in mouse brain, *Biochem. Pharmacol.* **23:**1817–1825.

Dubinsky, B., Robichaud, R. C., and Goldberg, M. E., 1973, Effects of (—) Δ^9-*trans*-tetrahydrocannabinol and its selectivity in several models of aggressive behavior, *Pharmacology* **9:**204–216.

Dykstra, L. A., McMillan, D. E., and Harris, L. S., 1975, Effects of Δ^9-THC and a water soluble ester of Δ^9-THC on schedule-controlled behavior, *Pharmacol. Biochem. Behav.* **3:**29–32.

Edery, H., and Gottesfeld, Z., 1975, The γ-aminobutyric acid system in rat cerebellum during cannabinoid-induced cataleptoid state, *Brit. J. Pharmacol.* **54:**406–408.

Edery, H., Grunfeld, Y., Porath, G., Ben-Zvi, Z., Shani, A., and Mechoulam, R., 1972, Structure-activity relationships in the tetrahydrocannabinol series, *Arzneim.-Forsch.* **22:**1995–2003.

Elsmore, T. F., 1972, Effects of delta-9-tetrahydrocannabinol on temporal and auditory discrimination performances of monkeys, *Psychopharmacologia* **26:**62–72.

Elsmore, T. F., and Fletcher, G. V., 1972, Δ^9-Tetrahydrocannabinol: Aversive effects in rat at high doses, *Science* **175:**911–912.

Estevez, V. S., Englert, L. F., and Ho, B. T., 1973, A new methylated metabolite of (—)-11-hydroxy-Δ⁸-tetrahydrocannabinol in rats, *Res. Comm. Chem. Pathol. Pharmacol.* **6**:821–827.

Estevez, V. S., Englert, L. F., and Ho, B. T., 1974, Effect of SKF-525-A on the metabolism of (—)-Δ⁹-tetrahydrocannabinol in the rat brain and liver, *Res. Comm. Chem. Pathol. Pharmacol.* **8**:389–392.

Fernandes, M., Warning, N., Christ, W., and Hill, R., 1973, Interactions of several cannabinoids with the hepatic drug metabolizing system, *Biochem. Pharmacol.* **22**:2981–2987.

Ferraro D. P., and Billings, D. K., 1972, Comparison of behavioral effects of synthetic (—)-Δ⁹-*trans*-tetrahydrocannabinol and marihuana extract distillate in chimpanzees, *Psychopharmacologia* **25**:169–174.

Ferraro, D. P., Lynch, W. C., and Grilly, D. M., 1972, Behavioral effects of small oral doses of marihuana extract in chimpanzees, *Pharmacology* **7**:273–282.

Ferraro, D. P., Gluck, J. P., and Herndon, G. B., 1974, Acquisition and extinction of variable interval schedule behavior by rats under Δ⁹-tetrahydrocannabinol, *Pharmacol. Biochem. Behav.* **2**:487–491.

Fetterman, P. S., and Turner, C. E., 1972, Constituents of *Cannabis sativa* L. I: Propyl homologs of cannabinoids from an Indian variant, *J. Pharm. Sci.* **61**:1476–1477.

Foltz, R. L., Fentiman, A. F., Jr., Leighty, E. G., Walter, J. L., Drewes, H. R., Schwartz, W. E., Page, T. F., Jr., and Truitt, E. B., Jr., 1970, Metabolite of (—)-*trans*-Δ⁸-tetrahydrocannabinol: Identification and synthesis, *Science* **168**:844–845.

Forney, R. B., 1971, Toxicology of marihuana, *Pharmacol. Rev.* **23**:279–284.

Frankenheim, J. M., 1974, Effects of repeated doses of 1-Δ⁸-*trans*-tetrahydrocannabinol on schedule-controlled temporally-spaced responding of rats, *Psychopharmacologia* **38**:125–144.

Frankenheim, J. M., McMillan, D. E., and Harris, L. S., 1971, Effects of 1-Δ⁹- and 1-Δ⁸-*trans*-tetrahydrocannabinol and cannabinol on schedule-controlled behavior of pigeons and rats, *J. Pharmacol. Exp. Ther.* **178**:241–252.

Friedman, E., and Gershon, S., 1974, Tetrahydrocannabinols: Inhibition in acetylcholine synthesis in regional rat brain slices, *Pharmacologist* **16**:286.

Gaoni, Y., and Mechoulam, R., 1964, Isolation, structure, and partial synthesis of an active constituent of hashish, *J. Amer. Chem. Soc.* **86**:1646–1647.

Gaoni, Y., and Mechoulam, R., 1971, The isolation and structure of Δ¹-tetrahydrocannabinol and other neutral cannabinoids from hashish, *J. Amer. Chem. Soc.* **93**:217–224.

Garriott, J. C., King, L. J., Forney, R. B., and Hughes, F. W., 1967, Effects of some tetrahydrocannabinols on hexobarbital sleeping time and amphetamine-induced hyperactivity in mice, *Life Sci.* **6**:2119–2128.

Garriott, J. C., Forney, R. B., Hughes, F. W., and Richards, A. B., 1968, Pharmacologic properties of some cannabis related compounds, *Arch. Int. Pharmacodyn.* **171**:425–434.

Gill, E. W., and Jones, G., 1972, Brain levels of Δ¹-tetrahydrocannabinol and its metabolites in mice—Correlation with behaviour, and the effect of the metabolic inhibitors SKF 525-A and piperonyl butoxide, *Biochem. Pharmacol.* **21**:2237–2248.

Gill, E. W., Paton, W. D. M., and Pertwee, R. G., 1970, Preliminary experiments in the chemistry and pharmacology of cannabis, *Nature* **228**:134–136.

Gill, E. W., Jones, G., and Lawrence, D. K., 1973, Contribution of the metabolite 7-hydroxy-Δ¹-tetrahydrocannabinol towards the pharmacological activity of Δ¹-tetrahydrocannabinol in mice, *Biochem. Pharmacol.* **22**:175–184.

Glick, S. D., and Milloy, S., 1972, Increased and decreased eating following THC administration, *Psychon. Sci.* **29**:6.

Grinspoon, L., 1971, *Marihuana Reconsidered,* Harvard University Press, Cambridge, Mass.

Grunfeld, Y., and Edery, H., 1969, Psychopharmacological activity of the active constituents of hashish and some related cannabinoids, *Psychopharmacologia* **14**:200–210.

Gurny, O., Maynard, D. E., Pitcher, R. G., and Kierstead, R. W., 1972, Novel *in vitro* metabolites of (—)-Δ⁸- and (—)-Δ⁹-tetrahydrocannabinol (THC), *5th Intl. Cong. Pharmacol.*, p. 92.

HAAVIK, C. O., and HARDMAN, H. F., 1973*a*, Evaluation of the hypothermic action of tetrahydrocannabinols in mice and squirrel monkeys, *J. Pharmacol. Exp. Ther.* **187**:568–574.

HAAVIK, C. O., and HARDMAN, H. F., 1973*b*, Hypothermic action of Δ⁹-tetrahydrocannabinol, 11-hydroxy-Δ⁹-tetrahydrocannabinol and 11-hydroxy-Δ⁸-tetrahydrocannabinol in mice, *Life Sci.* **13**:1771–1778.

HARRIS, R. T., WATERS, W., and MCLENDON, D., 1972, Behavioral effects in rhesus monkeys of repeated intravenous doses of Δ⁹-tetrahydrocannabinol, *Psychopharmacologia* **26**:297–306.

HINE, B., FRIEDMAN, E., TORRELIO, M., and GERSHON, S., 1975*a*, Morphine-dependent rats: blockade of precipitated abstinence by tetrahydrocannabinol, *Science* **187**:443–445.

HINE, B., FRIEDMAN, E., TORRELIO, M., and GERSHON, S., 1975*b*, Tetrahydrocannabinol-attenuated abstinence and induced rotation in morphine-dependent rats: Possible involvement of dopamine, *Neuropharmacology* **14**:607–610.

HO, B. T., FRITCHIE, G. E., KRALIK, P. M., ENGLERT, L. F., MCISAAC, W. M., and IDANPAAN-HEIKKILA, J., 1970, Distribution of tritiated-1-Δ⁹-tetrahydrocannabinol in rat tissues after inhalation, *J. Pharm. Pharmacol.* **22**:538–539.

HO, B. T., ESTEVEZ, V., ENGLERT, L. F., and MCISAAC, W. M., 1972*a*, Δ⁹-Tetrahydrocannabinol and its metabolites in monkey brains, *J. Pharm. Pharmacol.* **24**:414–416.

HO, B. T., TAYLOR, D., FRITCHIE, G. E., ENGLERT, L. F., and MCISAAC, W. M., 1972*b*, Neuropharmacological study of Δ⁹- and Δ⁸-1-tetrahydrocannabinols in monkeys and mice, *Brain Res.* **38**:163–170.

HO, B. T., ESTEVEZ, V. S., and ENGLERT, L. F., 1973*a*, The uptake and metabolic fate of cannabinoids in rat brains, *J. Pharm. Pharmacol.* **25**:488–490.

HO, B. T., ESTEVEZ, V. S., and ENGLERT, L. F., 1973*b*, Effect of repeated administration on the metabolism of (—)-Δ⁹-tetrahydrocannabinols in rats, *Res. Comm. Chem. Path. Pharmacol.* **5**:215–218.

HO, B. T., TAYLOR, D., and ENGLERT, L. F., 1973*c*, The effect of repeated administration of (—)-Δ⁹-tetrahydrocannabinol on the biosynthesis of brain amines, *Res. Comm. Chem. Path. Pharmacol.* **5**:851–854.

HOCKMAN, C. H., PERRIN, R. G., and KALANT, H., 1971, Electroencephalographic and behavioral alterations produced by Δ¹-tetrahydrocannabinol, *Science* **172**:968–970.

HOLLISTER, L. E., 1971, Hunger and appetite after single doses of marihuana, alcohol, and dextroamphetamine, *Clin. Pharmacol. Therap.* **12**:44–49.

HOLTZMAN, D., LOVELL, R. A., JAFFE, J. H., and FREEDMAN, D. X., 1969, 1-Δ⁹-Tetrahydrocannabinol: neurochemical and behavioral effects in the mouse, *Science* **163**:1464–1467.

HOWES, J. F., 1970, A study of two water soluble derivatives of Δ⁹-tetrahydrocannabinol, *Pharmacologist* **12**:758.

JARBE, T. U. C., and HENRIKSSON, B. G., 1973, Effects of Δ⁸-THC, and Δ⁹-THC on the acquisition of a discriminative positional habit in rats, *Psychopharmacologia* **31**:321–332.

JARBE, T. U. C., and HENRIKSSON, B. G., 1974, Discriminative response control produced with hashish, tetrahydrocannabinols (Δ⁸-THC and Δ⁹-THC), and other drugs, *Psychopharmacologia* **40**:1–16.

JOHNSON, K. M., and DEWEY, W. L., 1975, Structure–activity relationships of the cannabinoids in blocking synaptosomal serotonin uptake, *Pharmacologist* **17**:182.

JUST, W. W., ERDMANN, G., THEL, S., WERNER, G., and WIECHMANN, M., 1975, Metabolism and autoradiographic distribution of Δ⁸- and Δ⁹-tetrahydrocannabinol in some organs of the monkey *Callithrix jacchus*, *N.-S. Arch. Pharmacol.* **287**:219–225.

KARBOWSKI, M., JAGODA, A., DEWEY, W. L., and HARRIS, L. S., 1975, Effect of Δ⁹-THC on the level and turnover of acetylcholine in mouse brain, *Pharmacologist* **17**:254.

KARLER, R., CELY, W., and TURKANIS, S. A., 1973, The anticonvulsant activity of cannabidiol and cannabinol, *Life Sci.* **13**:1527–1531.

KARLER, R., CELY, W., and TURKANIS, S. A., 1974*a*, Anticonvulsant properties of Δ^9-tetrahydrocannabinol and other cannabinoids, *Life Sci.* **15:**931–947.

KARLER, R., CELY, W., and TURKANIS, S. A., 1974*b*, A study of the development of tolerance to an anticonvulsant effect of Δ^9-tetrahydrocannabinol and cannabidiol *Res. Comm. Chem. Pathol. Pharmacol.* **9:**23–39.

KARLER, R., CELY, W., and TURKANIS, S. A., 1974*c*, A study of the relative anticonvulsant and toxic activities of Δ^9-tetrahydrocannabinol and its congeners, *Res. Comm. Chem. Pathol. Pharmacol.* **7:**353–358.

KARNIOL, I. G., and CARLINI, E. A., 1973*a*, Comparative studies in man and in laboratory animals on Δ^8- and Δ^9-*trans*-tetrahydrocannabinol, *Pharmacology* **9:**115–126.

KARNIOL, I. G., and CARLINI, E. A., 1973*b*, Pharmacological interaction between cannabidiol and Δ^9-tetrahydrocannabinol, *Psychopharmacologia* **33:**53–70.

KARNIOL, I. G., TAKAHASHI, R. N., and MUSTY, R. E., 1974, Effects of Δ^9-tetrahydrocannabinol and cannabinol on operant performance in rats, *Arch. Int. Pharmacodyn. Ther.* **212:**230–237.

KAYAALP, S. O., KAYMAKCALAN, S., VERIMER, T., ILHAN, M., and ONUR, R., 1974, *In vitro* neuromuscular effects of Δ^9-*trans*-tetrahydrocannabinol (THC), *Arch. Int. Pharmacodyn. Ther.* **212:**67–75.

KAYMAKCALAN, S., and DENEAU, G. A., 1971, Some pharmacological effects of synthetic Δ^9-tetrahydrocannabinol, *Pharmacologist* **13:**247.

KAYMAKCALAN, S., TURKER, R. K., and TURKER, M. N., 1974, Analgesic effect of Δ^9-tetrahydrocannabinol in the dog, *Psychopharmacologia* **35:**123–128.

KILLAM, K. F., and KILLAM, E. K., 1972, The action of tetrahydrocannabinol on EEG and photomyoclonic seizures in the baboon, 5th Intl. Cong. Pharmacol., p. 124.

KING, L. J., and FORNEY, R. B., 1967, The absorption and excretion of the marihuana constituents, cannabinol and tetrahydrocannabinol, *Fed. Proc.* **26:**540.

KLAUSNER, H. A., and DINGELL, J. V., 1971, The metabolism and excretion of Δ^9-tetrahydrocannabinol in the rat, *Life Sci.* **10:**49–59.

KLAUSNER, H. A., WILCOX, H. G., and DINGELL, J. V., 1971, Studies on the interaction of Δ^9-tetrahydrocannabinol with plasma lipoproteins, *Acta Pharmaceut. Suecica* **8:**705–706.

KLAUSNER, H. A., WILCOX, H. G., and DINGELL, J. V., 1975, The use of zonal ultracentrifugation in the investigation of the binding of Δ^9-tetrahydrocannabinol by plasma lipoproteins, *Drug Metab. Disp.* **3:**314–319.

KOSERSKY, D. S., MCMILLAN, D. E., and HARRIS, L. S., 1974, Δ^9-Tetrahydrocannabinol and 11-hydroxy-Δ^9-tetrahydrocannabinol: Behavioral effects and tolerance development, *J. Pharmacol. Exp. Ther.* **189:**61–65.

KREUZ, D. S., and AXELROD, J., 1973, Delta-9-tetrahydrocannabinol: Localization in body fat, *Science* **179:**391–393.

KUBENA, R. K., 1970, Behavioral and physiological effects of delta-1-tetrahydrocannabinol, Ph.D. Thesis, University of Pittsburgh, pp. 82–86.

KUBENA, R. K., and BARRY, H., III, 1970, Interactions of Δ^1-tetrahydrocannabinol with barbiturates and methamphetamine, *J. Pharmacol. Exp. Ther.* **173:**94–100.

KUBENA, R. K., and BARRY, H., III, 1972, Stimulus characteristics of marihuana components, *Nature* **235:**397–398.

LAPA, A. J., SAMPAIO, C. A. M., TIMO-IARIA, C., and VALLE, J. R., 1968, Blocking action of tetrahydrocannabinol upon transmission in the trigeminal system of the cat, *J. Pharm. Pharmacol.* **20:**373–376.

LEMBERGER, L., SILBERSTEIN, S. D., AXELROD, J., and KOPIN, I. J., 1970, Marihuana: Studies on the disposition and metabolism of delta-9-tetrahydrocannabinol in man, *Science* **170:**1320–1322.

LEMBERGER, L., CRABTREE, R. E., and ROWE, H. M., 1972, 11-Hydroxy-Δ^9-Tetrahydrocannabinol: Pharmacology, disposition, and metabolism of a major metabolite of marihuana in man, *Science* **177:**62–64.

LEMBERGER, L., MCMAHON, R. E., ARCHER, R. A., MATSUMOTO, K., and ROWE, H., 1973, The *in vitro* and *in vivo* metabolism of $\Delta^{6a,10a}$ dimethyl heptal tetrahydrocannabinol (DMHP), *J. Pharmacol. Exp. Ther.* **187:**169–175.

LEONARD, B. E., 1971, The effect of $\Delta^{1,6}$-tetrahydrocannabinol on biogenic amines and their amino acid precursors in the rat brain, *Pharmacol. Res. Comm.* **3:**139–145.

LIPPARINI, F., SCOTTI DE CAROLIS, A., and LONGO, V. G., 1969, A neuropharmacological investigation of some *trans*-tetrahydrocannabinol derivatives, *Physiol. Behav.* **4:**527–532.

LIU, R. K., 1974, Hypothermic effects of marihuana, marihuana derivatives and chlorpromazine in laboratory mice, *Res. Comm. Chem. Path. Pharmacol.* **9:**215–228.

LOEV, B., BENDER, P. E., DOWALO, F., MACKO, E., and FOWLER, P. J., 1973, Cannabinoids. Structure-activity studies related to 1,2-dimethylheptyl derivatives, *J. Med. Chem.* **16:**1200–1206.

LOEWE, S., 1946, Studies on the pharmacology and acute toxicity of compounds with marihuana activity, *J. Pharmacol. Exp. Ther.* **88:**154–161.

LOMAX, P., 1971, Acute tolerance to the hypothermic effect of marihuana in the rat, *Res. Comm. Chem. Pathol. Pharmacol.* **2:**159–167.

MAITRE, L., 1971, Effects of some cannabinols on biosynthesis of brain amines and on pituitary response in the rat, *Acta Pharmaceut. Suecica* **8:**693–694.

MAITRE, L., STAEHELIN, M., and BEIN, H. J., 1970, Effect of an extract of cannabis and of some cannabinols on catecholamine metabolism in rat brain and heart, *Agents and Actions* **1:**136–143.

MANNING, F. J., MCDONOUGH, J. H., JR., ELSMORE, T. F., SALLER, C., and SODETZ, F. J., 1971, Inhibition of normal growth by chronic administration of Δ^9-tetrahydrocannabinol, *Science* **174:**424–426.

MARIHUANA AND HEALTH, Fourth Report to the United States Congress, From the Secretary of Health, Education and Welfare, United States Government Printing Office, 1974, pp. 15–29.

MASUR, J., and KHAZAN, N., 1970, Induction by *Cannabis sativa* (marihuana) of rhythmic spike discharges overriding REM sleep electrocorticogram in the rat, *Life Sci.* **9:**1275–1280.

MAYNARD, D. E., GURNY, O., PITCHER, R. G., and KIERSTEAD, R. W., 1971, (—)-Δ^8-Tetrahydrocannabinol: Two novel *in vitro* metabolites, *Experientia* **27:**1154–1155.

MCCAUGHRAN, J. A., JR., CORCORAN, M. E., and WADA, J. A., 1974, Anticonvulsant activity of Δ^8- and Δ^9-tetrahydrocannabinol in rats, *Pharmacol. Biochem. Behav.* **2:**227–233.

MCMILLAN, D. E., HARRIS, L. S., FRANKENHEIM, J. M., and KENNEDY, J. S., 1970, 1-Δ^9-*trans*-Tetrahydrocannabinol in pigeons: Tolerance to the behavioral effects, *Science* **169:**501–503.

MCMILLAN, D. E., FORD, R. D., FRANKENHEIM, J. M., HARRIS, R. A., and HARRIS, L. S., 1972, Tolerance to active constituents of marihuana, *Arch. Int. Pharmacodyn. Ther.* **198:**132–144.

MCMILLAN, D. E., DEWEY, W. L., TURK, R. F., HARRIS, L. S., and MCNEIL, J. H., JR., 1973, Blood levels of ^3H-Δ^9-tetrahydrocannabinol and its metabolites in tolerant and nontolerant pigeons, *Biochem. Pharmacol.* **22:**383–397.

MECHOULAM, R., 1970, Marihuana chemistry, *Science* **168:**1159–1166.

MECHOULAM, R., 1973, *Marijuana Chemistry, Pharmacology, Metabolism and Clinical Effects*, Academic Press, New York.

MIKES, F., HOFMANN, A., and WASER, P. G., 1971, Identification of (—)-Δ^9-6a,10a-*trans*-tetrahydrocannabinol and two of its metabolites in rats by use of combination gas chromatography-mass spectrometry and mass fragmentography, *Biochem. Pharmacol.* **20:**2469–2476.

MIKURIYA, T. H., 1969, Marijuana in medicine: Past, present and future, *Calif. Med.* **110:**34–40.

MORETON, J. E., and DAVIS, W. M., 1970 Effects of Δ^9-tetrahydrocannabinol on locomotor activity and on phases of sleep, *Pharmacologist* **12:**258.

NAHAS, G. G., 1973, *Marihuana—Deceptive Weed,* Raven Press, New York.

NILSSON, I. M., AGURELL, S., NILSSON, J. L. G., OHLSSON, A., SANDBERG, F., and WAHLQVIST, M., 1970, Δ^1-Tetrahydrocannabinol: Structure of a major metabolite, *Science* **168:**1228–1229.

NILSSON, I. M., AGURELL, S., NILSSON, J. L. G., OHLSSON, A., LINDGREN, J.-E., and MECHOULAM, R., 1973*a*, Metabolism of 7-hydroxy-$\Delta^{1(6)}$-tetrahydrocannabinol in the rabbit, *Acta Pharmaceut. Suecica* **10:**97–106.

NILSSON, I., AGURELL, S., NILSSON, J. L. G., WIDMAN, M., and LEANDER, K., 1973*b*, Two cannabidiol metabolites formed by rat liver, *J. Pharm. Pharmacol.* **25:**486–487.

NORDQVIST, M., and WIDMAN, M., 1975, Metabolism of Δ^1-tetrahydrocannabinol by lung and liver from dog, *Sixth Intl. Cong. Pharmacol.,* p. 266.

NORDQVIST, M., AGURELL, S., BINDER, M., *et al.* Nilsson, I. M., 1974, Structure of an acidic metabolite of Δ^1-tetrahydrocannabinol isolated from rabbit urine, *J. Pharm. Pharmacol.* **26:**471–473.

PAGE, J. G., and WEST, L. E., 1975, Acute tolerance to hypothermia in rats produced by *dl*-3-(1,1-dimethylheptyl)-6aβ, 7, 8, 10, 10aα hexahydro-1-hydroxy-6,6-dimethyl-9H-dibenzo b,d pyran-9-One (Lilly Compound 109514), *Pharmacologist* **17:**211.

PARS, H. G., GRANCHELLI, F. E., RAZDAN, R. K., KELLER, J. K., TEIGER, D. G., ROSENBERG, F. J., and HARRIS, L. S., 1976, Drugs derived from cannabinoids—Part I. Nitrogen analogs: benzopyranopyridines and benzopyranopyrroles, *J. Med. Chem.* **19:**445–454.

PATON, W. D. M., 1975, Pharmacology of marijuana, *Ann. Rev. Pharmacol.* **15:**191–220.

PATON, W. D. M., and CROWN, J., 1972, *Cannabis and Its Derivatives, Pharmacology and Applied Psychology,* Oxford Univ. Press, London.

PETRZILKA, T., and SIKEMEIER, C., 1967, Compounds of hashish. II. Synthesis of (−)-delta-6,1-3,4 *trans*-tetrahydrocannabinol and (+)-delta-6,1-3,4 *trans*-tetrahydrocannabinol, *Helv. Chim. Acta* **50:**2111–2113.

PHILLIPS, R. N., BROWN, D. J., and FORNEY, R. B., 1971*a*, Enhancement of depressant properties of alcohol or barbiturate in combination with aqueous suspended Δ^9-tetrahydrocannabinol in rats, *J. Forensic Sci.* **16:**152–161.

PHILLIPS, R. N., NEEL, M. A., BROWN, D. J., and FORNEY, R. B., 1971*b*, Enhancement of caffeine or methamphetamine stimulation in mice with aqueous-suspended Δ^9-tetrahydrocannabinol, *Pharmacologist* **13:**297.

PHILLIPS, R. N., BROWN, D. J., MARTZ, R., HUBBARD, J. D., and FORNEY, R. B., 1972, Subacute toxicity of aqueous-suspended Δ^9-tetrahydrocannabinol in rats, *Tox. Appl. Pharmacol.* **22:**45–49.

RATING, E., BROERMANN, I., HONECKER, H., KLUWE, S., and COPER, H., 1972, Effect of subchronic treatment with (−) Δ^8-*trans*-tetrahydrocannabinol (Δ^8-THC) on food intake, body temperature, hexobarbital sleeping time and hexobarbital elimination in rats, *Psychopharmacologia* **27:**349–357.

RAZDAN, R. K., HANDRICK, G. R., DALZELL, H. C., HOWES, J. F., WINN, M., PLOTNIKOFF, N. P., DODGE, P. W., and DREN, A. T., 1976*a*, Drugs derived from cannabinoids, IV: Effect of alkyl substitution in sulfur and carbocyclic analogs, *J. Med. Chem.* **19:**552–554.

RAZDAN, R. K., ZITKO TERRIS, B., HANDRICK, G. R., DALZELL, H. C., PARS, H. G., HOWES, J. F., PLOTNIKOFF, N., DODGE, P., DREN, A., KYNCL, J., SHOER, L., and THOMPSON, W. R., 1976*b*, Drugs derived from cannabinoids, III: Sulfur analogs: thiopyranobenzopyrans and thienobenzopyrans, *J. Med. Chem.* **19:**549–551.

RAZDAN, R. K., ZITKO TERRIS, B., PARS, H. G., PLOTNIKOFF, N. P., DODGE, P. W., DREN, A. T., KYNCL, J., and SOMANI, P., 1976*c*, Drugs derived from cannabinoids, II: Basic esters of nitrogen and carbocyclic analogs, *J. Med. Chem.* **19:**454–461.

RYRFELDT, A., and RAMSAY, C. H., 1973, Whole-body autoradiography of Δ^1-tetrahydrocannabinol and $\Delta^{1(6)}$-tetrahydrocannabinol in mouse, *Acta Pharmaceut. Suecica* **10:**13–28.

SAMPAIO, C. A. M., LAPA, A. J., and VALLE, J. R., 1967, Influence of cannabis, tetrahydrocannabinol and pyrahexyl on the linguomandibular reflex of the dog, *J. Pharm. Pharmacol.* **19:**552–554.

SASMAN, M., 1938, Cannabis indica in pharmaceuticals, *J. Med. Soc. N.J.* **35:**51–52.

SCHECKEL, C. L., BOFF, E., DAHLEN, P., and SMART, T., 1968, Behavioral effects in monkeys of racemates of two biologically active marijuana constituents, *Science* **160:**1467–1469.

SCHILDKRAUT, J. J., and EFRON, D. H., 1971, The effects of Δ^9-tetrahydrocannabinol on the metabolism of norepinephrine in rat brain, *Psychopharmacologia* **20:**191–196.

SEGAL, M., 1974, Central implantation of cannabinoids: Induction of epileptiform discharges, *Europ. J. Pharmacol.* **27:**40–45.

SEGAL, M., and KENNEY, A. F., 1972, Δ^1- and $\Delta^{1(6)}$-Tetrahydrocannabinol: Preliminary observations on similarities and differences in central pharmacological effects in the cat, *Experientia* **28:**816–819.

SEGELMAN, A. B., SOFIA, R. D., SEGELMAN, F. P., HARAKAL, J. J., and KNOBLOCH, L. C., 1974, *Cannabis sativa* L. (marijuana) V: Pharmacological evaluation of marijuana aqueous extract and volatile oil, *J. Pharm. Sci.* **63:**962–964.

SIEMENS, A. J., and KALANT, H., 1974, Metabolism of Δ^1-tetrahydrocannabinol by rats tolerant to cannabis, *Can. J. Physiol. Pharmacol.* **52:**1154–1166.

SIEMENS, A. J., and KALANT, H., 1975, Metabolism of Δ^1-tetrahydrocannabinol by the rat *in vivo* and *in vitro*, *Biochem. Pharmacol.* **24:**755–762.

SIEMENS, A. J., KALANT, H., KHANNA, J. M., MARSHMAN, J., and HO, G., 1974, Effect of cannabis on pentobarbital-induced sleeping time and pentobarbital metabolism in the rat, *Biochem. Pharmacol.* **23:**477–488.

SIEMENS, A. J., DE NIE, L. C., KALANT, H., and KHANNA, J. M., 1975, Effects of various psychoactive drugs on the metabolism of Δ^1-tetrahydrocannabinol by rats *in vitro* and *in vivo*, *Europ. J. Pharmacol.* **31:**136–147.

SIGG, E. B., KEIM, K. L., KOVACS, J. L., and SIGG, T. D., 1973, Selective effect of psychotropic agents on preganglionic sympathetic outflow in cat, *Fed. Proc.* **32:**221.

SJODEN, P.-O., JARBE, T. U. C., and HENRIKSSON, B. G., 1973, Influence of tetrahydrocannabinols (Δ^8-THC and Δ^9-THC) on body weight, food, and water intake in rats, *Pharmacol. Biochem. Behav.* **1:**395–399.

SOFIA, R. D., 1972, A paradoxical effect for Δ^1-tetrahydrocannabinol on rectal temperature in rats, *Res. Comm. Chem. Path. Pharmacol.* **4:**281–288.

SOFIA, R. D., 1974, The lethal effects of Δ^9-tetrahydrocannabinol in mice enhanced by pretreatment with SKF 525-A or chloramphenicol, *Europ. J. Pharmacol.* **26:**383–385.

SOFIA, R. D., and BARRY, H., III, 1970, Depressant effect of Δ^1-tetrahydrocannabinol enhanced by inhibition of its metabolism, *Europ. J. Pharmacol.* **13:**134–137.

SOFIA, R. D., and BARRY, H., III, 1972, The influence of SKF 525-A on the analgesic actions of Δ^1-tetrahydrocannabinol, *Fed. Proc.* **31:**506.

SOFIA, R. D., and BARRY, H., III, 1973, Interactions of chronic and acute Δ^1-tetrahydrocannabinol pretreatment with zoxazolamine and barbiturates, *Res. Comm. Chem. Path. Pharmacol.* **5:**91–98.

SOFIA, R. D., and BARRY, H., III, 1974, Acute and chronic effects of Δ^9-tetrahydrocannabinol on food intake by rats, *Psychopharmacologia* **39:**213–222.

SOFIA, R. D., and KNOBLOCH, L. C., 1973, The interaction of Δ^9-tetrahydrocannabinol pretreatment with various sedative–hypnotic drugs, *Psychopharmacologia* **30:**185–194.

SOFIA, R. D., and KNOBLOCH, L. C., 1974, The effect of Δ^9-tetrahydrocannabinol pretreatment on ketamine, thiopental or CT-1341-induced loss of righting reflex in mice, *Arch. Int. Pharmacodyn. Ther.* **207:**270–281.

SOFIA, R. D., and KNOBLOCH, L. C., 1976, Comparative effects of various naturally occurring cannabinoids on food, sucrose and water consumption by rats, *Pharmacol. Biochem. Behav.* **4:**591–599.

SOFIA, R. D., DIXIT, B. N., and BARRY, H., III, 1971*a*, The effect of Δ^1-tetrahydrocannabinol on serotonin metabolism in the rat brain, *Life Sci.* **10:**425–436.

SOFIA, R. D., ERTEL, R. J., DIXIT, B. N., and BARRY, H., III, 1971*b*, The effect of Δ^1-tetrahydrocannabinol on the uptake of serotonin by rat brain homogenates, *Europ. J. Pharmacol.* **16:**257–259.

SOFIA, R. D., NALEPA, S. D., HARAKAL, J. J., and VASSAR, H. B., 1973, Anti-edema and analgesic properties of Δ^9-tetrahydrocannabinol (THC), *J. Pharmacol. Exp. Ther.* **186:**646–655.

SOFIA, R. D., SOLOMON, T. A., and BARRY, H., III, 1976, Anticonvulsant activity of Δ^9-tetrahydrocannabinol compared with three other drugs, *Europ. J. Pharmacol.* **35:**7–16.

SOFIA, R. D., VASSAR, H. B., and KNOBLOCH, L. C., 1975, Comparative analgesic activity of various naturally occurring cannabinoids in mice and rats, *Psychopharmacologia* **40:**285–295.

STARK, P., and ARCHER, R. A., 1975, Preclinical pharmacologic profile of a psychoactive cannabinoid, *Pharmacologist* **17:**210.

STOELTING, R. K., MARTZ, R. C., GARTNER, J., CREASSER, C., BROWN, D. J., and FORNEY, R. B., 1973, Effects of delta-9-tetrahydrocannabinol on halothane MAC in dogs, *Anesthesiology* **38:**521–524.

TEN HAM, M., and VAN NOORDWIJK, J., 1973, Lack of tolerance to the effect of two tetrahydrocannabinols on aggressiveness, *Psychopharmacologia* **29:**171–176.

TEN HAM, M., and DE JONG, Y., 1974, Tolerance to the hypothermic and aggression-attenuating effect of Δ^8- and Δ^9-tetrahydrocannabinol in mice, *Europ. J. Pharmacol.* **28:**144–148.

TEN HAM, M., and DE JONG, Y., 1975, Absence of interaction between Δ^9-tetrahydrocannabinol (Δ^9-THC) and cannabidiol (CBD) in aggression, muscle control and body temperature experiments in mice, *Psychopharmacologia* **41:**169–174.

TEN HAM, M., LOSKOTA, W. J., and LOMAX, P., 1975, Acute and chronic effects of Δ^9-tetrahydrocannabinol on seizures in the gerbil, *Europ. J. Pharmacol.* **31:**148–152.

TRUITT, E. B., JR., 1971, Biological disposition of tetrahydrocannabinols, *Pharmacol. Rev.* **23:**273–278.

TRUITT, E. B., JR., and BRAUDE, M. C., 1974, Preclinical pharmacology of marihuana, in *Research Advances in Alcohol and Drug Problems,* Vol. 1 (R. J. Gibbins, Y. Israel, H. Kalant, R. E. Popham, W. Schmidt, and R. G. Smart, eds.), pp. 199–242, Wiley, New York.

VITEZ, T. S., WAY, W. L., MILLTER, R. D., and EGER, E. I., II, 1973, Effects of delta-9-tetrahydrocannabinol on cyclopropane MAC in the rat, *Anesthesiology* **38:**525–527.

VREE, T. B., BREIMER, D. D., VAN GINNEKEN, C. A. M., and VAN ROSSUM, J. M., 1972, Identification in hashish of tetrahydrocannabinol, cannabidiol and cannabinol analogues with a methyl side-chain, *J. Pharm. Pharmacol.* **24:**7–12.

WAHLQVIST, M., NILSSON, I. M., SANDBERG, F., AGURELL, S., and GRANSTRAND, B., 1970, Binding of Δ^1-tetrahydrocannabinol to human plasma proteins, *Biochem. Pharmacol.* **19:**2579–2584.

WALL, E., 1971, The *in vitro* and *in vivo* metabolism of tetrahydrocannabinol (THC), *Ann. N.Y. Acad. Sci.* **191:**23–29.

WALL, M. E., BRINE, D. R., and PEREZ-REYES, M., 1975, Metabolism and excretion of cannabidiol and cannabinol in man, *Sixth International Congress of Pharmacology,* p. 450.

WALLACH, M. B., and GERSHON, S., 1973, The effects of Δ^8-THC on the EEG, reticular multiple unit activity and sleep of cats, *Europ. J. Pharmacol.* **24:**172–178.

WELCH, B. L., WELCH, A. S., MESSIHA, F. S., and BERGER, H. J., 1971, Rapid depletion of adrenal epinephrine and elevation of telencephalic serotonin by (−)-*trans*-Δ^9-tetrahydrocannabinol in mice, *Res. Comm. Chem. Path. Pharmacol.* **2:**382–391.

WIDMAN, M., NILSSON, I. M., NILSSON, J. L. G., AGURELL, S., and LEANDER, K., 1971, Metabolism of cannabis. IX. Cannabinol: Structure of a major metabolite formed in rat liver, *Life Sci.* **10:**157–162.

WIDMAN, M., NILSSON, I. M., NILSSON, J. L. G., AGURELL, S., BORG, H., and GRANSTRAND, B., 1973, Plasma protein binding of 7-hydroxy-Δ^1-tetrahydrocannabinol: An active Δ^1-tetrahydrocannabinol metabolite, *J. Pharm. Pharmacol.* **25:**453–457.

WIDMAN, M., AGURELL, S., EHRNEBO, M., and JONES, G., 1974*a*, Binding of (+)- and (−)-Δ^1-tetrahydrocannabinols and (−)-7-hydroxy-Δ^1-tetrahydrocannabinol to blood cells and plasma proteins in man, *J. Pharm. Pharmacol.* **26:**914–916.

WIDMAN, M., NORDQVIST, M., AGURELL, S., LINDGREN, J.-E., and SANDBERG, F., 1974*b*, Biliary excretion of Δ^1-tetrahydrocannabinol and its metabolites in the rat, *Biochem. Pharmacol.* **23:**1163–1172.

WILLINSKY, M. D., SCOTTI DE CAROLIS, A., and LONGO, V. G., 1973, EEG and behavioral effects of natural, synthetic and biosynthetic cannabinoids, *Psychopharmacologia* **31:**365–374.

WILLINSKY, M. D., KALANT, H., MERESZ, O., ENDRENYI, L., and WOO, N., 1974, Distribution and metabolism *in vivo* of ^{14}C-tetrahydrocannabinol in the rat, *Europ. J. Pharmacol.* **27:**106–119.

WILSON, R. S., and MAY, E. L., 1975, Analgesic properties of the tetrahydrocannabinols, their metabolites, and analogs, *J. Med. Chem.* **17:**700–703.

WINN, M., ARENDSEN, D., DODGE, P., DREN, A., DUNNIGAN, D., HALLAS, R., HWANG, K., KYNCL, J., LEE, Y.-H., PLOTNIKOFF, N., YOUNG, P., ZAUGG, H., DALZELL, H., and RAZDAN, R. K., 1976, Drugs derived from cannabinoids, V: Δ6a,10a-tetrahydrocannabinol and heterocyclic analogs containing aromatic side chains, *J. Med. Chem.* **19:**461–471.

ZITKO, B. A., HOWES, J. F., RAZDAN, R. K., DALZELL, B. C., DALZELL, H. C., SHEEHAN, J. C., PARS, H. G., DEWEY, W. L., and HARRIS, L. S., 1972, Water-soluble derivatives of Δ^1-tetrahydrocannabinol, *Science* **177:**442–444.

ZUNIN, L. M., 1969, Marijuana: The drug and the problem, *Mil. Med.* **134:**104–110.

ZINBERG, N. E., 1980, Marijuana: The drug and the problem, *Mil. Med.* 134:104–110.

7

MARIHUANA: HUMAN EFFECTS

Reese T. Jones

1. ACUTE EFFECTS

A person ingesting or smoking cannabis experiences a fairly predictable sequence of physiologic and psychologic changes that last a few hours and then gradually disappear. Although dose administered and individual differences in personality, expectations, setting, and past drug experience all contribute to varied consequences from a given dose of cannabis, the variability in acute effects from cannabis seems no greater than with any other psychoactive drug. Recently, a number of reviews and collections of papers have appeared that attempt to cover the vast amount of information accumulating about the acute and chronic effects of cannabis (Bech *et al.*, 1974; Brecher, 1975; Committee on Drugs, 1975; Edwards, 1974; Hollister, 1974*a*; Kalant and Kalant, 1974; Kaymakcalan, 1975; Lemberger and Rubin, 1975; McGlothlin, 1975; Mechoulam *et al.*, 1976; Miller, 1974; Nahas, 1975*a*, *b*). Some authors have attempted to consider the research findings in the context of political–social decisions (Edwards, 1974; Pillard, 1974) and point out the lacunae in the data as well as the well-established facts (Edwards, 1974). Other reviews tend to emphasize possible adverse effects (Nahas, 1975*a*, *b*; Kaymakcalan, 1975), legal versus health issues (Brecher, 1975), or the chemistry of cannabis (Lemberger and Rubin, 1975; Mechoulam *et al.*, 1976). The continuing research efforts this past year have attempted to fill some of the gaps. Research papers on cannabis are appearing at an average

Reese T. Jones • Langley Porter Neuropsychiatric Institute, University of California, San Francisco, California 94143. This chapter was adapted from a review written for the 1977 report to Congress on marihuana.

rate of more than one per day and about a third of them deal with effects in humans. Thus, a single detailed review of the literature is becoming an almost impossible task.

1.1. Activity of Natural and Synthetic Cannabinoids

Detailed pharmacokinetic studies of Δ^8-THC in man using mass fragmentographic techniques indicate a similar time course and clearance pattern to that seen with Δ^9-THC (Agurell *et al.,* 1976). A very rapid α phase was followed by a slower phase. While blood levels did not always predict physiological and psychological effects, they paralleled heart-rate changes well.

DMHP ($\Delta^{6a,10a}$-dimethylheptyltetrahydrocannabinol), a synthetic cannabinoid, differs from Δ^9-THC by having a double bond in the 6a, 10a positions. Intravenous administration in man produced profound cardiovascular effects but only minimal psychological effects (Lemberger *et al.,* 1976). As is the case with natural cannabinoids, hydroxylation seemed to be the major metabolic pathway.

A report of an early phase I clinical trial of Nabilone, a synthetic cannabinoid-like compound, is probably one of the first of many investigations with drugs of novel chemical structures that resemble cannabinoids (Lemberger and Rowe, 1975). Nabilone and other synthetics such as a series of benzopyrans (Mechoulam *et al.,* 1976), have many advantages over natural cannabinoids in terms of stability, water solubility, etc. Most importantly, they have more specific pharmacologic actions. That is, it seems possible to develop compounds with more cardiovascular effects and less central nervous system effects or vice versa. Compounds with analgesic, sedative, hypnotic, and anticonvulsant activity are undergoing preclinical and early clinical trials. If there is any clinical application of cannabinoid-like drugs, it is likely it will come from these newer synthetics rather than from the administration of *Cannabis sativa* to people.

1.2. Metabolism of Cannabinoids and Biochemistry

1.2.1. Metabolites

Although studies of a major metabolite of Δ^9-THC, 11-hydroxy-THC, indicate it is pharmacologically active, some question remains as to whether it is the only metabolite or whether Δ^9-THC needs to be hydroxylated to 11-hydroxy-THC before the THC is active (Hollister and Gillespie, 1975*a*; Lemberger and Rubin, 1975; Mechoulam *et al.,* 1976). In an attempt to clarify these issues, Hollister and Gillespie sorted people into fast and slow hydroxylators on the basis of antipyrine and phenylbutazone plasma disappearance rates. THC and these drugs are metabolized by the same liver microsomal enzyme system (Wall *et al.*, 1976). There was no difference in speed of onset, intensity, or duration of effects after intravenous injection of Δ^9-THC when the two groups were compared. Such results suggest 11-hydroxy-THC may not be the sole source of Δ^9-THC effects. Another group of investigators found 11-hydroxy-THC to leave the plasma more rapidly than THC, suggesting that THC may, in fact, be more potent (Perez-Reyes *et al.*, 1976).

A number of additional marihuana metabolites have been reported in a series of studies (Kanter *et al.*, 1974*a*, *b*, 1975) and for the first time, unchanged Δ^9-THC was identified in the urine using conventional thin-layer chromatographic techniques in amounts estimated at 0.01–0.005% of the dose (Hollister *et al.*, 1974). New extraction procedures revealed a previously ignored fraction containing abundant metabolites (Kanter *et al.*, 1974*b*) including many polar metabolites (Kanter *et al.*, 1974*a*). The exact identity and activity has yet to be determined. In a review of structure–activity relationships of cannabinoids in humans, Hollister (1974*b*) concluded that the potency of the THC molecule is altered by changing the length of side chains, or by metabolic hydroxylations. No material has yet been formed in nature, in cannabis itself, or in THC metabolites that differs qualitatively from THC. There is now evidence indicating that the human small intestinal mucosa, as well as the liver, can hydroxylate THC (Greene and Saunders, 1974).

1.2.2. *Cannabinoid Interactions*

Studies of the possible interaction between Δ^9-THC and the other two major cannabinoids of marihuana—cannabinol (CBN) and cannabidiol (CBD)—are not completely consistent in their conclusions. Hollister and Gillespie (1975*a*) found only slight interaction between THC and CBD. After administration of CBD, there was a delayed onset and prolonged effects of THC that were slightly more intense. The magnitude of the interactions was so small as to be clinically insignificant. A similar study using smoked plant material found diminished euphoria when CBD was mixed with THC, as well as a trend toward decreased THC effects on psychomotor impairments (Dalton *et al.*, 1976). CBD smoked alone was inactive. Other experiments in man with samples of marihuana plant material containing varied amounts of CBN and CBD found differences in effects possibly owing to differing proportions of CBN, CBD, and THC (Carlini *et al.*, 1974). In subsequent studies by the same group, large doses of CBD blocked many of the effects of THC (Karniol *et al.*, 1974), and oral doses of CBN slightly increased THC effects on some physiological and psychological processes (Karniol *et al.*, 1975). One possible complicating factor in cannabinoid interaction studies is the question of relative stability of various synthetic and naturally occurring cannabinoids (Turner and Henry, 1975). Some are more stable than others.

There is little question that interactions occur, although at this point they seem to be inconsistent and of limited magnitude.

1.2.3. Interactions with Other Drugs

Besides CBD and CBN, other drug interactions with THC have been investigated in man. Secobarbital and smoked marihuana had additive effects on subjective responses and psychomotor impairment (Dalton *et al.*, 1975). Subjects had difficulty distinguishing 150 mg of secobarbital from 25 μg of THC per kilogram. When the effects of amphetamine and smoked marihuana were combined, additive effects of heart rate and blood pressure and subjective symptoms were observed, but no interaction effect on psychomotor performance was found (Evans *et al.*, 1974). Based on the assumption that THC interferes with cholinergic brain mechanisms, physostigmine was administered after THC and decreased the tachycardia and conjunctival injection, but had little effect on psychological changes (Freemon *et al.*, 1975). Little potentiation of narcotic drug effects was noted in a study evaluating THC as a preanesthetic agent (Johnstone *et al.*, 1974). Animal studies indicate that whatever the drug combination, the depressant effects of THC tend to predominate (Pryor, 1976). Effects of alcohol and cannabis were similar in their impairment of a divided attention performance task (MacAvoy and Marks, 1975). When combined the drugs had synergistic effects in nonusers, at least at lower doses of alcohol.

1.2.4. Assay Techniques

A great deal of effort has gone into the development of practical assays of cannabinoid levels in man. Such measures are needed not only for research purposes, but they would be useful clinically and in law enforcement (particularly in cases where intoxication while driving an automobile is an issue). A number of techniques using saliva and THC with mass spectrometry (Just *et al.*, 1974), radioimmunoassay of blood and urine (Marks *et al.*, 1975; Teale *et al.*, 1974), and gas chromatography of blood (McCallum, 1974) have been developed. The problems regarding sensitivity, specificity, and reliability of assays have been partially solved, and some methods can now be employed in a routine manner. The tight binding of THC to plasma protein (Widman *et al.*, 1974) is only one of the many problems in the development of sensitive, reliable tissue-level assays.

A report, *Cannabinoid Assays in Humans,* from a recent conference sponsored by the National Institute on Drug Abuse describes the tremendous progress in assay techniques made over the past few years (Willette, 1976). Investigators from ten different laboratories in the United States and abroad reported on the results of a variety of analytic techniques—radioimmunoassays, high-pressure gas chromatography, thin-layer chromatography, and gas chromatography/mass spectrometry. No single technique is best, each having advantages or disadvantages depending on the purpose of the analysis, the type of body fluid or tissue, the drug levels of interest, etc. The monograph describes many of the characteristics of cannabinoids that make sensitive, specific, and reliable assays difficult. Cannabinoids are lipophilic drugs, tightly bound to lipoproteins; selected antibodies for the various cannabinoids are difficult to obtain as are radioligands with high specificity. Unidentified factors in human plasma appear to interfere with assays even though animal studies are satisfactory. Interlaboratory comparisons are risky since sensitivity to test conditions is great and standardized test procedures are just developing. The most precise and sensitive techniques still require cumbersome and expensive equipment. The radioimmunoassays may ultimately be ideal for routine clinical tests but they still have not lived up to their potential. However, the monograph, written for those with highly specialized backgrounds, reports a number of optimistic studies indicating that practical and sensitive assays will soon be available for routine application in clinical, research-oriented, and medical–legal situations.

1.3. Cardiovascular Effects

Cannabis has long been known to have marked cardiovascular effects (Clark, 1975; Savary *et al.*, 1974). Previous reports reviewed preliminary data that resulted in some expressed concern about electrocardiographic changes during acute intoxication. The subsequent publication of a number of studies where cardiovascular dynamics were studied some time after administration of large doses of THC indicates that cannabis produces only minimal EKG changes in young healthy subjects (Benowitz and Jones, 1975; Clark *et al.*, 1974; Johnstone *et al.*, 1974; Malit *et al.*, 1975). Nonspecific P or T changes are most commonly noted. Occasional premature beats also occur. Tachycardia continues to be the most common and prominent physiological response to acute doses (Schaefer *et al.*, 1975*b*). In a study of prolonged administration of oral doses of 30 mg Δ^9-THC given every 4 hr, heart-rate slowing and blood-pressure drops developed (Benowitz and Jones, 1975). Blunting of peripheral vascular reflexes developed along with plasma volume expansion. Although tolerance developed to the orthostatic hypotension, the supine hypotensive effects persisted throughout the period of drug administration. These changes commonly seen in laboratory animals but not previously noted in man suggest a biphasic action of THC in humans with an increase in sympathetic activity involving the heart and peripheral blood vessels at low doses and centrally mediated sympathetic inhibition at higher doses (Hardman *et al.*, 1976). Similar biphasic cardiovascular effects were noted after intravenous THC was given as a premedication for oral surgery (Gregg *et al.*, 1976*a*). The slightly increased supine blood pressure following drug administration would be consistent with this mechanism (Clark *et al.*, 1974; Johnstone *et al.*, 1974; Malit *et al.*, 1975). Forearm blood flow increases and total peripheral resistance decreases slightly with acute doses (Malit *et al.*, 1975; Johnstone *et al.*, 1974) consistent with β-adrenergic stimulation. The great individual variability in response to large intravenous doses has, however, led one group to suggest an indirect episodic activation of the sympathetic system secondary to psychological arousal in addition to the β-adrenergic stimulation (Malit *et al.*, 1975). Cardiovascular and psychological mechanisms of action may be independent, as is suggested by the observation that DMHP, a synthetic cannabinoid, produces profound cardiovascular but few psychological effects (Lemberger *et al.*, 1976).

A study with hospitalized volunteers investigated cardiovascular responses to isoproterenol, phenylephrine, atropine, and propranolol before and after 14 days of chronic cannabis intoxication (Benowitz and Jones, 1977). There was no significant change in response to isoproterenol or phenylephrine. Heart-rate and blood-pressure increase after atropine was greater during THC ingestion. The pattern of changes suggested enhanced parasympathetic activity along with sympathetic insufficiency. The interaction with atropine may represent a clinically significant event in chronic high-dose cannabis users presenting as patients. Such an interaction might explain the prolonged postoperative tachycardia in marihuana smokers given atropine prior to general anesthesia (Gregg *et al.*, 1976*a*).

A series of reports on the cardiovascular effects of cannabis smoking in persons with coronary disease are consistent with the preliminary report cited several years ago (Angelico and Brown, 1974; Aronow and Cassidy, 1975; Prakash *et al.*, 1975). Smoking either marihuana or high-nicotine cigarettes decreased exercise performance prior to the onset of angina by increasing myocardial oxygen demand and decreasing myocardial oxygen delivery (Aronow and Cassidy, 1975). Cardiovascular hemodynamics were evaluated by echocardiography (Prakash *et al.*, 1975). After marihuana, stroke index and ejection fraction decreased. Elevated carboxyhemoglobin levels probably produced some changes after both smoked marihuana and placebo. There was some disagreement between experts as to the explanation for the observed cannabis effects. One group favored an explanation in which the diminished cardiac performance was secondary to THC-induced increase in heart rate and afterload rather than a direct negative inotropic effect of THC (Kanakis, 1976) and cited data from cannabis studies with normal people suggesting enhanced cardiac performance and an increase in cardiac index (Kanakis *et al.*, 1976*a,b*; Malit *et al.*, 1975). The group that did the original study with coronary diseased patients remains concerned about negative inotropic effects of THC (Prakash and Aronow, 1976). Whatever the mechanism, these studies demonstrate that marijuana effects may differ in individuals with preexisting disease from those in normals. Most cannabis research thus far has, of course, been done on youthful, carefully selected, normal volunteers. Effects in various disease states cannot always be predicted from studies in health populations of research subjects.

1.4. Pulmonary Effects

Because smoking is the most common means of cannabis consumption in this country, the effects of cannabinoids and marihuana smoke on pulmonary function have been of continuing interest. The Fifth Marihuana and Health Report described bronchodilating effects with possible therapeutic implications after marihuana smoking. Previous reports have described mainly adverse findings in frequent and chronic cannabis smokers including bronchitis, obstructive pulmonary defects, and chronic cough (Abramson, 1974).

Two groups have published reports of cannabis's effects in people with asthma (Shapiro and Tashkin, 1976; Tashkin *et al.*, 1974, 1976*a*; Vachon *et al.*, 1976). In these studies, acute administration of either smoked marihuana or oral doses of THC produced statistically significant increases in bronchodilation and reversed experimentally induced bronchospasm in young adults with bronchial asthma (Tashkin *et al.*, 1974, 1976*a*; Vachon *et al.*, 1976). Indications are that the mechanism is independent of β-adrenergic or antimuscarinic effects (Shapiro and Tashkin, 1976). In contrast to these promising reports, a British group (Davies *et al.*, 1975; Graham *et al.*, 1976) found that measures of forced vital capacity, peak expiratory flow rate, and other clinically useful measures of pulmonary function did not improve in a group of patients with reversible airway obstruction given 10 mg doses of oral THC. One possible reason for these discrepant findings may be that the groups reporting cannabis-induced bronchodilation (Shapiro and Tashkin, 1976; Tashkin *et al.*, 1974) used whole body plethysmography, an exceedingly sensitive measure that will detect very small changes in pulmonary function, whereas the less optimistic reports came from a group using less sensitive, although clinically relevant, measurement techniques.

Chronic smoking may produce different and less useful effects than acute administration, as indicated by pulmonary function changes during periods of chronic administration. Mendelson *et al.* (1974*b*) found significant impairments in pulmonary function tests (vital capacity, or FEV 1.0) in a group of chronic marihuana smokers. Further reduction in pulmonary function test performance developed during this study in which the volunteers smoked 3–10 marijuana cigarettes daily for 21 days. Using more sophisticated measures, another group found decreases in maximal midexpiratory flow rates and specific airway conductance after 6 to 8 weeks of heavy cannabis smoking (Tashkin *et al.*, 1975, 1976*b*). Although still within the limits of normality, the changes persisted at least 1 week after smoking and suggest that a longer period of smoking could lead to clinically important changes. An outpatient study of young adults with varying tobacco cigarette habits found more improvement in pulmonary function during an 8-week period of no smoking in the cannabis smoker subgroup (Backhouse, 1975). An *in vitro* study suggests that the water-soluble components of marihuana smoke may contain substances toxic to the defense network of the lung other than Δ^9-THC or other cannabinoids (Cutting *et al.*, 1974). Studies using high doses of THC given intravenously noted only modest changes in minute ventilation and the ventilatory response to CO_2 equivalent to that produced by 5-mg doses of morphine (Johnstone *et al.*, 1974; Malit *et al.*, 1975). However, a more sensitive technique produced evidence of a small degree of respiratory depression (Wiberg *et al.*, 1975).

Another study of the respiratory effects of smoked marihuana and orally ingested Δ^9-THC has examined the effects of the drugs on the respiratory response curve. Both the synthetic and natural material produced a respiratory depression in a group of previously chronic users. Although the effect was found to be slight, the authors recommended further study because of the possible relevance of this effect to patients with chronic lung disease or central nervous system impairment of respiratory regulation (Bellville *et al.*, 1975*b*).

A clinical study of patients with pneumomediastinum identified a small group of patients who had a common history of repeated and sustained Valsalva's maneuvers during marihuana smoking or heroin injection and no other obvious explanation for the mediastinal or cervical emphysema (Mattox, 1976). The author suggested that the forceful Valsalva's maneuver used during marihuana smoking may have been an etiologic factor.

1.5. Endocrine and Metabolic Effects

The report of depressed plasma testosterone levels in chronic marihuana smokers (Kolodny *et al.*, 1974*a*) and the report of a failure to find such a change in marihuana smokers receiving the drug daily over a 21-day period (Mendelson *et al.*, 1974*a*) or in a sample of college student smokers (Cushman, 1975) have led to further studies and discussion (Friedman, 1975; Koff, 1974; Kolodny, 1975*a*, *b*; Kolodny *et al.*, 1974*b*, 1976; Lemberger *et al.*, 1975). Kolodny (1975*a*) reviewed the numerous problems confounding the study of drug effects on the hypothalamic–pituitary–testicular axis in man and discussed possible biologic implications of lowered testosterone levels. He presented data (Kolodny, 1975*b*; Kolodny *et al.*, 1976) showing significant drops in plasma testosterone levels and luteinizing hormone levels 2 and 3 hr after smoking a single marihuana cigarette. In a chronic administration study, subjects showed no significant drop in levels after the first 4 weeks of daily marihuana smoking; but with continued smoking they had significant drops in luteinizing hormone, followed by falling testosterone levels and follicle stimulating hormone levels. Thus, the data from research finding no marihuana-related hormone changes (Cushman, 1975; Hembree *et al.*, 1976; Koff, 1974; Mendelson *et al.*, 1974*a*; Schaefer *et al.*, 1975*a*) are quite consistent with studies that do (Kolodny, 1975*b*; Kolodny *et al.*, 1974*a*, 1976) if the different time periods of marihuana use are taken into account. The biological significance of these changes is unclear, and Kolodny (1975*a*) is appropriately cautious in his interpretation of their importance. In most cases the plasma hormone levels remain well within the usually accepted normal limits. However, a recent study (Hembree *et al.*, 1976) confirmed a decreased sperm count in otherwise normal marihuana smokers. Such hormone alterations might be expected to be more important for prepubertal or pubertal males or males with already impaired sexual functioning. Corresponding endocrine changes in females have not been studied. There might also be adverse effects on sexual differentiation of the fetus of expectant mothers using cannabis. In the absence of clinical evidence for these consequences, such concern is at present only speculative. Since recent reports (Gordon *et al.*, 1976; Stimmel, 1975) suggest alcohol may have similar effects, interpretation of many clinical findings will be complicated, since cannabis and alcohol are usually both used by cannabis users.

One surgeon has attempted to link such hormonal changes to the development of gynecomastia in male marihuana users (Harmon and Aliapoulios, 1974; Hill, 1975). He was able to stimulate the development of rat breast tissue by Δ^9-THC administration (Harmon and Aliapoulios, 1974). Other investigators (Lemberger *et al.*, 1975) have not found changes in serum prolactin levels in men given THC experimentally. The absence of prolactin changes is surprising since many centrally acting drugs alter prolactin levels. The reported gynecomastia was postulated to result from a prolactin-dependent mechanism.

Hollister and Reaven (1974) described glucose intolerance in a small group of subjects given intravenous doses of Δ^9-THC. A lower dose of THC given as smoked hashish had no effect on blood glucose though blood lactic acid decreased (Papadakis *et al.*, 1974). Glucose efflux from human erythrocytes was inhibited by THC and cannabidiol, suggesting some drug effects on glucose transport mechanisms (Schurr *et al.*, 1974). It would, however, be quite speculative to try to relate these changes to the craving for sweets often reported by cannabis users. A more recent study (Permutt *et al.*, 1976) found no changes in carbohydrate metabolism in marihuana users.

A depressed growth hormone and cortisol response to insulin hypoglycemia was found after a period of prolonged THC ingestion in hospitalized volunteers (Benowitz *et al.*, 1976). As was the case with the testosterone changes described above, the decreased growth hormone levels were still within acceptable limits of normality. The findings are consistent with others suggesting suppression of the hypothalamic–pituitary axis after prolonged THC administration.

1.6. Sexual Functioning

Reports discussed in Section 1.5 describe sex hormone changes related to cannabis use. Although anecdotal accounts describe cases of sexual dysfunction possibly associated with such changes, properly controlled studies are needed to confirm them (Kolodny, 1975*a*; Kolodny *et al.*, 1976). A number of accounts report enhanced sexual activity associated with cannabis use (Brill and Christie, 1974; Chausow and Saper, 1974; Fisher and Steckler, 1974; Hager, 1975; Koff, 1974). However, the psychological, social, and pharmacologic factors associated with sexual activity probably interact in complicated ways as is true with most other drug effects on sexual behavior (Chausow and Saper, 1974; Ellinwood and Rockwell, 1975; Hollister, 1976; Koff, 1974). For example, with cannabis, as with alcohol, dose is important. Small to moderate doses appear to be most effective as releasers of inhibitions (Koff, 1974). Larger doses and/or chronic use of marihuana may actually diminish sexual interest and potency in males. Adequate data elucidating the effect of marihuana use on sexual functioning are not yet available.

1.7. Neurological Effects

Perceptual, cognitive, and mood changes are presumably reflected in changes in nervous system activity. Thus, there is no question as to the presence of neurological effects. As with any psychoactive drug, however, simple one-to-one correlations between behavioral changes and brain activity are rare (Jones, 1973). The most important questions have to do with how long the effects persist: for hours, days, or weeks, or even permanently.

Most recently, two studies have been conducted in Missouri (Co *et al.*, 1977) and Massachusetts (Kuehnle *et al.*, 1977) of two samples of young men with histories of heavy cannabis smoking using computerized transaxial tomography (CTT), a brain scanning technique for visualizing the anatomy of the brain. In this technique the head is scanned by a narrow beam of X-rays in a series of "slices." Computer processing of the data obtained from a large number of measurements makes it possible to reconstruct the anatomy of the brain in a more detailed manner and with greater precision than pneumoencephalography.

In the St. Louis study, 12 young male subjects, aged 20–30 (mean age, 24.1) who had smoked at least 5 joints a day (mean number, 9.0/day) for 5 or more years (mean years, 6.6) were compared to 34 neurologically normal young men of similar age who did not indicate drug use. In the Cambridge study 19 heavily using young male marihuana smokers, whose use was verified on a closed research ward, were matched with a control series of nonusing males of similar age.

In both studies, the resulting brain scans were read blindly by experienced neuroradiologists. In neither study was there any evidence of cerebral atrophy. Despite these negative findings, several additional points should be emphasized. Neither study rules out the possibility that more subtle changes of brain function may occur as a result of heavy and continued marihuana smoking. It is entirely possible to have impairment of brain function from toxic or other causes that is not apparent on gross examination of the brain in the living organism. Nevertheless, virtually all studies completed to date (early 1977) show no evidence of impaired neuropsychologic test performance in humans at dose levels studied so far.

Other recent studies are extensions of or attempts to replicate findings reported previously. Smoked cannabis produces acute, reversible, dose-related changes in brain waves as measured by computer-analyzed EEG (Fink *et al.*, 1976; Klonoff and Low, 1974). Following ordinarily used doses, the changes are modest, consisting mostly of α-wave slowing and are not indicative of any particular pathology. Cannabis does not appear to have unique qualities among CNS active drugs as measured by scalp EEGs. Changes in EEG recorded from deep brain structures, consisting of slow-wave and spiking activity, have not, however, been seen with any other drug (Heath, 1976). These changes have been well described in monkeys. Similar changes have been reported in a small number of humans (Heath, 1976). The behavioral significance of these lasting neurological changes is yet to be determined (Jones, 1973). Drew and Miller (1974), in a review of possible neural mechanisms of cannabis, suggest the hippocampus and other deep structures may be important sites of action, at least in animals.

Scalp EEG and evoked potentials showed marked changes in subjects given very large smoked doses of THC or marihuana (Tassinari *et al.*, 1974, 1976). Alpha abundance increased with posterior slow-wave activity becoming prominent. Ataxia, hypersomnia, increased deep tendon reflexes, tremor, tonic muscle contractions, and myoclonus followed these 1 mg/kg doses of THC. In contrast, Seyfeddininpur (1975) administered 2 mg of hashish to subjects and found no pathological changes in scalp EEG even though the dose produced profound hypotension, anxiety, and ataxia.

Loss of REM sleep appears to be a predictable effect of cannabis (Tassinari *et al.*, 1974, 1976). Total sleep time increases, while stage 4 or slow-wave sleep is relatively unaffected. In this respect, cannabis is unlike any sedative–hypnotic drug studied thus far (Feinberg *et al.*, 1975). When the drug is stopped after a period of prolonged administration, REM sleep stage and eye movement show a rebound above baseline levels. In contrast to the relatively small changes in waking EEGs after the drug is given, sleep EEG changes are very dramatic and large—both when the drug is acutely or chronically administered (Feinberg *et al.*, 1975, 1976).

Changes in the slow cortical potentials recorded from the scalp (contingent negative variation or CNV) after cannabis are of particular interest since this measure is said to be sensitive to changes in motivation and attention deployment, among other factors. A recent study of the CNV (Braden *et al.*, 1974) obtained somewhat different results from those reported earlier. Like many neurophysiologic measures, it appears the CNV is far more complicated than was originally assumed. It appears that the CNV may get larger or smaller after cannabis or it may not change at all (Roth *et al.*, 1977), depending on the level of intoxication, the task demands, the motivation of the subject, and changes in attention. The group originally reporting CNV changes associated with cannabis intoxication now reports another EEG-evoked potential component, P300 or the positive going wave at about 300 msec after the stimulus, as being the component most sensitive to cannabis and ethanol (Roth *et al.*, 1977). The researchers suggest that P300 is sensitive to both subjective probability judgments and response set attention. Both cannabis and alcohol intoxication were associated with decreased P300 waves. However, their own work as well as other reports suggest that to view the cannabis-induced CNV or P300 changes as any direct measure of attention deployment or motivation is probably an oversimplification (Braden *et al.*, 1974).

Coleman *et al.*, (1976) reported cranial nerve damage, specifically, a paresis of the fourth cranial nerve leading to superior oblique muscle weakness, headache, and hyperphoria. The only common denominator of the 83% of drug treatment clinic patients showing this somewhat unusual condition was heavy cannabis use. The investigator thought the trochlear nerve may be more sensitive to toxic drug effects because of its anatomy. A study of peripheral nerve function using electrostimulation produced no evidence of conduction defects in marihuana smokers (DiBenedetto, 1976).

1.8. Effects on Cell-Mediated Immunity

Conflicting opinions as to the possible effects of cannabis on the cell-mediated immune response continue to appear (Segelman *et al.*, 1974). It has been observed that chronic marihuana users had decreased *in vitro* lymphocyte response to allogeneic cells and to a mitogen (Nahas *et al.*, 1976). This original observation led to extensive *in vitro* and animal studies. Related studies in humans published in the past few years provide partial support for the notion of an immune-system- or thymus-derived cell alteration in people who smoke marihuana (Cushman *et al.*, 1974; Cushman and Khurana, 1975; Nahas *et al.*, 1976; Petersen *et al.*, 1974, 1975*a,b*). However, Silverstein and Lessin (1976), using an *in vivo* skin testing procedure, found no evidence of impairment of cell-mediated immunity in chronic marihuana users. Petersen *et al.* (1974) found that marihuana smokers had less T cell response to phytohemagglutin stimulation and decreased PMH phagocytic capacity; however, they caution that the clinical significance of these findings is uncertain. In possibly related *in vivo* studies, the white blood cells from both cannabis users and nonusers showed similar dose-related inhibition of migration when exposed to THC and extracts of cannabis (Schwartzfarb *et al.*, 1974). However, substances other than THC in the crude extract may have effects on this test system.

Administration of THC or cannabis to controlled populations, with before and after testing, is underway and may provide useful information in clarifying the etiology of the cell-mediated immune effects (Nichols *et al.*, 1974), as was the case with the supposed chromosome breakage. One such controlled study with hospitalized volunteers found no alterations in lymphocyte responses to phytohemagglutinin after subjects received a substantial oral dose of THC for 18 days (Lau *et al.*, 1976).

The problem of interpreting data from groups of cannabis users indicating high rates of infection arises from the possibility that uncontrolled factors such as living habits and shared drugs may contribute to such events rather than some defect in the immune system (Drachler, 1975).

1.9. Other Physiologic Effects

Cannabis has many effects on the eye and on visual functioning (Dawson, 1976). Previous findings associated cannabis intoxication with decreases in intraocular pressure. Studies in normal volunteer subjects indicate a non-dose-related pressure drop from 4 to 5 hr (Hepler *et al.*, 1976; Purnell and Gregg, 1975). The magnitude of the eye pressure decrease (about 30%) was the same whether the person smoked 1 or 22 marihuana cigarettes. Effects on other aspects of eye physiology (acuity, refractive error, biomicroscopy, fundus changes, visual fields, ophthalmodynamometry, electroretinography, and orthoptic evaluation) were minimal or absent. Other investigators concluded that the observed eye pressure decreases were more likely a consequence of drug-induced relaxation and sedation rather than specific cannabis effects on the eye, since other sedative drugs produced similar changes in eye pressure (Flom *et al.*, 1975). Results of studies of the effects of smoked marihuana on galvanic skin response are consistent with drug-induced reduction in level of autonomic nervous system arousal (Cohen *et al.*, 1975). However, recent findings seem to contradict this interpretation.

Intravenous administration of water infusions of cannabis plant material fortunately seems to be rarely used (Farber and Huertas, 1976; Payne and Brand, 1975). In the few cases reported, gastroenteritis, hypoalbuminemia, hepatitis, and many cardiovascular changes secondary to hypovolemia or renal insufficiency, thrombocytopenia, and rhabdomyolysis are severe and require vigorous treatment (Payne and Brand, 1975). The syndrome is quite different from that following intravenous administration of medically pure and sterile cannabis components. Many of the consequences of injections of crude extracts seem to be more the effect of injected foreign plant material, particulate matter, and bacteremia.

Given the probable potency of marihuana plant material as allergins, there are surprisingly few reports of allergic reactions associated with the handling of the substance (Shapiro *et al.*, 1975; Lewis and Slavin, 1975).

1.10. Acute Effects on Mental and Psychomotor Performance

As in previous years, a host of studies have reported impaired functioning on a variety of cognitive and performance tasks while marihuana intoxicated. For the most part, impairments were dose related. As research designs become more sophisticated, evidence is accumulating that interactions between dose and task difficulty are such that performance on some cognitive tasks might even improve when low doses are used (Weckowicz *et al.*, 1975). This study also looked for selective brain laterality effects and surprisingly found more impairment on nondominant-hemisphere-related tasks.

Greater appreciation has developed for the need to study a range of doses on a variety of cognitive tasks before trying to describe the effect of cannabis. There are apt to be multiple cannabis effects depending on dose and the exact demands of the task. Prior practice on a task (Beautrais and Marks, 1976; Peeke *et al.*, 1976) may or may not alter the effects of given doses of cannabis depending on the type of task. Incentives to perform well (more money for correct responses) can decrease some marihuana effects (Casswell, 1975).

In general, investigators using the smallest doses of marihuana have reported the fewest effects. Impaired memory (Borg and Gershon, 1975; Darley *et al.*, 1974; Domino *et al.*, 1976; Dornbush, 1974; Vachon *et al.*, 1974), altered time sense (Borg and Gershon, 1975; Vachon *et al.*, 1974), and decrements in performance on a number of tasks—such as those involving reaction time, concept formation, learning, perceptual motor coordination, attention, and signal detection—are commonly described in the literature (Borg and Gershon, 1975; Cohen and Rickles, 1974; Cohen *et al.*, 1975; Dalton *et al.*, 1975; DeSouza *et al.*, 1974; Dittrich *et al.*, 1975; Linton *et al.*, 1975; Milstein *et al.*, 1974, 1975*b*; Moskowitz and McGlothlin, 1974; Moskowitz *et al.*, 1973, 1974; Roth *et al.*, 1975; Salvendy and McCabe, 1975; Sharma and Moskowitz, 1974; Steadward and Singh, 1975; Stoller *et al.*, 1976; Thoden *et al.*, 1974).

A number of discussions on the locus of the memory impairment are available (Darley *et al.*, 1974; Dornbush, 1974; Tinklenberg and Darley, 1976). There is a growing consensus that the memory defect is a result of an alteration in storage rather than acquisition or retrieval. In most laboratory studies, the duration of measurable memory alterations is a few hours after a smoked marihuana cigarette. However, preliminary study by Gianutsos and Litwack (1976) suggests lasting problems with transfer of new information into long-term memory storage for some marihuana smokers.

There has been concern that cannabis may increase the suggestibility of those using it. In laboratory studies marihuana smoking had no effect on hypnotic susceptibility (Beahrs *et al.*, 1974).

1.11. Effects on Sensory Function

One of the more commonly reported effects of cannabis is a subjective change in sensation, often a feeling of enhanced sensations. A number of groups investigated drug effects on various aspects of sensory functioning. None has reported improved or enhanced sensitivity. Although subjective impressions of changes in skin sensitivity are commonly associated with cannabis intoxication, no objective or measurable change in cutaneous sensitivity using a number of measures was noted (Milstein *et al.*, 1974). The decrease in auditory signal detection while intoxicated appeared to be caused by a decrease in sensitivity rather than a change in criteria (Moskowitz and McGlothlin, 1974). This finding contrasts with the usual subjective reports of enhanced auditory sensitivity. The characteristics of preferred tone frequency were shifted while intoxicated (DeSouza *et al.*, 1974).

A number of aspects of visual functioning seem to be altered by cannabis. Visual acuity for detection of a small moving target was decreased by smoked marihuana (Brown *et al.*, 1975). Alcohol had an even greater effect, however. Reduced dynamic acuity may be a factor in traffic accidents. Static visual acuity, an easier task, was not altered by alcohol or cannabis (Adams *et al.*, 1975). Significant dose-related impairments in color discrimination were produced by both alcohol and smoked cannabis (Adams *et al.*, 1976). The transient changes were similar to those seen in retinal disease and were of a magnitude such that tasks where stable color perception is important could be affected by the drugs.

THC given to patients suffering from pain demonstrated mild analgesic effects, but 20-mg doses administered orally produced many unpleasant side effects—somnolence, dizziness, ataxia, blurred vision, etc. (Noyes *et al.*, 1975*a,b*). The experience of experimentally induced pain in normal subjects was also diminished by smoked marihuana (Milstein *et al.*, 1975*a*; Payer, 1974). Pain secondary to spinal cord injury was decreased by cannabis use (Dunn and Davis, 1974).

1.12. Automobile Driving Performance

More evidence has accumulated indicating that driving ability and related skills are impaired by cannabis at doses likely to be commonly used in the United States (Erlich, 1974; Isrealstam and Lambert, 1974; Klonoff, 1974*a,b*; Moskowitz, 1976; Moskowitz *et al.*, 1973). Despite their commonly expressed belief that their driving ability is impaired when intoxicated (Dalton *et al.*, 1975; Klonoff, 1974*b*; Thompson, 1975), more cannabis users appear to drive today while intoxicated than was the case a few years ago. In limited surveys, 60–80% of the users questioned reported driving soon after marihuana use (Klonoff, 1974*b*; Smart, 1974). The use of alcohol in combination with marihuana before driving was reported by 64% of one sample and during driving by 20% of the sample (Klonoff, 1974*b*). As the risks of arrest for possession decrease, one might expect that more users will take the chance of being caught while intoxicated and driving (Smart, 1974).

A recent study of drivers involved in fatal accidents in the greater Boston area was conducted by the Boston University Accident Investigation Team for the National Highway Traffic Safety Administration (NHTSA). The study found that marihuana smokers were over-represented in fatal highway accidents when compared with a control group of nonsmokers of similar age and sex (Sterling-Smith, 1976).

A more detailed report of a Canadian driving study (Klonoff, 1974*a,b*) revealed data that clearly demonstrated that marihuana, in relatively low doses (cigarettes containing approximately 5 and 8 mg of THC), typically had a detrimental effect on driving skills and performance not only on a test course but also under more usual city driving conditions. However, as is true with alcohol, effects were not uniform with all drivers. Some, particularly at the lower dose, actually improved their performance. Thus, the problem of individual differences that has complicated developing and enforcing "drunk driving" laws will probably recur when medical and legal discussions of the minimal allowable dose or blood level of cannabinoids begin.

Compared with most of the behavioral tasks studied in the laboratory, automobile driving is more complex. The relative importance of the various perceptual, cognitive, and psychomotor functions in determining driving ability is not completely understood. For example, in some situations the cognitive impairment produced by cannabis may have only limited impact on actual driving performance resulting from concomitant drug-induced changes in risk acceptance or feelings of aggression. In a laboratory simulation of driving, cannabis-intoxicated subjects took longer to decide whether to pass another car, seemed less likely to accept the risks of passing, and seemed less aggressive than alcohol-intoxicated subjects (Dott, 1974; Ellingstad *et al.*, 1973). Other laboratory simulator studies have found that, while some driving skills are relatively unaffected by marihuana, there is a dose-related impairment in the ability to attend to peripheral stimuli while driving (Moskowitz *et al.*, 1973, 1976). Such an impairment might interfere with such things as a driver's response to a car suddenly emerging from a side street even though tracking and car control are not impaired.

Because of the many inherent inadequacies of laboratory driving simulator studies (Klonoff, 1974*b*), cannabis-related driving risks will ultimately have to be assessed on the basis of studies of actual accident rates for users compared with nonusers. This has been difficult in the study of alcohol. It promises to be still more difficult with cannabis because of the problems of measuring tissue levels of the cannabinoids, the longer excretion times, the more complicated metabolism, and the often combined use of cannabis and alcohol while driving, making the relative contribution of either drug uncertain (Garriott and Latman, 1976; Klonoff, 1974*b*; Smart, 1974).

Blood and urine analysis for cannabinoids revealed extremely high levels in an automobile driver killed in a head-on collision (Teale and Marks, 1976). Cannabis leaf and a pipe were found in the car. No alcohol was found in the blood, nor were other explanations found for the erratic driving prior to the accident. How common this pattern of event is can only be determined when practical assays for cannabinoids in body fluids become available.

Flying an airplane demands still more complex skills than does driving. There is little information concerning possible pilot error or impairment in performance as a result of having used marihuana (Zeller, 1975). Several studies have shown that under flight simulator test conditions experienced pilots showed marked deterioration in performance following smoking marihuana containing 6 mg of THC (Meacham *et al.*, 1974), 0.9 mg/kg Δ^9-tetrahydrocannabinol (Janowsky *et al.*, 1976*a*), and 2.1% Δ^9-tetrahydrocannabinol in 0.09 mg/kg (Janowsky *et al.*, 1976*b*). More detailed studies are planned to follow up these initial observations.

1.13. Nonpharmacologic Determinants of Subjective Response

Sociocultural factors (Adamec *et al.*, 1976; Klonoff and Clark, 1976; Orcutt and Biggs, 1975) appear to interact with such pharmacologic aspects as dose and route of administration so as to modify marihuana's subjective effects. To some extent, what happens during cannabis intoxication is determined by the individual's expectations, as is the case with most psychoactive drugs. Sometimes even students in a professional health field are misinformed as to what can happen (Seiden *et al.*, 1975). Some of these factors were explored in previous studies.

Laboratory studies are often criticized because a sterile, scientific laboratory setting may alter the response to the drug so that findings have little relevance to more typical conditions of use. This does not necessarily seem to be the case. Hollister *et al.* (1975) randomly assigned a group of subjects to smoke marihuana (16 mg THC) either in a typical medical research laboratory or in a private living room designed to facilitate a pleasurable drug experience. Although there were great differences between subjects in their subjective responses to the smoked marihuana, the effect of the very different settings was negligible. A similar study using only a subjective level of intoxication as an index of drug effects found a psychedelic environment was associated with greater intoxication at intermediate dose levels, but not at the highest (16 mg THC) dose employed (Cappell and Kuchar, 1974). Another attribute of the setting in which cannabis is often used is the possible effect other intoxicated friends have on a person's "high." However, in a study testing the effect of modeling, subjects smoking marihuana for the first time were relatively unaffected by the presence of an actor modeling a marihuana high (Carlin *et al.*, 1974). The results of this study suggest that previous experience with cannabis is a complicated socialization process in which individuals learn from friends and others to discriminate and label various aspects of the drug state (Carlin *et al.*, 1974).

The mood one is in before smoking is sometimes thought to interact with the drug effects to produce varied outcomes. A laboratory study found no difference in subjective response to low doses of smoked marihuana and no difference in level of anxiety in groups of subjects made anxious by exposure to laboratory stresses (Pillard *et al.*, 1974). Finally, Cappell and Pliner (1974) found that the dose of cannabis consumed in an experimental laboratory setting was determined by many factors (size of cigarettes, past drug experience) other than pharmacologic potency of the drug. A similar study by the same group (Cappell and Kuchar, 1974) found that controlling the amount of drug consumed in accord with its varying strength was difficult for subjects, again suggesting that nonpharmacologic considerations are important in affecting the amounts consumed.

2. CANNABIS AND PSYCHOPATHOLOGY

The association of cannabis use with psychiatric illness raises complex questions for which no completely satisfactory answers are yet available. Two reviews of past research point out the many methodological and theoretical shortcomings of existing work (Halikas, 1974; Meyer, 1975). A variety of psychiatric disorders are clearly associated with the use of cannabis; however, whether the psychopathology is an antecedent to use, a consequence, or a mere coincidence is still very much open to question. There are some hints that those using cannabis with therapeutic intent experience more adverse reactions (Naditch, 1974). A "best guess" is that cannabis use, like that of many other psychoactive drugs, will sometimes be an antecedent, a consequence, or a coincidence psychopathology, depending on the person and many other variables (Abruzzi, 1975; El Guebaly, 1975; Kroll, 1975; Meyer, 1975; Segal and Merenda, 1975; Stefanis *et al.*, 1976*b*; Tennant *et al.*, 1975; Westermeyer and Walzer, 1975).

As is often true in medicine, the ambiguity in diagnostic classification and definitions adds to the confusion concerning adverse psychological reactions associated with cannabis use. The classification of the subsections below has been adopted to impose some order on the literature (Halikas, 1974; Meyer, 1975).

2.1. Acute Panic Anxiety Reactions

The acute panic anxiety reaction has been noted by many reviewers to be the most common adverse reaction to cannabis use (Halikas, 1974; Meyer, 1975). The symptoms and signs are usually exaggerations of normal cannabis effects more generally described by users. Anxiety is often focused on fears of "going crazy." This reaction appears most likely to occur in novices and after consuming more potent materials. Personality variables that make for poorer coping skills play a role. The symptoms diminish with authoritative reassurance or in a few hours when the immediate drug effects have worn off. A number of reports illustrate these considerations (Ablon and Goodwin, 1974; Keeler and Moore, 1974; Mirin and McKenna, 1975; Naditch, 1974; Noyes *et al.*, 1975*a*; Tinklenberg and Darley, 1976; Tylden, 1974).

Patients with chronic pain (Noyes *et al.*, 1975*a*) and depression (Ablon and Goodwin, 1974; Regelson *et al.*, 1976) given low doses of THC in therapeutic trials had far more dysphoric and acute panic episodes than would be expected if the same doses were given to typically youthful cannabis users. These older people presumably found it difficult to accept the drug-induced mental changes as desirable. Younger, but equally inexperienced, "cannabis experimenters" often react similarly (Mirin and McKenna, 1975; Tinklenberg and Darley, 1976) as do people under stress (Bridger, 1975; Gregg *et al.*, 1976*b*).

Cannabis-induced mild paranoid feelings in student and "counterculture" users of marihuana are common and are usually not a source of undue concern to them (Keeler and Moore, 1974). About two-thirds of a student group and 95% of a counterculture group studied described suspicion of being subjected to a police raid or having friends tricking them while intoxicated. Inability to test reality concerning these suspicions was reported by over half of the subjects. Another field survey found that individuals with a tendency to use paranoid defense mechanisms experienced fewer acute anxiety reactions after cannabis (Naditch, 1974). The authors thought that the more sophisticated defenses represented in paranoid functioning may be effective in preventing acute adverse reactions. The same study found that persons with high scores on the schizophrenia subscale of the MMPI tended to have more problems with adverse psychological reactions indicating (as have a host of previous studies) that preexisting psychopathology is an important factor in such reactions. The same survey (Naditch *et al.*, 1975) suggested that the setting in which the drug is consumed may be a less important determinant of adverse reactions.

2.2. Cannabis-Induced Acute Brain Syndrome or Toxic Delirium

The clinical features of the acute brain syndrome associated with cannabis intoxication—such as clouding of mental processes, disorientation, confusion, and marked memory impairment—are similar to those produced by other exogenous toxins (Halikas, 1974; Meyer, 1975). The syndrome is most likely to occur at high doses and to be dose related, whereas the panic reactions may occur at any dose unfamiliar to the user (Halikas, 1974; Jones, 1975; Meyer, 1975). The toxic delirium is likely to follow the time course of other drug effects. This syndrome appears to be relatively rare in the United States.

A 4-year-old child presumably ate some cannabis resin (up to 1.5 g) and was found thereafter alternately stuporous and excited with inappropriate laughing and ataxia. Body temperature was markedly lowered and respiration rate was decreased. Residue on the child's teeth was identified as cannabis material. All symptoms and signs cleared in about a day (Bro *et al.*, 1975). Two cases from Nigeria involved children given smoked cannabis (Binitie, 1975). One child was perspiring and restless and could not sleep. Hyperactive and destructive behavior continued for 4 months. The second child manifested more of a toxic psychosis with hyperactivity lasting for some weeks. One must assume that a large dose was involved in these latter cases in addition to preexisting problems, given the duration of symptoms. Such case reports are rarely definitive, but can point the way for more controlled surveys and clinical studies.

In clinical studies where patients were given substantial intravenous doses of THC prior to surgery, many experienced dysphoria and psychotic-like shifts from euphoria to dysphoria, panic, and paranoid thinking (Gregg *et al.*, 1976*b*). The stress of surgery was, of course, a factor as was the large dose of intravenous THC, but the study does point out that such reactions are possible and even common under certain conditions, even with healthy, relatively well-adjusted people.

2.3. Prolonged Reactions

Possible prolonged psychological effects of cannabis use are an area of serious concern and much controversy. These include not only psychotic reactions but also personality change, change in life-style, a possible "amotivational syndrome," "flashbacks," and a possible causal relationship between marihuana use and use of other drugs. Here it is even more difficult to establish precise cause and effect because the close temporal relationship between ingestion of the drug and acute effects is lacking.

Descriptions of a specific long-lasting cannabis psychosis appear largely in the Eastern literature, and, thus, are largely drawn from a culture where use is generally more frequent, and at higher dose levels, than is typical for the United States. This acute "cannabis psychosis" is generally associated with very frequent use and reportedly lasts 1 to 6 weeks or longer (Halikas, 1974; Meyer, 1975). Recent studies abroad, in Jamaica (Rubin and Comitas, 1975), Greece (Stefanis *et al.*, 1976*a*), and Costa Rica (Coggins, 1976), where frequent users of high-potency cannabis were examined, failed to document the existence of a specific cannabis psychosis. However, small sample sizes were involved and a relatively rare occurrence could well have been missed.

In contrast, a clinical study done in India contrasted the features of a paranoid psychosis arising in the course of long-term cannabis use with paranoid schizophrenia (Thacore and Shukla, 1976). The study compared 25 consecutive admissions for each diagnosis. The majority of cannabis users had used bhang daily for 5 or more years in doses up to several grams, gradually increasing dose. The cannabis psychosis, in contrast to the paranoid schizophrenia, was characterized by more bizarre behavior, more violence and panic, an absence of schizophrenic thought disorder, and more insight. The cannabis psychosis cleared rapidly after hospitalization and phenothiazine treatment. Patients relapsed only when cannabis administration was reinitiated.

A few years ago a clinical report by Kolansky and Moore (1971) described eight psychotic reactions in a group of 39 marihuana smokers in this country and attempted to demonstrate a cause-and-effect relationship to their marihuana use. A more recent clinical study demonstrates how correlations between various behaviors and subsequent psychiatric disorders can be misleading (Altman and Evenson, 1973). Consecutive first admissions to a psychiatric hospital were evaluated. Thirty-eight patients who had used marihuana prior to the onset of psychiatric problems were studied. Indeed, apathy, poor judgment, confusion, and depression followed marihuana smoking, but the correlations between marihuana use and subsequent illness was less than with such presumably causally unrelated variables as having masturbated, having experienced sex education, and having drunk beer. In this clinical study marihuana use could not be singled out as a prime factor leading to psychiatric illness.

Marihuana flashbacks—spontaneous recurrences of feelings and perceptions similar to those produced by the drug—continue to be reported (Brown and Stickgold, 1974). Data from a survey of drug users in the Army indicate that flashbacks attributed to marihuana occur among infrequent as well as frequent users and are experienced by people who have never had LSD (Stanton *et al.*, 1976). The etiology of such flashbacks remains obscure, but most of those who experience them seem to require minimal treatment, if any.

2.4. Nonpsychotic Prolonged Adverse Reactions

Surveys of user and nonuser populations provide some information as to neuropsychological changes, changes in life-style, and the so-called amotivational syndrome associated by some with cannabis use. When discussing issues related to marihuana use, it is difficult to distinguish between antecedents and consequences of cannabis use. Therefore, the question of causality remains unresolved in many studies. In an all too rare prospective study, Culver and King (1974) compared groups of LSD–mescaline users with marihuana–hashish users and non-drug-using controls. The investigators used a sophisticated psychological test battery including the Halsted–Reitan tests, the Wechsler Adult Intelligence Scale, and tests of spatial perceptual abilities. When tested a year later, the LSD–mescaline group scored least well on the trail-making test, but the performance of all three groups fell within normal limits. No evidence could be found for the existence of a neuropsychological deficit with either light or frequent cannabis use. Another study of heavy drug users using a similar test battery arrived at similar conclusions (Bruhn and Maage, 1975). However, the authors of that study remind their readers that one should not conclude that no organic changes occurred since psychological test data are inferential and definitive statements as to organic changes can only be based on radiological or pathological evidence. One study of multiple drug users in the Navy (Gunderson *et al.*, 1975) found a large number of psychiatric symptoms reported by them on the Cornell Medical Index; but because of the variety of drugs habitually used, it was impossible to single out marihuana use as an important factor.

The possible effects of cannabis on student performance have been a major concern because of the extensive use by that group. A longitudinal study of a sample of 1,970 college students examined the relationship between cannabis use and psychosocial adaptation and academic performance (Brill and Christie, 1974). Users and nonusers did not differ in grade point average or in educational achievement, but the marihuana users seemed to have more difficulty in deciding on career goals and dropped out of college more often to reassess goals. A smaller percentage of regular users planned to seek advanced or professional degrees. There was, in the opinion of the users themselves, a poorer academic adjustment among the most frequent users than among infrequent or nonusers. Only 6% of nonusers reported a worsening of their emotional state since beginning college but 20% of the long duration users reported negative changes in emotional state. A problem with the study was that a significant percentage of the initial sample was lost over the 3-year period. If the loss was from the group who failed out or dropped out, those most likely to show loss of motivation or intellectual functions may have been automatically excluded from the study. Also, the study merely reported the students' own assessment of their adaptation since no interviews were attempted.

Investigations of why people stop using marihuana can give hints as to possible adverse effects. In a follow-up on the longitudinal survey of marihuana quitters described above, continuing users and never users were compared (Pack *et al.*, 1976). The quitters had used marihuana less frequently than the continuing users. It was used more often as a mild intoxicant than a consciousness alterer. More had experienced adverse effects. Fear of punishment was not a reason for quitting. Quitters had more experience with psychotherapy. For one group of quitters, cannabis use was mostly a social accident; they were in the right place at the right time to obtain the drug. A second type was the ex-rebel who changed identity and quit. A third group seemed to be emotionally fragile people who were psychologically threatened by the drug.

Other questionnaire surveys reported differences between users and nonusers but the question of causation remains and the mental health significance of some of the findings is unclear. In a study of high school students marihuana users were intermediate between nonusers and hard drug users on grades, absenteeism, suspensions, and likelihood of graduation (Smith and Fogg, 1976). Another study found little difference between marihuana users and nonusers in terms of their responses on personality inventories, although users of other drugs differed from nonusers (Richek *et al.*, 1975). Simon (1974) found that nonusers scored higher on need for achievement and order and, thus, not surprisingly, had higher grades. Other surveys found marihuana users to be more dissatisfied, disillusioned and alienated (Cunningham *et al.*, 1974), more oriented toward the past (King and Manaster, 1975), but, also, to be more creative and adventuresome (Grossman *et al.*, 1974). They also had lower levels of achievement (Carlin and Post, 1974), and heavy users dropped out of school more often (Kahn and Kulick, 1975).

A comparison of 850 chronic cannabis users and 839 non-cannabis-using controls recruited from Egyptian prisons revealed slower psychomotor performance, defective visual–motor coordination, and impaired memory for designs in the cannabis users (Soueif, 1975). Most were presumably not using the drug at the time of testing. When literate and illiterate and urban and rural users and nonusers were compared, Soueif (1976) found more evidence of drug-induced impairment in the subjects with literate and urban backgrounds. He presents a working hypothesis and some data suggesting that there is less functional impairment after cannabis use in the illiterate, rural, and older subjects. Of course, if such a hypothesis proves true, then the results of studies of chronic users in less sophisticated and more rural countries (Rubin and Comitas, 1975) may not apply to other populations—particularly in highly literate, urban, and young populations.

The ability of cannabis users to work in nonacademic contexts has been examined in attempts to see if a measurable "amotivational syndrome" exists (Mendelson *et al.*, 1976*a,b*; Miles *et al.*, 1974). In a study of frequent and infrequent users smoking cannabis while living on a research ward, work output decreased as marihuana consumption increased (Mendelson *et al.*, 1976*a,b*). However, the investigators noted that "motivation" is a function of situational variables as well as drug factors. These authors reasoned that to term the decrement in work output "amotivational" would imply that the users in the experiment had lost interest in working for money. However, if the work decrement resulted from a drug-induced impairment of performance, it would not be proper to term it a motivational effect. They found the change in work output to be caused more by the latter than the former drug effects. In a similar Canadian study (Miles *et al.*, 1974), a decrease in productivity (making stools) followed the smoking of cannabis. The decreased productivity appeared to be due to less time spent working rather than to reduced efficiency. The authors interpret this as indicative of an "amotivational syndrome," present at least during the period of drug use. To the extent that these types of studies involve artificial work conditions and tasks dissimilar to more usual employment, it is hazardous to draw more general conclusions regarding the role of cannabis in a more generalized amotivational picture. Moreover, these studies involved intensive daily use. The relationship of their findings to episodic or less frequent use in altering motivation is unknown. However, uncontrolled clinical reports from countries where cannabis is readily available continue to report decreased work output and initiative in chronic cannabis users (Sharma, 1975). Thus, further studies are important.

An assumed relationship between cannabis use and the use of other drugs (mainly opiates) has been a source of concern. The best predictor of marihuana and other illicit drug use may be early (before age 12) tobacco and alcohol use (Tennant and Detels, 1976). The progression hypothesis is a good example of a theoretical construct repeated so many times by so many people that it has become verified by repetition rather than by facts (Tec, 1974). The patterns of the shifts from one drug to another seem to be changing with more of a "progression" to "polydrugs," excluding heroin (Gould and Kleber, 1974). In both military and civilian populations, the pattern of drug use and selection of drugs were determined more by availability, peer pressure, and drug use fads than by pharmacologic or personality variables (Nace *et al.*, 1975; Tzeng and Skafidas, 1975). Cannabis users are, however, very likely to use other licit and illicit drugs with a positive correlation between level of cannabis use and the variety of drugs used (Mullins *et al.*, 1975).

2.5. Criminal and Aggressive Behavior

The often discussed possible link between cannabis use and crime or aggressive behavior has been the topic of reviews (Goode, 1974; Knudten and Meade, 1974) and experimental studies (Colaiuta and Breed, 1974; McGuire and Megargee, 1974; Salzman *et al.*, 1975). Both reviews concluded that evidence showing marihuana to cause crime is virtually nonexistent. McGuire and Megargee (1974) compared young prisoners who varied in their degree of marihuana use on a number of personality measures (e.g., MMPI, CPI). Nonusers and occasional users had typical criminal profiles. Regular users of only marihuana were better socialized and adjusted, though more deviant than collegiate marihuana users. Prisoners who used marihuana plus other drugs were the most deviant.

In addition to concern about marihuana use and criminality, the association between marihuana intoxication and hostile human behavior has been a topic of great interest and discussion. Surveys of California adolescents noted that aggressive and sexually assaultive behavior was more commonly associated with ethanol intoxication even though the adolescents used marihuana almost as frequently (Tinklenberg, 1974). The results of observation and self-reports of hostile, aggressive feelings from subjects acutely or chronically intoxicated with cannabis in laboratory experiments suggest that the usual effects are to decrease expressed and experienced hostility (Jones and Benowitz, 1976; Mendelson *et al.*, 1974*b*; Salzman *et al.*, 1975). In one laboratory study, college undergraduates were placed in a situation in which they could aggressively interact with another person. Those intoxicated with alcohol instigated more intense aggression than similar students intoxicated with THC (Taylor *et al.*, 1976). Yet, in other cultures, for example, in India, violent behavior is commonly associated with cannabis psychosis (Thacore and Shukla, 1976).

3. CHRONIC EFFECTS

3.1. Tolerance

Marked tolerance to the effects of cannabis doses commonly consumed in this country is not usually evident, presumably because of relatively infrequent use and the generally low doses of active material. However, as data accumulate from countries where more frequent use of high doses is common (Coggins, 1976; Fink *et al.*, 1976; Rubin and Comitas, 1975; Stefanis *et al.*, 1976a), it is apparent that tolerance must develop to many of the psychological and physiological effects. In controlled experimental situations where prolonged administration of THC or marihuana to volunteer subjects has been undertaken, what appears to be dose-related tolerance develops rapidly (Benowitz and Jones, 1975; Cohen *et al.*, 1976; Jones and Benowitz, 1976; Mendelson *et al.*, 1974*b*, 1976*b*), as judged by behavioral, psychologic, and physiologic measures. At lower doses (one cigarette per day) a longer period of administration (27 days) is necessary for clear-cut tolerance to develop (Gibbins *et al.*, 1976).

In outpatient studies where frequent and infrequent users or other populations with differing drug histories are compared in their response to a given dose of cannabis, the results are less consistent. Marked tolerance to measured effects is rarely obvious, if evident at all (Dornbush and Kokkevi, 1976; Perez-Reyes *et al.*, 1974; Renault *et al.*, 1974; Stefanis *et al.*, 1976*a*). However, when sensitive and reliable measures are used, even infrequent use may produce evidence of some degree of tolerance on outpatient laboratory tests (Borg and Gershon, 1975; Cohen and Rickles, 1974). Tolerance in humans is apparently a dose-related effect as it is in animals (Dewey *et al.*, 1976). Although tolerance regularly develops when cannabis is given experimentally for periods of time, changes in drug-seeking behavior do not seem to be clearly related to degree of tolerance (Babor *et al.*, 1975). The determinants of just how many cigarettes per day are smoked appear to be altered by many factors besides the presence or absence of drug tolerance.

3.2. Dependence

When volunteers were given 30 mg doses of THC orally every 4 hr for 10–20 days, sudden cessation of the drug was associated with the appearance of irritability, restlessness, decreased appetite, marked sleep disturbance (including sleep EEG alterations), sweating, salivation, tremor, weight loss, nausea and vomiting, diarrhea, and, in general, a clinical picture similar to that following chronic administration at moderate doses of many sedative-hypnotic drugs (Benowitz and Jones, 1975; Feinberg *et al.*, 1975; Jones and Benowitz, 1976). Such psychologic and physiologic changes have not been commonly observed in other chronic administration studies in this country, although it has been reported once in a German paper (Kielholz and Ladewig, 1970). Restlessness, anorexia, and a sudden 12-lb weight loss were reported by one group in an inpatient volunteer study at the end of a 21-day smoking period (Mendelson *et al.*, 1974*b*; Greenberg *et al.*, 1976). Drug-seeking behavior has not been associated with the withdrawal syndrome, but the presence or absence of such behavior is difficult to assess in the laboratory. A withdrawal syndrome has not been described in recent investigations of chronic users abroad (Coggins, 1976; Fink *et al.*, 1976; Rubin and Comitas, 1975).

3.3. Field Studies of Chronic Users

Several field studies of populations of frequent long-term users have searched for possible adverse or other effects associated with chronic use (Coggins, 1976; Fink *et al.*, 1976; Dornbush and Kokkevi, 1976; Rubin and Comitas, 1975). These were all concerned with users in countries in which high potency cannabis is more readily available than in the United States.

The results of a chronic user study were recently published in book form (Rubin and Comitas, 1975). The 30 experimental subjects had been smoking high potency cannabis almost daily for 10 years or more. Many of the noncannabis smokers in the control groups did use cannabis tea. This type of drug use was not controlled for; thus, both cannabis smokers and many nonsmokers were cannabis users. Few psychological or physiological differences between the cannabis smokers and nonsmokers were evident. There was no evidence for liver, kidney, or cardiovascular malfunction. While no differences in chromosomal abnormalities were found, the results must be regarded as inconclusive because of various technical deficiencies of the study. Modest decreases in pulmonary function and altered hemoglobin levels were the only physiologic differences evident. The impact of tobacco use by the subjects on these findings is uncertain. After smoking cannabis, a small group of workers produced less work (weeding, hoeing, digging) with more movements but otherwise showed no evidence of "amotivation." The importance of cultural differences in the interpretation of drug effects is evident in that people in Jamaica did not find their appetite increased by cannabis and, in fact, seemed often to use it to decrease appetite. This is, of course, not the expected effect in the United States (Abel, 1975). They did not think their hearing was enhanced nor their time sense altered and, in fact, said they used cannabis to work better. Although reassuring, the findings should also be judged in perspective. They were derived from a small group of selected users, so that rare consequences (if they did occur) such as brain atrophy or psychosis might not have been detected. The subjects were laborers and farmers in a very different culture, so that intellectual impairment may have been relatively difficult to detect. Soueif (1976) has argued that such subjects may show fewer cannabis effects than urban and literate subjects.

A similar although larger and more complex study is underway in Costa Rica. Coggins (1976) presented a preliminary report. Eighty daily marihuana users and matched non-cannabis-using controls were evaluated with extensive medical examinations; laboratory studies; X-rays; and EEG, EKG, and neuropsychological testing. Although the study is still in progress, no evidence for a greater incidence of disease or deterioration among the cannabis users has yet been found.

In the studies of Greek chronic hashish users approximately 47 chronic users were compared with 40 control nonusers on a variety of EEG, echoencephalographic, neuropsychologic, and experimental laboratory tests (Fink *et al.*, 1976; Dornbush and Kokkevi, 1976; Stefanis *et al.*, 1976*a*). Conventional clinical measures of brain damage (EEG, echo-EEG) showed no evidence of abnormality in the chronic users. Tolerance to administered doses rapidly developed on the EEG indices. No evidence of withdrawal symptoms after 3 days of chronic administration was evident. When given high doses of THC, some of these very experienced subjects developed unpleasant psychological symptoms when their tolerance level was exceeded. These were all outpatients so no precise control over drug use outside of the laboratory was possible. A slightly higher incidence of personality disorders in the hashish-using group was better explained by psychosocial variables than by marihuana use.

Thus, these three field studies of users abroad do not report brain damage, psychosis, or an "amotivational syndrome." However, the cultures are different, and the sample populations are relatively small so such drug effects cannot be ruled out. Such adverse effects may be simply uncommon or difficult to measure, should they exist.

3.4. Chronic Effects—Laboratory Studies

A number of groups have studied the effects of daily cannabis use in paid volunteer subjects consuming cannabis for up to 72-day periods while hospitalized (Benowitz and Jones, 1975; Feinberg *et al.*, 1975; Cohen *et al.*, 1976; Jones and Benowitz, 1976; Mendelson *et al.*, 1974*b*, 1976*b*; Miles *et al.*, 1974). Although even 72 days is not really chronic use, such studies complement the more commonly performed acute outpatient studies. In general, in all these chronic or subchronic studies, subjects have tolerated the drug treatment phase well and very few dropouts, psychoses, or other blatant manifestations of distress were revealed. Except for the pulmonary function impairment noted in two studies (Mendelson *et al.*, 1974*b*; Tashkin *et al.*, 1975, 1976*b*), drug effects on mental, behavioral, and physiologic functions seem to disappear rapidly on cessation of drug administration and have been, in general, similar to those seen in acute studies. Tolerance is evident at lower doses (Babor *et al.*, 1975; Bellville *et al.*, 1975*a*; Cohen *et al.*, 1976; Mendelson *et al.*, 1974*b*) and obvious at higher doses (Jones and Benowitz, 1976).

4. REFERENCES

Abel, E. L., 1975, Cannabis: Effects on hunger and thirst, *Behav. Biol.* **15**:255–281.

Ablon, S. L., and Goodwin, F. K., 1974, High frequency of dysphoric reactions to tetrahydrocannabinol among depressed patients, *Am. J. Psychiat.* **131**(4):448–453.

Abramson, H. A., 1974, Respiratory disorders and marijuana use, *J. Asthma Res.* **11**(3):97.

Abruzzi, W., 1975, Drug-induced psychosis—or schizophrenia?, *Am. J. Psychoanal.* **35**(4):329–342.

Adamec, C., Pihl, R. O., and Leiter, L., 1976, An analysis of the subjective marijuana experience, *Int. J. Addict.* **11**(2):295–307.

Adams, A. J., Brown, B., Flom, M. C., Jones, R. T., and Jampolsky, A., 1975, Alcohol and marijuana effects on static visual acuity, *Am. J. Optom. Physiol. Opt.* **52**:729–735.

Adams, A. J., Brown, B., Hagerstrom-Portnoy, G., Flom, M. C., and Jones, R. T., 1976, Evidence for acute effects of alcohol and marijuana on color discrimination, *Percept. Psychophys.* **20**(2):119–124.

Agurell, S., Levander, S., Binder, M., Bader-Bartfai, A., Gustafsson, B., Leander, K., Lindgren, J. E., Ohlsson, A., and Tobisson, B., 1976, Pharmacokinetics of delta-8-THC in man after smoking: Relations to physiological and psychological effects, in: *Pharmacology of Marihuana* (M. C. Braude and Szara, eds.), pp. 49–61, Raven Press, New York.

Altman, H., and Evenson, R. C., 1973, Marijuana use and subsequent psychiatric symptoms: A replication, *Comp. Psychia.*, **14**:415–420.

Angelico, I., and Brown, J., 1974, Marihuana and angina pectoris, *N. Engl. J. Med.* **191**(15):800.

Aronow, W. S., and Cassidy, J., 1975, Effect of smoking marihuana and of a high-nicotine cigarette on angina pectoris, *Clin. Pharmacol. Therap.* **17**(5):549–554.

Babor, T. F., Mendelson, J. H., Greenberg, I., and Kuehnle, J. C., 1975, Marijuana consumption and tolerance to physiological and subjective effects, *Arch. Gen. Psychiat.* **32**(12):1548–1552.

BACKHOUSE, C. I., 1975, Peak expiratory flow in youths with varying cigarette smoking habits, *Brit. Med. J.* **1**:360–362.

BEAHRS, J. O., CARLIN, A. S., and SHEHORN, J., 1974, Impact of psychoactive drugs on hypnotizability, *Am. J. Clin. Hypn.* **16**(4):267–269.

BEAUTRAIS, A. L., and MARKS, D. F., 1976, A test of state dependency effects in marihuana intoxication for the learning of psychomotor tasks, *Psychopharmacologia* **46**(1):37–40.

BECH, P., RAFAELSEN, L., and RAFAELSEN, O. J., 1974, Cannabis: A psychopharmacological review, *Dan. Med. Bull. (Copenhagen)*, **21**(3):106–120.

BELLVILLE, J. W., GASSER, J. C., MIYAKE, T., and AQLEH, K., 1975*a*, Tolerance to the respiratory depression of marijuana, *Pharmacologist (Abst.)* **17**(2):180.

BELLVILLE, J. W., SWANSON, G. D., and KAMEL, A. A., 1975*b*, Respiratory effects of delta-9-tetrahydrocannabinol, *Clin. Pharmacol. Therap.* **17**(5):541–548.

BENOWITZ, N. L., and JONES, R. T., 1975, Cardiovascular effects of prolonged delta-9-tetrahydrocannabinol ingestion, *Clin. Pharmacol. Therap.* **18**:287–297.

BENOWITZ, N. L., and JONES, R. T., 1977, Prolonged delta-9-tetrahydrocannabinol ingestion: Effects of sympathomimetic amines and autonomic blockades, *Clin. Pharmacol. Therap.* **21**(3):336–342.

BENOWITZ, N. L., JONES, R. T., and LERNER, C. B., 1976, Depression of growth hormone and cortisol response to insulin-induced hypoglycemia after prolonged oral delta-9-tetrahydrocannabinol administration in man, *J. Clin. Endocrinol. Metab.* **42**(5):938–941.

BINITIE, A., 1975, Psychosis following ingestion of hemp in children. *Psychopharmacologia* **44**(3):301–302.

BORG, J., and GERSHON, S., 1975, Dose effects of smoked marihuana on human cognitive and motor functions, *Psychopharmacologia (Berlin)*, **42**:211–218.

BRADEN, W., STILLMAN, R. C., and WYATT, R. J., 1974, Effects of marijuana on contingent negative variation and reaction time, *Arch. Gen. Psychiat.* **31**(4):537–541.

BRECHER, E. M., 1975, Marijuana: The health questions/the legal question. *Contemp. Drug Prob.* **4**(2):115–140.

BRIDGER, W. H., 1975, Good trip or bad trip: The roles of tolerance and stress in hallucinogenic drug action, *Adv. Biochem. Psychopharmacol.* **13**:287–298.

BRILL, N. Q., and CHRISTIE, R. L., 1974, Marihuana use and psychosocial adaptation. Follow-up study of a collegiate population, *Arch. Gen. Psychiat.* **31**(5):713–719.

BRO, P., SCHOU, J., and TOPP, G., 1975, Cannabis poisoning with analytical verification, *N. Engl. J. Med.* **293**(20):1049–1050.

BROWN, A., and STICKGOLD, A., 1974, Self-diagnosed marihuana flashbacks, *Clin. Res.* **22**(3):316A.

BROWN, B., ADAMS, A. J., HAGERSTROM-PORTNOY, G., JONES, R. T., and FLOM, M. C., 1975, Effects of alcohol and marijuana on dynamic visual acuity: I. Threshold measurements, *Percept. Psychophys.* **18**(6):441–446.

BRUHN, P., and MAAGE, N., 1975, Intellectual and neuropsychological functions in young men with heavy and long-term patterns of drug abuse, *Am. J. Psychiat.* **132**(4):397–401.

CAPPELL, H., and KUCHAR, E., 1974, Pharmacologic and nonpharmacologic factors in marijuana intoxication, *Clin. Toxicol.* **7**(3):315.

CAPPELL, H., and PLINER, P., 1974, Regulation of the self-administration of marijuana by psychological and pharmacological variables, *Psychopharmacologia (Berlin)* **40**(1):65–76.

CARLIN, A. S., and POST, R. D., 1974, Drug use and achievement, *Int. J. Addict.* **9**(3):401–410.

CARLIN, A. S., POST, R. D., BAKKER, C. B., and HALPERN. I. M., 1974, The role of modeling and previous experience in the facilitation of marijuana intoxication, *J. Nerv. Ment. Dis.* **159**(4):275–281.

CARLINI, E. A., KARNIOL, I. G., RENAULT, P. F., and SCHUSTER, C. R., 1974, Effects of marijuana in laboratory animals and in man, *Br. J. Pharmacol.* **50**:229–309.

CASSWELL, S., 1975, Cannabis intoxication: Effects of monetary incentive on performance, a controlled investigation of behavioral tolerance in moderate users of cannabis, *Percept. Mot. Skills* **41**(2):423–434.

CASTILLO, J. D., ANDERSON, M., and RUBOTTOM, G. M., 1975, Marijuana, absinthe and the central nervous system, *Nature (London)* **253**:365–366.

CHAUSOW, A. M., and SAPER, C. B., 1974, Marihuana and sex, *N. Engl. J. Med.* **291**(6):308.

CLARK, S. C., 1975, Marihuana and the cardiovascular system, *Pharmacol. Biochem. Behav.* **3**:299–306.

CLARK, S. C., GREENE, C., KARR, G. W., MACCANNELL, K. L., and MILSTEIN, S. L., 1974, Cardiovascular effects of marihuana in man, *Canad. J. Physiol. Pharmacol. (Ottawa)* **52**(3):706–719.

CO, B. T., GOODWIN, D. W., GADO, M., MIKHAEL, M., and HILL, S. Y., 1977, Absence of cerebral atrophy in chronic cannabis users by computerized transaxial tomography, *JAMA* **237**(12):1229–1230.

COGGINS, W. J., 1976, The general health status of chronic cannabis smokers in Costa Rica, in: *Pharmacology of Marijuana* (S. Szara and M. Braude, eds.), Raven Press, New York.

COHEN, M. J., and RICKLES, W. H., JR., 1974, Performance on a verbal learning task by subjects of heavy past marijuana usage, *Psychopharmacologia (Berlin)* **37**:323–330.

COHEN, M. J., RICKLES, W. H., and NALIBOFF, B. D., 1975, Marijuana influenced changes in GSR activation peaking during paired-associate learning, *Pharmacol. Biochem. Behav.* **3**:195–200.

COHEN, S., LESSIN, P. J., HAHN, P. M., and TYRRELL, E. D., 1976, A 94-day cannabis study, in: *Pharmacology of Marihuana* (M. C. Braude and S. Szara, eds.), pp. 621–626, Raven Press, New York.

COLAIUTA, V., and BREED, G., 1974, Development of scales to measure attitudes toward marijuana and marijuana users, *J. Appl. Psychol.* **59**(3):398–400.

COLEMAN, J. H., TACKER, H. L., EVANS, W. E., LEMMI, H., and BRITTON, E. L., 1976, Neurological manifestations of chronic marijuana intoxication. Part I: Paresis of the fourth cranial nerve, *Dis. Nerv. Sys.* **37**(1):29.

COMMITTEE ON DRUGS, AMERICAN ACADEMY OF PEDIATRICS, 1975, Effects of marihuana on man, *Pediatrics* **56**:134–144.

CULVER, C. M., and KING, F. W., 1974, Neuropsychological assessment of undergraduate marihuana and LSD users, *Arch. Gen. Psych.* **31**:707–711.

CUNNINGHAM, W. H., CUNNINGHAM, I. C. M., and ENGLISH, W. D., 1974, Sociopsychological characteristics of undergraduate marijuana users, *J. Genet. Psychol.* **125**:3–12.

CUSHMAN, P., 1975, Plasma testosterone levels in healthy male marijuana smokers, *Am. J. Drug. Alc. Abuse* **1**(2):269–275.

CUSHMAN, P., and KHURANA, R., 1975, Marijuana smoking and T-lymphocyte rosette formation *in vitro*, *J. Clin. Pharmacol.* **15**(7):556–557.

CUSHMAN, P., GRIECO, M., and GUPTA, S., 1974, Impaired rosette forming T-cells in chronic marijuana smokers, *Int. J. Clin. Pharmacol., Therap. Toxicol. (Munich)* **10**(2):154.

CUTTING, M., GOODENOUGH, S., SIMMONS, G., WATSON, A., LAGUARDA, R., and ANDHUBER, G., 1974, Marijuana and pulmonary antibacterial defenses: Depression of alveolar macrophage function following experimental exposure to marijuana smoke, *Chest* **66**(3):321–322.

DALTON, W. S., MARTZ, R., LEMBERGER, L., RODDA, B. E., and FORNEY, R. B., 1975, Effects of marijuana combined with secobarbital, *Clin. Pharmacol. Therap.* **18**(3):298–304.

DALTON, W. S., MARTZ, R., LEMBERGER, L., RODDA, B. E., and FORNEY, R. B., 1976, Influence of cannabidiol on delta-9-tetrahydrocannabinol effects, *Clin. Pharmacol. Therap.* **19**(3):300–309.

DARLEY, C. F., TINKLENBERG, J. R., ROTH, W. T., and ATKINSON, R. C., 1974, The nature of storage deficits and state-dependent retrieval under marihuana, *Psychopharmacologia (Berlin)* **37**:139–149.

Davies, B. H., Radcliffe, S., Seaton, A., and Graham, J. D. P., 1975, A trial of oral Δ-1-(trans)-tetrahydrocannabinol in reversible airways obstruction, *Thorax* **30:**80–85.
Dawson, W. W., 1976, Cannabis and eye function, *Invest. Ophthalmol.* **15**(4):243–245.
De Souza, M. R. C., Karniol, I. G., and Ventura, D. F., 1974, Human tonal preferences as a function of frequency under delta-8-tetrahydrocannabinol, *Pharmacol., Biochem. Behav.* **2**(5):607–611.
Dewey, W. L., Martin, B. R., and Harris, L. S., 1976, Chronic effect of delta-9-THC in animals: Tolerance and biochemical changes, in: *Pharmacology of Marihuana* (S. Szara and M. Braude, eds.), Raven Press, New York.
DiBenedetto, M., 1976, Electrodiagnostic evidence of subclinical disease states in drug abusers, *Arch. Phys. Med. Rehab.* **57**(2):62–66.
Dittrich, A., Bickel, P., and Zimmer, D., 1975, Effekte von (−)delta-9-*trans*-tetrahydrocannabinol (delta-9-THC) auf Psychotizismus-Tests, *Psychopharmacologia (Berlin)* **40:**351–358.
Domino, E. F., Rennick, P., and Pearl, J. H., 1976, Short term neuropsychopharmacological effects of marijuana smoking in experienced male users, in: *Pharmacology of Marihuana* (S. Szara and M. Braude, eds.), Raven Press, New York.
Dornbush, R. L., 1974, Marijuana and memory: Effects of smoking on storage, *Trans. N. Y. Acad. Sci., Ser. II* **36**(1):94–100.
Dornbush, R. L., and Kokkevi, A., 1976, The acute effects of various cannabis substances on cognitive, perceptual and motor performance in very long-term hashish users, in: *Pharmacology of Marihuana* (M. C. Braude and S. Szara, eds.), pp. 421–427, Raven Press, New York.
Dott, A. B., 1974, Effect of marijuana on aggression and risk acceptance in an automotive simulator, *Clin. Toxicol.* **7**(3):289.
Drachler, D. H., 1975, Hashish and the transmission of hepatitis, *N. Engl. J. Med.* **293**(13):667.
Drew, W. G., and Miller, L. L., 1974, Cannabis: Neural mechanisms and Behavior—A theoretical review, *Pharmacology* **11**(1):12–32.
Dunn, M., and Davis, R., 1974, The perceived effects of marijuana on spinal cord injured males, *Paraplegia (London)* **12**(3):175.
Edwards, G., 1974, Cannabis and the criteria for legalisation of a currently prohibited recreational drug: Groundwork for a debate, *Acta Psychi. Scand. Suppl.* **251:**1–62.
Ehrlich, D., 1974, Marijuana smoking young drivers more accident prone: ARF study, *The Journal (Addiction Research Foundation) (Toronto)* **3**(1):5.
El Guebaly, N., 1975, Manic depressive psychosis and drug abuse, *Canad. Psych. Assoc. J.* **20:**595–598.
Ellingstad, V. S., McFarling, L. H., and Struckman, D. L., 1973, Alcohol, marijuana and risk taking, Contract No. DOT-HS-191-2-301, University of South Dakota, Vermillion.
Ellinwood, E. H., and Rockwell, W. J., 1975, Effect of drug use on sexual behavior, *Med. Asp. Human Sex.* **9**(3):10–32.
Evans, M., 1974, Cannabis and cerebral atrophy, *Roy. Soc. Health J. (London)* **94**(1):15–18.
Evans, M. A., Martz, R., Lemberger, L., Rodda, B. E., and Forney, R. B., 1974, Clinical effects of marihuana dextroamphetamine combination, *Pharmacologist* **16**(2):281.
Farber, S. J., and Huertas, V. E., 1976, Intravenously injected marihuana syndrome, *Arch. Int. Med.* **136**(3):337–339.
Feinberg, I., Jones, R., Walker, J. M., Cavness, C., and March, J., 1975, Effects of high dosage delta-9-tetrahydrocannabinol on sleep patterns in man, *Clin. Pharmacol. Therap.* **17**(4):458–464.
Feinberg, I., Jones, R. T., Walker, J., Cavness, C., and Floyd, T., 1976, Marijuana extract and THC: Similarity of effects on EEG sleep patterns in man. *Clin. Pharmacol. Therap.* **19:**782–794.
Fink, M., 1976, Cerebral effects of acute and chronic inhalation of hashish, marijuana, and

delta-9-THC, in: *Pharmacology of Marihuana* (S. Szara and M. Braude, eds.), Raven Press, New York.

FINK, M., VOLAVKA, J., PANAGIOTOPOULOS, C. P., and STAFANIS, C., 1976, Quantitative EEG studies of marihuana, delta-9-THC and hashish in man. in: *Pharmacology of Marihuana* (M. C. Braude and S. Szara, eds.), pp. 383–392, Raven Press, New York.

FISHER, G., 1974, Harmful effects of marihuana use: Experiences and opinions of current and past marihuana users, *Br. J. Addict. (Oxford)* **69**(1):75–84.

FISHER, G., and STECKLER, A., 1974, Psychological effects, personality and behavioral changes attributed to marijuana use, *Int. J. Addict.* **9**(1):101–126.

FLOM, M. C., ADAMS, A. J., and JONES, R. T., 1975, Marijuana smoking and reduced pressure in human eyes: Drug action or epiphenomenon?, *Invest. Opthalmol.* **14**(1):52–55.

FRANK, I. M., LESSIN, P., HAHN, P., COHEN, S., and SZARA, S., 1976, The 94-day marihuana study, in: *Pharmacology of Marihuana* (S. Szara and M. Braude, eds.), Raven Press, New York.

FREEMON, F. R., ROSENBLATT, J. E., and EL-YOUSEF, M. K., 1975, Interaction of physostigmine and delta-9-tetrahydrocannabinol in man, *Clin. Pharmacol. Therap.* **17**(2):121–126.

FRIEDMAN, J. G., 1975, Marihuana and testosterone levels, *N. Engl. J. Med.* **292**(9):484.

GARRIOTT, J. C., and LATMAN, N., 1976, Drug detection in cases of "drving under the influence," *J. For. Sci.* **21**(2):398–415.

GIANUTSOS, R., and LITWACK, A. R., 1976, Chronic marijuana smokers show reduced coding into long-term storage, *Bull. Psychon. Soc.* **7**(3):277–279.

GIBBINS, R. J., McDOUGALL, J., MILES, C. G., and MARSHMAN, J. A., 1976, Tolerance to marijuana-induced tachycardia in man, *Acta Pharmacol. Toxicol.* **39**:65–76.

GOODE, E., 1974, The criminogenics of marijuana, *Addict. Dis.* **1**(3):297–322.

GORDON, G. G., ALTMAN, K., SOUTHREN, A. L., RUBIN, E., and LIEBER, C. S., 1976, Effect of alcohol (ethanol) administration on sex hormone metabolism in normal men, *N. Engl. J. Med.* **295**(15):793–797.

GOULD, L. C., and KLEBER, H. D., 1974, Changing patterns of multiple drug use among applicants to a multimodality drug treatment program, *Arch. Gen. Psychiat.* **31**:408–413.

GRAHAM, J. D. P., DAVIES, B. H., and SEATON, A., 1976, Bronchodilator action of cannabis and delta-9-THC, in: *Pharmacology of Marihuana* (S. Szara and M. Braude, eds.), Raven Press, New York.

GREENBERG, I., KUEHNLE, J., MENDELSON, J. H., and BERNSTEIN, J. G., 1976, Effects of marihuana use on body weight and caloric intake in humans, *Psychopharmacology* **49**:79–84.

GREENE, M. L., and SAUNDERS, D. R., 1974, Metabolism of tetrahydrocannabinol by the small intestine, *Gastroenterology* **66**(3):365–372.

GREGG, J. M., CAMPBELL, R. L., LEVIN, K. J., GHIA, J., and ELIOTT, R. A., 1976*a*, Cardiovascular effects of cannabinol during oral surgery, *Anesth. Analg.* **55**(2):203–213.

GREGG, J. M., SMALL, E. W., MOORE, R., RAFT, D., and TOOMEY, T. C., 1976*b*, Emotional response to intravenous delta-9-tetrahydrocannabinol during oral surgery, *J. Oral Surg.* **34**(4):301–313.

GROSSMAN, J. C., GOLDSTEIN, R., and EISENMAN, R., 1974, Undergraduate marijuana and drug use as related to openness to experience, *Psych. Quart.* **48**(1):86–92.

GUNDERSON, E. K. E., NAIL, R. L., and KOLB, D., 1975, Health status of drug abusers as measured by the Cornell Medical Index, *J. Commun. Psychol.* **3**(1):58–67.

HAGER, M., 1975, To enhance sex, marijuana is "unparalleled." *The Journal (Addiction Research Foundation) (Toronto)* **4**(2):1, 5.

HALIKAS, J. A., 1974, Marijuana use and psychiatric illness, in: *Marijuana: Effects on Human Behavior* (L. L. Miller, ed.), Chap. 2, Academic Press, New York.

HARDMAN, H. F., HOSKO, M. J., and LAHIRI, P. K., 1976, Cardiovascular pharmacology of cannabis, in: *Pharmacology of Marihuana* (S. Szara and M. Braude, eds.), Raven Press, New York.

HARMON, J. W., and ALIAPOULIOS, M. A., 1974, Marijuana-induced gynecomastia: Clinical and laboratory experience, *Surg. For.* **25**:423–425.

HEATH, R. G., 1976, Marihuana and delta-9-THC: Acute and chronic effects on brain function of monkeys, in: *Pharmacology of Marihuana* (S. Szara and M. Braude, eds.), Raven Press, New York.

HEMBREE, W., 1975, Effects of marihuana on gonadal function in man. Paper presented at the Satellite Symposium on Marihuana of the Sixth International Congress of Pharmacology, Helsinki, Finland, July 26–27, 1975.

HEMBREE, W. C., NAHAS, G. G., ZEIDENBERG, P., and DYRENFURTH, I., 1976, Marihuana effects upon the human testis, *Clin. Res.* (Abst.) **24**(3):272A.

HEPLER, R. S. FRANK, I. M., and PETRUS, R., 1976, Ocular effects of marijuana, in: *Pharmacology of Marihuana* (S. Szara and M. Braude, eds.), Raven Press, New York.

HILL, T. W., 1975, Breast growth for male pot smokers, *The Journal (Addiction Research Foundation) (Toronto)* **4**(1):1, 2.

HOLLISTER, L., 1976, Drugs and sexual behavior in man, *Life Sci.* **17**:661–668.

HOLLISTER, L. E., 1974*a*, Clinical pharmacology of marihuana, in: *Research Advances in Alcohol and Drug Problems* (R. J. Gibbons, Y. Israel, R. E. Kalant, R. E. Popham, W. Schmidt, and R. G. Smart, eds.), Wiley, New York.

HOLLISTER, L. E., 1974*b*, Structure–activity relationships of cannabis constituents in man, *Clin. Pharmacol. Therap.* **15**(2):208–209.

HOLLISTER, L. E., and GILLESPIE, H. K., 1975*a*, Interactions in man of delta-9-tetrahydrocannabinol. II. Cannabinol and cannabidiol, *Clin. Pharmacol. Therap.* **18**(1):80–83.

HOLLISTER, L. E., and GILLESPIE, H. K., 1975*b*, Action of delta-9-tetrahydrocannabinol (THC): An approach to the active metabolite hypothesis. Personal communication.

HOLLISTER, L. E., and REAVEN, G. M., 1974, Delta-9-tetrahydrocannabinol and glucose tolerance, *Clin. Pharmacol. Therap.* **16**(2):297–302.

HOLLISTER, L. E., KANTER, S. L., BOARD, R. D., and GREEN, D. E., 1974, Marihuana metabolites in urine of man. III. Unchanged delta-9-tetrahydrocannabinol, *Res. Commun. Chem. Pathol. Pharmacol.* **8**(4):579–584.

HOLLISTER, L. E., OVERALL, J. E., and GERBER, M. L., 1975, Marihuana and setting. *Arch. Gen. Psych.* **32**:798–801.

ISREALSTAM, S., and LAMBERT, S., eds., 1975, *Alcohol, Drugs, and Traffic Safety*, Proceedings of the Sixth International Conference on Alcohol, Drugs and Traffic Safety, Toronto, September 8–13, 1974. Toronto: Addiction Research Foundation of Ontario, 1975.

JANOWSKY, D. S., MEACHAM, M., BLAINE, J., SCHORR, M., and BOZZETTI, L., 1976*a*, Simulated flying performance after marihuana intoxication, *Aviat. Space Environ. Med.* **47**(2):124–128.

JANOWSKY, D. S., MEACHAM, M. P., BLAINE, J. D., SCHORR, M., and BOZZETTI, L. P., 1976*b*, Marijuana effects on simulated flying ability, *Am. J. Psych.* **133**(4):384–388.

JOHNSTONE, R. E., LIEF, P. L., KULP, R. A., and SMITH, T. C., 1974, Combination of delta-9-tetrahydrocannabinol with oxymorphone or pentobarbital: Effects on ventilatory control and cardiovascular dynamics, *Anesthesiology* **42**(6):674–684.

JONES, R. T., 1973, Drug models of schizophrenia—cannabis, in: *Psychopathology and Psychopharmacology* (J. O. Cole, A. M. Freedman, and A. J. Friedhoff, eds.), Johns Hopkins Press, Baltimore.

JONES, R. T., 1975, Does cannabis affect the minds of people? in: *Marihuana and Health Hazards: Methodological Issues in Current Marihuana Research* (J. R. Tinklenberg, ed.), Academic Press, New York.

JONES, R. T., and BENOWITZ, N., 1976, The 30-day trip—Clinical studies of cannabis tolerance and dependence, in: *Pharmacology of Marihuana* (S. Szara and M. Braude, eds.), Raven Press, New York.

JUST, W. W., FILIPOVIC, N., and WERBER, G., 1974, Detection of delta-9-tetrahydrocannabinol in saliva of men by means of thin-layer chromatography and mass spectometry, *J. Chromatogr.* **96**:189–194.

KAHN, M., and KULICK, F., 1975, Relationship of drug involvement to dropping out of college, *Psychol. Rep.* **37**(3, part 2):1095–1098.

KALANT, H., and KALANT, O. J., 1974, Cannabis—Some new answers to old questions, *Addictions* **21**(3):48–61.

KANAKIS, C., 1976, Effects of marijuana in coronary disease *Clin. Pharmacol. Therap.* **19**(1):94.

KANAKIS, C., POUGET, J. M., and ROSEN, K. M., 1976*a*, The effects of delta-9-tetrahydrocannabinol (cannabis) on cardiac performance with and without beta blockade, *Circulation* **53**(4):703–707.

KANAKIS, C., POUGET, J. M., and ROSEN, K. M., 1976*b*, Effects of delta-9-tetrahydrocannabinol (cannabis) on cardiac performance as measured by echocardiography, *Clin. Res.* **24**(3):255A.

KANTER, S. L., HOLLISTER, L. E., MOORE, F., and GREEN, D. E., 1974*a*, Marihuana metabolites in urine of man. IV. Extraction procedures using diethyl ether, *Res. Commun. Chem. Pathol. Pharmacol.* **9**(2):205–213.

KANTER, S. L., HOLLISTER, L. E., MOORE, F., and GREEN, D. E., 1974*b*, Marihuana metabolites in urine of man. II. Undescribed metabolite following oral ingestion of delta-9-tetrahydrocannabinol, *Res. Commun. Chem. Pathol. Pharmacol.* **7**:79–84.

KANTER, S. L., HOLLISTER, L. E., and MOORE, F., 1975, Marihuana metabolites in urine of man. V. Characterization and separation of polar metabolites of delta-9-tetrahydrocannabinol, *Res. Commun. Chem. Pathol. Pharmacol.* **10**(2):215–219.

KARNIOL, I. G., SHIRAKAWA, I., KASINSKI, N., PFEFERMAN, A., and CARLINI, E. A., 1974, Cannabidiol interferes with the effects of delta-9-tetrahydrocannabinol in man, *Europ. J. Pharmacol.* **28**:172–177.

KARNIOL, I. G., SHIRAKAWA, I., TAKAHASHI, R. N., KNOBEL, E., and MUSTY, R. E., 1975, Effects of delta-9-tetrahydrocannabinol and cannabinol in man, *Pharmacology* **13**:502–512.

KAYMAKCALAN, S., 1975, Potential dangers of cannabis, *Int. J. Addict.* **10**(4):721–735.

KEELER, M. H., and MOORE, E., 1974, Paranoid reactions while using marijuana, *Dis. Nerv. Sys.* **35**(11):535–536.

KIELHOLZ, P., and LADEWIG, E., 1970, Uber Drogenabhangigkeit bei Jugendlichen. *Deutsche Med. Wochensch.* **95**:101–105.

KING, M. R., and MANASTER, G. J., 1975, Time perspective correlates of collegiate marijuana use, *J. Consult. Clin. Psychol.* **43**(1):99.

KLONOFF, H., 1974*a*, Marijuana and driving in real-life situations, *Science* **186**:317–324.

KLONOFF, H., 1974*b*, Effects of marijuana on driving in a restricted area and on city streets: Driving performance and physiologic changes, in: *Marijuana: Effects on Human Behavior* (L. L. Miller, ed.), Chap. 14, Academic Press, New York.

KLONOFF, H., and CLARK, C., 1976, Drug patterns in the chronic marijuana user, *Int. J. Addict.* **11**(1):71–80.

KLONOFF, H., and LOW, M. D., 1974, Psychological and neurophysiological effects of marijuana in man: An interaction model, in: *Marijuana: Effects on Human Behavior* (L. L. Miller, ed.), Chap. 6, Academic Press, New York.

KNUDTEN, R. D., and MEADE, A. C., 1974, Marijuana and social policy, *Addict. Dis.* **1**(3):323–351.

KOFF, W., 1974, Marijuana and sexual activity, *J. Sex Res.* **10**(3):194–204.

KOKKEVI, A., and DORNBUSH, R. L., 1976, The acute effects of various cannabis substances on cognitive, perceptual, and motor performance in very long-term hashish users, in: *Pharmacology of Marihuana*, (S. Szara and M. Braude, eds.), Raven Press, New York.

KOLANSKY, H., and MOORE, W. T., 1971, Effects of marihuana on adolescents and young adults, *JAMA* **216**:486–492.

KOLODNY, R. C., 1975*a*, Research issues in the study of marihuana and male reproductive physiology in humans, in: *Marijuana and Health Hazards: Methodological Issues in Current Research* (J. R. Tinklenberg, ed.), Academic Press, New York.

KOLODNY, R. C., 1975*b*, Paper presented at the International Academy of Sex Research meeting, Stonybrook, New York.

KOLODNY, R. C., MASTERS, W. H., KOLODNER, R. M., and TORO, G., 1974*a*, Depression of plasma testosterone levels after chronic intensive marihuana use, *N. Engl. J. Med.* **290:**872–874.

KOLODNY, R. C., MASTERS, W. H., and TORO, G., 1974*b*, Marihuana and sex, *N. Engl. J. Med.* **291**(6):310.

KOLODNY, R. C., LESSIN, P., TORO, G., MASTERS, W. H., and COHEN, S., 1976, Depression of plasma testosterone with acute marihuana administration, in: *Pharmacology of Marihuana* (S. Szara and M. Braude, eds.), Raven Press, New York.

KROLL, P., 1975, Psychoses associated with marijuana use in Thailand, *J. Nerv. Ment. Dis.* **161**(3):149–156.

KUEHNLE, J., MENDELSON, J. H., DAVIS, K. R., and NEW, P. F. J., 1977, Computerized tomographic examination of heavy marihuana smokers, *JAMA* **237**(12):1231–1232.

LAU, R. J., TUBERGEN, D. G., BARR, M., DOMINO, E. F., BENOWITZ, N., and JONES, R. T., 1976, Phytohemagglutin-induced lymphocyte transformation in humans receiving delta-9-tetrahydrocannabinol, *Science* **192:**805–807.

LEMBERGER, L., and ROWE, H., 1975, Clinical pharmacology of nabilone, a cannabinol derivative, *Clin. Pharmacol. Therap.* **18**(6):720–726.

LEMBERGER, L., and RUBIN, A., 1975, The physiologic disposition of marihuana in man, *Life Sci.* **17**(11):1637–1742.

LEMBERGER, L., CRABTREE, R., ROWE, H., and CLEMENS, J., 1975, Tetrahydrocannabinols and serum prolactin levels in man, *Life Sci.* **16**(8):1339–1343.

LEMBERGER, L., MCMAHON, R., and ARCHER, R., 1976, The possible role of metabolic conversion on the mechanism of action of cannabinoids, in *Pharmacology of Marihuana* (S. Szara and M. Braude, eds.), Raven Press, New York.

LEWIS, C. R., and SLAVIN, R. G., 1975, Allergy to marijuana: A clinical and skin testing study, *J. All. Clin. Immunol.* **55**(2):131–132.

LINTON, P. H., KUECHENMEISTER, C. A., WHITE, H. B., and TRAVIS, R. P., 1975, Marijuana: Heart rate and EEG response, *Res. Commun. Chem. Pathol. Pharmacol.* **10:**201–214.

MACAVOY, M. G., and MARKS, D. F., 1975, Divided attention performance of cannabis users and non-users following cannabis and alcohol, *Psychopharmacologia* **44**(2):147–152.

MALIT, L. A., JOHNSTONE, R. E., BOURKE, D. I., KULP, R. A., KLEIN, V., and SMITH, T. C., 1975, Intravenous delta-9-tetrahydrocannabinol: Effects on ventilatory control and cardiovascular dynamics, *Anesthesiology* **42**(6):666–673.

MARKS, V., TEALE, D., and FRY, D., 1975, Detection of cannabis products in urine by radioimmunoassay, *Br. Med. J.* **3:**348–349.

MATTOX, K. L., 1976, Pneumomediastinum in heroin and marijuana users, *J. Amer. Coll. Emerg. Phys.* **5**(1):26–28.

MCCALLUM, N. K., 1974, The determination of cannabinol levels in the blood and interpretation of their significance, *Pharmacology* **11:**33–37.

MCGLOTHLIN, W. H., 1975, Drug use and abuse, *Ann. Rev. Psychol.* **26:**45–64.

MCGUIRE, J. S., and MEGARGEE, E. I., 1974, Personality correlates of marijuana use among youthful offenders, *J. Consult. Clin. Psychol.* **42**(1):124–133.

MEACHAM, M. P., JANOWSKY, D. S., BLAINE, J. D., BOZZETTI, L. P., JR., and SCHORR, M., 1974, Effects of marihuana on flying ability, *JAMA* **230**(9):1258.

MECHOULAM, R., MCCALLUM, N. K., and BERNSTEIN, S., 1976, Recent advances in the chemistry and biochemistry of cannabis, *Chem. Rev.* **76**(1):75–112.

MENDELSON, J. H., KUEHNLE, J., ELLINGBOE, J., and BABOR, T. F., 1974*a*, Plasma testosterone levels before, during and after chronic marihuana smoking, *N. Engl. J. Med.* **291** (20):1051–1055.

MENDELSON, J. H., ROSSI, A. M., and MEYER, R. E. (eds.), 1974*b*, *The Use of Marihuana, A Psychological and Physiological Inquiry,* Plenum, New York.

MENDELSON, J. H., KUEHNLE, J. C., GREENBERG, I., and MELLO, N., 1976*a*, Operant acquisition of marihuana in man, *J. Pharmacol. Exper. Therap.* **198**(1):42–53.

MENDELSON, J. H., KUEHNLE, J. C., GREENBERG, I., and MELLO, N., 1976*b*, Marihuana, use, work and motivation, in: *Pharmacology of Marihuana* (S. Szara and M. Braude, eds.), Raven Press, New York.

MEYER, R. E., 1975, Psychiatric consequences of marihuana use: The state of the evidence, in: *Marijuana and Health Hazards: Methodologic Issues in Current Research* (J. R. Tinklenberg, ed.), Academic Press, New York.

MILES, C. G., CONGREVE, G. R. S., GIBBINS, R. J., MARSHMAN, J., DEVENYI, P., and HICKS, R. C., 1974, An experimental study of the effects of daily cannabis smoking on behaviour patterns, *Acta Pharmacol. Toxicol. (Copenhagen)* **34**(*Suppl. 1*):1–44.

MILLER, L. L. (ed.), 1974, *Marijuana. Effects on Human Behavior,* Academic Press, New York.

MILSTEIN, S. L., MACCANNELL, K. L., KARR, G., and CLARK, S., 1974, Marijuana-produced changes in cutaneous sensitivity and affect: Users and nonusers, *Pharmacol. Biochem. Behav.* **2**(3):367–374.

MILSTEIN, S. L., MACCANNELL, K., KARR, G., and CLARK, S., 1975*a*, Marijuana-produced changes in pain tolerance. Experienced and non-experienced subjects, *Int. Pharmacopsych.* **10**(3):177–182.

MILSTEIN, S. L., MACCANNELL, K., KARR, G., and CLARK, S., 1975*b*, Marijuana-produced impairments in coordination, *J. Nerv. Ment. Dis.* **161**(1):26–31.

MIRIN, S. M., and MCKENNA, G. J., 1975, Combat zone adjustment: The role of marijuana use, *Mil. Med.* **140**(7):482–485.

MORISHIMA, A., and NAHAS, G. G., 1976, Effects of cannabinoids on replication of human lymphocytes, in: *Pharmacology of Marihuana* (S. Szara and M. Braude, eds.), Raven Press, New York.

MOSKOWITZ, H., 1976, Marihuana and driving, *Acc. Anal. Prevent.* **8**(1):21–26.

MOSKOWITZ, H., and MCGLOTHLIN, W., 1974, Effects of marihuana on auditory signal detection, *Psychopharmacologia (Berlin)* **40**(2):137–145.

MOSKOWITZ, H., MCGLOTHLIN, W., and HULBERT, S., 1973, The effects of marijuana dosage on driver performance. Contract No. DOT-HS-150-2-236, University of California, Los Angeles.

MOSKOWITZ, H., SHEA, R., and BURNS, M., 1974, Effect of marihuana on the psychological refractory period, *Percept. Mot. Skills* **38**:959–962.

MOSKOWITZ, H., HULBERT, S., and MCGLOTHLIN, W. H., 1976, Marihuana: Effects on simulated driving performance, *Acc. Anal. Prevent.* **8**(1):45–50.

MULLINS, C. J., VITOLA, B. M., and MICHELSON, A. E., 1975, Variables related to cannabis use, *Int. J. Addict.* **10**(3):481–502.

NACE, E. P., MEYERS, A. L., ROTHBERG, J. M., and MALESON, F., 1975, Addicted and nonaddicted drug users—A comparison of drug usage patterns, *Arch. Gen. Psychiat.* **32**:77–80.

NADITCH, M. P., 1974, Acute adverse reactions to psychoactive drugs, drug usage, and psychopathology, *J. Abnorm. Psychol.* **83**(4):394–403.

NADITCH, M. P., 1975, Relation of motives for drug use and psychopathology in the development of acute adverse reactions to psychoactive drugs, *J. Abnorm. Psychol.* **84**(4):374–385.

NADITCH, M. P., ALKER, P. C., and JOFFE, P., 1975, Individual differences and setting as determinants of acute adverse reactions to psychoactive drugs, *J. Nerv. Ment. Dis.* **161**(5):326–335.

NAHAS, G. G., 1975*a*, Marihuana, *JAMA* **233**(1):80.

NAHAS, G. G., 1975*b*, *Marihuana—Deceptive Weed,* Raven Press, New York.

NAHAS, G. G., DESOIZE, B., ARMAND, J. P., HSU, J., and MORISHIMA, A., 1976, Natural cannabinoids: Apparent depression of nucleic acids and protein synthesis in cultured human lymphocytes, in: *Pharmacology of Marihuana* (M. C. Braude and S. Szara, eds.), pp. 177–186, Raven Press, New York.

NICHOLS, W. W., MILLER, R. C., HENEEN, W., BRADT, C., HOLLISTER, L., and KANTER, S., 1974, Cytogenetic studies on human subjects receiving marihuana and delta-9-tetrahydrocannabinol, *Mut. Res. (Amsterdam)* **26**(5):413–417.

NOYES, R., JR., BRUNK, S. F., AVERY, D. H., and CANTER, A., 1975*a*, The analgesic properties of delta-9-tetrahydrocannabinol and codeine, *Clin. Pharmacol. Therap.* **18**(1):84–89.

NOYES, R., JR., BRUNK, S. F., BARAM, D. A., and CANTER, A., 1975*b*, Analgesic effect of delta-9-tetrahydrocannabinol, *J. Clin. Pharmacol.* **15**(2&3):139–143.

ORCUTT, J. D., 1975, Social determinants of alcohol and marijuana effects: A systematic theory, *Int. J. Addict.* **10**(6):1021–1033.

ORCUTT, J. D., and BIGGS, D. A., 1975, Recreational effects of marijuana and alcohol: Some descriptive dimensions *Int. J. Addict.* **10**(2):229–239.

PACK, A. T., BRILL, N. Q., and CHRISTIE, R. L., 1976, Quitting marijuana, *Dis. Nerv. Sys.* **37**(4):205–209.

PAPADAKIS, D. P., MICHAEL, C. M., KEPHALAS, T. A., and MIRAS, C. J., 1974, Effects of cannabis smoking in blood lactic acid and glucose in humans, *Experientia* **30**(10):1183–1184.

PAYER, L., 1974, Marijuana increases pain tolerance, *The Journal (Addiction Research Foundation) (Toronto)* **3**(12):4.

PAYNE, R. J., and BRAND, S. N., 1975, The toxicity of intravenously used marijuana, *JAMA* **233**(4):351–354.

PEEKE, S. C., JONES, R. T., and STONE, G. C., 1976, Effects of practice on marijuana induced changes in reaction time, *Psychopharmacology* **48:**159–163.

PEREZ-REYES, M., TIMMONS, M. C., and WALL, M. E., 1974, Long-term use of marijuana and the development of tolerance or sensitivity to delta-9-tetrahydrocannabinol, *Arch. Gen. Psychiat.* **31:**89–91.

PEREZ-REYES, M., WAGNER, D., BRINE, D., CHRISTENSEN, H. D., and WALL, M. E., 1976, The rate of plasma disappearance of tetrahydrocannabinols in humans and their rate of penetration to the brain of mice, in: *Pharmacology of Marihuana* (S. Szara and M. Braude, eds.), Raven Press, New York.

PERMUTT, M. A., GOODWIN, D. W., SCHWIN, R., and HILL, S. Y., 1976, The effect of marijuana on carbohydrate metabolism, *Am. J. Psychiat.* **133**(2):220–221.

PETERSEN, B. H., GRAHAM, J., LEMBERGER, L., and DALTON, B., 1974, Studies of the immune response in chronic marihuana smokers, *Pharmacologist* **16**(2):259.

PETERSEN, B. H., GRAHAM, J., and LEMBERGER, L., 1975*a*, Marihuana, tetrahydrocannabinol and T-cell formation, *Clin. Res.* **23**(4):477A.

PETERSEN, B. H., LEMBERGER, L., GRAHAM, J., and DALTON, B., 1975*b*, Alterations in the cellular-mediated immune responsiveness of chronic marihuana smokers, *Psychopharmacol. Commun.* **1**(1):67–74.

PILLARD, R. C., 1974, Marihuana is not a public health menace: It is time to relax our social policy, in: *Controversy in Internal Medicine II* (F. J. Ingelfinger, M. Finland, A. Relman, and R. Elbert, eds.), pp. 762–768, Saunders, Philadelphia.

PILLARD, R. C., MCNAIR, D. M., and FISHER, S., 1974, Does marijuana enhance experimentally induced anxiety?, *Psychopharmacologia (Berlin)* **40**(3):205–210.

PRAKASH, R., and ARONOW, W. S., 1976, Effects of marijuana in coronary disease. Reply, *Clin. Pharmacol. Therap.* **19**(1):94–95.

PRAKASH, R., ARONOW, W. S., WARREN, M., LAVERTY, W., and GOTTSCHALK, L. A., 1975, Effects of marihuana and placebo marihuana smoking on hemodynamics in coronary disease, *Clin. Pharmacol. Therap.* **18**(1):90–95.

PRYOR, G. T., 1976, Acute and subacute behavioral and pharmacological interactions of delta-9-THC with other drugs, *Pharmacology of Marihuana* (S. Szara and M. Braude, eds.), Raven Press, New York.

PURNELL, W. D., and GREGG, J. M., 1975, Delta-9-tetrahydrocannabinol, euphoria and intraocular pressure in man, *Ann. Ophthalmol.* **7**(7):921–923.

REGELSON, W., BUTLER, J. R., SCHULZ, J., KIRK, T., PEEK, L., and GREEN, M. L., 1976, Delta-nine-tetrahydrocannabinol (delta-9-THC) as an effective antidepressant and appetite-stimulating agent in advanced cancer patients, *Pharmacology of Marihuana* (S. Szara and M. Braude, eds.), Raven Press, New York.

RENAULT, P. F., SCHUSTER, C. R., FREEDMAN, D. X., SIKIC, B., DE MELLO, D. N., and HALARIS, A., 1974, Repeat administration of marihuana smoke to humans, *Arch. Gen. Psychiat.* **31**:95–102.

RICHEK, H. G., ANGLE, J. F., MCADAMS, W. S., and D'ANGELO, J., 1975, Personality/mental health correlates of drug use by high school students, *J. Nerv. Ment. Dis.* **160**(6):435–442.

ROTH, W. T., ROSENBLOOM, M. J., DARLEY, C. F., TINKLENBERG, J. R., and KOPELL, B. S., 1975, Marijuana effects on TAT form and content, *Psychopharmacologia* **43**:261–266.

ROTH, W. T., TINKLENBERG, J. R., and KOPELL, B. S., 1977, Ethanol and marijuana effects on event related potentials in a memory retrieval paradigm, *Electroencephalogr. Clin. Neurophysiol.* **42**(3):381–388.

RUBIN, V., and COMITAS, L., 1975, Ganja in Jamaica: A medical anthropological study of chronic marihuana use. The Hague, Mouton.

SALVENDY, G., and MCCABE, G. P., JR., 1975, Marijuana and human performance, *Hum. Fact.* **17**:229–235.

SALZMAN, C., VAN DER KOLK, B. A., and SHADER, R. I., 1975, Marijuana and hostility in a small group setting. Presented at the American Psychiatric Association Meeting (May, 1975).

SAVARY, P., LAURENCEAU, J. L., DE LEAN, A., ROY, P., and MARQUIS, Y., 1974, Acute cardiovascular effects of inhaled *Cannabis sativa* smoke in man. *Int. J. Clin. Pharmacol. Ther. Toxicol. (Munich)* **10**(2):150.

SCHAEFER, C. F., GUNN, C. G., and DUBOWSKI, K. M., 1975*a*, Normal plasma testosterone concentrations after marihuana smoking, *N. Engl. J. Med.* **292**(16):867–868.

SCHAEFER, C. F., GUNN, C. G., and DUBOWSKI, K. M., 1975*b*, Marihuana dosage control through heart rate, *N. Engl. J. Med.* **293**(2):101.

SCHNOLL, S. H., 1975, Male sex organ function in drug users, *N. Engl. J. Med.* **293**(4):202.

SCHURR, A., SHEFFER, N., GRAZIANI, Y., and LIVNE, A., 1974, Inhibition of glucose efflux from human erythrocytes by hashish components, *Biochem. Pharmacol.* **23**:2005–2009.

SCHWARTZFARB, L., NEEDLE, M., and CHAVEZ-CHASE, M., 1974, Dose-related inhibition of leukocyte migration by marihuana and delta-9-tetrahydrocannabinol (THC) *in vitro*, *J. Clin. Pharmacol.* **14**(1):35–41.

SEGAL, B., and MERENDA, P. F., 1975, Locus of control, sensation seeking, and drug and alcohol use in college students, *Drug For.* **4**(4):349–369.

SEGELMAN, A. B., SEGELMAN, F. P., NAHAS, G. G., SUCIU-FOCA, N., DESOIZE, B., ARMAND, J. P., and MORISHIMA, A., 1974, Possible noninhibition of cellular-mediated immunity in marihuana smokers, *Science* **185**(4150):543–544.

SEIDEN, R. H., TOMLINSON, K. R., and O'CARROLL, M., 1975, Patterns of marijuana use among public health students, *Am. J. Pub. Health.* **65**(6):613–621.

SEYFEDDININPUR, N., 1975, Clinical and electroencephalographic observations during the acute action of hashish, *Munch. Med. Wochenschr.* **117**(12):477–482.

SHAPIRO, B. J., and TASHKIN, D. P., 1976, Effects of beta-adrenergic blockage and muscarinic stimulation upon cannabis bronchodilation, *Pharmacology of Marihuana* (S. Szara and M. Braude, eds.), Raven Press, New York.

SHAPIRO, C. M., ORLINA, A. R., UNGER, P. J., TELFER, M., and BILLINGS, A. A., 1975, Marihuana-induced antibody response and laboratory correlates, *Clin. Res.* **23**(4):488A.

SHARMA, B. P., 1975, Cannabis and its users in Nepal, *Br. J. Psychiat.* **127**:550–552.

SHARMA, S., and MOSKOWITZ, H., 1974, Effects of two levels of attention demand on vigilance performance under marihuana, *Percept. Mot. Skills* **38**(3, Part 1):967–970.

SILVERSTEIN, M. J., and LESSIN, P. J., 1976, DNCB skin testing in chronic marijuana users, *Pharmacology of Marihuana* (S. Szara and M. Braude, eds.), Raven Press, New York.

SIMON, W. E., 1974, Psychological needs, academic achievement and marijuana consumption, *J. Clin. Psychol.* **30**(4):496–498.

SIMON, W. E., SIMON, M. G., PRIMAVERA, L. H., and ORNDOFF, R. K., 1974, A comparison of marijuana users and nonusers on a number of personality variables. *J. Consult. Clin. Psychol.* **42**(6):917–918.

SMART, R. G., 1974, Marihuana and driving risk among college students, *J. Safety Res.* **6**(4):155–158.

SMITH, G. M., and FOGG, C. P., 1976, High school performance and behavior before and after initiation of illicit drug use, *Fed. Proc.* **35**(3):564.

SOUEIF, M. I., 1976, Some determinants of psychological deficits associated with chronic cannabis consumption, *Bull. Narc.* **28**(1):25–42.

SOUEIF, M. I., 1975, Chronic cannabis users: Further analysis of objective test results, *Bull. Narc.* **27**(4):1–26.

STANTON, M. D., MINTZ, J., and FRANKLIN, R. M., 1976, Drug flashbacks. II. Some additional findings. *Int. J. Addict.* **11**(1):53–69.

STEADWARD, R. D., and SINGH, M., 1975, The effects of smoking marihuana on physical performance, *Med. Sci. Sports* **7**(4):309–311.

STEFANIS, C., BOULOUGOURIS, J., and LIAKOS, A., 1976*a*, Clinical and psychophysiological effects of cannabis in long term users, *Pharmacology of Marihuana* (S. Szara and M. Braude, eds.), Raven Press, New York.

STEFANIS, C., LIAKOS, A., BOULOUGOURIS, J., FINK, M., and FREEDMAN, A. M., 1976*b*, Chronic hashish use and mental disorder, *Am. J. Psychiat.* **133**(2):225–227.

STERLING-SMITH, R. S., 1976, A special study of drivers most responsible in fatal accidents. Summary for Management Report, Contract No. DOT HS 310-3-595.

STIMMEL, B., 1975, Male sex organ function in drug users, *N. Engl. J. Med.* **293**(4):202.

STOLLER, K., SWANSON, G. D., and BELLVILLE, J. W., 1976, Effects on visual tracking of delta-9-tetrahydrocannabinol and pentobarbital, *J. Clin. Pharmacol.* **16**(5–6):271–275.

TASHKIN, D. P., SHAPIRO, G. J., and FRANK, I. M., 1974, Acute bronchial effects of smoked marijuana (MJ) and oral delta-9-tetrahydrocannabinol (THC) in asthmatic subjects, *Clin. Res.* **22**(3):512A.

TASHKIN, D. P., SHAPIRO, B. J., ROSENTHAL, D., and MCLATCHIE, C., 1975, Chronic effects of heavy marijuana smoking on pulmonary function and sputum cytology in healthy, young men, *Am. Rev. Resp. Dis.* **111**(6):895.

TASHKIN, D. P., SHAPIRO, B. J., and FRANK, I. M., 1976*a*, Acute effects of marijuana on airway dynamics in spontaneous and experimentally induced bronchial asthma, *Pharmacology of Marihuana* (S. Szara and M. Braude, eds.), Raven Press, New York.

TASHKIN, D. P., SHAPIRO, B. J., LEE, Y. E., and HARPER, C. E., 1976*b*, Subacute effects of heavy marihuana smoking on pulmonary function in healthy men, *N. Engl. J. Med.* **294**(3):125–129.

TASSINARI, C. A., PERAITA-ADRADOS, M. R., AMBROSETTO, G. and GASTAUT, H., 1974, Effects of marihuana and delta-9-THC at high doses in man. A polygraphic study, *Electroencephalogr. Clin. Neurophysiol. (Amsterdam)* **36**(1):94.

TASSINARI, C. A., AMBROSETTO, G., and GASTAUT, H., 1976, Clinical and polygraphic studies during wakefulness and sleep of high doses of marihuana and delta 9-THC in man, *Pharmacology of Marihuana* (S. Szara and M. Braude, eds.), Raven Press, New York.

TAYLOR, S. P., VARDARIS, R. M., RAWTICH, A. B., GAMMON, C. B., CRANSTON, J. W., and LUBETKIN, A. I., 1976, The effects of alcohol and delta-9-tetrahydrocannabinol on human physical aggression, *Aggress. Behav.* **2**:153–161.

TEALE, D., and MARKS, V., 1976, A fatal motor car accident and cannabis use: Investigation by radioimmunoassay, *Lancet* **1**(7965):884–885.

TEALE, J. D., KING, L. J., FORMAN, E. J., and MARKS, V., 1974, Radioimmunoassay of cannabinoids in blood and urine, *Lancet* **2**(7880):553–555.

TEC, N., 1974, Marihuana and other illegal drugs, *Int. J. Soc. Psych. (London)* **20**(3–4):173–179.

TENNANT, F. S., and DETELS, R., 1976. Relationship of alcohol, cigarette, and drug abuse in adulthood with alcohol, cigarette, and coffee consumption in childhood, *Prevent. Med.* **5**(1):70–77.

Tennant, F. S., Detels, R., and Clark, V., 1975, Some childhood antecedents of drug and alcohol abuse, *Am. J. Epidemiol.* **102**(5):377–385.

Thacore, V. R., and Shukla, S. R. P., 1976, Cannabis psychosis and paranoid schizophrenia, *Arch. Gen. Psychiat.* **33**(3):383–386.

Thoden, J. S., Mosher, R., MacConaill, M., and Ling, G., 1974, Effects of marihuana on treadmill performance, *Med. Sci. Sports* **6**(1):81.

Thompson, P., 1975, "Stoned" driving is unpleasant, say marijuana smokers, *The Journal (Addiction Research Foundation) (Toronto)* **4**(1):13.

Tinklenberg, J. R., 1974, Marijuana and human aggression, in: *Marijuana: Effects on Human Behavior* (L. L. Miller, ed.), pp. 339–357, Academic Press, New York.

Tinklenberg, J. R., and Darley, C. F., 1976, A model of marihuana's cognitive effects, *Pharmacology of Marihuana* (S. Szara and M. Braude, eds.), Raven Press, New York.

Turner, C. E., and Henry, J. T., 1975, Constituents of *Cannabis sativa* L. IX: Stability of synthetic and naturally occurring cannabinoids in chloroform, *J. Pharm. Sci.* **64**(2):357–359.

Tylden, E., 1974, The clinical features of cannabis use, *Practitioner (London)* **212**(1272):810–814.

Tzeng, O. C. S., and Skafidas, T., 1975, Differentiation of psychoactive drug users and non-users and prediction of their using intention, *J. Drug Ed.* **5**(3):261–273.

Vachon, L., Sulkowski, A., and Rich, E., 1974, Marihuana effects on learning, attention and time estimation, *Psychopharmacologia (Berlin)* **39**(1):1–11.

Vachon, L., Mikus, P., Morrissey, W., Fitzgerald, M., and Gaensler, E., 1976, Bronchial effect of marihuana smoke in asthma, *Pharmacology of Marihuana* (S. Szara and M. Braude, eds.), Raven Press, New York.

Wall, M. E., Brine, D. R., and Perez-Reyes, M., 1976, Metabolism of cannabinoids in man, *Pharmacology of Marihuana* (S. Szara and M. Braude, eds.), Raven Press, New York.

Weckowicz, T. E., Fedora, O., Mason, J., Radstaak, D., Bay, K. S., and Yonge, K. A., 1975, Effect of marijuana on divergent and convergent production cognitive tests, *J. Abnorm. Psychol.* **84**(4):386–398.

Westermeyer, J., and Walzer, V., 1975, Sociopathy and drug use in a young psychiatric population, *Dis. Nerv. Syst.* **36**(12):673–677.

Wiberg, D. M., Swanson, G. D., and Bellville, J. W., 1975, Respiratory effects of marijuana characterized by dynamic end-tidal forcing, *Pharmacologist* **17**(2):180.

Widman, M., Agurell, S., Ehrnebo, M., and Jones, G., 1974, Binding of (plus)- and (minus)-delta-1-tetrahydrocannabinols and (minus)-7-hydroxy-delta-1-tetrahydrocannabinol to blood cells and plasma proteins in man, *J. Pharm. Pharmacol. (London)* **26**(11):914–916.

Willette, R. E. (ed.), 1976, Cannabinoid assays in humans, National Institute on Drug Abuse Research Monograph #7, U. S. Government Printing Office, Washington, D. C.

Zeller, A. F., 1975, Joint committee on aviation pathology: IX. Alcohol and other drugs in aircraft accidents, *Aviat. Space Environ. Med.* **46**(10):1271–1274.

INDEX

MIX
Papier aus verantwortungsvollen Quellen
Paper from responsible sources
FSC® C105338

If you have any concerns about our products,
you can contact us on
ProductSafety@springernature.com

In case Publisher is established outside the EU,
the EU authorized representative is:
Springer Nature Customer Service Center GmbH
Europaplatz 3, 69115 Heidelberg, Germany

Printed by Libri Plureos GmbH
in Hamburg, Germany